Ophthalmic Echography 13

Documenta Ophthalmologica Proceedings Series

VOLUME 55

Ophthalmic Echography 13

Proceedings of the 13th SIDUO Congress, Vienna, Austria, 1990

Edited by
PETER TILL

Springer Science+Business Media, B.V.

Library of Congress Cataloging-in-Publication Data

SIDUO Congress (13th : 1990 : Vienna, Austria)
   Ophthalmic echography 13 : proceedings of the 13th SIDUO Congress,
Vienna, Austria, 1990 / edited by P. Till.
       p.   cm. -- (Documenta ophthalmologica. Proceedings series ; v.
55)
   Includes index.
   ISBN 0-7923-1808-0 (HB : alk. paper.
   1. Ultrasonics in ophthalmology--Congresses.   I. Till, P.
II. Title. III. Series.
   [DNLM: 1. Eye Diseases--ultrasonography--congresses.   W3 DO637
v.55 / WW 141 S569 1990o]
RE79.U4S5   1990
617.7'1543--dc20
DNLM/DLC
for Library of Congress   92-19775

ISBN 978-0-7923-1808-8   ISBN 978-94-011-1846-0 (eBook)
DOI 10.1007/978-94-011-1846-0

Printed on acid-free paper

Table of contents

Preface   XI

PART ONE: OPTIC NERVE AND EXTRAOCULAR MUSCLES

1. Standardized echography of the optic nerve. *Jules François*   3
   Memorial Lecture. K.C. Ossoinig (Iowa City, USA)
2. CSF dynamic parameters and changes of optic nerve diameters
   measured by standardized echography   101
   C. Tamburrelli, C. Anile, A. Mangiola, B. Falsini & P. Palma
   (Rome, Italy)
3. Functional echographic biometry of extraocular muscles   111
   C. Tamburrelli (Rome, Italy)
4. Standardized A-scan echography of the optic nerve in a patient
   with leukemic meningeosis and papilledema   117
   A. Stanowsky (Augsburg, Germany)
5. Optic nerve anomalies in childhood   123
   Á. Szabó, Zs. Pelle, J. Németh & M. Janáky (Szeged and
   Budapest, Hungary)
6. A case of bilateral chronic myositis with compressive optic
   neuropathy   127
   V. Juvan (Varaždin, Croatia)

PART TWO: ORBITAL AND PERIORBITAL LESIONS

7. Results of standardized echography in orbital diseases: A review
   of 311 cases   135
   G. Hasenfratz & U. Lewan (Munich, Germany)
8. Lacrimal gland amyloidosis: Characteristics in standardized
   A-scan echography   145
   A. Stanowsky (Augsburg, Germany)
9. Standardized echography in adenoid-cystic carcinomas of the
   orbit   151
   P. Till (Vienna, Austria)

10. Two cases of benign lacrimal gland tumors: Correlation between
    echographic and histopathologic findings   161
    J. Fukiyama, N. Nao-i, F. Maruiwa & A. Sawada (Miyazaki, Japan)
11. Bilateral orbital and adnexal lymphoma   179
    L. Henč-Petrinovic (Zagreb, Croatia)
12. Unusual orbital mucocele   185
    J. McAdam, W.A.J. van Heuven & K.S. Held (San Antonio,
    USA)
13. Importance of ultrasound diagnostics in lacrimal sac diseases   193
    M. Végh & J. Németh (Szeged and Budapest, Hungary)
14. Standarized echography in a case of orbital varix   199
    H.R. Atta (Aberdeen, UK)
15. A case of orbital phlebectasy   205
    A. Cantalloube & J. Poujol (Paris, France)
16. The diagnosis of intracranial AV malformation with orbital
    involvement by B-scan, color Doppler and CT-scan   209
    Z. Wu, Y. Mo, Y. Pang, J. Lian & Q. Zeng (Guangzhou,
    China) & J.S. Kennerdell (Pittsburgh, USA)
17. Traumatic carotid-cavernous fistula affecting the orbit   217
    K. Janev, K. Spahiu, N. Salihu and D. Perović-Stamenković
    (Pristina, Servia)
18. Standardized A-scan examination of the eye and orbit in a
    newborn child after forceps delivery   221
    E. Frieling & A. Stanowsky (Augsburg, Germany)
19. Standardized echography in a case of congenital oculodermal
    melanocytosis with orbital melanoma   227
    P. Till (Vienna, Austria)
20. Glomus tumor of the eyelid and anterior orbit: Echographic and
    histological features   233
    D. Doro, E. Mantovani & L. Bergamo (Padua, Italy)
21. Microphthalmus with congenital orbital cyst   239
    M. Lohmeyer & K.B. Mellin (Essen, Germany)

PART THREE: INTRAOCULAR TUMORS

22. Choroidal melanoma: Zonal relationship between echographic
    tracing and cellularity   247
    R. Sampaolesi, J.F. Casiraghi & J.O. Zarate (Buenos Aires,
    Argentina)
23. The role of echography in small-sized melanomas   251
    P. Perri, V. Mazzeo, L. Ravalli, M. Chiarelli & P. Monari
    (Ferrara, Italy)
24. Ultrasonography in the diagnosis and follow-up of Ruthenium-
    treated malignant melanomas   257
    F. Goes, J.P. Huyghe, H. Verbraeken, P. Brabant &
    J.J. De Laey (Antwerp and Ghent, Belgium)

25. Choroidal malignant melanoma masquerading as posterior
    scleritis   265
    P.G. Wolff-Kormann, G. Hasenfratz, F.H. Stefani &
    K.G. Riedel (Munich, Germany)
26. Standardized A-scan diagnosis of bilateral choroidal osteoma in
    a 4½-year-old girl   273
    A. Stanowsky (Augsburg, Germany)
27. Metastatic choroidal lesions: A retrospective study   277
    G. Cennamo, N. Rosa, T. Foà & A. Mele (Naples, Italy)
28. Three cases of choroidal metastases with rapid growth and
    atypical echographic characteristics   285
    L. Ravalli, P. Perri, P. Monari, M. Chiarelli,
    M. Ziosi & V. Mazzeo (Ferrara, Italy)
29. Echographical examinations of patients with Coat's disease   291
    J. Damjanovich & L. Kolozsvári (Debrecen, Hungary)
30. Different echographic aspects of retinoblastoma in two members
    of a family   297
    L. Pierro, C. Capoferri, R. Magni & R. Brancato (Milano,
    Italy)
31. Dysplastic retina and persistent primary vitreous simulating a
    retinoblastoma   301
    R. Sampaolesi & J.O. Zarate (Buenos Aires, Argentina)
32. Tumours of the choroid: Three unusual cases examined by
    ultrasound   307
    H.C. Fledelius, J.U. Prause & E. Scherfig (Hillerød and
    Copenhagen, Denmark)
33. Echographic differential diagnosis of small choroidal solid
    lesions   313
    G. Marchini & R. Tosi (Verona, Italy)
34. Contribution of standardized echography to diagnostic work-up
    of intraocular lymphoma   319
    D. Doro, E. Midena, E. Mantovani, M. Sala & F. Moro
    (Padua, Italy)

PART FOUR: INTRAOCULAR DISORDERS

35. Hemorrhagic and degenerative vitreal interfaces   329
    V. Mazzeo, P. Perri & L. Ravalli (Ferrara, Italy)
36. Is B-scan ultrasound useful in predicting the source of vitreous
    hemorrhage?   333
    R.C. Bosanquet & J.A. Bell (Newcastle Upon Tyne, UK)
37. Echography in the study of vitreo-retinal interface pathology   337
    T. Avitabile, L. Franco, C. Marino, A. Pappalardo, A. Longo,
    R. Ghirlanda & A. Reibaldi (Catania, Italy)
38. Tamponade substances in vitreo-retinal surgery: A
    echographical study   345

A. Reibaldi, T. Avitabile, A. Pappalardo, G. Cascone,
L. Franco & S. Sileci (Catania, Italy)
39. Retinoschisis: Our echographic experience   351
    L. Kolozsvári (Debrecen, Hungary)
40. Further indications for the evaluation of the prescleral layer   355
    N. Rosa & G. Cennamo (Naples, Italy)
41. Recognition of retinal pigmentepithelium   361
    S. Clemens & H. Busse (Münster, Germany)
42. Effect of intraocular pressure on ocular wall volume   369
    J. Nemeth (Budapest, Hungary)
43. Ultrasonography in cryopexy of the retina   375
    H. Gerding & S. Clemens (Münster, Germany)
44. Ultrasonography in cases of phthisis bulbi   381
    Zs. Lampé & L. Kolozsvári (Debrecen, Hungary)
45. Posterior pole configurations in progressive myopia   385
    V. Hidasi, L. Kolozsvári & Z. Nagy (Debrecen, Hungary)
46. Choroidal thickness in general anesthesia   393
    P. Rademacher, S. Clemens & Ch. Radig (Münster, Germany)
47. Echographic study of an episcleral reabsorbable explant   395
    F.A. Rodriguez, R.R. Gosalbez & R.B. Marti (Barcelona,
    Spain)
48. Ultrasound elaboration: Our position and results   399
    L. Falco, F. Andreuccetti & S. Esente (Florence, Italy)

PART FIVE: ANTERIOR SEGMENT

49. Echographic evaluation of experimental cataractogenesis in
    rabbits by radio frequency signal   405
    F. Cennamo, G. Cennamo, T. Libondi, G. Iaccarino, N. Rosa
    & G. Auricchio (Naples, Italy)
50. Corneal thickness measured by ultrasound: A study of its
    variation with or without contact lens use   411
    E. Moragrega, P. Garcia-Reza & C. Velasco (Mexico City,
    Mexico)
51. Corneal graft and echography   415
    G. Cennamo, A. Loffredo, N. Rosa, A. Pezone & E. Guida
    (Naples, Italy)
52. Diagnostic ultrasonography of the anterior segment of the eye   421
    A.M. Verbeek (Nijmegen, The Netherlands)
53. Ultrasonography of the posterior lens capsule in trauma   431
    S. Clemens & K.-H. Emmerich (Münster, Germany)

PART SIX: INSTRUMENTATION

54. A newly developed A- and B-scan device for ophthalmic
    ultrasonography   439

A. Sawada, J. Fukiyama, F. Maruiwa & Y. Baba (Miyazaki,
Japan)
55. Power spectrum analysis of ultrasonic radio-frequency signals on
cataracts   445
S. Tane, M. Hashimoto & Y. Kimura (Kawasaki, Japan)
56. Three-dimensional display and its application to stereoscopic
representation   451
Y. Sugata, K. Murakami, M. Ito, T. Shiina & Y. Yamamoto
(Tokyo, Japan)
57. From computer-assisted echography to a multielement linear
curtain ultrasonic system: Our experiences   459
S. Guerriero, G. Minerva, L. Cardia, F. Nirchio,
G. Pasquariello & N. Veneziani (Bari, Italy)
58. Telediagnoses by faxed ophthalmic ultrasonogram   475
S. Tane & M. Hashimoto (Kawasaki, Japan)
59. The differential diagnosis of endobulbar tumors by means of
false colors   483
T. Avitabile, G. Cascone, C. Marino, C. Gagliano,
O. Bonaccorsi, F. Marano & C. Buccheri (Catania, Italy)
60. Usefulness of simultaneous display of four different B-scan
images in ocular diagnosis   489
A. Sawada, J. Fukiyama, F. Maruiwa & Y. Baba (Miyazaki,
Japan)
61. Area and volume calculation by three-dimensional echography
of the eye   495
E. Motolese, M. Burroni, G. Addabbo, G. Dell'Eva,
B. D'Aniello & N. Paterra (Siena, Italy)

PART SEVEN: BIOMETRY

62. Extracapsular cataract extraction with posterior chamber lens
implantation: Comparison between preoperative lens power
calculation and postsurgical refraction   501
F. Sayegh, Z. Shamayleh, G. Jayyousi & A. Shaheen (Amman,
Jordan)
63. Clinical results of preoperative intraocular lens power
calculation by the Binkhorst formula   507
P. Lewandowski & M. Skurczyński (Warsaw, Poland)
64. Ultrasound biometry and deprivation myopia   511
H.C. Fledelius & E. Goldschmidt (Hillerød, Denmark)
65. Postoperative disappointment in emmetropic patients   515
H.J. Shammas (Lynwood, USA)
66. Biometric measurement in the evaluation of pathological myopia   517
L. Pierro, F.I. Camesasca, M. Mischi & R. Brancato (Milan,
Italy)

x

PART EIGHT: DOPPLER METHODS

67. Analysis of ocular circulatory kinetics in glaucoma using the
    ultrasonic Doppler method   525
    S. Tane, M. Hirata & M. Hashimoto (Kawasaki, Japan)
68. Angiodinography: Ultrasound technique for the study of normal
    and abnormal vascularization of the eye and orbit   533
    L. Falco, S. Esente, F. Fanfani & S. Fanfani (Florence, Italy)
69. The effect of intracranial diseases on ophthalmic artery
    circulation   537
    E. Balász, L. Rózsa & S. Szabó (Debrecen, Hungary)

Authors Index   543

Subject Index   547

Preface

This Volume of the Documenta Ophthalmoligica Proceeding Series presents the scientific papers read during the 13th Congress of SIDUO, the International Society for Ultrasonic Diagnosis in Ophthalmology, held in Vienna in the Summer of 1990. It was the second time that SIDUO had selected Vienna as a site for its biennial congresses in the 28 years of its existence. Previously, the 3rd SIDUO Meeting had taken place as part of the 1st World Congress for Ultrasonic Diagnosis in Medicine organized by Karl C. Ossoinig in 1969. Ossoinig, the pioneer of Standardized Echography opened the scientific sessions of SIDUO 13 with the First Jules François Memorial Lecture on the Optic Nerve reviewing the modern examination techniques for precise measurements of the orbital optic nerve and its various sheaths and for an accurate diagnosis and differential diagnosis of diseases affecting the optic nerve, highlighting the new field of prophylactic recognition of early optic nerve compression (e.g., in Graves' orbitopathy) and the important confirmation of CON in the presence of other conditions affecting the optic nerve functions.

The first scientific session then dealt with a variety of interesting conditions of the optic nerve and of the extraocular muscles ranging from inflammatory diseases such as optic neuritis and orbital myositis to congenital anomalies, from glaucomatous changes to IIH, and from normal anatomical (dynamic) findings to malignant tumors such as lymphomas and leucemic meningeosis. The following section on orbital and periorbital lesions deals with a number of frequently encountered conditions such as benign and malignant lymphocytic tumors, orbital mucoceles, varices, and A-V fistulas, as well as with rare lesions such as amyloidosis, a glomic tumor and an adenoid-cystic carcinoma of the lacrimal gland.

The subsequent section deals with the diagnosis of lesions of the posterior eye segment ranging from Vogt-Koyanagi-Harada's syndrome to retinal necrosis, from benign reactive lymphoid hyperplasia to diabetic vitreo-retinopathy. A large section then deals with intraocular tumors and their diagnosis and management. Cell type of malignant melanomas as well as the effects of radio-active plaque therapy on melanomas, diagnostically difficult situations such as a masquerading posterior scleritis, choroidal osteomas and metastatic carcinomas, and many other challenging and important neoplasms and their echographic diagnosis are all contained in this section. Further fascinating contributions deal with new concepts in instrumentation including computerized techniques, with the diagnosis of lesions of the anterior eye segment.

These proceedings offer a wealth of new information on Diagnostic Ultrasound in Ophthalmology, covering particularly well the field of Standardized Echography, but equally well the methods of B-scan Echography, of Doppler Ultrasound and of Computerized Methods.

As is already tradition, this latest Volume of SIDUO Proceedings adds another fascinating and important chapter to the library that is a must for every echographer in ophthalmolgy.

The financial support of Alcon/Biophysic Medical to SIDUO for the publication of this volume is gratefully acknowledged.

PROF. DR. PETER TILL

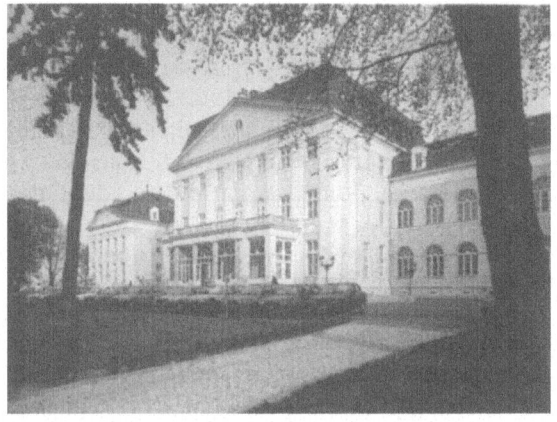

Schlos Wilhelminenberg, Vienna, Austria
Venue of the 13th Biennial SIDUO Congress.

PART ONE

Optic nerve and extraocular muscles

1. Standardized echography of the optic nerve*
Jules François Memorial Lecture

KARL C. OSSOINIG
(Iowa City, USA)

1. INTRODUCTION

Standardized Echography, a special advanced method of diagnostic ultrasound in ophthalmology (Ossoinig [21]) has become an effective, clinically very useful and, at times, indispensable diagnostic aid in the evaluation of the orbital portion of the optic nerve. Standardized Echography provides by far the most precise and accurate measurements of the thicknesses of the optic nerve and its sheaths throughout their orbital course. This method also provides a unique opportunity to study the in vivo dynamics of the subarachnoidal fluid surrounding the optic nerve and thus gives invaluable insight into the mechanism of compressive optic neuropathy and of BIH, and adds tremendously to the clinical differential diagnosis of optic nerve and related disorders.

Standardized Echography combines the uses of A-scan, B-scan and Doppler instrumentation and techniques for: (1) the evaluation of topographic (location, borders, shape and special relationship of normal as well as abnormal structures), quantitative (internal structure, reflectivity and sound absorption) and kinetic data (consistency, motility, pulsations and bloodflow). (2) The precise measurements of the thickness of the optic nerve (maximal pial diameter), of the amount of perineural fluid (maximal arachnoidal diameter), and of the thickness of the dura (half the difference between maximal arachnoidal and maximal dural diameters), anywhere within the orbit, i.e., at any site between the globe and the optic nerve canal.

Standardized Echography utilizes specially designed, highly sophisticated real-time A-scan technology, which allows easy and reliable extraction of quantitative data and eliminates falsification of such data by otherwise unavoidable and in part prohibitive artefacts. Together with high-resolution real-time B-scan instrumentation, this A-scan technology is applied with special techniques called topographic, quantitative and kinetic echography. Both the special A-scan technology and the A-scan as well as the B-scan and Doppler examination techniques are standardized thus representing a single

* This study was supported in part by an unrestricted grant from Research to Prevent Blindness, Inc.

P. Till (ed.), Ophthalmic Echography 13, pp. 3–99.
© 1993 *Kluwer Academic Publishers*.

optimal ultrasonic language and providing invaluable, understandable, comparable and repeatable results. This standardization gives the method its name.

Historically, Standardized Echography was developed mainly during the 1960's and was first presented (then under the name of ophthalmic clinical echography; Ossoinig [15, 16]) in its different facets during the 1st World Congress on Ultrasonic Diagnosis in Medicine, held in Vienna in 1969. In the 1970s the full range of clinical applications of Standardized Echography including the optic nerve examinations was realized and publicized (Ossoinig [21]). The diagnosis and differential diagnosis of optic nerve lesions was consolidated in the 1980's. While the first in vivo B-scan displays of the optic nerve were initiated as early as 1957, and were published, by Baum [2], the in vivo A-scan displays of the optic nerve were initiated in 1972, and were first published, by Ossoinig [17]. Many others performing Standardized Echography have contributed much to our today's knowledge and to the state of the art in the imaging of the optic nerve and its disorders with Standardized Echography [1, 3–8, 10–14, 27–36].

A-scan vs. B-scan
The orbital optic nerve consists – for practical purposes – of two major compartments, which will be treated separately: the optic disk and the (orbital) optic nerve. While the optic disk is evaluated mostly with the B-scan method, the optic nerve (from its retrobulbar portion back into the orbital apex) is evaluated primarily with the standardized A-scan method.

For this study, the Kretztechnik 7200 MA model (the first standardized A-scan instrument), the Sono–Kretz module designed for the Ocuscan 400 of Sonometrics, the Ophthascan-S of Biophysic and, for the last 3 years, the most advanced digital Standardized A-scan instrument, the Mini A-scan by Biophysic/Alcon (all instruments were developed by the author with the respective companies) have been used for the A-scan examinations of the optic disk and the optic nerve. All A-scan echograms shown in the figures of this report, which are not designated otherwise, were obtained with the Mini A-scan and at the standardized tissue sensitivity, according to the rules of Standardized Echography.

For the B-scan examinations, first the Kretz 7900 S was used together with binocular immersion goggles. This instrument, developed by the author with Kretztechnik in the 1960s [8], was the first combined A-scan and B-scan instrument commercially available in ophthalmology (the A-scan part was the prototype of the Kretz 7200 MA). Next, in the early 1970s, the first real-time contact B-scan developed by Bronson-Turner, and later the Ocuscan 400 of Sonometrics, the analog B-scan instrument of Cooper-Vision, the Mini B-scan of Biophysic/Alcon, and in recent years predominantly the Ophthascan S (the standardized version of the Ophthascan B) of the same company, were utilized. Both the Mini B-scan and the Ophthascan S were developed by the author together with Biophysic Medical. All B-scan echograms shown in the figures of this report, which are not designated otherwise, were obtained with the Ophthascan S at optimized sensitivity settings according to the rules of Standardized Echography.

Basis and purpose of this study
The typical echographic patterns and the clinical applications and uses of Standardized Echography as presented and discussed in this study are based on nearly 12,000 orbital patient examinations, performed with Standardized Echography during the past 20 years in the Echography Service of the Department of Ophthalmology at the University of Iowa. The purpose of this report is not only the review of the wide range of applications, the remarkable effectiveness and the invaluable clinical usefulness of this powerful tool for the diagnosis and management of disorders affecting or involving the optic nerve. This report also explains the anatomical, physiological and pathological basics of Standardized Echography of the optic nerve. And, most important, it communicates to the novice how to perform Standardized Echography of the optic nerve and how to skillfully and successfully apply it, avoiding the more common pitfalls.

2. THE OPTIC DISK

The echographic evaluation of the optic disk and its various lesions is a domain of real-time high-resolution B-scan. The A-scan method is sometimes useful and occasionally necessary to make a diagnosis in this area.

2.1 Glaucomatous excavation of the optic disk

Glaucomatous optic disk excavation is among the optic disk lesions more frequently encountered by Standardized Echography. Excavation of the disk is evaluated and documented exclusively with high-resolution real-time B-scan. While it defies direct precise measurement of either depth or width of the cupping by echography, careful B-scan examination can be very helpful in (a) detecting or ruling out significant optic disk excavation in an eye with opaque media; (b) accurately comparing such a disk excavation with the excavation of the disk in the fellow eye and thus quantitating the excavation, provided the disk in the fellow eye is visible; (c) estimating the cup/disk ratio with an accuracy of better than ±0.15, in deeper cups; and (d) establishing a trend by accurately comparing cup sizes over time in eyes with opaque media, thus following up the natural course of hypertension/glaucoma or the effectiveness of the treatment of glaucoma, especially in infantile glaucoma.

Standard sections
Figure 1 demonstrates standard B-scan sections through a left optic disk with total glaucomatous excavation following early childhood trauma. Signs of adequate B-scan displays of an optic cup are clear delineations of the cup margins and a distinct line representing the cribriform plate. In this aphakic

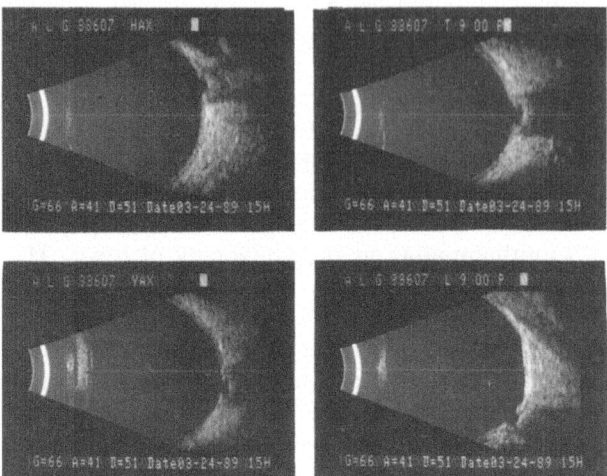

Fig. 1. Standard B-scan sections demonstrate total glaucomatous excavation of the left optic disk in a 22-year old female patient with absolute glaucoma following trauma. *Top left:* horizontal axial section (HAX) through macula and optic disk (probe placed horizontally over center of cornea with marker pointing nasally so that upper margin of B-scan corresponds to nasal end of acoustic section). *Bottom left:* vertical axial section (VAX) through optic disk centered at fundus just above the disk (probe placed vertically over center of cornea with marker pointing upwards so that upper edge of echogram corresponds with upper end of scan). *Top right:* transverse section (T) through the disk at 9:00; to obtain it, the probe was placed across the 3:00 meridian of the left globe just behind the limbus in a vertical fashion so that the acoustic section bypassed the lens (avoiding its absorptive and refractive distortion) and was centered at the disk; the marker of the probe pointed upwards so that the upper end of the B-scan corresponds with the upper end of the acoustic section. *Bottom right:* longitudinal section (L) through the disk at 9:00; the probe was placed horizontally along the 3:00 meridian with half of it overlying the cornea and the other half extending behind the limbus; the marker was pointing toward the center of the cornea so that the upper edge of the echogram corresponds with the anterior end of the acoustic section; therefore the optic disk (lying posteriorly within the section) appears near the lower end of the echogram.

eye the horizontal and vertical axial scans provided optimal documentation. Often, however, a transverse (vertical) section directed across, and a longitudinal (horizontal) section lined up with, the horizontal nasal meridian of the fundus (right echograms in Figure 1), provide optimal documentation. These pairs of transverse and longitudinal, or horizontal axial and vertical axial, B-scan sections provide a three-dimensional record of the disk cupping by documenting two planes that are perpendicular to each other and centered over the disk excavation.

Besides precise centering of an optic cup within the acoustic section, the choice of an optimal system sensitivity is crucial for recording diagnostically meaningful and valid scans (Figure 2). The best approach is to start displaying an optic disk at the maximum sensitivity setting of the instrument, that barely avoids showing noise signals on the screen. Noise would spoil the quality of

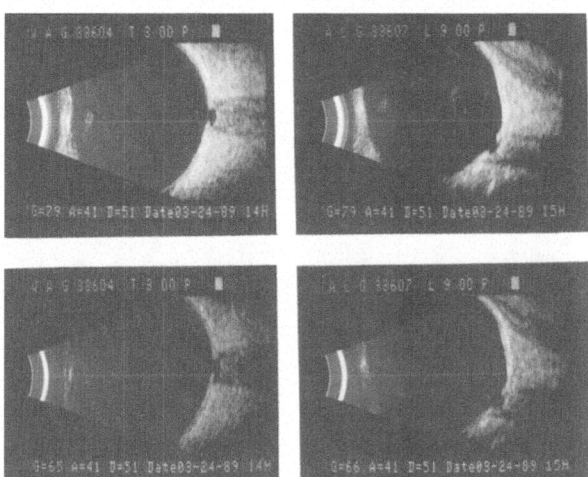

Fig. 2. Transverse sections through a right optic disk showing a very large and deep excavation in a 16-month-old male patient with infantile glaucoma (*left echograms*) and longitudinal sections through the left optic disk of the patient depicted in Figure 1 (*right echograms*). The top echograms obtained with close to maximum system sensitivity are looking good, but the bottom echograms recorded with reduced (optimal) sensitivity settings are diagnostically more useful.

a B-scan at higher than these 'maximal' sensitivity settings. After centering the cup within the displayed acoustic section at that maximum sensitivity setting, instrument sensitivity is then reduced to a minimum which still allows the display of the cribriform plate; in this way the slightly overhanging edges of the cup will be displayed in minimum signal widths thus avoiding or at least minimizing the artefact of overemphasizing that overhanging. This artefact caused by increased sound beam widths at high sensitivity settings may lead to an underestimation of the cup width. The reduced sensitivity setting allows a more reliable estimation of the cup width (without, however, ever achieving precise measurements with the B-scan).

Comparison of both sides

The careful and meticulous comparison between the right and left optic disks of a patient (Figure 3) is of great importance for the meaningful and useful echographic evaluation of disk cupping. The top echograms in Figure 3 compare the minimal cupping of the right optic disk (*left*) with the total glaucomatous excavation in the left eye (*right*) in the patient who has been described in Figure 1.

The bottom echograms of Figure 3 show the optic disk cuppings in the two eyes of a patient with long-standing glaucoma secondary to a slow-flow carotid cavernous sinus fistula: the right disk (bottom left echogram in Figure 3), which was not visualized ophthalmoscopically due a bullous keratopathy of this eye, was judged echographically to have a total or nearly total glauco-

8

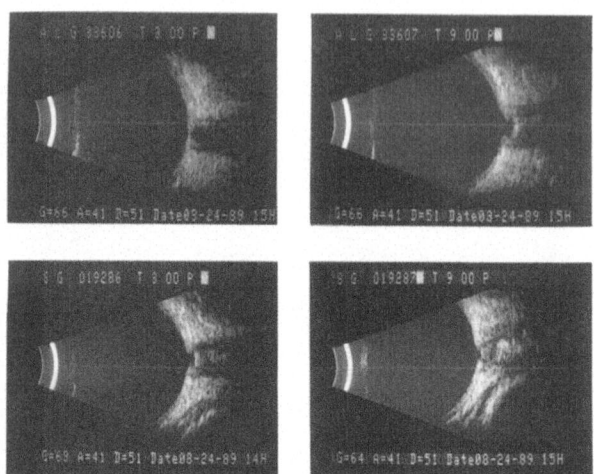

Fig. 3. Comparison of optic disk excavations between the right eyes (left echograms) and the left eyes (right echograms) of two patients. *Top:* post-traumatic absolute glaucoma OS (described in Figure 1). *Bottom:* 64-year-old female patient with bilateral glaucoma secondary to a slow-flow arteriovenous fistula.

matous excavation, through the comparison with the left optic disk (bottom right echogram) which was known to have an 0.8 cup/disk ratio from ophthalmoscopy. For a reliable comparison between right and left optic disk cups, the same types of acoustic sections must be used at the same or at comparable system sensitivity levels of the instrument.

Add axial eye length measurements in infantile glaucoma

In congenital or infantile glaucoma, A-scan axial eye length measurements performed with the immersion ring technique can add immensely to the information obtained by B-scan about the cupping. These A-scan measurements are the most accurate means of checking and following up the effectiveness of treatment in this type of glaucoma (Sampaolesi [27]). Figure 4 depicts such a case of congenital glaucoma. The longer axial eye length (28.8 mm) is found in the left eye (vs. 28.3 mm OD; normal axial eye length for this age is 21.6 mm). Fittingly the left eye also features the larger excavation of the disk.

2.2 Optic disk coloboma / morning glory syndrome / optic pit

Figure 5 illustrates the B-scan and A-scan echograms from an eye with optic disk coloboma. While even total cupping of the disk is still too small to allow it to be displayed and thus measured by A-scan, colobomas are usually large enough to be demonstrated and evaluated with A-scan. By comparing the two precise A-scan measurements shown in Figure 5, one indicating the

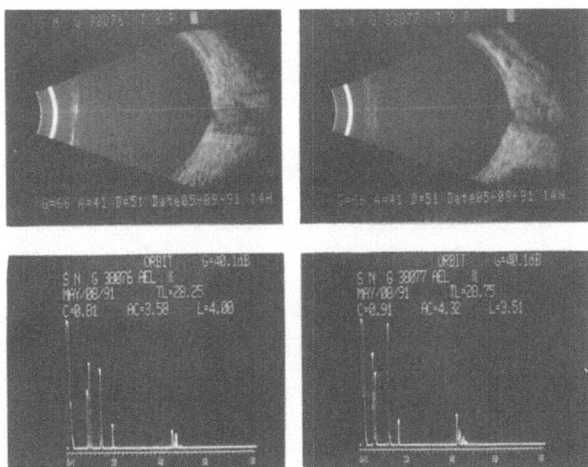

Fig. 4. B-scans showing the optic cups, and immersion A-scans indicating the axial eye lengths, of the right (left echogram) and left (right echogram) eyes of a 2-year-old female infant with congenital glaucoma (post-surgical follow-up examination).

distance between the tip of the probe and the fundus at the edge of the coloboma (20.55 mm, top echogram) and the other showing the distance between the probe and the bottom of the coloboma (29.23 mm, bottom echogram), the exact depth of the coloboma can be calculated to be 8.68 mm.

Figure 6 displays longitudinal sections from an optic disk with a unilateral temporal pit in an otherwise normal globe of a young male patient (left). On the right of this figure, sections from an optic disk coloboma in a morning glory syndrome are shown. Huge funnel-shaped tissue is noted to emanate from the edges and the bottom of the coloboma.

2.3 Optic disk drusen

Without a doubt, the most frequently encountered optic disk lesions are buried drusen, the small calcified deposits in the deeper layers of the optic disk resembling tiny foreign bodies. Drusen of the optic disk are frequently accidental findings during echographic examinations of a globe, usually performed for a reason other than that of detecting or confirming disk drusen.

B-scan signs
Figure 7 illustrates the typical B-scan echograms of a conglomerate of small buried drusen in the left eye of an elderly male patient. Because a disk drusen is calcified, a strong foreign body-like B-scan signal originates from it signalizing its presence through a much brighter dot in the disk pattern. In B-scan echograms, the drusen become most obvious at reduced system sensitivities (right B-scans in Figure 7).

Similar to foreign bodies, drusen cast shadows; unlike most foreign bodies

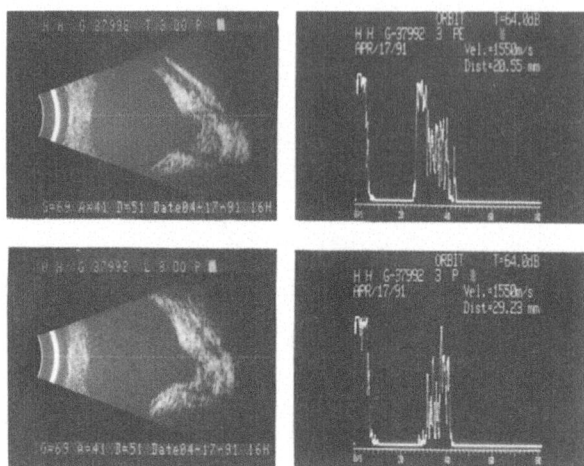

Fig. 5. Echograms from an optic disk coloboma (right eye of a 2-month-old female infant with dense cataract). The two B-scans were obtained along the two standard optic disk planes (which are perpendicular to each other), i.e., a transverse section across the nasal horizontal meridian (3:00 in OD), and a longitudinal section along this meridian. The top A-scan echogram was obtained by aiming the acoustic beam perpendicularly at the inner retinal surface near the edge of the coloboma; by electronic measurement this surface was located at a distance of 20.55 mm from the probe (electronic gates placed at the left end of the echogram and over the peak of the retinal spike). When the beam was angled into the depth of the coloboma, the bottom A-scan echogram was received. The highest spike on the right corresponds to the surface at the bottom of the coloboma reached by a perpendicular beam, located at a distance of 29.23 mm from the probe. The preceding low to medium high spikes (rising in height from left to right and being located between the 28 and the 37 microsecond marks of the scale underneath the echogram), were recorded from the sloping lateral wall of the coloboma. The lowest (*left*) of these spikes originated when the beam periphery reached a more anterior portion of the sloping wall almost tangentially, whereas the higher (*right*) of these spikes were generated when more central portions of the beam periphery struck more posterior areas of the sloping wall at smaller and increasingly more favorable angles of incidence.

their shadowing is caused by strong sound absorption (calcium). In the standard sections, however, the shadows cast by a drusen coincide with the optic nerve pattern (acoustic void) and therefore have no diagnostic significance. This is why B-scans always suggest, but not always prove, the presence of drusen; A-scans obtained with oblique beams from the area of the disk are sometimes needed to clinch the diagnosis, and are always useful to safeguard the diagnosis.

A-scan signs – oblique beam technique
The presence of optic disk drusen can always be detected with B-scan echography. Short of looking for drusen with this B-scan technique, however, drusen are often discovered by accident during routine basic A-scanning; during this examination, the beam reaches the optic disk at times in a

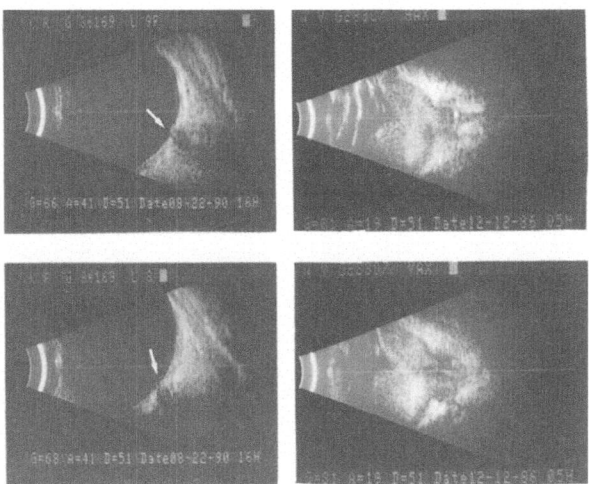

Fig. 6. Left: B-scans from left eye with small optic pit (arrow) in a 29-year-old male patient. These echograms were obtained with longitudinal scans along the 9:00 (top) and 3:00 (*bottom*) meridians. Because of the slightly slanted direction of the pit, the transverse sections did not show it as well as these two longitudinal sections. As is typical, the optic pit is located near the temporal edge of the disk. *Right:* B-scans from the painful, blind (since birth) left eye of a 22-year-old female patient with optic disk coloboma and morning glory sydrome. In contrast to the simple optic disk coloboma as shown in Figure 5, dense irregularly structured tissue emanates from the depth of the coloboma and extends forward into the vitreous cavity in a morning glory fashion.

direction oblique to the large surfaces of the disk and the surrounding ocular wall letting the drusen 'light up' through their strong signals like a beacon in the dark.

Figure 7 (bottom echograms) and especially Figure 8 illustrate this 'lighting up' of (usually unexpected) optic disk drusen during such A-scanning: as the beam is angled from a direction perpendicular to the fundus behind the equator (top echogram in Figure 8) posteriorly, getting closer to the posterior pole, the beam slightly deviates from ideal perpendicularity and the retinal and choroidal signals become slightly weaker (second and third echograms from top). At the same time the beam periphery reaches the drusen whose signals rise in front of the retinal spike (second echogram from the bottom). The reason for this 'displacement' of the drusen signals which appear to come from the vitreous cavity, is the following situation: the low (displaced) drusen signals are generated by the weak beam periphery which arrives at the site of the drusen prior to the arrival of the strong central beam portion at the curved fundus next to the drusen (oblique beam). This phenomenon is seen whenever a strongly reflecting small echo source, e.g., a foreign body, a scleral buckle (implant), or a drusen are reached by the periphery of an oblique beam (oblique toward the large strongly reflecting surface of the fundus) and is not yet centered in the beam axis.

12

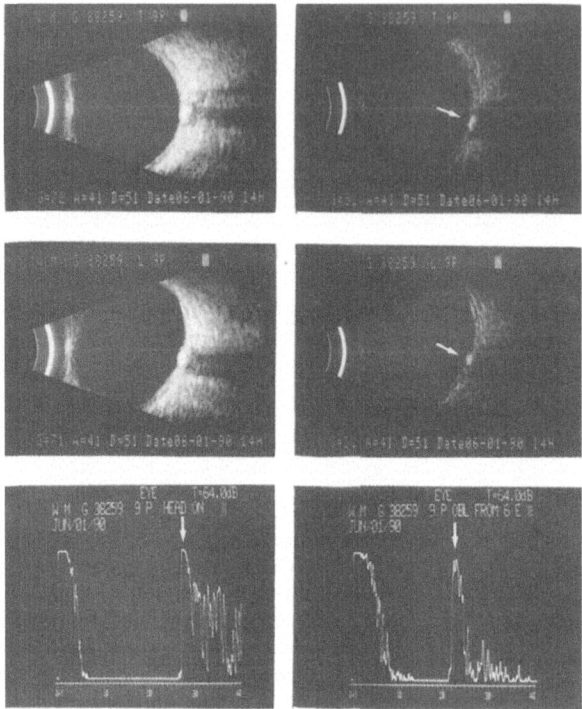

Fig. 7. Echograms from buried optic disk drusen (arrows) in the left eye of a 68-year-old male patient. The foreign body-like properties of the calcified drusen make them more obvious in the B-scan echograms obtained at markedly reduced system sensitivities (*right*) and in the A-scan echogram when centered within an oblique beam (*right*).

As the beam centers on the drusen, the drusen spike becomes maximally high suggesting its presence (see also left bottom echogram of Figure 7); in the absence of a drusen the disk area simply does not produce such a strong echo signal. Once the examiner notices this suggestive A-scan signal or when the objective is to confirm B-scan signs of a disk drusen, extremely oblique beams are directed toward the optic disk to prove the presence of drusen (Figure 9; see also Figure 11): the acoustic beam is aimed at the optic disk in an oblique direction thus avoiding perpendicular sound incidence at the large surfaces of the various layers of the posterior ocular wall (i.e., retinal, choroidal, scleral and disk surfaces, as well as the cribriform plate) which like the drusen would produce strong signals when exposed to a perpendicular beam. However, in contrast to the drusen the large ocular wall surfaces remain unimpressive and thus do not interfere with the diagnosis of drusen, during oblique beam incidence. Like foreign bodies, drusen produce maximally strong echoes when they are centered in the sound beam regardless of the sound beam direction.

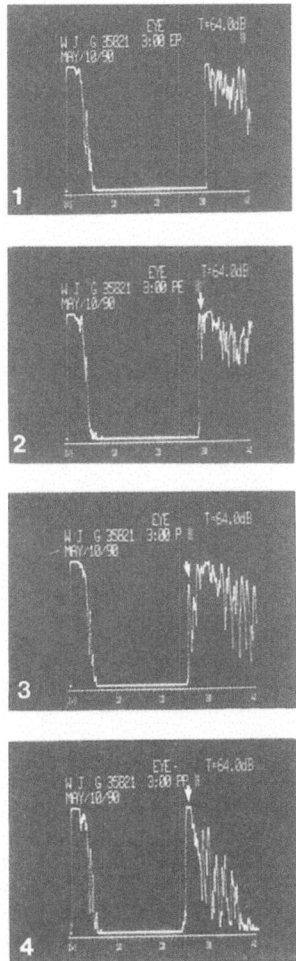

Fig. 8. Sequence of A-scan echograms obtained from the left eye of a 47-year-old male patient with large buried optic disk drusen during a basic A-scanning along the horizontal meridian. *Echogram 1:* the beam reaches the retina perpendicularly behind the equator of the 3:00 meridian in this left eye. *Echogram 2:* closer to the disk, the beam is angled slightly away from perpendicularity allowing the signals from the retina and choroid (arrow) to weaken enough to be clearly distinguishable from the scleral signals at the maintained high tissue sensitivity of the Standardized A-scan instrument. *Echogram 3:* as the beam periphery reaches the strongly scattering drusen, a group of spikes rises in front of the fundus signals (arrow). *Echogram 4:* once the drusen is centered within the beam, these additional signals become very strong and foreign body-like (arrow) suggesting the presence of drusen. Normal disk tissues produce much weaker signals under these conditions.

14

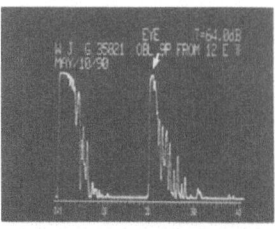

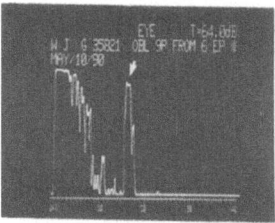

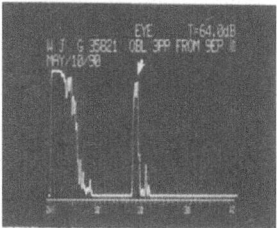

Fig. 9. A-scan echograms obtained from the optic disk drusen in the same eye as depicted in Figure 8, this time through planned very oblique sound beams. The probe was placed near the equator at 12 o'clock and the beam was directed toward the disk to display the top echogram. The probe was placed behind the equator at 6:00 for the display of the drusen in the center echogram, and the probe was placed at 9:00 behind the equator to obtain the bottom echogram. In each of these three echograms the optic disk drusen stands out through its much higher signal (arrow), while the large ocular wall surfaces produce only weak and insignificant signals, when exposed to such an oblique sound beam. In the absence of drusen an echogram similar to the bottom right A-scan in Figure 11 would have resulted in each of the three oblique beam examinations performed in this case, and no such distinctly higher foreign body-like spike would have been displayed as can be seen in the echograms of Figure 9.

Pseudo-drusen

The very large drusen displayed in Figure 10, is large and deep enough to be safely diagnosed with B-scan alone; the A-scans confirming them through the oblique beam approach are reassuring but not absolutely needed in this case. Note that there is a stronger point-like signal in front of the drusen in each of the B-scans: they originated at a point of the large and more reflective optic disk surface which was reached by the focussed B-scan beam in a perpendicular direction. To identify such a point-like stronger echo source as part of a large irregularly shaped strongly reflecting surface such as the disk surface and differentiate it from a smaller or more superficially located

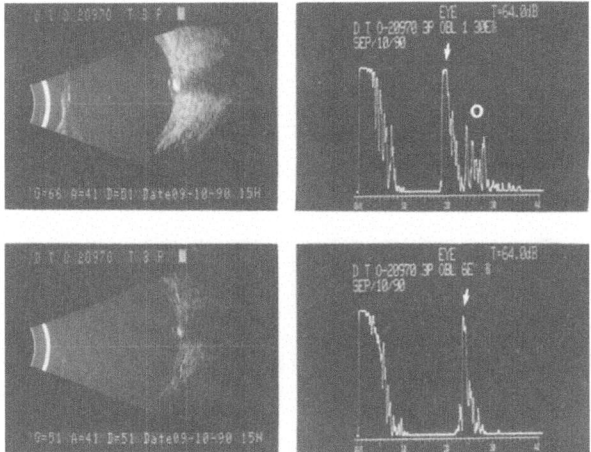

Fig. 10. B-scan and A-scan echograms from the right eye with large buried disk drusen in a 16-year-old male patient. The A-scans were recorded with strongly oblique sound beams: while the drusen signal 'lights up' like a beacon in the dark (arrow), the ocular wall and disk signals (o) remain low and unimpressive (top A-scan) or fail to show up altogether (bottom A-scan).

optic disk drusen is not possible with B-scan alone. There A-scans obtained with the oblique sound beam approach are required to safely diagnose or rule out such smaller drusen and to differentiate them from 'pseudo-drusen' (Figure 11). Small portions of large irregular surfaces, which happen to be reached by a small portion of the wide and parallel A-scan beam will never generate the strong signal a drusen does, during an oblique beam approach.

2.4 Optic disk tumors / pseudotumors

Most tumors occurring at the optic disk can be seen ophthalmoscopically and can be differentiated clinically at least into groups, e.g., pigmented tumors vs. non-pigmented tumors, or highly vascular vs. non-vascular tumors. This is often sufficient to allow Standardized Echography to play an important complementary role in clarifying the nature of the lesion underlying a disk elevation.

Melanocytomas, for instance, differ echographically from malignant melanomas clearly by their irregular internal acoustic structure and their high reflectivity, which both contrast the homogenous low-reflective structure of *malignant melanomas*. In addition, melanomas are clearly vascular on echographic examination, whereas melanocytomas are not. Clinically, malignant melanomas may appear like optic disk tumors whether they in fact originate there or are just overlying the disk. If they are not pigmented, they may easily be confused with *hemangiomas* because of their vascularity.

16

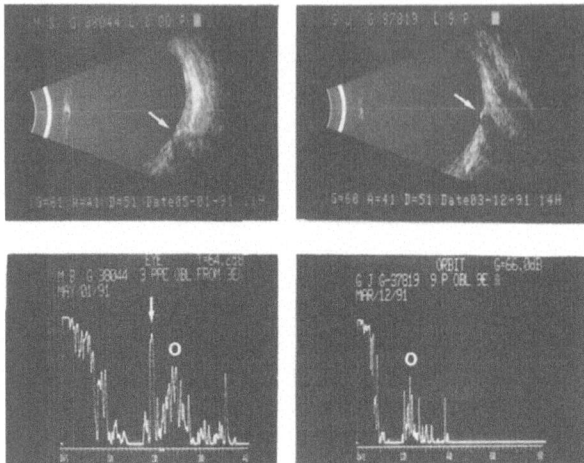

Fig. 11. B-scan and A-scan echograms from a right optic disk with a small buried peripheral drusen (see arrow) in a 26-year-old male patient (left echograms) and from a normal left optic disk in a 37-year-old male patient (right echograms). In the latter case a small portion of the disk surface was reached by a perpendicular beam producing the pattern of a 'pseudodrusen' (mimicking a small superficial drusen, see arrow in right top B-scan). In cases like these, the A-scans obtained with an oblique sound beam easily distinguish the small true drusen (arrow in bottom left echogram) from the pseudodrusen (bottom right echogram: "o" = weak signals from optic disk tissues and neighboring ocular wall).

Echographically, however, the hemangiomas are high-reflective and cannot be mixed up with melanomas.

Gliomas of the optic nerve may include the optic disk tissues and then appear to be optic disk tumors. Echographically the underlying optic nerve glioma with its typical acoustic features is easy to detect (see p. 80).

Papilledema can echographically be differentiated from other types of disk swellings first of all through the detection of increased amounts of orbital subarachnoidal fluid (see p. 43). Secondly, papilledema tends to continuously expand into the surrounding retinochoroidal layer in a tapering fashion (see Figures 21, 23 A, 37A and 40A), whereas tumors are usually clearly delineated toward the surrounding fundus.

If opaque ocular media prevent an optic disk tumor to be evaluated ophthalmoscopically, Standardized Echography still provides important information for a farreaching differentiation. Whether optic disk tumors can be seen or not, echography provides the most reliable and precise means of measuring their maximal elevation.

2.5 Optic disk trauma

As in any other place within and around the eye ball, foreign bodies (metallic or other materials) can easily and reliably be detected and localized when imbedded in or around the optic disk, with the oblique beam technique; see p. 10). Their usually irregular shape and larger size, and the fact that they are protruding beyond the surface and other boundaries of the disk allow their differentiation from optic disk drusen. Also, tell-tale signs such as a foreign body tract within the vitreous cavity pointing toward, or inserting at, the site of the foreign body, in addition to the known history of an eye injury make a confusion of a disk foreign body with an optic disk drusen extremely unlikely.

An evulsion of the optic nerve, during its acute phase, causes a rather typical ring-like, very elevated choroidal hematoma surrounding the disk. This hematoma lets the disk itself appear like the bottom of a very deep total glaucomatous excavation if not of a deep coloboma, except that everything is located in front of the surrounding scleral wall. This echographic finding together with total loss of vision in the affected eye following trauma is pathognomonic for an evulsion of the optic nerve.

In Terson's syndrome early on a subretinal and then a subvitreal hematoma develop next to the optic disk which in addition may be swollen, usually in both eyes. An optic nerve sheath distension by fluid blood (low-reflective) may be detected at this time. Later on, a dense mobile vitreous hemorrhage with extensive, if not total, posterior vitreous detachment is usually seen in these eyes together with a typical thin and smooth, dome-shaped or shallow preretinal membrane located in front of the posterior pole (Ossoinig et al. [25]). This membrane is clearly less reflective than detached retina and represents the internal limiting membrane in some cases, and a part of the posterior vitreous membrane separated through schisis (vitreoschisis), in others.

3. THE OPTIC NERVE

The echographic evaluation of the orbital portion of the optic nerve (from its insertion into the globe back to the orbital apex) and the detection and differential diagnosis of optic nerve alterations and lesions is a domain of the (real-time and high-resolution) standardized A-scan method. The B-scan method is sometimes helpful and occasionally necessary to make a diagnosis in this area.

3.1 Examination techniques, normal optic nerve echograms and dynamics of subarachnoidal fluid

3.1.1 *Basic A-scan examination and normal echograms*

Figure 12 illustrates the examination technique for the A-scan evaluation of the optic nerve and the resulting optic nerve A-scan echograms which represent true cross-sections of the optic nerve in its different segments between globe and orbital apex. Usually the A-scan probe is placed on the anesthet-

18

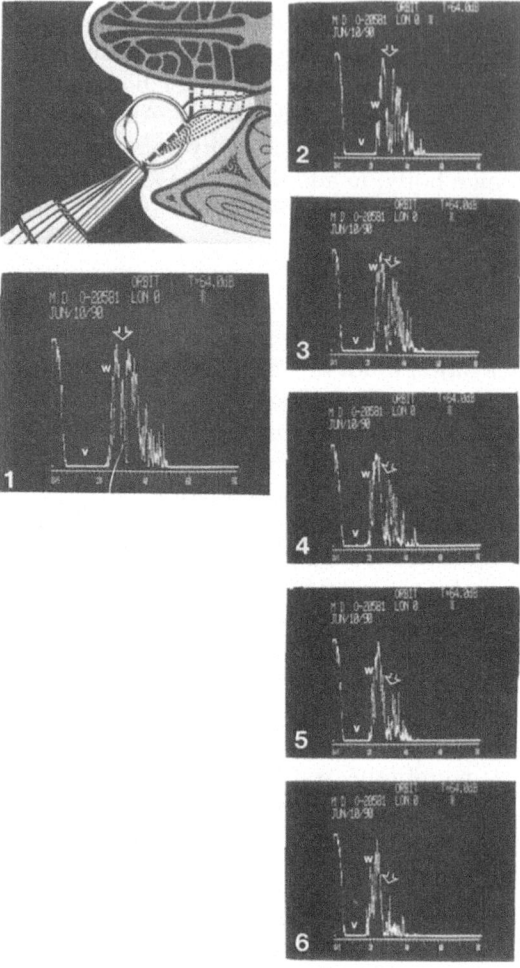

Fig. 12. A-scanning of optic nerve: schematic drawing explaining the basic A-scan screening of a normal left optic nerve and typical cross-sectional echograms obtained from the optic nerve during such scanning, ranging from the immediately retrobulbar area (echogram 1) to the orbital apex (echogram 6). Arrows point at the 'defect' in the orbital echogram representing the optic nerve cross-section. v = vitreous line; w = weakened posterior ocular wall signals (oblique exposure to sound beam); for details see Figure 13B.

ized bulbar conjunctiva in the temporal meridian behind the limbus. The beam is aimed, through the globe, first toward the inserting tendon of the medial rectus muscle (Figure 13A); then the beam is angled posteriorly gliding along the medial rectus muscle into the posterior orbit. Thereby the beam is intercepted by the optic nerve (echogram 3 of Figure 13A). At this point the optic nerve is centered within the beam through minimal angling of the probe (echogram 4 in Figure 13A). From there on the optic nerve is the guiding structure and is always centered in the beam while the beam is

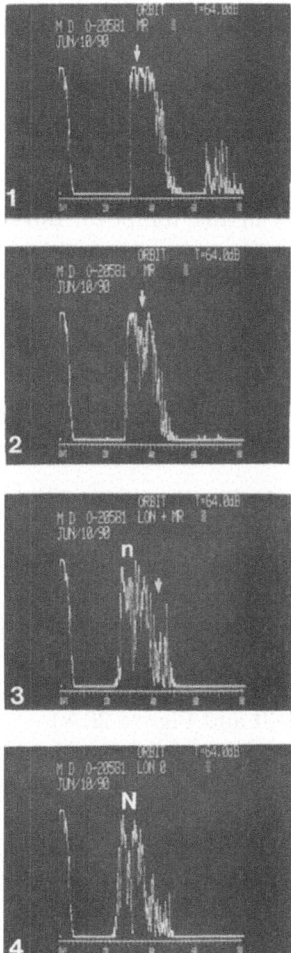

Fig. 13A. How to find the optic nerve during an A-scanning: the sound beam is first directed toward the inserting tendon of the medial rectus muscle (echogram 1, arrow). Then it is angled posteriorly into the anterior belly of this muscle (echogram 2, arrow) and further into the muscle's posterior belly (echogram 3, arrow). In echogram 3 the most anterior portion of the optic nerve is cut by the acoustic beam (n). Through minimal further angling the most anterior optic nerve cross-section is centered in the beam (echogram 4; N = normal retrobulbar optic nerve cross-section).

continuously angled posteriorly toward the orbital apex (Figure 12). During such optic nerve scanning with the A-scan method, the medial optic nerve sheaths can frequently be noted to pulsate indicating the area of entry of the central retinal artery. These pulsations translate into vertical pulsing changes in the height of the right optic nerve surface spike in the live echogram.

Display of true maximum optic nerve cross-sections – a matter of refraction
It is the refraction of the (parallel) acoustic A-scan beam at the outer layers
of the dura, which bends the beam toward the center of the optic nerve,
enough to let it trace a true cross-section of the nerve. Obviously the beam
is continuously and strongly refracted as it passes through the progressively
denser outer dural layers until it becomes perpendicular to the remaining
large surfaces of the optic nerve. This refraction is the stronger, the more
obliquely the beam arrives at the temporal dural surface (usually at more
posterior segments of the optic nerve). Once refracted enough to be perpendicular to one of the deeper layers of the temporal dura, the beam then stays
on its track perpendicular to the other, subsequently reached, large optic
nerve surfaces, i.e., the arachnoidal and pial surfaces on the temporal side
of the nerve, and the pial, arachnoidal and dural surfaces on the nasal side
of the nerve, allowing their signals to be displayed in maximal height. The
returning echoes follow the track of the incident beam (see schematic drawing
in Figure 12).

By minimally angling and adjusting the probe and beam, and by displaying
maximally high signals from the relevant optic nerve surfaces (see Figure
14B) the examiner achieves beam perpendicularity at the important large
surfaces of the optic nerve and thus guarantees the display of true cross-
sections of the optic nerve and its sheaths. As will be demonstrated and
explained later, the focused B-scan beam is not refracted enough to allow the
display of true cross-sections of the optic nerve in other than just immediately
retrobulbar planes (see p. 40 and Figure 20A).

Proof of refraction
At a first glance, the refraction as pictured in the schematic drawing of Figure
12 appears strange, if not unacceptable. That this refraction at the outer
dural layers of the optic nerve really takes place in the pictured way, however,
is proven through the application of basic rules of physics, through the
measurement of optic nerve patterns during clinical investigations, and experimentally.

(a) Maximally high, steeply rising and falling, single-peaked spikes indicate perpendicular sound beam exposure of large reflecting surfaces. It is
physically impossible to display such maximal spikes with the parallel A-scan
beam being oblique to these surfaces. When such maximal spikes are displayed from both arachnoidal surfaces of an optic nerve, the beam must
have been refracted before reaching the temporal arachnoidal surface to the
extent of being perpendicular there. The same holds true of both pial surfaces, the nasal dural surface and a large surface within the temporal dura,
once the spikes from these interfaces too are maximized.

(b) The maximal pial diameters of a normal optic nerve, measured at
different stages during an antero-posterior scanning of the nerve (see Figure
12), remain always the same (with less than 0.1 mm variations). Thus the
same maximal optic nerve thickness is measured throughout the orbit be-

tween globe and apex. This proves that even in the orbital apex where the beam certainly reaches the temporal dura obliquely, a true cross-section of the optic nerve is traced and measured. Clearly longer measurements would result from an oblique beam traversal of the optic nerve there. One could argue, that the refraction of the beam may take place at a different, may be more plausible place such as the obliquely traversed ocular wall, rather than at the outer dural layers. During the antero-posterior angling of the beam as performed in the optic nerve scanning (see Figure 12) the beam would then traverse always the same (retrobulbar) segment of the optic nerve explaining the constancy of the measurements. That this is absolutely not the case and that the apical portion of the optic nerve is indeed reached and measured when the beam is angled there, has been proven over and over again when isolated apical optic nerve thickenings (as documented with CT or MRI, or proven surgically) were clearly and without difficulty detected through echographic measurements.

(c) When measuring the maximal dural diameters of dry optic nerves first in straight gaze ('0 degree') and then in abduction ('30 degree'), the results differ slightly: the 30 degree measurement yields a slightly greater (usually by 0.3 to 0.9 mm greater) diameter than the 0 degree measurement. This is explained by the fact, that in a straight gaze the ultrasonic beam reaches the temporal dural surface more obliquely so that more of the outer dural layer is needed to refract the beam toward the perpendicular (thus being excluded from the cross-sectional measurement), than in a 30 degree examination when the beam arrives at much smaller angles of incidence to begin with (see Figure 30B). Therefore a few tenths of a mm of dural thickness are lost to the 0 degree measurement. It should be emphasized again, that an oblique traversal of the beam in straight gaze measurements would result in longer rather than the shorter measurements that, in fact, are obtained.

(d) Experimental evidence was obtained (Ossoinig [24]) that the parallel A-scan beam as used for the optic nerve measurements produced maximal single-peaked, steeply rising and falling signals from large surfaces (smooth mirror-like as well as coarsened plexiglass surfaces in a water bath) only when aimed at these surfaces perpendicularly. Finally, Hasenfratz [10] proved the refraction to occur at the outer dural layers experimentally in vitro by using particularly long optic nerves still attached to enucleated human eye bank eyes and eyes from cattle.

The height of maximum optic nerve spikes varies
(a) With the beam direction at ocular wall: When displaying the optic nerve cross-sections as illustrated in Figure 12, the maximum height of the optic nerve surface signals and the overall height of the optic nerve and orbital patterns decrease as the beam is aimed more posteriorly (see echograms 2–6 in Figure 12). This is due to sound attenuation caused by two factors: first of all, more acoustic energy is absorbed as the beam has to travel longer distances through the orbital tissues in order to reach more posterior optic

nerve portions (see the drawing in Figure 12). The same holds true of the returning echoes. Secondly, shadowing of the posterior ocular wall also weakens the advancing beam and the returning echoes. This shadowing is caused by total reflection of the portion of the beam, which reaches the curved ocular wall obliquely enough (above a critical angle of incidence) not to traverse it.

The drawing in Figure 12 illustrates that as the beam is aimed more posteriorly into the orbit, it reaches the ocular wall more obliquely and an increasing portion of the beam is totally reflected at the ocular wall. The ocular wall then casts denser acoustic shadows thus weakening the echoes returning from the orbit and optic nerve.

(b) With the positioning of the probe: For the same reason the position of the probe on the globe also determines the maximum height of the optic nerve surface signals and the overall height of the orbital and optic nerve patterns: the closer to the limbus the probe is placed, the smaller is the angle of incidence of the ultrasonic energy at the ocular wall and the higher are the orbital and optic nerve spikes as a consequence. The farther posterior the location of the probe on the globe is, the more obliquely the beam and echoes cross the ocular wall and the more of the ultrasonic energy is prevented from reaching the orbit, and from returning to the probe, respectively; this results in lower echo spikes from the optic nerve and retrobulbar tissues. These considerations are crucial for a correct assessment of lesion reflectivity during quantitative echography.

The positioning of the probe on the globe and the obliqueness of the beam at the ocular wall can be assessed retrospectively on the basis of the length of the vitreous line (signal-free zone of the echogram corresponding to the beam length within the acoustically clear vitreous body) that precedes the orbital and optic nerve spikes: the more peripherally the beam traverses the vitreous cavity and the more obliquely the beam arrives at the posterior ocular wall at the moment the echogram is documented, the shorter is the vitreous line. In Figure 12, for instance, the vitreous line appears continously shorter as the beam is angled more posteriorly (echograms 2–4). For the registration of echogram 5 the probe was repositioned more anteriorly on the globe so that the resulting vitreous line is similar to that in echogram 4 although for echogram 5 the beam was angled more posteriorly. The vitreous line in echogram 6 further decreases in length as a result of angling the beam further back yet, in order to display an optic nerve cross-section in the orbital apex (without repositioning of the probe on the globe). It should be noted, however, that all the optic nerve surface signals as observed in the echograms 1–6 of Figure 12 (although of decreasing height due to the increasingly oblique orientation of the beam toward the ocular wall) are still the maximum signals available under the conditions and thus indicate exposure of the optic nerve surfaces to a perpendicular beam. Each of these echograms, therefore, represents a true maximal cross-section of a different segment of the optic nerve ranging from an immediately retrobulbar location (echogram 1) to the orbital apex (echogram 6).

3.1.2 *Electronic measurements*

Once an optimal optic nerve cross-sectional A-scan echogram is displayed and frozen on the screen (for instance the echogram 1 in Figure 12), the arachnoidal, dural and pial diameters can be measured precisely with the help of two dot-like electronic gates which are placed over the peaks of the two relevant surface signals (the two arachnoidal spikes, the two dural signals or the two pial spikes, respectively; see Figure 13B). The diameter thus measured is digitally displayed in mm on the screen of the instrument together with the frozen echogram and the gate settings.

An electronic gate is set precisely over the peak of the relevant spike by

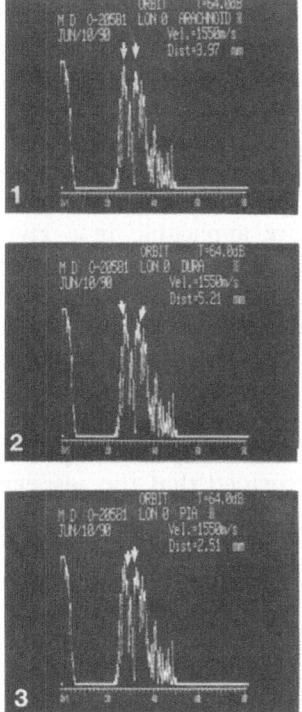

Fig. 13B. Cross-section of the retrobulbar optic nerve centered in the acoustic beam (as seen in echogram 4 of Figure 13A). By placing electronic gates for a 2-point measurement over the peaks of the two maximized arachnoidal spikes (arrows in echogram 1) the true maximum arachnoidal cross diameter is measured (3.97 mm). In echogram 2 the gates were placed over the peaks of the two maximized dural spikes (arrows) measuring the maximal dural diameter as 5.21 mm. In echogram 3 the electronic gates were placed over the peaks of the maximized pial spikes (arrows) measuring a pial diameter of 2.51 mm. Due to the excentric course of the optic nerve within the fluid-filled bag of meninges, this pial diameter, however, is not the maximal (central), but rather a peripheral one. See text on pp. 29 & 58 for technique how to measure the maximal pial diameter.

Table 1. In vivo optic nerve measurements of normals – preliminary data obtained with the Mini A-scan

Measurement	Range (mm)	Mean (mm)	Difference RON vs. LON (mm)
Maximal pial diameter	2.8–3.1	2.95	0.0–0.1
Maximal arachnoidal diameter	3.1–4.5		0.0–0.7
Maximal dural diameter	3.8–5.3		0.0–0.9
Maximal dural thickness	0.3–0.8	0.5	0.0–0.2

No significant differences between different age groups (range from birth to 91 years of age), sexes or races were noted in the normal optic nerve measurements.

shifting the live (blinking) gate over the peak coming from the left ascending limb. As soon as the gate has (barely) passed the peak (the peak is barely cleared of the gate which now is located at the top end of the right descending limb of the spike) the gate is moved minimally back to the left in order to include the peak. This way one makes sure that the peak is used as the actual reference point for the measurement and not a section of the ascending left limb next to the peak.

For the calculation of the diameters a sound velocity of 1,550 m/sec is automatically used by the Mini A-scan instrument. However, any sound velocity that might be more applicable in a given situation, may be set manually for the calculation.

Table 1 lists the ranges of maximum measurements for the pial, the arachnoidal, and the dural diameters of the normal optic nerve. It should be remembered, that only maximum measurements represent truely cross-sectional diameters. Therefore the usual statistical criteria do not apply. If, for instance, serial measurements of a pial diameter result in 2.71, 2.85, 2.95, 2.70, 2.98, 2.34, and 3.01 mm, the maximum pial diameter measured in this optic nerve is 3.01 mm, provided that the respective echogram fulfills the criteria of optimal beam alignment (maximally high pial spikes with clear-cut single peaks that do not allow any other alignment of the electronic gates than the ones which were used to obtain the 3.01 mm result). It would be misleading and useless, to calculate and list as result the mean value or a standard deviation of all these measurements, since it is known that the other lesser results are inaccurate and do not represent the true cross diameter of this optic nerve. The ranges of normal (maximal) measurements listed in the table were obtained from more than 200 patients of all age groups whose orbits were examined with the Mini A-scan instrument for a variety of orbital symptoms but without evidence of optic nerve disease, or whose optic nerves in the normal fellow orbits contributed the normal maximal measurements. The figures resulting from these measurements and listed in the table differ only slightly from our previous long-term experience in optic nerve measurements with the Kretz 7200 MA instrument.

In general, those 7200 MA measurements were shorter since the upper segments of the inner limbs (descending limbs of the left sheath signals and ascending limbs of the right surface spikes) rather than the peaks had to be used for the measurements. The reason for this shortcoming of the 7200 MA instrument is the fact, that the peaks of the optic nerve surface spikes were usually 'overloaded' and thus distorted when the high Tissue Sensitivity was used with this instrument. The Mini A-scan provides much more precise echogram tracings which can be measured electronically with greater precision and accuracy. In Mini A-scan displays of optic nerve patterns, the peaks of the important surface spikes are well defined and clearly identifiable, even at Tissue Sensitivity. This is important since the peaks are the only parts of the surface spikes which truly represent the optic nerve surfaces displayed. Therefore the optic nerve measurements obtained with the Mini A-scan (see Table 1) are more realistic and accurate than the ones that were available in the past through Kretz 7200 MA instruments. Since the Mini A-scan is real-time and provides a high picture repetition frequency, the display of the maximal surface spikes is easier and more reliable with this instrument than with the Ophthascan S, which is more difficult to handle and less accurate because of its low picture frequency.

In addition to the normal ranges of the various maximal optic nerve diameters, the mean values for the optic nerves as found in the patient population evaluated as well as the range of differences found between the measurements of the right and left optic nerves in those patients with bilaterally normal nerves, are also presented in Table 1. The normal values listed in the table apply to persons of all age groups and races as well as of both genders.

3.1.3 *Morphological basics*

In order to be able to recognize, to optimally display and to accurately as well as precisely measure the various diameters of optic nerve cross-sections, the examiner needs to know the acoustic qualities of the three optic nerve surfaces and to master the techniques designed to identify and display them.

Figures 14A–C show gross histological sections of the optic nerve and its sheaths in comparison with the surrounding orbital tissues explaining their acoustic properties, which together with the instrument design and the examination techniques determine the appearance and clinical value of the optic nerve echograms.

Figure 14A illustrates the finer overall structuring of the optic nerve causing its lower reflectivity, in contrast to the coarser structuring of the surrounding orbital tissues, resulting in their higher reflectivity. The tiny trabeculae separating the nerve fiber bundles are the main echo source in the normal optic nerve; they only weakly scatter the ultrasonic energy, whereas the larger surfaces of fat lobules, vessels and nerves within the surrounding tissues more strongly scatter the ultrasound. That is why at tissue sensitivity the optic nerve, similar to the extraocular muscles, shows up as a 'defect' in the orbital echogram (see Figure 13A). The optic nerve pattern is further enhanced by the maximum signals from the optic nerve

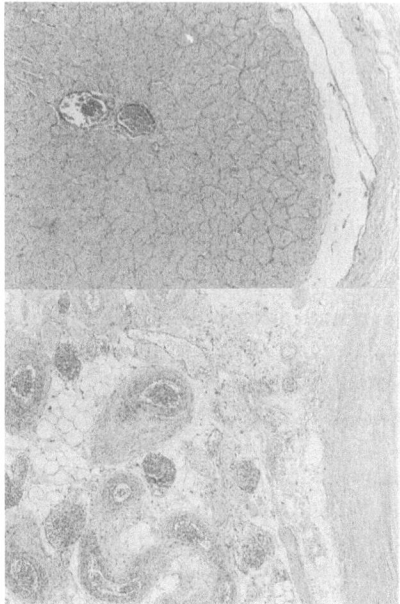

Fig. 14A. Gross histological cross-sections of a normal optic nerve and its sheaths (top) and the surrounding normal orbital tissues (bottom). Identical magnification is used for both sections. Note the clear difference between these two tissue types with regard to structure and consequent acoustic reflectivity (optic nerve is more homogenous and lower reflective than surrounding tissues creating a 'defect' in spike height in the A-scan pattern at tissue sensitivity, and an echo-free zone in B-scan patterns at optimal system sensitivity).

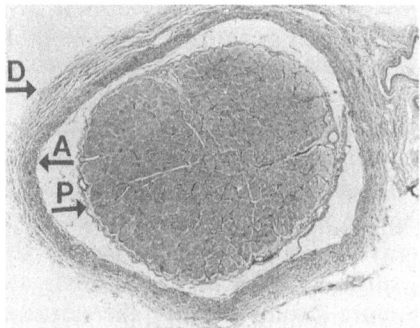

Fig. 14B. Gross histological section across normal optic nerve and meninges: D = dural surface; A = arachnoidal surface; P = pial surface.

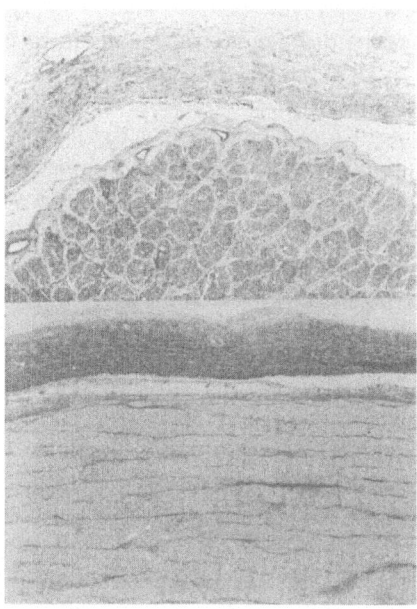

Fig. 14C. Gross histological cross-section (*top*) and long-section (*bottom*) through part of a normal optic nerve and its meninges. Note that the arachnoidal surface is fairly smooth along both the longitudinal and the transverse dimensions, whereas the pial surface appears quite bumpy (because of the longitudinal ripples created by the nerve fiber bundles) along the transverse section, but appears smooth along the longitudinal section. Therefore the simultaneous display of 2 maximal arachnoidal spikes requires absolute perpendicularity on both sides of the nerve guaranteeing true maximal cross-sections of the arachnoidal bag. In contrast, the simultaneous display of two maximal pial spikes only guarantees that the beam was directed straight across the nerve but does not indicate whether the diameter is maximal, i.e., central, or smaller than maximal because only peripheral (perpendicularity on the surface of two of the longitudinal ripples, not necessarily two exactly opposite ripples).

sheaths, which during adequate examination techniques (exposure of the large, strongly reflecting surfaces of the optic nerve sheaths to a perpendicular sound beam) produce the towering signals which most clearly separate the optic nerve echo pattern from the signals of the surrounding tissues (see Figure 13B).

Figure 14B shows a gross histological cross-section of the optic nerve and its meninges stressing the importance of the large sheath surfaces for the echographic display of the optic nerve. As is the rule for the display of all large acoustic surfaces in Standardized A-scan echography, a perpendicular sound beam exposure of the optic nerve sheaths, i.e., the arachnoidal, dural and pial surfaces, is required to record their landmark signals in maximum height and to optimize the optic nerve echograms for most accurate and precise results in the measurement of the various optic nerve (sheath) diameters and in the differential diagnosis of optic nerve lesions.

Dural, arachnoidal, and pial surfaces
Figure 14B elucidates the three echographically most important large surfaces of the optic nerve:

(a) The dura is a tunic of dense collagenous tissue which surrounds the optic nerve more like a loose bag than a tight tube. Although it is clearly non-elastic, it is wrapped around the nerve so loosely that it allows the nerve to sweep widely throughout the soft orbital tissues with eye movements, or to be stretched extensively, be it physiologically during extreme gaze directions, or pathologically by marked exophthalmus. The normal dural thickness ranges from 0.3 to 0.8 mm. The dura fuses anteriorly with the sclera and posteriorly, in the orbital apex, with the periosteum of the optic nerve canal. The outer surface, called simply 'dural surface', delineates the optic nerve sheaths from the surrounding orbital tissues. Like the outer scleral surface, the dural surface is normally indistinct, in a way continuously changing into the surrounding tissues, and has a relatively weak reflectivity. In Graves' orbitopathy and in the presence of optic nerve tumors such as meningiomas and gliomas, the dural surface becomes both more distinct and reflective.

(b) The inside surface of the dural sheath is lined by a very thin layer of the arachnoid. This is called the 'arachnoidal surface'. The arachnoidal surface is especially smooth and highly reflective. It has numerous delicate trabular connections with the pia of the optic nerve; both the small actual sizes of these trabeculae and their radial direction make them virtually silent in acoustic terms. They do not usually interfere with the clarity of the arachnoidal surface signals.

Wet and dry optic nerves
Usually the arachnoidal surface is separated from the pia by the subarachnoidal fluid. Such an optic nerve is called 'wet'. If the subarachnoidal fluid is scarce or absent altogether, the optic nerve is called 'dry'. In a dry nerve the arachnoidal and pial surfaces form one and the same acoustic interface which resembles the pial surface and is much less distinct and reflective then the arachnoidal surface in a wet nerve. Since this common interface resembles the pial surface of the wet nerve in terms of reflectivity and bumpiness, it continues to be called the pial surface in the dry nerve (with the arachnoidal surface practically disappearing in the absence of the subarachnoidal fluid).

(c) The pia lines the surface of the optic nerve molding the longitudinal ridges or ripples caused by the optic nerve fiber bundles and blends with the trabecular septal system separating the nerve fiber bundles. The outer surface of the pia is called the 'pial surface'. Like the dural surface, the pial surface is much less reflective than the arachnoidal surface. Unless the optic nerve is stretched maximally and its surface is smoothened as a consequence (e.g., in extreme lateral gaze), the pial surface is coarse.

The pial surface, while smooth along the longitudinal plane of the nerve (bottom part of Figure 14C), is quite bumpy in a transverse direction because of its longitudinal ripples (top part of Figure 14C). Therefore it is inconceivable to measure too long (obliquely anterior/posterior) sections of the optic nerve, when optimal, i.e. maximal, surface spikes are simultaneously displayed from both the temporal and nasal pial surfaces of the wet or dry optic nerve. Within the plane of an optic nerve cross-section, however, different pathways of the beam may all produce maximal pial spikes. Because of the bumps modelled by the optic nerve fiber bundles and their trabecular septa, there are several directions in which the beam may reach the pial surface perpendicularly. Thus shorter more peripheral diameters of the optic nerve cross-section may be measured (falsely suggesting optic atrophy) instead of the maximum central true optic nerve diameter (proving normal optic nerve thickness).

Optic nerve needs to be dried out
before maximal pial diameter is measured
Since the pial surface signals are less distinct and therefore much more difficult to isolate and display optimally in a wet nerve than are the arachnoidal signals, the basic rule is to always first try to dry out the nerve and eliminate the arachnoidal surfaces before measuring the maximal pial diameter. This drying out is done by extremely stretching the nerve (usually through maximum abduction of the globe), which also smoothens out the pial surface and makes perpendicular beam alignment on both optic nerve surfaces identical with the display of a true maximum cross-section of the optic nerve. Only such cross-sections will tell the examiner beyond a doubt whether an optic nerve is normal in thickness (see Figure 28, center right echogram), slightly thickened (e.g., in AION, see Figure 40B, center echogram) or thinned indicating optic nerve atrophy (see Figure 27, bottom right echogram, or Figure 28, center left echogram).

In the wet optic nerve (see Figure 15, top) the arachnoidal surface stands out acoustically through its distinctness caused by its smoothness and particularly by its high reflectivity, just like the inner scleral surface does among the ocular wall surfaces of the normal globe. Through slight angling of the probe and beam, the examiner can maximize the arachnoidal spikes fairly easily, much easier than the pial or dural spikes. In order to display the two signals from the arachnoidal surface on both the temporal and nasal sides of the optic nerve simultaneously in maximum height (as done in the echogram 4 of Figure 13A, and in the echograms of Figure 13B), the ultrasonic beam must cross through the center of the fluid-filled bag outlined by the arachnoidal surface and must hit this surface perpendicularly on both sides. Thus a true maximum cross-section of the arachnoidal bag is displayed and a maximum arachnoidal diameter is measured, when both arachnoidal spikes are simultaneously displayed in maximum height. So, in wet optic nerves, the important rule is to always display both arachnoidal surface spikes simultaneously in maximum height, which is relatively easy to do. It needs to be emphasized, that in displaying the maximal arachnoidal and dural diameters the widest sheath distension must be searched for by scanning the optic nerve throughout the orbit. In normal optic nerves, in Graves' orbitopathy and in many cases of compressive optic neuropathy, the maximum sheath diameters are found in the immediate retrobulbar area, wheras the maximum diameter is located halfway between the globe and orbital apex in cases of increased intracranial pressure. In contrast, the maximum pial diameters are identical throughout the entire orbit in normal optic nerves and in many cases of optic atrophy.

Once the arachnoidal spikes are maximized it is then easy to also recognize the lower dural and pial spikes of the optic nerve pattern (Figure 13B). The pial spikes, however, may drop out of site, if the optic nerve courses eccentrically within the fluid-filled arachnoidal bag within the cross-section from which the echogram is recorded. This is especially the case when excessive fluid is present (see Figures 24A, B and 25A).

Application of the same principle to the display and measurement of maximum dural or pial diameters, i.e., to display the two dural or the two pial spikes simultaneously in maximum height, is a more difficult (dural diameters) or at times even impossible (pial diameters) undertaking as long as the optic nerve is wet. In normal optic nerves it is usually the arachnoidal spikes which tower above all other signals and tend to come up, not the dural or pial spikes. On the other hand, the simultaneous display of both pial spikes in maximum height does not mean that the maximum pial diameter is displayed for measurement (see discussions of the display and measurement of peripheral pial diameters above and on p. 58).

In order to display the maximum optic nerve cross-section (true maximal pial diameter), the nerve first needs to be stretched to smoothen out the ripples and avoid maximum signals to originate in any other than central beam direction. In addition, the stretching must be pursued long enough to dry the optic nerve out and to eliminate the misleading and distracting (much easier maximized) arachnoidal signals. Thus, only after prolonged maximal abduction of the eye has provided a dry optic nerve, a safe and meaningful measurement of the maximal pial diameter can be achieved, which is the only reliable way of diagnosing mild thickening of the nerve or mild optic atrophy.

3.1.4. *Dynamics of subarachnoidal fluid*

The normal situation
Figure 15 illustrates the dynamics of the subarachnoidal fluid of the wet optic nerve during and following a period of extreme gaze directions (optic nerve "exercise") in the normal person. The top drawing in the figure indicates the distribution of subarachnoidal fluid which surrounds the optic nerve within the bag provided by the meninges in straight gaze ("O degree") direction. This fluid protects the optic nerve from mechanical damage during eye movements (similar to the protection of the brain by the subarachnoidal intracranial fluid). The drawings in Figure 15 somewhat exaggerate the amount of fluid surrounding the normal optic nerve, and also disregard the fact that most of this fluid is collected in the subarachnoidal space behind

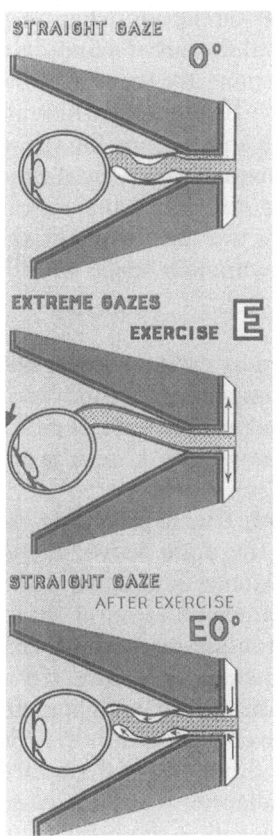

Fig. 15. Schematic drawings illustrating the course and topographic relationship of the optic nerve and its meninges as well as the distribution of the orbital subarachnoidal fluid and its communication with the intracranial subarachnoidal space through the bony optic canal, as they apply to straight gaze ("O"; top drawing), to thirty degree gaze, which actually means maximal gaze toward temporal ("E"; central drawing), and in straight gaze after exercise ("EO"; bottom drawing). "E" stands for "exercise" and means a 3-minute course of extreme gaze directions (especially toward temporal) which effects the fluid shift from the orbit into the brain.

the globe where the lack of closeness of the extraocular muscles and of the orbital bone, as well as an excess in optic nerve sheath size, allow it to pool. The drawing, however, realistically shows the relative straightness of the sheaths as compared to the meandering course of the nerve within the fluid-filled bag, caused by the surplus length of the nerve which in turn allows the nerve to stretch during physiologic eye movements and on the other hand allows even exorbitant exophthalmus to occur pathologically without being torn apart. This explains why the optic nerve is rarely located centrally within the bag of meninges and why the arachnoidal and pial surfaces often do not course concentrically in a 0-gaze direction. The meninges, however, become concentric in extreme gaze directions when the optic nerve is maximally stretched. Then, however, all the subarachnoidal fluid is eliminated from the orbit and the nerve has become dry (central drawing in Figure 15).

The drawings in Figure 15 also illustrate how the dural optic nerve sheaths continue as sclera anteriorly and as bony lining (periosteum) within the optic canal posteriorly. The subarachnoidal fluid-filled space around the optic nerve communicates through the optic canal (being reduced there to a narrow "spongy" tissue resembling the meshwork in the anterior chamber angle) with the intracranial subarachnoidal space where the subarachnoidal orbital fluid originates.

What determines the amount of orbital subarachnoidal fluid?
The amount of orbital subarachnoidal fluid varies from person to person, from one orbit to the other in the same person, and from time to time in the same orbit of the same person. It results from the combined effect of several influential factors:

(a) Intracranial pressure. The higher it is, the more fluid is displaced into the orbit surrounding the optic nerve. In patients with severely raised intracranial pressure, for instance in patients with severe 'benign' intracranial hypertension (BIH), the arachnoidal/dural sheaths may be distended to a maximum of close to 8 mm in the mid-orbit (see Figure 24A). On the other hand, with a rather low intracranial pressure, the optic nerve may be virtually dry in a normal person (even during straight gaze).

(b) Resistance to fluid exchange within the optic canal. A valve mechanism may also be involved at either end of the optic canal (possibly conditioned by the topography of the adjacent brain tissues or the annulus zinnii as well as by the shape of the bony wall in the orbital apex). This could explain the differences in the amount of subarachnoidal orbital fluid, which were observed in the same examinee when examined in different positions (prone vs. supine).

(c) Soft tissue pressure within the orbit. This factor is influenced by the volume of orbital tissues relative to the size of the bony orbit; by the blood supply to, and drainage from, the orbit; by the thicknesses of the extraocular muscles, the periorbita and the arachnoidal as well as dural sheaths of the optic nerve themselves; and by the tightness of the lids. All these factors influence the amount of the subarachnoidal fluid present in an orbit.

Optic nerve exercise and '30 degree test'
Through the optic canal, the subarachnoidal fluid may shift into and out of the orbit, and in fact does so on a regular basis. This occurs especially with eye movements and intracranial pressure changes:

During extreme gaze directions, especially in maximal abduction of the eye, the optic nerve and its sheaths are maximally stretched and the orbital subarachnoidal fluid is squeezed out of the orbit entirely and shifted into the intracranial space. This is effected by the stretching of the non-elastic dural sheaths and the compression of the subarachnoidal space through pressuring by the stretched and contracted horizontal or vertical rectus muscles. This action is called 'exercise' of the optic nerve ("E"; center drawing in Figure 15). It is used to dry out the orbital optic nerve. The drying of the optic nerve may occur quickly within seconds or more slowly within a few minutes.

The exercise may be performed by letting the patient look extremely to the lateral side for 15 to 20 seconds and then repeating extreme gaze directions in other directions (especially in medial and also in superior ones) for similar time intervals. The alternation in gaze direction allows the patient to more forcefully do the stretching while changing to other gaze directions before getting tired and letting up. This exercise is performed for a total of at least three minutes. Or, when measurements on a completely dry optic nerve are to be performed (e.g., for measuring the maximal pial diameter to determine, for example, optic atrophy or optic nerve swelling in optic neuritis), the optic nerve is examined while the patient has assumed an extreme lateral gaze direction. An optic nerve examination during this maximal abduction of the eye is called the 30 degree test (Ossoinig et al. [22]). This name was adopted toward the end of the 1970s, when the optic nerve structures were evaluated in an exactly 30 degree abduction of the globe – in addition to the basic evaluation in primary ('0' degree) gaze (see also discussion on p. 47). When the 30 degree standard was omitted in the mid 1980s as it became obvious that the exact angle of gaze deviation did not matter, and a maximum abduction was often more effective than the 30 degree gaze direction, the name continued to be used signifying maximal lateral gaze direction, however.

What happens after the exercise?
After the exercise, the patient is given sufficient time of rest (at least three minutes) with closed eyes allowing the subarachnoidal fluid, which was shifted from the orbit during the exercise, to return into the orbit. The return of the original amount of orbital subarachnoidal fluid may take from a few seconds to a few minutes depending on the factors that also determine the amount of subarachnoidal fluid found in the orbit to begin with (see above).

In the normal person, the original amount of orbital subarachnoidal fluid will be restored as indicated in the bottom drawing of Figure 15, which illustrates the situation in straight gaze after the exercise ('EO'), at the latest after the three minutes of rest have passed.

It should be mentioned that the resulting equilibrium between all these factors is re-established in a wave-like fashion with undulating maximal arachnoidal diameters being measured during the period of restauration. This undulation is obviously caused by the kinetics involved. Thus more than the originally measured and finally restored amount of subarachnoidal fluid may be measured temporarily (see Figure 25B).

The intracranial pressure may be too high (as evidenced by extreme distension of the optic nerve sheaths), or the effect of the muscle contraction and the stretching of the optic nerve may be too weak (usually when the ocular motility is limited, but also after surgical decompression of the orbit)

34

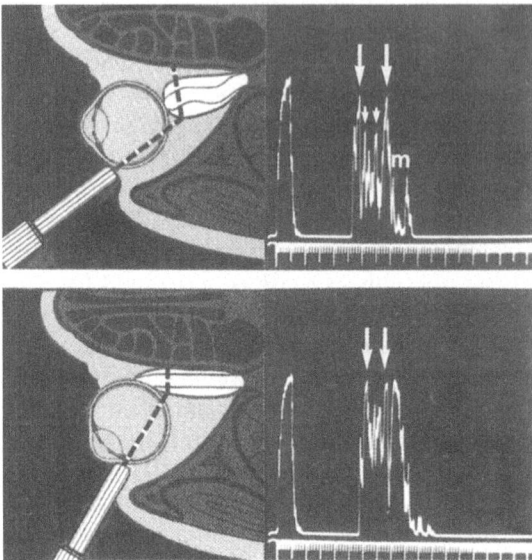

Fig. 16. Distribution and dynamics of orbital subarachnoidal fluid in BIH: the schematic draw-ings and corresponding A-scan echograms (Kretz 7200 MA instrument) in a case of BIH demonstrate the marked distension of the arachnoidal bag caused by increased amounts of subarachnoidal fluid in straight gaze (top) and the reduced distension and amount of fluid at 30 degree gaze (bottom). Large arrows point out the arachnoidal surfaces, small arrows mark the pial surfaces; m = medial rectus muscle. Note that the muscle too is being stretched and thus thinned during the 30 degree testing.

in order to completely dry out an optic nerve (e.g., case of BIH as illustrated in Figure 16). As long as a decrease in the maximal arachnoidal diameter of at least 5% can be shown during an attempted 30 degree test in such cases, the fact that the distension of the optic nerve sheaths is caused by increased subarachnoidal fluid is proven (see also p. 47). When attempting to differenti-ate between fluid and solid distension of the optic nerve sheaths with the help of the 30 degree test or through exercise, one needs, however, to consider the simultaneous presence of increased fluid and of thickening of the optic nerve (e.g., glioma, see Figures 43, 44B) or simultaneous fluid distension and thickening of the optic nerve sheaths (e.g., meningioma, see Figures 45B and 46A).

Valsalva's procedure
Figure 17 illustrates another facet of the hydrodynamics of subarachnoidal fluid. During a Valsalva's test the optic nerve sheaths may expand dramat-ically as seen in the figure, obviously as a consequence of increased intra-cranial pressure. While a Valsalva's test for obvious reasons can be dangerous in certain conditions, especially in an old patient, and therefore should be restricted to rare necessary indications (i.e., to prove the presence of an

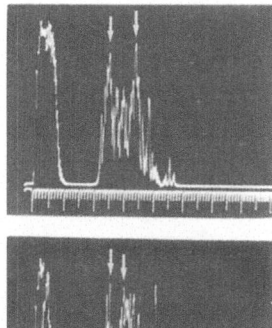

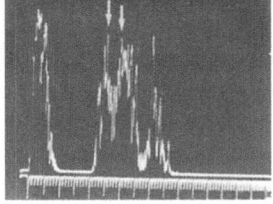

Fig. 17. Effect of a Valsalva's test on the amount of orbital subarachnoidal fluid: Standardized A-scan echograms (Kretz 7200 MA instrument) demonstrate the maximal arachnoidal diameter in straight gaze during a Valsalva's procedure (top) and before or after the Valsalva's test (bottom) in a normal optic nerve. Arrows mark the arachnoidal surfaces. Note that during the Valsalva's procedure the arachnoidal diameter has more than doubled over the normal diameter in this person.

orbital varix – after other lesions, especially aneurysms and A-V fistulas have been ruled out), it may on occasion be useful in re-introducing increased subarachnoidal fluid after exercise has expelled it from the orbit, in order to prove compressive optic neuropathy (see discussion on pp. 37, 62). While a positive Valsalva's test in this situation can be very helpful, a negative test does not mean much, since it may be caused by markedly increased volume of orbital soft tissues (especially of the extraocular muscles) which may be overwhelming enough to prevent the excess subarachnoidal fluid to collect within the orbit, under the special conditions of a Valsalva's test. It all depends on whether the increased intracranial pressure succeeds in overcoming the compression and in pumping fluid into the orbital subarachnoidal space before orbital blood congestion and swelling of orbital tissues (especially that of extraocular muscles but also that of the arachnoidal and pial sheaths) prevent the subarachnoidal fluid from streaming into the orbit.

Optic nerve compression
Figure 18 demonstrates the hydrodynamics in cases of compression of the optic nerve, which provide the morphological basis for the diagnosis of compressive optic neuropathy (both abbreviated CON). The top echogram shows the presence of increased subarachnoidal fluid anteriorly. It gets there usually during sleeping periods. It stays there being caught in the anterior orbit unable to pass through the zone of compression until it is squeezed back through this zone by 'exercise'.

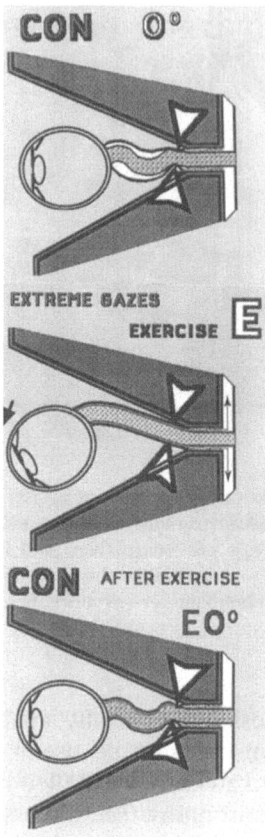

Fig. 18. The distribution and dynamics of orbital subarachnoidal fluid in CON caused by severe Graves' orbitopathy: the *top drawing* indicates the increased subarachnoidal fluid during O-gaze prior to the exercise. The *center drawing* illustrates the drying out of the optic nerve during exercise. The *bottom drawing* indicates that because of the optic nerve compression (example of Graves' orbitopathy) at the orbital apex (arrows), the optic nerve remains dry after the exercise (compare with the physiological restitution of orbital subarachnoidal fluid in the normal person as illustrated in the bottom drawing of Figure 15).

It must be postulated that during the sleeping period of a person the intracranial pressure rises temporarily high enough to displace greater amounts of subarachnoidal fluid into the orbit overcoming the obstacle placed by the compression zone. While after such spikes in intracranial pressure, the excess orbital fluid in a normal person returns into the intracranial space spontaneously re-establishing the previous balance, this fluid remains caught in the orbit of a patient with CON (see Figures 31A, 31B, 32, 33 and 35B).

The compression zone is often located in the orbital apex, as is the case with Graves' orbitopathy (optic nerve surrounded by a cuff of swollen tissues) or in the presence of large, posteriorly and nasally situated orbital tumors which push the optic nerve against the temporal rim of the optic canal entrance. At other times the compression zone lies within the optic canal, e.g., in cases of optic neuritis caused by sphenoidal sinusitis. Or the compression zone is located within the mid- to posterior orbits, e.g., when optic nerve tumors such as gliomas and meningiomas obliterate the subarachnoidal space.

During the exercise some or, as illustrated in the center echogram of Figure 18, all of the orbital subarachnoidal fluid is pushed out of the orbit and into the intracranial subarachnoidal space by temporarily overcoming the obstacle of the compression zone. Following the exercise, the orbital portion of the optic nerve remains dry (bottom echogram of Figure 18) or shows a reduced amount of orbital subarachnoidal fluid as compared to the situation prior to the exercise (depending on how much fluid was shifted from the orbit during the exercise). At times the exercise fails to dry out a compressed optic nerve or even to result in a significant decrease of the subarachnoidal fluid. Then a second or even third round of exercise may be needed to yield a clear-cut result decreasing the amount of orbital subarachnoidal fluid significantly (see Figures 32 and 35B) or to finally result in a dry optic nerve.

Morphological proof of CON
Optic nerve compression is proven, when initially present orbital subarachnoidal fluid (which may be present in a normal quantity or may be clearly augmented) decreases during an exercise or dissappears altogether resulting in a dry optic nerve, and when this fluid fails to fully return or to return at all during the resting period of at least 3 minutes, which follows the exercise (Figures 32, 33, and 35B). The failure of the displaced fluid to return spontaneously indicates that there is a lack of free communication between the intracranial and the orbital subarachnoidal spaces, i.e., compression of the optic nerve.

Effectiveness of the exercise in CON
There is a wide range of responses to exercise in cases of CON: sometimes even one brief set of extreme eye movements, as performed during testing of ocular motility, or an applanation tonometry done in a patient with Graves' disease, with the patient being directed to look somewhat higher than normal, is sufficient to permanently dry out an optic nerve or at least rid the nerve of a significant amount of its orbital subarachnoidal fluid. In other cases two or three courses of 3-minute exercises are necessary to achieve a noticeable effect. The ease or difficulty of expelling orbital subarachnoidal fluid in cases of CON depends on several factors: the ability of a patient to perform extreme gaze directions; the effectiveness of the contraction and/or extension of the muscles involved in squeezing the orbital subarachnoidal fluid out; the degree to which the manoeuvre stretches the optic nerve; the rigidity and thickness of the optic nerve sheaths and their part in expelling the fluid from

the orbit; the resistence of the intracanalicular tissues to fluid exchange and, of course, the severity of compression exerted upon the optic nerve.

The ease or the difficulty, with which fluid is expelled from the orbit, are no reliable indicators of the severity of CON
The discussion of the effectiveness of an exercise (above) makes it understandable, that the ease or difficulty with which subarachnoidal fluid may be expelled from the orbit, does not allow direct conclusions upon the severity of the optic nerve compression. Experience has shown, however, that great amounts of orbital subarachnoidal fluid present in compressed optic nerves prior to an exercise always indicate severe compression.

An exception to this rule has been experienced by us in a case of combined Graves' orbitopathy (with CON) and BIH: both optic nerves in this patient showed marked fluid sheath distension prior to an exercise. Following the exercise, the fluid returned promptly and completely in one nerve, whereas it returned incompletely and at a very slow pace over a period of 10 minutes to the other. In this case the great amount of sheath distension was caused by the increased intracranial pressure and did not necessarily indicate severe CON. The extremely slow fluid exchange in the compressed nerve (as proven by the incomplete return of the fluid after the exercise in our case) may be a valid indicator of CON in cases of severe BIH should no fluid deficit result from an exercise at all. In plain BIH, the fluid always returns to the orbits in a matter of seconds (on the side with the greater fluid distension) and a couple of minutes (on the side of the lesser fluid distension) as illustrated in Figures 25A and B.

Need for baseline measurement prior to any exercise
It is also understandable from the above discussion on the effectiveness of an exercise, that any type of exercise must be avoided prior to an echographic evaluation for CON on the day of such examination. It is therefore preferable to do the echographic evaluation during the morning hours rather than late in the day; it is absolutely necessary to do the echographic test prior to any other type of eye examination including checking the visual acuity or doing an applanation tonometry, etc. By the same token, the initial straight gaze optic nerve measurements must be done prior to any other echographic evaluations such as a basic examination of the orbit. Unless these rules are observed, a lack of (increased) orbital subarachnoidal fluid (dry optic nerve or optic nerve with minimal amounts of subarachnoidal fluid on the outset) does not rule out the possibility of CON.

3.1.5 *Basic B-scan examination*

Standard cuts
Figure 19 illustrates the capacity of B-scan for demonstrating the exact location of the optic disk and of the retrobulbar course of the optic nerve as it inserts into the globe, whenever this is clinically useful. Posterior longitudi-

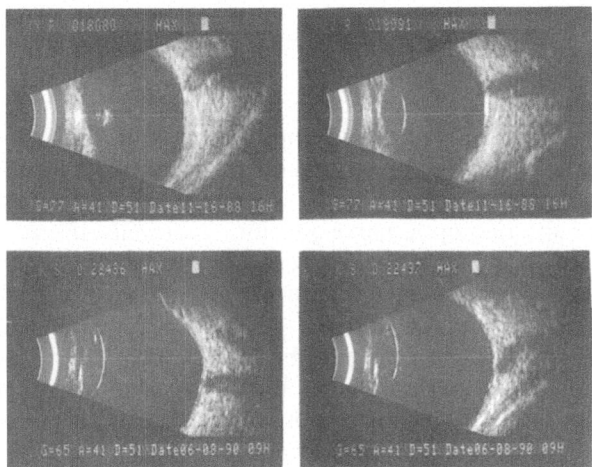

Fig. 19. Inverse optic nerve insertion: horizontal axial B-scan echograms from both eyes and orbits of two persons, one (top echograms) with an inverse optic nerve insertion OD (top left) and another one (bottom echograms) with an inverse optic nerve insertion OS (bottom right). The optic nerves of the fellow orbits (top right and bottom left) insert regularly. Note that the inversely inserting optic nerves approach the globe from the nasal side.

nal scans through the optic disk, especially those along the nasal horizontal meridians (3:00 meridian in the right orbit, 9:00 meridian in the left orbit) and posterior transverse sections through the optic disk across these meridians (see Figures 2 and 31A) are the preferred B-scan techniques for the documentation of the optic disk location and of the topography of the retrobulbar optic nerve portion. In addition, vertical axial sections through the optic disk or horizontal axial cuts through the optic disk and macula (as utilized for the echograms in Figure 19) are useful for B-scan documentation.

Artefacts
For the B-scan display of long-sections of the optic nerve, the acoustic beam reaches the surfaces of the optic nerve and its sheaths at large angles of incidence if not tangentially, which causes strong shadowing (total reflection of a significant portion of the ultrasonic energy at these surfaces). This artefact together with the lower reflectivity of the optic nerve (as compared to the surrounding tissues) causes the artefactitious cone-shape of the optic nerve pattern in many B-scan echograms (narrow pattern next to the globe, progressively wider patterns more posteriorly) and limit the B-scan display of the optic nerve to the anterior half of its orbital extent (see also the bottom right echogram in Figure 21).

Inverse insertion of the optic nerve
In Figure 19, the right (left echograms) and left (right echograms) optic

nerves of two patients are displayed in horizontal axial B-scan sections. One optic nerve in each patient inserts regularly, wheras the fellow optic nerve in the other orbit inserts inversely. In the usual insertion, the optic nerve is seen to approach the posterior ocular wall straight from behind or slightly more from temporal. In contrast, the optic nerve with the 'inverse' insertion curves steeply from the nasal side as it inserts into the globe. This "inverse" insertion necessitates a change in the A-scan approach for evaluating and measuring the anterior optic nerve portion. Normally the A-scan probe is placed on the temporal meridian between limbus and equator and the beam is aimed at the optic nerve from temporal (see Figure 12). In the case of an inverse optic nerve insertion into the globe, this temporal approach turns out to be difficult or impossible; the beam then would approach the optic nerve surfaces almost tangentially so that even massive refraction cannot bend the beam into a direction that is perpendicular to these surfaces. In this situation the probe is placed between limbus and equator of the nasal meridian and the optic nerve is beamed at from the nasal side. An inverse optic nerve insertion as well as any other oblique insertion may, in some globes, cause choroidal folds (see Figure 21).

Cross-sectional display limited to retrobulbar area

Figures 20A and B illustrate two major drawbacks of B-scan echography in the documentation of the optic nerve and in the measurement and differential diagnosis of its lesions. The well-focussed beam required for B-scan echography is not refracted as readily toward the optic nerve when arriving obliquely at the nerve's outer dural surface, as is the case with the parallel A-scan beam (see discussion on p. 20). Therefore, a true cross-section may only be displayed from a small portion of the optic nerve lying immediately behind the globe. More posterior portions of the optic nerve may usually be shown as long-sections only, resulting in the artefacts described above.

In Figure 20A, 6 acoustic sections of the retrobulbar portion of an optic nerve are shown. They were obtained by minimally angling the transverse acoustic sections through the optic nerve from a more nasal anterior direction toward temporal and posterior (echograms 1–6), similar to the angling of the A-scan beam as demonstrated in Figure 12. For echogram 1, the vertical acoustic section was aimed at a nasal fundus portion adjacent to the disk, barely touching the disk margin while reaching a nasally located more posterior section of the optic nerve. Echograms 2 and 3 were obtained by minimally angling the acoustic section more posteriorly and temporally (i.e., toward and into the optic disk). Echogram 2 shows a partial, and echogram 3 displays a complete (maximal) cross-section of a portion of the optic nerve that is located immediately behind the globe.

When attempting to show a more posterior B-scan cross-section of the optic nerve by angling the acoustic section more posteriorly yet, the cross-section quickly turns into a long-section with the corresponding acoustic artefacts described above. Echogram 4 shows how the cross-section opens

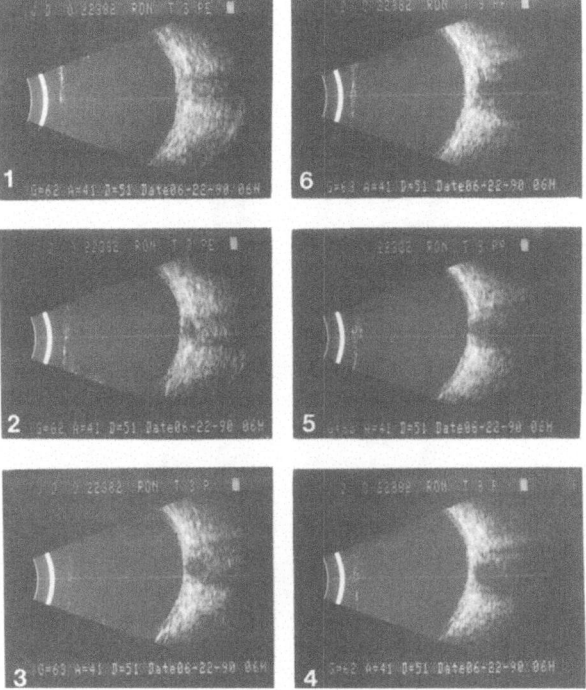

Fig. 20A. How to display a B-scan cross-section of the retrobulbar optic nerve portion. *Echogram 1:* transverse B-scan section through a normal right optic nerve, cutting through the nasal disk margin. A stepwise (minimal) angling of the acoustic section (not of the proximal end of the probe which is angled nasally) toward temporal results in the *echograms 2, 3, 4* and finally in the *echogram 5,* when the center of the disk is reached. Only with the sound beam direction chosen for *echogram 3* a true maximum cross-section of the optic nerve at a site immediately behind the globe is achieved. When angling on, the cross-section quickly turns into a long-section due to lack of sufficient refraction of the focussed B-scan beam toward the nerve center (compare with the strong refraction of the parallel A-scan beam as illustrated in Figure 12). Echogram 3 shows the true maximal cross-section of the retrobulbar optic nerve only because the probe was shifted more posteriorly on the globe for a more favorable direction of the acoustic section upon arrival at the nerve's surface. For the display of *echogram 6* the probe was angled posteriorly in an attempt to repeat the cross-sectional view of the optic nerve at a more posterior site; this did not succeed, however, since the acoustic section met the posterior optic nerve surface too obliquely for a cross-sectional cut and a long-sectional cut resulted instead.

up posteriorly into a long-section; echogram 5 resulted from the acoustic section reaching the center of the disk.

This is in contrast to the A-scan beam which is parallel and therefore much more refracted toward the optic nerve center (see Figure 12). Since the refraction of the A-scan beam is the stronger, the more obliquely the beam arrives at the outer surface of the dural sheath, true maximal A-scan

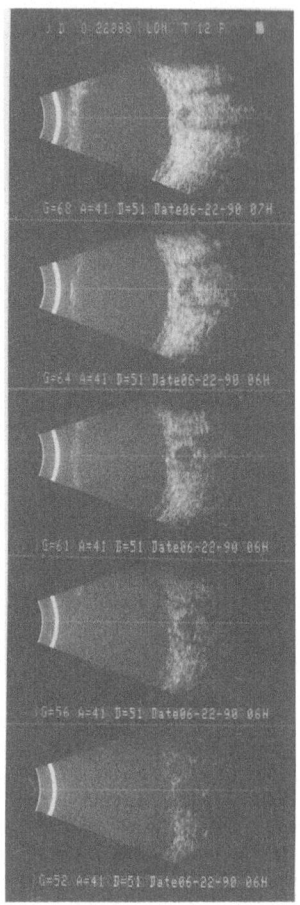

Fig. 20B. "Blooming" prevents B-scans from being useful for optic nerve measurements: series of cross-sectional B-scans of the same retrobulbar portion of a normal left optic nerve at various system sensitivities (decreasing from top to bottom: settings of 68, 64, 61, 56 and 52 decibels) demonstrating the "blooming" artefact of B-scan displays. Note how the optic nerve diameter appears progressively larger as system sensitivity decreases.

cross-sections may be obtained with ease even from the apical portion of the optic nerve.

If one attempted to show a more posterior B-scan cross-section of the nerve by shifting (rather than angling) the probe and thus the acoustic section more posteriorly (echogram 6), a more posterior long-section of the optic nerve is usually obtained instead of a more posterior cross-section. Thus the area from which a true B-scan cross-section of the optic nerve may be obtained is very small and limited to the retrobulbar area. The best placement of the B-scan probe on the globe, i.e., the best meridian across which the acoustic section is aimed in order to obtain an optimal cross-sectional display of the optic nerve, depends on the course the optic nerve assumes behind the globe and thus also on the gaze direction during the echographic display.

The 'blooming' artefact
In Figure 20B the same retrobulbar cross-section of the optic nerve is displayed at high system sensitivity of the B-scan instrument (echogram 1, top) and at progressively lower system sensitivities (echograms 2–5, below). The dark-appearing disk-like echo-free zone representing a retrobulbar cross-section of the optic nerve clearly increases in size with decreasing echo signal intensities (system sensitivities). This is another artefact of B-scan, called 'blooming', which renders B-scan displays virtually useless for measurements of the optic nerve cross-diameter. Blooming of the signals is caused by the fact, that with increasing echo intensities (or increasing amplification of the echo signals), not only the brightness of the displayed signals increases but also their sizes on the screen. Thus the echo-free zone representing the nerve cross-section, decreases in size with increasing system sensitivities (signal intensities) falsely giving the impression of optic atrophy. In order to realistically display a true cross-section of the optic nerve, the system sensitivity would have to be reduced to the point where the B-scan would lose its two-dimensional characteristics and thus any clinical advantage over the A-scan. In addition, such a B-scan display would lack the reliability of the A-scan display in measuring the maximal diameter of the optic nerve (B-scan displays lack sensitive indicators for maximal signals and thus perpendicular sound beam incidence).

For these reasons, B-scan is neither useful for the display of optic nerve cross-sections (except for a tiny zone behind the globe) nor for measurements of the optic nerve. Since B-scan is also very limited in indicating the internal structure and reflectivity of optic nerve lesions and equally limited in demonstrating the hydrodynamics of the subarachnoidal fluid, it is much less useful for the evaluation of optic nerve disorders than the A-scan method. Nevertheless, B-scan, at times, adds important information to the standardized A-scan findings in certain cases.

3.2 Optic nerve lesions

3.2.1 *Benign intracranial hypertension (BIH) or idiopathic intracranial hypertension (IIH)*

Papilledema
A swollen optic nerve head, particularly when the swelling is mild or appears to be unilateral, can be a great challenge for the clinician. Clarification of its underlying cause may require a battery of expensive or uncomfortable tests ranging from neuro-imaging procedures to lumbar puncture; some of these may be entirely unnecessary.

By easily and quickly answering the one question that arises first in these cases, i.e., whether or not a swollen disk represents true papilledema, Standardized Echography is of great help: by simply measuring the arachnoidal diameter, echography indicates whether the subarachnoidal fluid is or is not abnormally increased and thus clarifies whether the disk swelling is true papilledema ("wet" disk swelling) or is caused by other local conditions such as ischemic events, buried drusen, etc., or whether it simply represents a disk anomaly ("dry" disk swelling).

This echographic measurement is an easy and quick clinical procedure that may involve only a single application of an anesthetic eye drop and may be completed in less than 3 minutes. In papilledema, the maximal arachnoidal diameter ranges from 5 to 8 mm. In the other causes of disk swelling, normal arachnoidal diameters (see Table 1) are found. In addition, Standardized Echography is helpful in directly identifying some of the conditions which cause swelling of the optic disk such as buried optic disk drusen (see p. 9) and anterior ischemic optic neuropathy (see p. 76).

Increased intracranial pressure vs. optic nerve compression
Since Standardized Echography also differentiates clearly and reliably between the two main causes of (wet) papilledema, i.e., increased intracranial pressure (BIH, intracranial tumors, Terson's syndrome) on the one hand, and optic nerve compression (e.g., Graves' orbitopathy, posterior ischemic optic neuropathy, posterior optic neuritis, optic nerve or other orbital tumors, sub-periosteal orbital hematomas, basal encephaloceles) on the other, this method deserves a place in the front line of diagnostic procedures applied for the clarification of the nature and cause of optic disk swelling. In fact, Standardized Echography is the easiest way of initially pointing out the probability of increased intracranial pressure (e.g., in a case of BIH) and is an easy, quick and inexpensive test for following the natural course of the condition or the effectiveness of its medical or surgical treatment during multiple visits of a patient.

In addition, Standardized Echography, has helped to better understand the dynamics of the subarachnoidal fluid flow in cases of increased intracranial pressure vs. optic nerve compression, and offers explanations for failure of papilledema to develop in one or both eyes inspite of increased intracranial pressure.

Standardized Echography – a reliable test to indicate increased intracranial pressure
G. Cennamo et al. [4, 5] demonstrated the immediate and prompt response of the optic nerve sheath width to changes of intracranial pressure in infants who underwent shunt procedures for hydrocephalus, while they were monitoring the optic nerve sheath diameters in these patients with Standardized Echography during general anesthesia and surgery.

Galetta et al. [8] reported a case of BIH, in whom they were able to show a significant decrease of orbital subarachnoidal fluid following lumbar puncture.

In our institution, with the assistance of T. Fisher, K. Itani, D. Reshef, G. Tamayo, and C. Tamburrelli, the maximal arachnoidal diameter was measured in 15 consecutive cases of BIH within a 24-hour period prior to lumbar punctures performed to determine the intracranial pressure. In all of these cases the maximal arachnoidal diameter was greater than 5 mm (the range was 5.04 to 8.00 mm, the mean was 6.24 mm). The opening pressure during lumbar puncture was greater than 200 mm of water in all of them (the range was from 238 to 570 mm, the mean was 384 mm). In 15 patients with a variety of conditions other than BIH, the maximal arachnoidal diameter was measured prior to a scheduled lumbar puncture, to match the BIH group. None of the patients in this control group had an abnormally wide maximal arachnoidal diameter (range was 3.1 to 3.49 mm, mean was 3.31 mm); none of these patients had an opening pressure of greater than 200 mm of water during the lumbar puncture that followed the echographic measurement (range was 60 to 182 mm, mean was 129 mm). In two of the BIH patients with marked sheath distension prior to the lumbar puncture, the maximal arachnoidal diameter was also measured during the procedure; in both cases the optic nerve dried out instantly as the cerebrospinal fluid was removed. The arachnoidal sheaths literally collapsed under the observation of the echographer. All optic nerve measurements in this study have been performed with the Kretztechnik 7200 MA standardized A-scan instrument.

B-scan signs of increased subarachnoidal fluid
Figure 21 shows B-scan images of optic nerves in eyes with papilledema and choroidal folds, both produced by marked optic nerve sheath distension due to increased subarachnoidal fluid behind the eye balls (left and top right). Because the nerve sheaths are excessively wide immediately behind the globe, more fluid is collected there giving the longitudinal B-scan images of the optic nerve their typical flying-bat appearance. Papilledema is also readily seen in B-scan sections through the optic disk in these eyes.

In the presence of increased subarachnoidal fluid, this fluid may not only be recognized from the flying-bat configuration in longitudinal cuts, but also from transverse B-scan sections placed through the retrobulbar optic nerve portion (left echograms in Figure 22A). As a matter of fact, careful and meticulous high-resolution B-scan techniques will even in the normal optic nerve always show signs of subarachnoidal fluid in its retrobulbar cross-sections as long as the nerve is wet. To obtain such cross-sectional B-scan images, the probe needs to be placed on the globe more posteriorly than is usually done. Such posterior cuts through the globe are necessary to allow the acoustic beam to arrive at the outer dural surface behind the globe in an almost perpendicular direction. Unlike the parallel A-scan beam (see Figure 12), the focussed B-scan beam is not deflected sufficiently by refraction at the outer dural surface to obtain true cross-sections of the subarachnoidal space and optic nerve, when it arrives there at larger angles of incidence. If

46

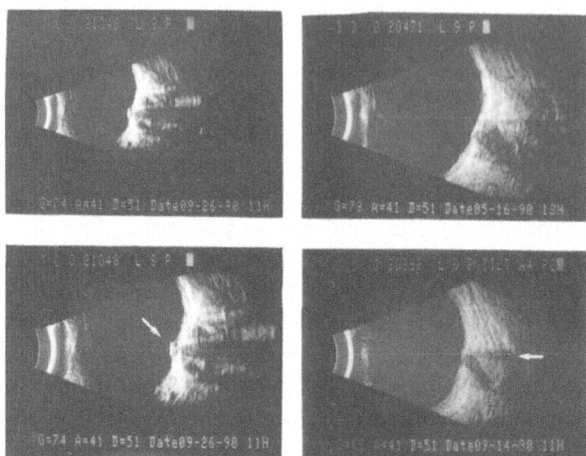

Fig. 21. B-scan signs of increased subarachnoidal fluid: *Left:* longitudinal B-scans of the right eye and orbit in a 20-year-old male patient with BIH showing marked papilledema (arrow) as well as a pronounced sheathing sign delineating the optic nerve (in this case caused by increased subarachnoidal fluid): two chains of echo signals correspond with the surface of the optic nerve as it is separated from the dural sheaths by copious amounts of fluid (both the subarachnoidal fluid and the optic nerve itself are low-reflective enough to appear as signal-free zones in the B-scan). Note the flying-bat configuration of the anterior optic nerve pattern (head looking left toward papilledema, the two wings seen above and below). It is important to display the optic nerve always at orbital expansion too to include signals from the deeper portion of the orbit (above), even though better detail display is obtained with the globe expansion (below). *Top right:* longitudinal B-scan from the left eye of a 41-year-old male patient with minimal papilledema and choroidal folds (both better recognizable in Figure 23A), both caused by marked fluid distension of the optic nerve sheaths behind this eye (see Figure 23B). Note the flying bat configuration of the anterior optic nerve pattern. *Bottom right:* longitudinal B-scan from the right eye of a 38-year-old female patient with choroidal folds, caused by a very oblique optic nerve insertion from temporal presumably indenting and thus flattening the posterior pole and producing the choroidal folds. The arrow points at an artefact caused by total reflection of the sound beam and not corresponding with any optic nerve sheath structure; the optic nerve can be seen to approach the globe obliquely from temporal (in the echogram from inferior).

a more antero-posterior beam approach is used for the transverse B-scan display by placing the B-scan probe near the limbus, flying-bat patterns similar to those in longitudinal scans (see Figure 21) may be obtained instead of the cross-sections seen in Figure 22A.

A-scan proof of subarachnoidal fluid (30 degree test)
A decrease in the amount of subarachnoidal fluid surrounding the optic nerve may be noticed to some extent upon 30 degree examination even in B-scan examinations (see Figures 22A and 31B). However, this decrease and the exact amount of subarachnoidal fluid are appreciated much better and are quantitated by precise electronic measurements with the A-scan display (Figures 16, 22A, 22B and 23B):

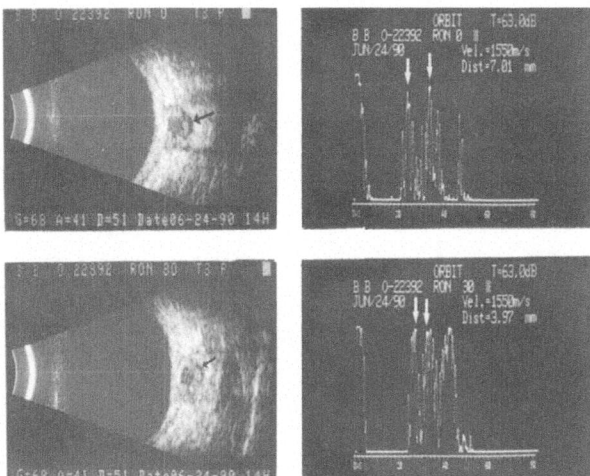

Fig. 22A. Optic nerve sheath distension by increased subarachnoidal fluid – effect of the 30 degree test: A-scan and transverse B-scan sections through a retrobulbar portion of the right optic nerve in a 50-year-old female patient with BIH, recorded in straight gaze direction (*top*) and at 30 degree gaze (*bottom*). The increased subarachnoidal fluid forms a dark ring around the cross-sectional view of the optic nerve in the B-scans (arrows); the decrease in retrobulbar fluid during the 30 degree test is recognizable in the B-scan, but much clearer in the A-scans which also allow to measure it with great precision: the point-like electronic gates were placed over the peaks (arrows) of the arachnoidal spikes in order to measure the retrobulbar maximal arachnoidal diameter (7.01 mm in straight gaze vs. 3.97 mm in 30 degree gaze, a decrease of 43%).

First the maximal arachnoidal diameter is measured in straight (0 degree) gaze. Then the maximal arachnoidal diameter is re-measured in maximal abduction of the eye (30 degree gaze). A decrease of the maximal arachnoidal diameter (as measured during the 30 degree test) of greater than 5% from the initial straight gaze measurement proves subarachnoidal fluid and differentiates this fluid distension of the optic nerve from either (a) solid thickening of the sheaths (e.g., in Graves' orbitopathy, in optic nerve sheath meningiomas, in neurogenic carcinomatosis or leucemic infiltrations of the optic nerve) or (b) swelling of the pial and arachnoidal sheaths with engorged vessels in cases of severe orbital congestion (e.g., in arteriovenous fistulas or in acute orbital inflammation). The maximal dural diameters increase slightly during the 30 degree test in cases of solid sheath thickening (see p. 21) or decrease by less than 5% (if at all) in cases of orbital congestion or leucemic infiltrations.

In addition to the 30 degree test, "visual pattern recognition" as performed so effectively with Standardized A-scan in tissue differentiation, also helps to recognize fluid within the optic nerve sheaths and to differentiate fluid distension from solid thickening of the sheaths. The typical appearances of the optic nerve surface spikes is discussed on pp. 21 and 27. Excessive amounts

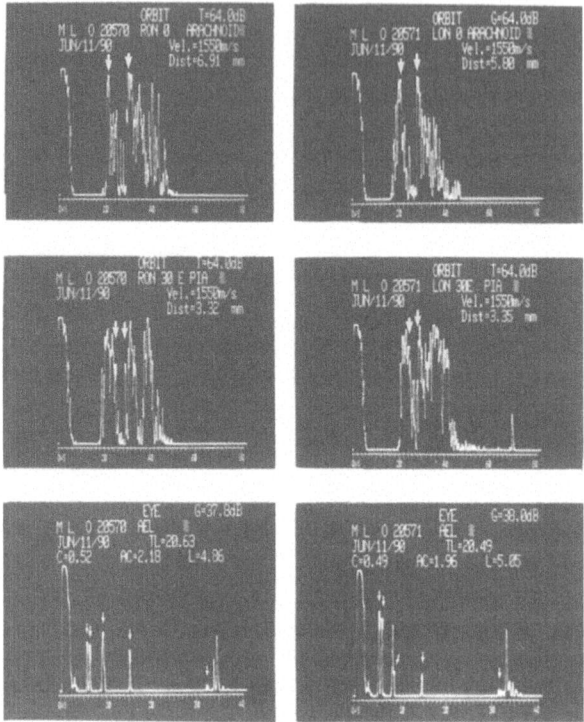

Fig. 22B. 48-year-old male patient with Alagille's syndrome: fluid-distended optic nerve sheaths. The maximal arachnoidal diameters are measured as 6.91 mm RON (top left echogram) and as 5.80 mm LON (top right echogram) in straight gaze direction. These measurements are clearly reduced during prolonged 30 degree testing, which showed the pial diameters to be larger than normal (3.32 mm OD and 3.35 mm OS). This amounts to a reduction of 52% in the RON and 42% in the LON. The immersion axial eye length measurements of OD (left bottom echogram) and OS (right bottom echogram) indicate short globes: 20.63 mm OD and 20.49 mm OS with rather shallow anterior chambers (2.18 mm OD and 1.96 mm OS) and thick lenses (4.86 mm OD and 5.05 mm OS). The arrows mark the electronic gates as they were placed over the peaks of the arachnoidal spikes (top echograms), of the pial spikes (center echograms) and of the spikes representing the two corneal, the two lens and the inner retinal surfaces (bottom echograms).

of subarachnoidal fluid even allow a short stretch of intact baseline to be seen between the pial and arachnoidal surface spikes proving the fluid (see Figure 31A).

Figure 22B presents the A-scan measurements of the arachnoidal diameters during initial straight gaze (top) indicating abnormally increased amounts of orbital subarachnoidal fluid (due to CON) in both optic nerves of a patient with Alagille's syndrome. The maximal arachnoidal diameters in both optic nerves decreased clearly (by more than the needed 5%) during the 30 test proving fluid.

In a recent study of 5 patients with Alagille's syndrome done in our department, all of them presented with moderate to marked fluid distension of their optic nerve sheaths probably caused by optic nerve compression. The maximal pial diameters were found to be increased slightly in these patients (center A-scans in Figure 22B). This thickening of the optic nerves presumably causes the optic nerve compression within the optic canals of these patients. The marked fluid distension behind the globes is the cause of the choroidal folds and the blurred disk margins that are frequently seen in patients with Alagille's syndrome. In the past, the choroidal folds were blamed on nanopthalmus also inherent in this disease.

Choroidal folds may also be caused by oblique optic nerve insertion without fluid distension of the sheaths (bottom right echogram in Figure 21), presumably caused through flattening of the posterior ocular wall by the pressuring optic nerve.

Figure 23A shows B-scan sections from a patient with left optic nerve sheath distension caused by increased subarachnoidal fluid producing mild unilateral papilledema as well as choroidal folds in this left eye. Fundus, optic disk and optic nerve were normal in the fellow eye of this patient. Figure 23B presents the A-scan measurements of both optic nerves in this patient during straight gaze and in 30 degree abduction of the eyes. Again, the decrease of the maximal arachnoidal diameter during the 30 degree test confirms fluid distension.

When the optic nerve sheaths are distended by large amounts of subarachnoidal fluid, they usually are stretched so that together with the subarachnoidal fluid they assume the form of a spindle-shaped bag with its maximum width located in the mid-orbit rather than in the retrobulbar space. In extreme cases the optic nerve sheaths are stretched so far as to produce maximum arachnoidal diameters of up to 8 mm in the mid-orbit (see right optic nerve of a patient with severe BIH and strictly unilateral papilledema as illustrated in Figure 24A; also see top left echogram in Figure 31B depicting the maximal arachnoidal diameter in a patient with severe CON caused by a basal encephalocele). Marked thickening of the extraocular muscles as present in severe Graves' orbitopathy, or large retrobulbar orbital tumors may prevent the formation of a spindle-shaped subarachnoidal space and the maximal arachnoidal diameters are then found in the retrobulbar area similar to normal optic nerves.

In cases of increased intracranial pressure, not all the orbital subarachnoidal fluid may be displaced from the orbit into the intracranial region during exercise even through prolonged maximal abduction or any other mode of exercise. The stretching of the optic nerve and the pressure exerted by both the stretched and the contracted extraocular muscles are insufficient in such cases to overcome the counterpressure from the intracranial subarachnoidal fluid. In the cases illustrated in Figures 24A and B, the reduction of the arachnoidal diameters during the 30 degree test was limited and the optic nerves remained wet even after prolonged exercise of the nerves. The reduc-

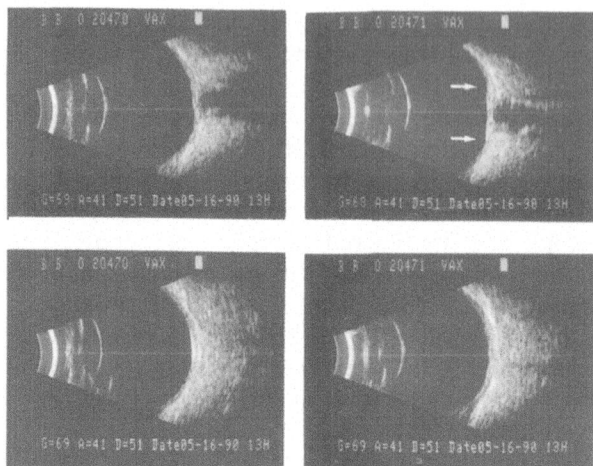

Fig. 23A. Papilledema and choroidal folds as a consequence of increased subarachnoidal fluid: vertical axial B-scan sections through the right normal eye (left echograms) and the left eye with posterior choroidal folds and mild papilledema caused by a marked fluid-distension of the optic nerve sheaths behind the left eye (right echograms) in a 41-year-old male patient. The top echograms represent sections through the optic disks, while the bottom echograms show sections through the maculae. Note the wide elevation (between arrows) of the optic disk tissues involving the surrounding retinochoroidal layer in the left eye (top right echogram) and the bumpy appearance of the retinal, choroidal as well as scleral signal lines in the right bottom echogram, corresponding to the ophthalmoscopically visible choroidal folds in this left eye (compare these curly lines with the straight smooth signal lines representing the normal posterior fundus and ocular wall in OD as seen in the bottom left echogram).

tion achieved is nevertheless sufficient for a differentiation clearly surpassing the needed 5% mark to prove fluid distension and rule out either solid optic nerve sheath thickening or sheath congestion.

When does papilledema develop? Unilateral papilledema
In cases of increased intracranial pressure just like in normals, the arachnoidal diameters return to the pre-exercise level after the exercise. As discussed on p. 33, they can be expected to surpass even the pre-exercise level temporarily by up to 1.0 mm (Figures 24B and 25B).

A certain minimal abnormal amount of subarachnoidal fluid (producing arachnoidal diameters above 5.5 mm) is necessary to produce, over time, papilledema. In the case depicted in Figure 24A, the increase in orbital subarachnoidal fluid of both optic nerves (maximal arachnoidal diameters were 7.66 RON and 6.42 LON in straight gaze) was high enough to produce papilledema in each eye. Similarly, the increase in subarachnoidal fluid surrounding the right optic nerve in the case depicted in Figure 24B (maximal arachnoidal diameter of 5.89 mm in straight gaze) was great enough to produce marked (unilateral) papilledema. In contrast, the subarachnoidal fluid

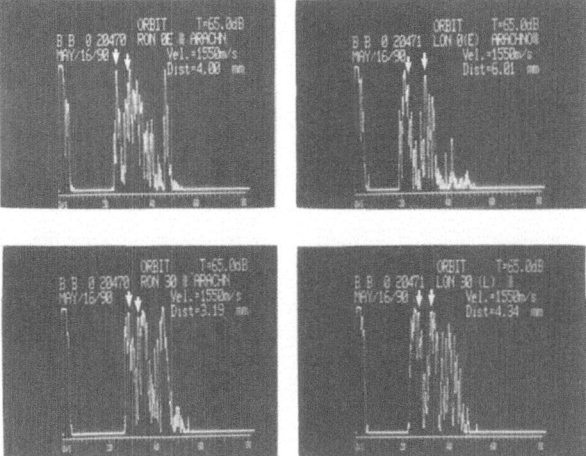

Fig. 23B. Proof and precise measurement of optic nerve sheath distension by increased subarachnoidal fluid: the same patient as in Figure 23A; A-scan measurements of the arachnoidal diameters in the right normal optic nerve (left echograms) and the left nerve with significant fluid distension of its sheaths (right echograms), in straight gaze (top echograms: 4.00 mm RON and 6.01 mm LON) and at 30 degree abduction of the eyes (bottom echograms: 3.19 mm RON and 4.34 mm LON). The reduction of the optic nerve sheath diameters during the 30 degree test is 20% in the RON and 28% in the LON, proving the fluid distension. The arrows indicate the positions of the two point-like electronic gates used for the measurements.

in the left optic nerve of this BIH patient (maximal arachnoidal diameter was measured at 4.59 mm, a borderline value) was not sufficient for a papilledema to develop in this left eye.

We observed in other cases that even great amounts of orbital subarachnoidal fluid did not produce papilledema, if the amount of fluid (and presumably the underlying intracranial pressure) was varying greatly and at times became much lower or even normal. Such variation was observed in the case illustrated in Figures 23A and B, and probably was the cause for the rather mild unilateral papilledema observed in this patient.

After exercise, the intracranial fluid gushes back into the orbit in a matter of seconds (e.g., right optic nerve depicted in Figure 25A) or slowly returns to the orbit over a period of a couple of minutes (see left optic nerve of the same patient as illustrated in Figure 25B), depending on the factors influencing the amount of orbital subarachnoidal fluid as discussed on p. 32, especially the resistance to fluid exchange as determined by the make-up of the perineural intracanalicular tissues. It is interesting to note, that the faster fluid exchange occurs, the wider the arachnoidal sheath diameter becomes.

Both fast fluid exchange and large arachnoidal diameters are usually linked to each other and both promote the development of papilledema. Slow fluid exchange, on the other hand, is usually coupled with a lesser fluid amount;

52

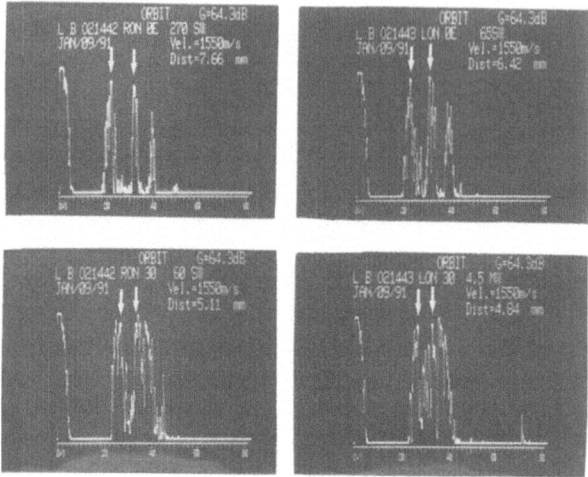

Fig. 24A. Bilateral papilledema: A-scan measurements of maximal arachnoidal diameters in a 27-year-old male patient with BIH, presenting with bilateral papilledema. The right arachnoidal diameter was measured as 7.66 mm in straight gaze (top left) and 5.11 mm in 30 degree gaze (bottom left), whereas the left arachnoidal diameter was measured as 6.42 mm in straight gaze (top right) and 4.84 mm in 30 degree gaze (bottom right). The reduction in the maximal arachnoidal diameter during 30 degree testing was 33% in the RON and 25% in the LON. Arrows point at the positions of the electronic gates.

both appear to be the reason that papilledema does not develop (e.g., left optic nerve in the BIH patient illustrated in Figures 25).

Effect of optic nerve sheath fenestration
Figure 26 demonstrates the measurements of arachnoidal diameters in a patient with severe BIH, following optic nerve sheath fenestration in the left orbit. Figure 26A shows the arachnoidal diameters of the left optic nerve immediately before (left) and 8 days after the left fenestration procedure (right). While fenestration produces a dry anterior optic nerve (anterior to, and at the site of, successful fenestration), the posterior nerve (posterior to the fenestration site) remains wet as long as the intracranial pressure stays high. During the immediate postoperative period, the amount of subarachnoidal fluid is also reduced posteriorly as the fenestration site continuously drains the cerebrospinal fluid into the surrounding orbital tissues (like a filtering blep after glaucoma surgery). Later on, usually after a few weeks, the tissues surrounding the fenestration site scar down ending the drainage and the optic nerve sheaths behind the fenestration site are blown up like a balloon once again. At any rate, as long as surgical optic nerve fenestration is successful, the papilledema on the operated side slowly dissipates as the subarachnoidal fluid no longer reaches the retrobulbar area.

During the initial phase of drainage at the fenestration site, the arachnoidal diameter of the (non-operated) fellow optic nerve also decreases in

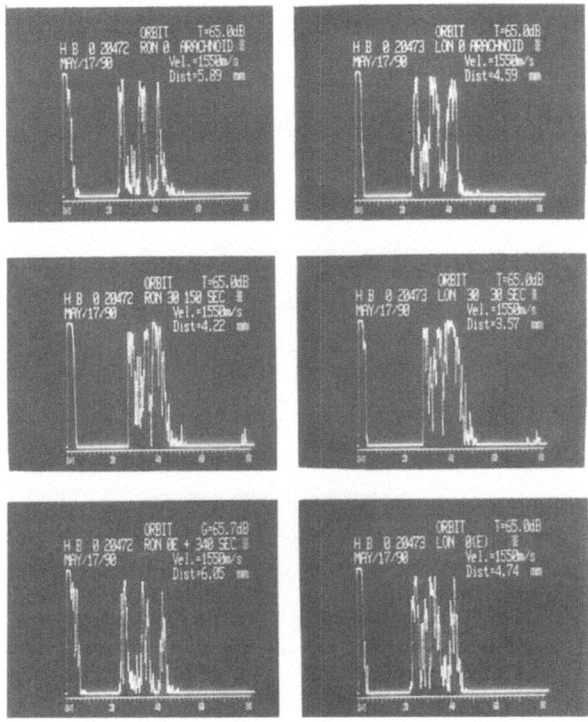

Fig. 24B. Unilateral papilledema: A-scan measurements of maximal arachnoidal diameters in both optic nerves of a 44-year-old female BIH patient with right, strictly unilateral papilledema, recorded in straight gaze before exercise (top echograms: "0"; 5.89 mm RON, 4.59 mm LON), in 30 degree gaze (center echograms: "30"; 4.22 mm RON, 3.57 mm LON), and in straight gaze after exercise (bottom echograms: "OE"; 6.05 mm RON, 4.74 mm LON). Note the slight (temporary) increase of the maximal arachnoidal diameters (0.16 mm RON, 0.15 mm LON) in straight gaze following the exercise. It is typical for increased intracranial pressure, that the subarachnoidal fluid promptly returns into the orbit after the exercise and that (presumably because of the kinetic energy involved) the post-exercise arachnoidal measurements temporarily overshoot the pre-exercise measurements.

size as a consequence of the reduction in intracranial pressure effected by the fenestration procedure (Figure 26 B). In the fellow optic nerve (from globe to apex) the amount of subarachnoidal fluid also returns to previous levels as the draining effect of the fenestration procedure ceases.

Similar changes in the amount of orbital subarachnoidal fluid can be observed during successful medical therapy of BIH, e.g., with Diamox. A-scan measurements are a reliable way of monitoring the course of BIH during such conservative treatment and relapses are easily and quickly proven by these measurements. Thus the non-invasive A-scan measurements of the optic nerve sheath diameters are a useful and clearly preferable alternative to observing the unreliable papilledema which is slow or failing to develop

54

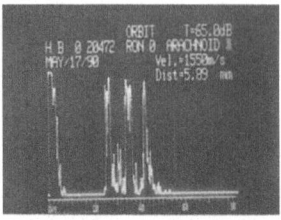

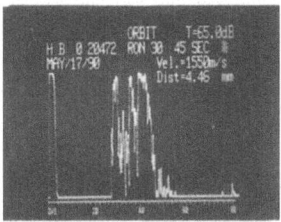

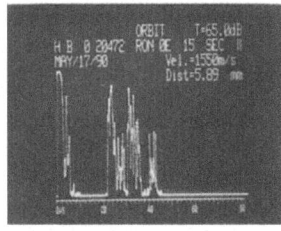

Fig. 25A. Fast fluid exchange in optic nerve with papilledema: A-scan measurements of the maximal arachnoidal diameter in the right eye (with papilledema) of the same patient illustrated in Figure 24B, recorded in straight gaze before exercise (top echogram: 5.89 mm), in 30 degree gaze during exercise (center echogram: 4.46 mm), and only 15 seconds after the exercise was ended, again in straight gaze (bottom echogram: 5.89 mm). Thus the fluid displaced during the exercise had returned fully in only 15 seconds.

and slow to disappear upon increases or decreases of intracranial pressure, and to the invasive lumbar puncture.

Conclusions
In summary, Standardized Echography is a quick and reliable test to (1) suggest increased intracranial pressure, (2) differentiate between papilledema and other causes of optic disk swelling, (3) differentiate between papilledema caused by increased intracranial pressure from that caused by optic nerve compression (see p. 61), (4) positively identify several of the conditions causing optic nerve compression or optic disk swelling other than papilledema; (5) Standardized A-scan Echography is an ideal test for following the natural course or the effectiveness of treatment of the different conditions, especially of BIH, and (6) gives insight into the dynamics of the subarachnoidal fluid in normal optic nerves as well as in the various disease processes. Regarding papilledema, and BIH patients in particular, Standardized Echog-

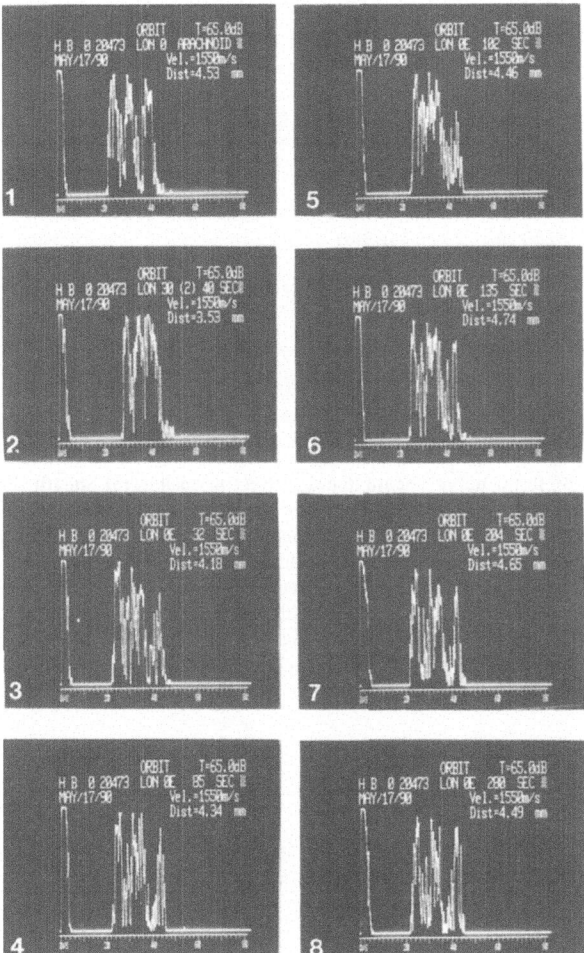

Fig. 25B. Slow fluid exchange in optic nerve without papilledema: A-scan measurements of the maximal arachnoidal diameter in the left eye (without papilledema) of the same patient depicted in Figures 24B and 25A, recorded in straight gaze before exercise (echogram 1: 4.53 mm), in 30 degree gaze during exercise (echogram 2: 3.53 mm) and then in increasing time intervals after the exercise ended (echograms 3–8: 4.18 mm–4.49 mm). Note that in this eye, which did not develop papilledema, the maximal arachnoidal diameter before the exercise was only border-line wide; when the exercise had ended, 102 seconds were not quite enough for the diameter to completely reach the pre-exercise value. Although it slowly expanded beyond the original size thereafter, it finally returned to its original value 280 seconds after the end of the exercise. Quite obviously, the fluid exchange in this optic nerve was considerably slower than in the right nerve with the papilledema.

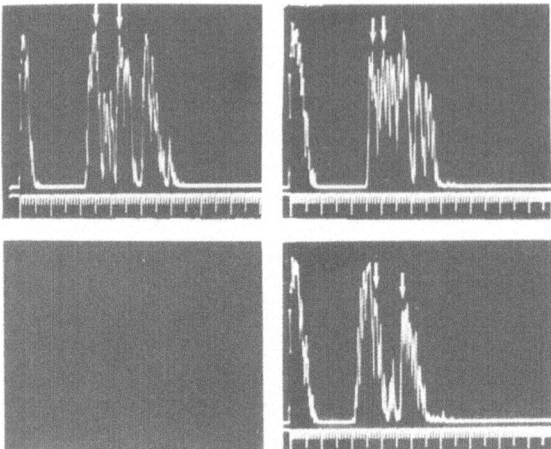

Fig. 26A. Effect of optic nerve sheath fenestration on ipsilateral sheath diameters: A-scan echograms (Kretztechnik 7200 MA) of the left optic nerve in a 25-year-old male patient with severe BIH, who underwent left optic nerve sheath fenestration. The left echogram indicates the maximal pre-operative arachnoidal sheath diameter in 0 degree gaze (5.9 mm). The right top echogram represents the dry anterior optic nerve portion 8 days after surgery (2.9 mm wide pial diameter) and the bottom right echogram illustrates the remaining fluid distension of the left optic nerve (6.3 mm) within the posterior orbit (also 8 days after surgery). The arrows point at the location of the peaks of the arachnoidal spikes (left and bottom right echograms) and of the pial spikes (right top echogram).

raphy is an ideal (both easy and reliable) test for both initiating the diagnosis and monitoring the course of the disease.

3.2.2 *Optic atrophy*

Decreased maximal pial diameter
Optic nerve atrophy is characterized by a less than normal maximal pial diameter, i.e., less than 2.8 mm (see Table 1 and discussion on p. 23). In conditions which cause thickening of the optic nerve such as Graves' orbitopathy (p. 73), even normal pial diameters may reflect mild optic atrophy (see Figure 36).

Usually the arachnoidal/dural diameters in atrophic nerves (primary atrophy or atrophy following ischemic optic neuropathy, glaucoma, chronic papilledema etc.) are within the normal range. This means that the A-scan patterns of these atrophic nerves show an enhanced sheathing sign which is caused by more fluid surrounding the thinner nerve (greater separation of the pial from the arachnoidal/dural surfaces than in the normal nerve). The additional fluid replaces the lost optic nerve substance. The optic nerve sheath diameters are, however, clearly increased if the optic atrophy is

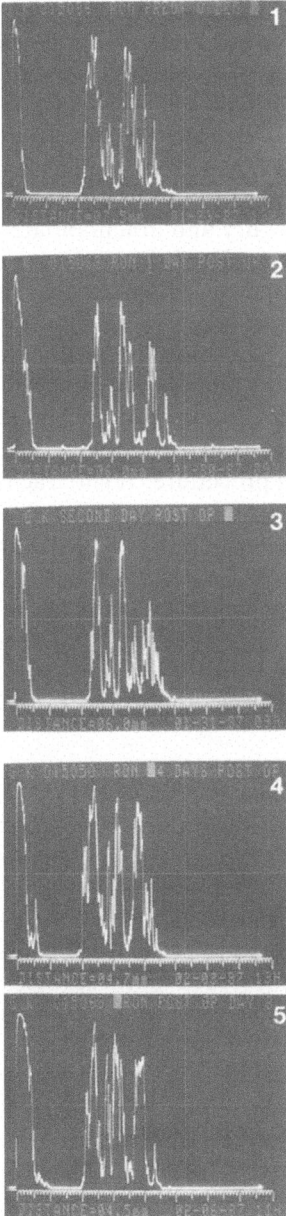

Fig. 26B. Effect of optic nerve sheath fenestration on contralateral sheath diameters: A-scan echograms (Ophthascan S) of the right not operated optic nerve in the same patient as illustrated in Figure 26A, demonstrating the indirect effect of the optic nerve sheath fenestration done in the left optic nerve on the optic nerve in the fellow orbit presumably reflecting a decrease of intracranial pressure effected by continuous drainage of the cerebrospinal fluid through the fenestration defect in the left optic nerve sheaths. Echogram 1 indicates the arachnoidal sheath diameter on the operating table prior to surgery (7.5 mm); echograms 2–5 show the decrease of the arachnoidal diameter in the days following surgery depicting the first (6.0 mm), the second (6.0 mm), the fifth (5.2 mm) and the eighth postoperative day (4.2 mm). Later on, the fenestration wound scarred down closing the drainage site and letting the intracranial pressure rise again as reflected by increased arachnoidal diameters along the entire orbital course of the right (not operated) optic nerve and the increased sheath diameters in the posterior portion of the left (operated) optic nerve.

secondary to lesions such as optic nerve meningiomas (see Figure 45A), optic sheath sarcoid, etc., at least in the area of those lesions, or if the optic atrophy is coexistent with ontgoing fluid sheath distension, such as in BIH.

Optic nerve must be dried out first
Maximal pial diameters can only be measured with reliability and high accuracy, when the optic nerve is dry and arachnoidal spikes do not distract from the effort to maximize the height of the pial signals as well as their distance (see p. 29). In optic nerve sheath tumors such as meningiomas, the optic nerve is dry at the site of the tumor so that the maximal pial diameter may be identified reliably and be measured there precisely in a straight gaze direction (Figures 45A and 47A). In other cases the optic nerve must be dried out first through vigorous exercise and must be measured in extreme lateral gaze ('30 degree' gaze) in order to avoid the appearance of arachnoidal spikes during the measuring procedure. If subarachnoidal fluid is still present, it is always easier to display and to maximize arachnoidal spikes instead of the pial spikes which may disappear from the display entirely or at least not be standing out as large surface spikes among the other optic nerve signals. It has proven advantageous to let the optic nerves dry out and to perform the measurement of maximal pial diameters by having the patient fixate a target on the ceiling above with the head turned as far as possible toward the contralateral side of the eye examined (e.g., head tilt left for examination of the right optic nerve).

Only the maximal pial diameter is meaningful
Because the pial surface of the optic nerve has little grooves and ridges running along the nerve surface in an antero-posterior direction (see discussion on p. 28 and Figure 14C), the display of maximal pial spikes (though necessary to prove truely cross-sectional echograms) does not by itself indicate and guarantee the display of true maximal (central) diameters of the optic nerve. The beam may reach both surfaces of the optic nerve in a direction perpendicular to the surfaces of the grooves or ridges producing maximal pial spikes, but at the same time not cross through the center of the optic nerve thus not tracing the maximal (central) cross diameter but rather cut through the nerve periphery displaying a peripheral (smaller than maximal) diameter (see Figure 14B). Therefore the examiner must – through meticulous, minimal angling of the probe and sound beam – attempt to display a maximal width of the optic nerve defect together with a maximal height of the pial spikes. During this procedure, arachnoidal spikes may turn up and prevail and then be mistaken for the pial signals if the optic nerve is not completely dried out thus obscuring optic atrophy and falsely procuring normal pial diameters.

In practice then, the examiner has to dry out an optic nerve entirely, has to display the optic nerve defect in maximal width, and, at the same time, the pial spikes in maximal height. In any event that a pial diameter slightly wider than normal (slightly larger than 3.1 mm) is measured, the examiner must attempt to prove, through meticulous minimal angling of the probe and beam in all possible directions, that both of the so-called pial spikes are really the pial surface signals and not arachnoidal signals instead, which were obtained from a persistently wet nerve. In doing so, the examiner attempts to bring up the real pial spikes within the optic nerve defect thus demonstrating that at least one of the previously maximized spikes was really an arachnoidal signal. Only if this attempt fails repeatedly, the diagnosis of mild optic nerve thickening is established.

By the same token, a slightly smaller than normal optic nerve diameter, i.e. a maximal pial diameter of slightly less than 2.8 mm may falsely indicate optic atrophy when in reality a smaller peripheral rather than the truly maximal (central) pial diameter was displayed and measured. In this case the examiner needs to attempt a wider measurement by angling the beam minimally across the optic nerve to find the maximal diameter. Only if this attempt fails repeatedly, the diagnosis of mild optic atrophy is established. It is these two opposing requirements, i.e., the one of displaying the widest possible optic nerve pattern and the other one of eliminating falsely wide patterns caused by wetness of the nerve, which makes the measurement of the true pial diameter in proving mild optic nerve thickening or mild optic atrophy the most difficult among all echographic tasks concerning the optic nerve. In contrast, the diagnoses of severe optic atrophy (maximal pial diameters of less than 2.5 mm) or of marked swelling of the optic nerve (maximal pial diameters of more than 3.5 mm) are easily and quickly accomplished and are reliable even without the meticulous adjusting and measuring approach explained above.

Figure 27 illustrates the optic nerve A-scan patterns of a right atrophic nerve. In straight gaze (left echograms), the arachnoidal spikes prevail indicating a normal arachnoidal diameter of 3.91 mm. The pial spikes are visible within the optic nerve pattern. Their distance does not reflect the maximal pial diameter but rather a peripheral (smaller) diameter of the nerve. Upon prolonged '30 degree' gaze direction (right echograms), the optic nerve has dried out and a true maximal pial diameter is displayed and measured at 2.36 mm indicating severe optic atrophy; normal maximal pial diameters are 2.8 to 3.1 mm (Table 1, p. 24).

Figure 28 compares the right atrophic optic nerve of an elderly patient with his left normal nerve and also shows that B-scan cannot be used to show differences of such a small degree. Even a lower system sensitivity, which may have been more appropriate to optimize the B-scan displays than the one used in this case, would not have made a difference. Again, a prolonged extreme lateral gaze direction had to be applied to surely dry out the optic nerves before a reliable measurement of the maximal pial diameter could be achieved with the Standardized A-scan. The difference in the measurements between right and left are similar for both the arachnoidal and the pial diameters. This may be due to the fact that the decrease in the right optic nerve substance was not made up for by increased subarachnoidal fluid (as is usually the case). On the other hand, differences of this small magnitude

60

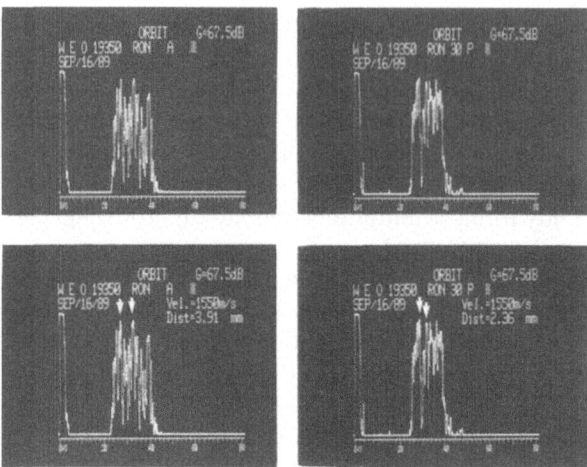

Fig. 27. Optic atrophy: A-scan measurements of a right severely atrophic optic nerve in an 89-year-old female patient with suspected old retinal vein occlusion. *Left:* optic nerve patterns in straight gaze. *Right:* optic nerve echograms in 30 degree gaze. *Top:* plain echograms for better recognition of the maximized spikes. *Bottom:* electronic gates (arrows) are placed over the peaks of the maximized arachnoidal spikes in the left wet nerve pattern (3.91 mm normal maximal arachnoidal diameter) and over the peaks of the maximized pial spikes in the right dried nerve pattern during the prolonged exercise proving severe optic atrophy (2.36 mm maximal pial diameter). Note that the pial diameter in straight gaze appears smaller (peripheral cross-section of the optic nerve) than the maximal pial diameter as correctly obtained from the dried optic nerve in prolonged 30 degree gaze direction (maximal central cross diameter).

are quite common in the arachnoidal (not the pial) diameters of the two optic nerves of a patient reflecting the differences in the resistance to the shift of fluid between the orbits and the brain and in the other factors that determine the amount of intraorbital subarachnoidal fluid present in any orbit at any time (see discussion on p. 32).

3.2.3 *Optic nerve hypoplasia*

Figure 29 shows the A-scans of the anterior optic nerve cross-sections in a male infant with optic nerve hypoplasia. The maximal pial/arachnoidal diameters measured only 2.5 mm in the RON and 1.9 mm in the LON. Ophthalmoscopically the optic disks also appeared very small. In contrast to optic atrophy, in optic nerve hypoplasia the optic nerves and their sheaths have stayed small during their development so that all optic nerve diameters, the pial as well as the arachnoidal and dural diameters, are much smaller than normal. Therefore no increased sheathing phenomenon is observed in this condition (no increased subarachnoidal fluid makes up for any loss in optic nerve volume).

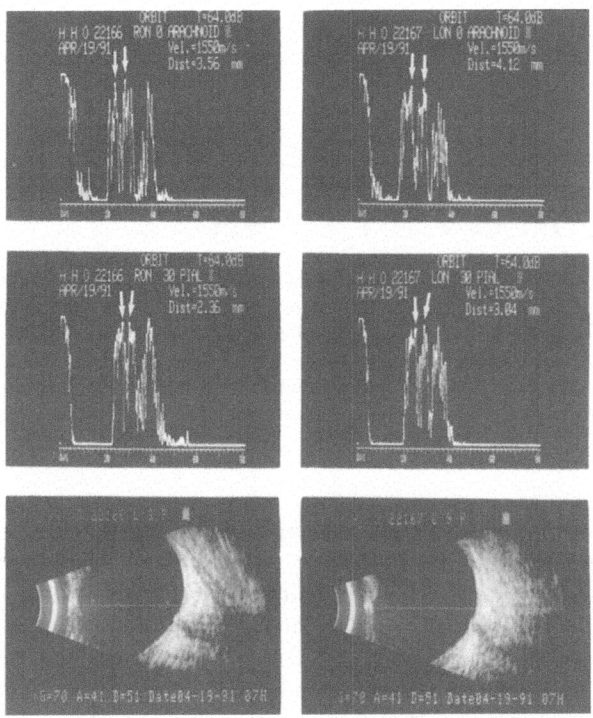

Fig. 28. Severe optic nerve atrophy OD in an 84-year-old male patient with old AION and count fingers vision OD: comparison of thicknesses of the right atrophic (left echograms) and the left normal (right echograms) optic nerves. The electronic gates (arrows) were placed over the peaks of the maximized arachnoidal spikes in the top A-scans obtained in straight gaze direction (maximal arachnoidal diameters were measured as 3.56 mm in the RON and as 4.12 mm in the LON). The electronic gates were positioned over the peaks of the maximized pial spikes in the central A-scans obtained in prolonged 30 degree gaze direction (maximal pial diameters of only 2.36 mm in the RON and of the normal 3.04 mm in the LON). The B-scan echograms shown at the bottom were obtained along the nasal meridians of each eye (longitudinal sections along the 3:00 meridian OD and along the 9:00 meridian OS); they are not useful in showing any reliable difference between the normal and the severely atrophic nerve, however.

3.2.4 *Compressive optic neuropathy (CON)*

Underlying causes

There are many different causes of optic nerve compression ranging from acute sub-periosteal hematomas (either spontaneous, e.g., during pregnancy especially during labor, or traumatic), subperiosteal abscesses, sinus infections (especially when located in the sphenoidal sinuses), orbital tumors (frequently when located in the nasal posterior muscle cone, e.g., cavernous hemangiomas), retro-orbital tumors such as sphenoidal mucoceles, osteomas, optic nerve tumors (again especially when located in the posterior orbit or in the optic canal; meningiomas, Figures 46 and 47; gliomas, Figure 41B;

62

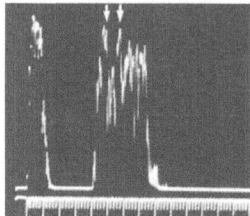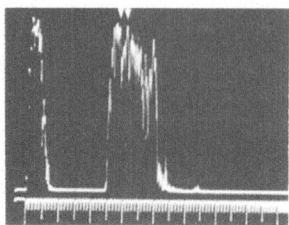

Fig. 29. A-scan echograms (Kretztechnik 7200 MA) demonstrating the maximal arachnoidal diameters of the right (left echogram) and left (right echogram) optic nerves in a 4-month-old male infant with bilateral optic nerve hypoplasia (clearly decreased optic disk sizes seen during ophthalmoscopy). The maximal arachnoidal diameters are reduced to 2.5 mm in the RON and to 1.9 mm in the LON (optic nerve diameters in normal newborns and infants compare well to those in normal adults, see Table 1, p. 24). The arrows point at the peaks of the arachnoidal spikes.

sarcoidosis; optic neuritis, Figures 37 and 39; ischemic optic neuropathy, Figures 40A and B; Alagille' syndrome, Figure 22B), basal encephaloceles (Figures 31A and B), and Graves' orbitopathy (Figures 30A, 32, 33, 34A and B, 35A and B). Graves' orbitopathy, although not causing the most dangerous, severe and acute forms of CON, is by far the single most frequent cause of CON and therefore is selected here to explain the mechanism and to illustrate the echographic (morphological) signs of CON.

Mechanism of CON in Graves' orbitopathy
In Graves' orbitopathy, excessive swelling of the posterior portions of the extraocular muscles is well known to cause compression of the optic nerve in the orbital apex. We have found, that it is particularly the combined posterior thickening of the superior rectus, the medial rectus and the superior oblique muscles, which causes such optic nerve compression (see Figures 34A, B; 35A, B). In addition, the thickening of the optic nerve sheaths themselves and the thickening of the periorbita all contribute significantly to the phenomenon of CON in Graves' orbitopathy. The shape and width of the bony orbital funnel is also an important factor in the development of CON.

Thus it is not surprising that the degree of exophthalmus as measured with the Hertel's instrument and heavily influenced by the length of the globe and the depth and spaciousness of the bony orbital funnel actually says very little about the probability for CON to develop in a given patient with Graves' orbitopathy. Patients with moderate or even minor exophthalmus may be prone to suffer CON if the above described circumstances apply. As a matter of fact, excessive exophthalmus infrequently co-exists with CON in Graves' disease and unilateral CON is not always found on the side with the greater exophthalmus. Standardized Echography provides precise measurements of the important factors that may lead to CON, i.e., the (posterior) thicknesses of the four straight and the superior oblique muscles (muscle profile of a patient as pictured in Figures 34A and B), and of the thicknesses of the periorbita and the optic nerve sheaths. Thus Standardized Echography, in addition to a safe diagnosis of the condition, provides an objective quantitative basis for the evaluation of Graves' patients with regard to their disposition to develop CON. Standardized Echography further provides the earliest indicator that compression of the optic nerve has developed, before the optic nerve function may be affected (case described in Figures 34A, B; 35A, B).

The morphological sign of CON
Optic nerve compression is morphologically confirmed, when (increased) subarachnoidal fluid is documented in an initial examination in straight gaze (Figures 30A, 31A), then driven out from the orbit by exercise, and proven to stay out of the orbit (Figures 32, 33, 35B), when tested again in straight gaze direction following the exercise, after an appropriate resting time of the eyes (see also discussion on p. 37 and Figure 18).

It is paramount, to document the initial straight gaze arachnoidal and dural A-scan measurements (see p. 38) before a patient is examined in any other way, be it for the visual acuity or ocular motility, the applanation pressure, a visual field, or a basic A-scan and B-scan examination of the eyes and orbits. By no means must a patient be subjected to any unnatural eye movements or gaze directions which the patient would not naturally assume during routine life situations, before the initial optic nerve measurements in straight gaze (in Graves' patients even in minimal downward gaze, at any rate in a relaxed gaze direction), are documented (see also discussion below).

Figure 30A presents initial A-scan measurements during straight gaze direction in three patients with severe Graves' orbitopathy complicated by CON, in whom inspite of the orbits being crowded by thickened muscles and swollen tissues (including markedly thickened optic nerve sheaths) fluid was noted to surround the anterior portion of the optic nerve suggesting the possibility of CON. In one of these patients the amount of fluid was minor (left echograms), whereas it was excessive in the other two (right echograms) illustrating the wide range of fluid distension of the anterior optic nerve sheaths that may occur with CON in Graves' orbitopathy.

Visual pattern recognition of signs
of fluid distension of the optic nerve sheaths
In each of these three echogram samples, the presence of fluid within the optic nerve sheaths is clear from the appearance of the surface spikes: (a) the arachnoidal spikes (their peaks are marked by arrows in the Figure 30A) are characterized by their sharp delineation toward the nerve pattern (right descending limb of the left vs. left ascending limb of the right arachnoidal spike) and by their lower inner base (base of spike on the side of the low inner optic nerve signals). (b) the clear presence of dural spikes next two the arachnoidal spikes. (c) if the amount of subarachnoidal fluid is sufficient, even a baseline representing the acoustically homogenous subarachnoidal

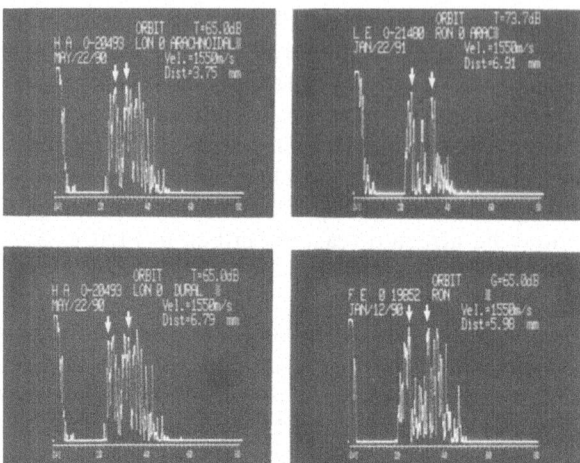

Fig. 30A. Severe Graves' orbitopathy with LON: *Left:* measurement of maximal arachnoidal (3.75 mm) and maximal dural (6.79 mm) diameters in the same echogram from the LON of a 52-year-old female patient with bilateral CON (see also Figure 33). *Top right:* maximal arachnoidal measurement (6.91 mm) from the RON of a 82-year-old female patient with right unilateral CON. This is an example of plentiful subarachnoidal fluid much of which was gone after exercise and stayed away from the orbit thereafter, proving CON. *Bottom right:* maximal arachnoidal diameter (5.98 mm) from the RON of a 84-year-old female patient with Graves' orbitopathy and bilateral CON. Arrows point at electronic gates as placed for the measurements.

fluid may be seen within the optic nerve sheath signals (see top left echogram in Figure 31A).

The characteristics of an arachnoidal spike may be obscured by the close-ness of the pial spike where the meandering nerve happens to come close to, or even touch, the arachnoidal surface (e.g., right arachnoidal signal in the left echograms of Figure 30A) and in those cases of Graves' orbitopathy where the reflectivity of the inner dural substance is markedly decreased so that the dural spikes resemble arachnoidal spikes by their sharp delineation toward the nerve center and their low inner base. Therefore subarachnoidal fluid in Graves' patients is proven or ruled out with a dynamic examination, i.e., the 30 degree test (see Figures 16 and 31B) and the straight gaze measurements after exercise (Figures 32, 33, 35B) rather than from evaluat-ing only the spike characteristics as noted during the initial straight gaze measurement (Figure 30A).

Figure 30B illustrates initially dry optic nerves in two patients with severe Graves' orbitopathy, but without CON. In one of these patients, the left optic nerve (top echogram in Figure 30B) displays thick dural sheaths which surround the optic nerve (dural surface spikes are marked by arrows) like a cuff very similar to optic nerve ring meningiomas (see Figure 45A). There are neither arachnoidal spikes present nor is there any fluid space between the pial surfaces and the dural sheaths. In the other patient the maximal

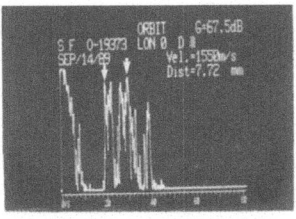

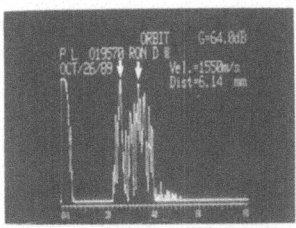

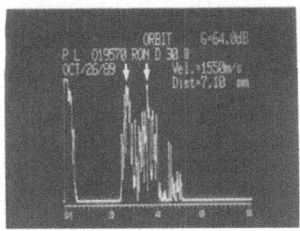

Fig. 30B. Severe Graves' orbitopathy without CON (initially dry optic nerves): Maximal dural diameter of a LON, documented and measured during initial examination in straight gaze direction (top echogram: 7.72 mm) in a 72-year-old male patient with severe Graves' orbitopathy and marked thickening of the dural sheaths, but without CON. Note the characteristic appearance of the dural spikes as marked by arrows: outer delineations (left ascending limb of left dural spike and right descending limb of right dural spike) drop sharply and way down to their lower outer bases (left in left spike, right in right spike). This is reversed from typical arachnoidal spikes which tend to drop deeply and sharply on the inside, i.e., the side facing the optic nerve defect. In another patient, a 75-year-old male with severe Graves' orbitopathy, but without CON, the maximal dural diameter of the right optic nerve with markedly thickened sheaths measured 6.14 mm initially in straight gaze (center echogram) and 7.10 mm during 30 degree gaze direction (bottom echogram). The reason for the slightly larger measurement in the 30 degree gaze is discussed and explained on p. 21. Arrows point at electronic gates set for the measurements.

(dural) sheath diameter as measured in initial primary gaze (center echogram of Figure 30B) increases from 6.14 to 7.10 mm during the 30 degree measurement (bottom echogram in Figure 30B). In addition to the appearance of the sheath surface spikes in this case which are atypical for arachnoidal spikes, the slight increase rather than decrease during the 30 degree measurement (see p. 21) proves that this right optic nerve in this patient was dry to begin with, ruling out CON.

Dry optic nerves are a frequent finding in patients with severe Graves' orbitopathy without CON since the fullness of the orbits and especially the

66

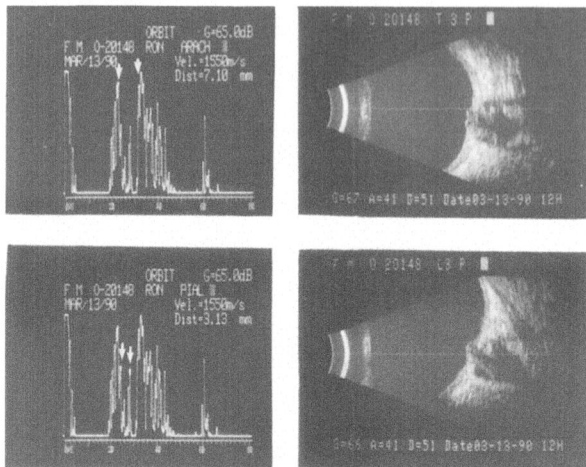

Fig. 31A. Basal encephalocele causing severe CON in a 35-year-old female patient. The A-scans demonstrate marked fluid distension of the optic nerve sheaths (note the clear separation of the right pial spike from the right arachnoidal surface spike in these echograms by a short baseline representing the homogenous non-reflective subarachnoidal fluid). The arrows point at the peaks of the arachnoidal spikes (top left echogram) and of the pial spikes (bottom left echogram). The B-scans too show this fluid distension as well as the papilledema; the longitudinal scan (bottom right echogram) displays the flying bat pattern.

constant gentle pressure by the thickened extraocular muscles as well as by the thickened optic nerve sheaths prevents any fluid from staying around the orbital portion of the optic nerve. It takes real compression of the optic nerve in the orbital apex, to trap fluid which has been pushed into the orbit during spikes of intracranial pressure while asleep, in the anterior subarachnoidal space of the optic nerves in severe Graves' orbitopathy.

Always document the maximal dural sheath diameter during the initial straight gaze examination too

During the initial straight gaze measurement, the maximal dural diameter should be documented in addition to the maximal arachnoidal diameter. After exercise all the fluid may be (and often enough is) gone and no more arachnoidal diameters may be displayed for comparison with the original ones obtained prior to the exercise (see Figure 33). If maximal dural diameters were documented before the exercise, they then can be compared directly with the maximal dural diameters documented after the exercise to prove CON. In the absence of CON any subarachnoidal fluid surrounding the nerve before the exercise will promptly return after the exercise always allowing a direct comparison of the arachnoidal diameters to rule out CON. If subarachnoidal fluid is present to an excessive degree (e.g., right echograms in Figure 30A) there is no need for initial dural measurements. If there is CON, the maximal dural diameter after the exercise will be smaller than the initial

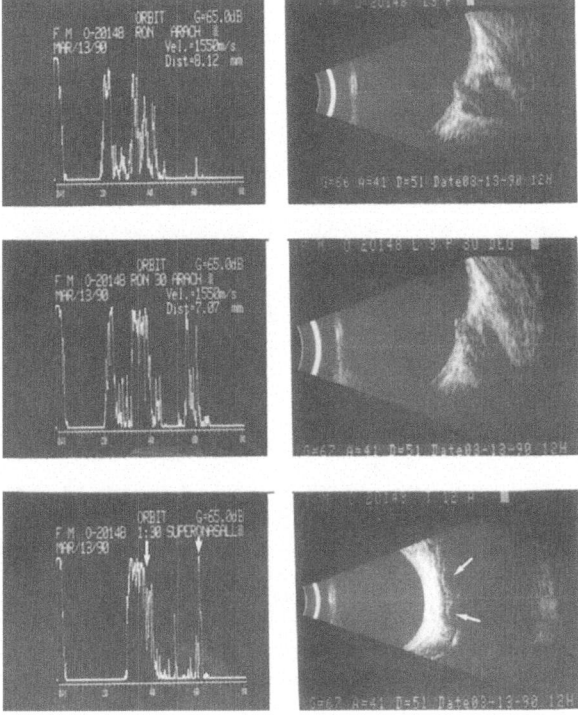

Fig. 31B. Basal encephalocele (same case as described in Figure 31A): the top A-scan recorded in straight gaze direction indicates a maximal arachnoidal diameter of 8.12 mm! The center A-scan, obtained in 30 degree gaze direction, indicates a slight but clear decrease in subarachnoidal fluid (arachnoidal diameter decreased to 7.07 mm). The top B-scan (a longitudinal section recorded in straight gaze) illustrates well the flying bat pattern of the retrobulbar optic nerve portion; the center B-scan (also a longitudinal scan) illustrates the stretching of the optic nerve and its sheaths during a 30 degree examination. The bottom A-scan, obtained in a sound beam direction through the globe towards superonasally, indicates the missing bony roof of the orbit (left arrow) recording typical brain signals (extremely low spikes from the brain tissue and single interspersed medium high to high signals from the larger brain surfaces intercepted by the beam (between the two arrows). During the live examination, marked pulsations of the dural and arachnoidal sheath signals separating the high orbital spikes from the low brain signals were observed (left arrow). The bottom B-scan represents an anterior transverse section through the globe, the orbital tissues, and the meninges across the 12:00 meridian. Again, pulsations were noted of the meningeal signals during the live examination (arrows).

arachnoidal diameter if the optic nerve is dried out, proving the CON. Or some of the fluid will remain in the orbit during the exercise allowing for a direct comparison between the arachnoidal diameters before and after the exercise. While it is occasionally possible to document and measure maximal arachnoidal and dural diameters in the same echogram (e.g., cases illustrated on the left in Figure 30A as well as in Figures 32 and 33), the display and documentation of maximal arachnoidal and dural diameters often has to be

68

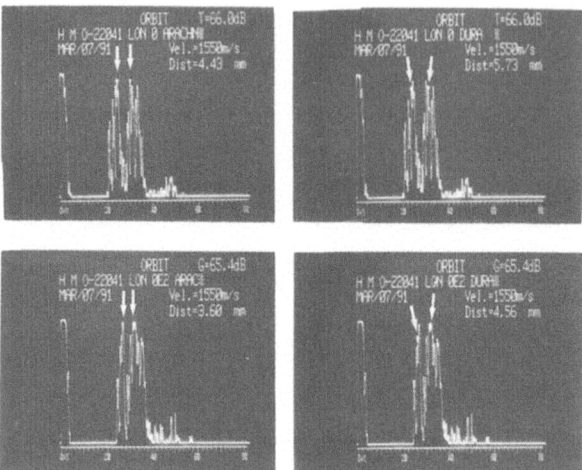

Fig. 32. Severe Graves' orbitopathy with CON: maximal arachnoidal (4.43 mm in top left echogram) and dural (5.73 mm in top right echogram) diameters of a LON, as documented and measured during the initial examination in straight gaze direction in a 51-year-old female patient with bilateral CON. The proof of CON required two courses of exercise after which the arachnoidal diameter in straight gaze had dropped to 3.60 mm (bottom left echogram) and the dural diameter was reduced to 4.56 mm (bottom right echogram). Only after a third course of exercise the left optic nerve dried out completely in this patient. The arrows point at the electronic gates set over the peaks of the arachnoidal spikes (left echograms) and dural spikes (right echograms), respectively.

done successively in different echograms displayed by the examiner while concentrating on one diameter at a time (while disregarding the other), since arachnoidal and dural surfaces are usually not ideally concentric due to irregular thickening of the dura.

As Figure 32 illustrates, the comparison of the maximal dural diameters as obtained prior to, and after, the exercise has confirming value in addition to the comparison of the arachnoidal diameters. Figure 33 takes up the case first shown on the left in Figure 30A to point out the importance of measuring the maximal dural diameter in addition to the maximal arachnoidal diameter during the first examination in primary gaze direction. As can be seen from Figure 33, no fluid whatsoever is left after the exercise in this case; nevertheless an accurate comparison can be made between the maximal dural diameters as measured before (6.7 mm) and after the exercise (4.49 mm) to prove CON in this case.

Quantitation of severity of morphological CON signs often not possible
The amount of orbital subarachnoidal fluid found in the orbit prior to an exercise does not necessarily indicate the severity of CON. While an excessive amount of fluid documented during the initial straight gaze examination

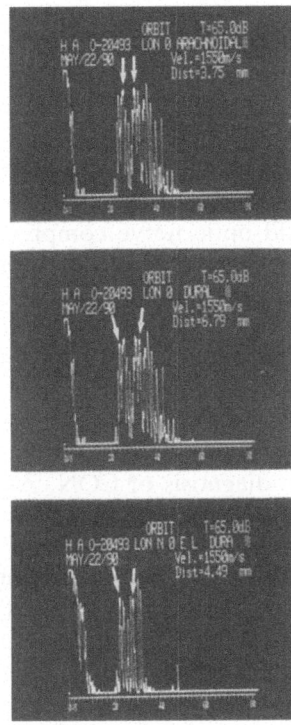

Fig. 33. CON with very small amount of initial subarachnoidal fluid – need for comparison of dural diameters: documentation and measurement of the maximal dural diameters of the LON in the same patient depicted in Figure 30A on the left. *Top:* maximal arachnoidal diameter measured during initial straight gaze direction is only 3.75 mm (normal range). Center: maximal dural diameter measured initially in straight gaze is 6.79 mm. Thus dural thickness is about 1.5 mm (normal is about 0.5 mm). *Bottom:* maximal dural diameter measured after prolonged exercise is only 4.49 mm proving CON. Note that the postexercise dural diameter is still clearly larger than the pre-exercise arachnoidal diameter. The arrows point at the electronic gates which were set for the measurements over the peaks of the arachnoidal spikes (top echogram) and of the dural spikes (center and bottom echograms).

usually indicates severe compression, a smaller amount of fluid can have its explanation in a number of factors:

a) there may have been inadvertant 'exercise' of the eyes prior to the echo-graphic examination which expelled a major portion of the increased subarachnoidal fluid;

b) there may be such high tissue pressure in the orbit, that only little amounts of fluid are pushed into the orbit through the compressed area during periods of spiking intracranial pressure that occur when the patient is asleep;

c) the amount of fluid pushed into the orbit depends on how great the promoting intracranial pressure spikes during the night before the examination were as well as on the resistance to fluid exchange as influenced by the factors outlined on p. 32;

d) severe compression may work in two opposite directions by either pre-venting greater amounts of fluid to filter into the orbit or by holding back greater amounts in the orbit.

Similarly, it is not possible to conclude from difficulties to expel the subar-achnoidal fluid from the orbit through exercise severe optic nerve com-pression or to assume mild optic nerve compression when the intraorbital subarachnoidal fluid is eliminated from the orbit with ease through only limited exercise. We have experienced cases in which the subarachnoidal fluid was expressed entirely by no more than performing a brief applanation tonometry or by testing the visual acuity (i.e., by making the patient look higher than done in a relaxed situation), and especially by checking the motility of the globes. On the other hand, up to three courses of exercise may be needed to expel a significant amount of the orbital subarachnoidal fluid in order to make the diagnosis of CON. All this depends so much on the intraorbital tissue pressure, the resistance to fluid exchange between orbit and brain, and the effectiveness of the exercise (squeezing action by the stretching of the optic nerve, by the contraction of the lateral rectus, and by the pushing of the extended medial rectus muscles) in putting pressure on the orbital subarachnoidal fluid. Figure 32 illustrates a case, in which 2 prolonged exercises were necessary to achieve the decrease in maximal arach-noidal diameter displayed. A third such exercise was needed to dry that optic nerve out entirely.

Graves' profiles
Figures 34A and B represent a complete "Graves' profile" of a patient who had been followed for moderately severe Graves' orbitopathy OU. Such a profile includes the maximal thickness measurements of all extraocular muscles in both orbits, the optic nerve patterns, the thicknesses of the periorbitae, and the sizes of the lacrimal glands. It takes a skilled examiner between 15 and 20 minutes to document such a complete profile.

Originally neither morphological nor functional signs of CON were noted in this patient. At the visit during which the profiles shown in Figures 34 were documented, not only marked, asymmetric, mostly posterior thickening of the extraocular muscles in both orbits together with all the other signs of more severe Graves' orbitopathy, i.e., significant thickening of the optic nerve sheaths and periorbitae and swelling of the lacrimal glands were found. In addition, however, the morphological signs of CON were detected in both optic nerves as illustrated in Figures 35A, B.

Muscle index
The muscle index (as calculated from the sum total of the six maximum muscle thicknesses in an orbit, divided by 6) indicated severe Graves' orbit-opathy in each orbit of this patient (muscle index is 7.42 OD and 6.97 OS). A muscle index of >6.5 in at least one orbit would qualify Graves' orbitopa-

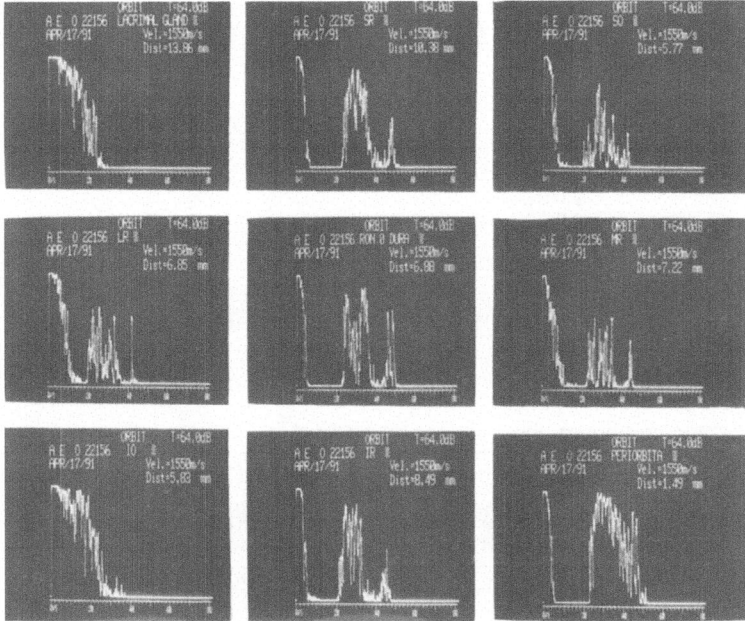

Fig. 34A. Graves' profile of the right orbit in a 73-year-old-female patient with severe Graves' orbitopathy who developed CON in both optic nerves. This profile includes the maximal dural diameter of the RON (center echogram: 6.88 mm); the maximal (posterior) thicknesses of the extraocular muscles pictured as the examiner looks at them facing the patient: medial rectus (middle row right, 7.22 mm); lateral rectus (middle left, 6.85 mm); superior rectus (top center, 10.38 mm); inferior rectus (bottom center, 8.49 mm); superior oblique (top right, 5.77 mm); and the inferior oblique (bottom left, 5.83 mm); the lacrimal gland size (top left, 13.86 mm) and the periorbita (bottom right, 1.49 mm). Note that the three key muscles with regard to the development of CON, i.e., the superior rectus, superior oblique and medial rectus muscles are all very thick in the posterior orbit (Superonasal Index = SNI = 7.79).

thy as severe, while indices between 5.5 and 6.5 (and between 4.5 and 5.5) would qualify the Graves' orbitopathy as moderate (and mild, respectively); a muscle index of <5.0 is normal.

It is noteworthy that this patient displayed the marked combined thickening of the superior and medial rectus, and of the superior oblique muscles in both posterior orbits, which is a hallmark of CON ("Superonasal Index" ≥ 7.0). At this visit, however, no functional signs of CON were noted. The patient returned three months later with worsened Graves' profiles and unchanged morphological signs of CON in both orbits and with clearly reduced optic nerve functions OU, but no papilledema. Medical treatment with high doses of systemic corticosteroids and low-grade radiation of both orbits was initiated immediately. It was the echographic detection of early CON which had prompted close follow-up of the patient's optic nerve func-

72

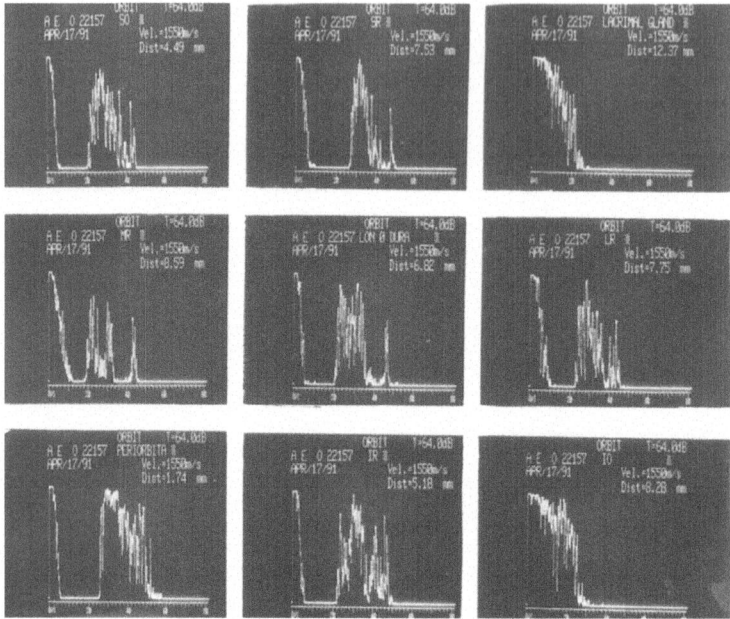

Fig. 34B. Graves' profile of the left orbit in the same patient depicted in Figure 34A. The measurements are: superior oblique (top left, 4.49 mm); superior rectus (top center, 7.53 mm); lacrimal gland (top right, 12.37 mm); medial rectus (middle left, 8.59 mm); dural diameter of optic nerve (middle center, 6.82 mm); lateral rectus (middle right, 7.75 mm); periorbita (bottom left, 1.74 mm); inferior rectus (bottom center, 5.18 mm); and inferior oblique muscle (bottom right, 8.28 mm). Note the differences between the right (Figure 34A) and left orbits. While the left superior rectus and superior oblique muscles are less thickened than their right counterparts, the left medial rectus is clearly thicker than the right one. All three of the left key muscles, which as a group concern the development of CON, are markedly thickened in the left orbit as well (SNI = 6.87).

tions and thus facilitated prompt treatment of the CON which was indicated by the decline of the optic nerve functions.

Optic atrophy in Graves' patients
One of the tasks of the optic nerve evaluation with Standardized Echography in patients with CON is to determine whether there is optic nerve atrophy or not. All that was discussed in the previous section on optic nerve atrophy applies. However, when dealing with Graves' patients, the examiner has to remember, that the maximal pial diameter in 'normal', i.e., non-atrophic optic nerves in this category of patients is increased over the pial diameter of a normal person due to thickening of the pia. The thicker the dural sheaths are noted to be in a Graves' patient, the wider the 'normal' pial diameter should be expected to be in this patient. Maximal pial diameters ranging from 3.1 to 3.8 mm can be expected in Graves' patients without optic atrophy

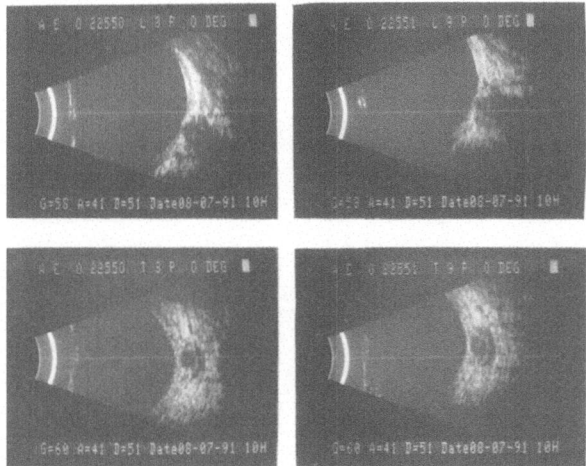

Fig. 35A. Severe Graves' orbitopathy with active CON (same patient as presented in Figures 34). *B-scans:* longitudinal (top echograms) and transverse (bottom echograms) standard B-scan cuts through the right (left echograms) and left (right echograms) retrobulbar optic nerves with fluid distension of the sheaths. Note the flying bat pattern of the longitudinal B-scans; the transverse B-scans were obtained with the probe placed posteriorly on the globes in order to show cross-sectional images of the optic nerves and surrounding fluid patterns.

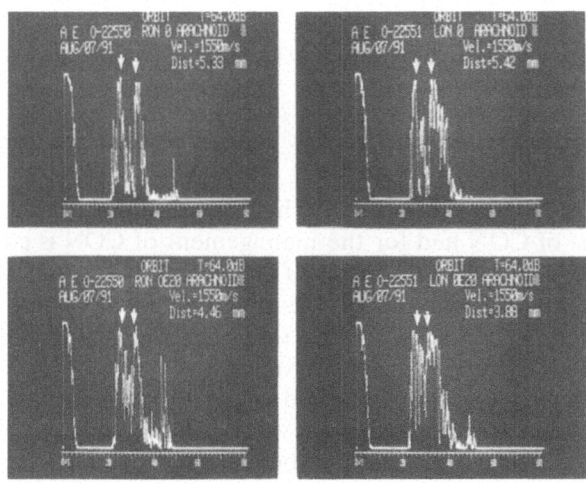

Fig. 35B. Severe Graves' orbitopathy with active CON (same patient as presented in Figures 34). *A-scans:* maximal arachnoidal diameters of the RON (left echograms) and of the LON (right echograms) as measured initially in straight gaze (top patterns: 5.33 mm RON and 5.42 mm LON) and after two courses of exercise (bottom patterns: 4.46 mm RON and 3.88 mm LON). The decrease in subarachnoidal fluid following the exercises is clear-cut and proves active CON. The arrows point at the electronic gates which were set over the peaks of the arachnoidal spikes.

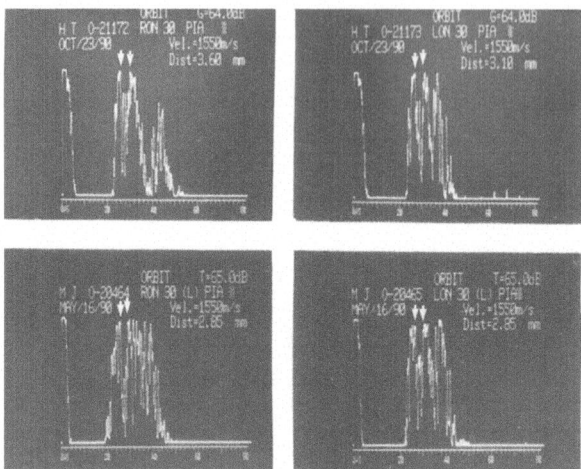

Fig. 36. Optic atrophy in severe Graves' orbitopathy: maximal pial diameters of RONs (left echograms) and LONs (right echograms) measured during prolonged 30 degree gaze directions in two patients suffering from severe Graves' orbitopathy (thick dural sheaths), one with 'normal' nerve thicknesses (top echograms: 3.6 mm RON and 3.1 mm LON) and the other with bilateral mild optic atrophy (bottom echograms: 2.85 mm pial diameter in both optic nerves). The arrows point at the electronic gates which were set over the peaks of the pial spikes.

(see top echograms in Figure 36). Maximal pial diameters of 2.8 to 3.1 mm, the range in normal persons, do then suggest some optic atrophy when measured in Graves' patients with clearly thickened dural sheaths (see bottom echograms in Figure 36).

Use of Standardized Echography in the management of Graves' orbitopathy (Figures 34 and 35)
(a) Early diagnosis and prophylaxis. The role of Standardized Echography in the diagnosis of CON and for the management of CON is comparable to the role of tonometry in the diagnosis of glaucoma: as an increased intraocular pressure (ocular hypertension) does not in itself make the diagnosis of glaucoma or require treatment, so does the morphological sign of optic nerve compression not make the diagnosis of treatable CON in itself. Just as patients with ocular hypertension need to be followed carefully regarding their optic disk appearances and their visual fields, so do patients with the morphological signs of CON need to be followed carefully regarding their optic nerve function and a development of papilledema. Because of the slow changes that occur in Graves' orbitopathy, Graves' patients do not usually need to be reevaluated more often than once a year. Patients need to be checked in much shorter intervals such as a few weeks or months, however, when they present with early morphological signs of CON.

(b) Confirmation of active CON. An impaired optic nerve function as confirmed through testing of visual acuity, visual fields, color vision and flicker fusion or through detection of a relative afferent pupillary defect, may either have occurred during a previous episode of CON, while at the time of its discovery no active CON may be present in this patient. Or the impaired optic nerve function may be caused by another condition coexisting with the Graves' orbitopathy. There is a host of such conditions ranging from macular disease to cataract, from ischemic optic neuropathy to hypertensive disease, from diabetes to glaucoma. It can then be difficult or impossible to identify the actual culprit for a failing visual function, to safely blame functional loss on compressive optic neuropathy and to initiate proper treatment at the proper time. It is in these cases in particular, that Standardized Echography offers a clear answer to the question of whether active optic nerve compression is present or not in such patients and whether therefore high-dosis systemic steroid therapy, or even more invasive radiation treatment or surgical orbital decompression should be contemplated or whether very different types of treatment for other conditions are needed instead.

(c) Monitoring of CON treatment. By the same token, Standardized Echography can be helpful in objectively indicating the end point of medical treatment by revealing the end or a continuation of CON at any time during the treatment. Function tests, although absolutely needed for good management of CON, again can be misleading for the reasons discussed above. Papilledema, if present at all, is slow to develop and slow to disappear and is a poor indicator of progress made or relapse suffered, during the management of patients with compressive optic neuropathy.

3.2.5 *Optic neuritis*

Optic neuritis causes primarily swelling of the optic nerve as evidenced by an increased pial diameter. The reflectivity of the swollen optic nerve is similar to the normal nerve, i.e., low, but its septa signals appear enhanced (medium high). At times, especially in chronic or recurrent cases the arachnoidal/dural sheaths are also slightly thickened. The swelling of the optic nerve (and of its sheaths) causes intrinsic compression of the nerve and, consequently, increased subarachnoidal fluid in the retrobulbar area, if the swelling occurs in the mid- to posterior orbits or in the optic canal. Upon exercise, at least some of this excess fluid disappears as is typically seen in CON. On the other hand, the optic nerve thickness remains unchanged, and the thickening of its sheaths may even increase slightly, during 30 degree examination, for the reasons given on p. 21.

Acute optic neuritis may cause overall thickening of the nerve structures in excess of 100% of normal optic nerve thickness. Thus on echographic grounds alone, it would be possible to confuse severe optic neuritis with a low-reflective optic nerve neoplasm (e.g., glioma). But the clinical history, the signs and the symptoms in these cases, all point clearly to optic neuritis rather than an orbital (optic nerve) neoplasm. The clinical findings may, however, leave open the possibility of other painful conditions such as orbital myositis and posterior scleritis, which secondarily can cause a reduction in

76

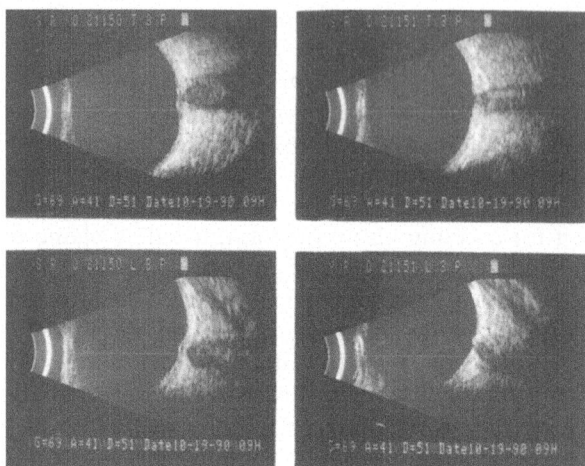

Fig. 37A. Optic neuritis with CON. B-scans: Transverse (top) and longitudinal (bottom) B-scan sections of both optic nerves (RON left, LON right) in a 48-year-old male patient with acute optic neuritis OD and hand-motion vision in this eye. The B-scans were directed so that the swollen disk of the right eye was centered for optimal documentation of the papilledema; as a consequence of this technical adjustment, the flying bat formation of the retrobulbar optic nerve sheath echogram as usually seen with increased subarachnoidal fluid is not well displayed (only suggested) in this transverse section. Because of the optic nerve swelling, the sheathing sign is suppressed in the right optic nerve patterns in contrast to the normal left transverse B-scan (top right) which shows it clearly. Note the overall widening of the right optic nerve patterns.

optic nerve functions. These other inflammatory orbital disorders are all easily and reliably identified and differentiated by Standardized Echography.

Figures 37A and B illustrate the CON component of a mostly posterior optic neuritis in the right orbit of a patient. The B-scans show the overall widening of the right optic nerve pattern (left echograms) in comparison to the normal left optic nerve (right echograms) as well as the signs of papilledema OD. The A-scan measurements demonstrate a definite but limited decrease of the retrobulbar arachnoidal diameter following exercise thus proving CON in this case.

Figure 38 conveys the marked increase in the maximal pial diameter of an inflamed right optic nerve (left echograms) in comparison with the normal left optic nerve (right echograms) in a young patient with severe optic neuritis OD. The swollen right nerve has low reflectivity and medium high, enhanced septa spikes; its thickness amounts to almost twice the thickness (5.7 mm) of the normal left normal nerve (3.04 mm).

Figure 39 illustrates a case of optic neuritis causing mild nerve swelling (maximal pial diamater of 3.50 mm) and minimal dural thickening (dural thickness of about 0.8 mm) confined primarily to the orbital apex. Inspite of the minor thickening of this optic nerve, clear-cut CON signs were docu-

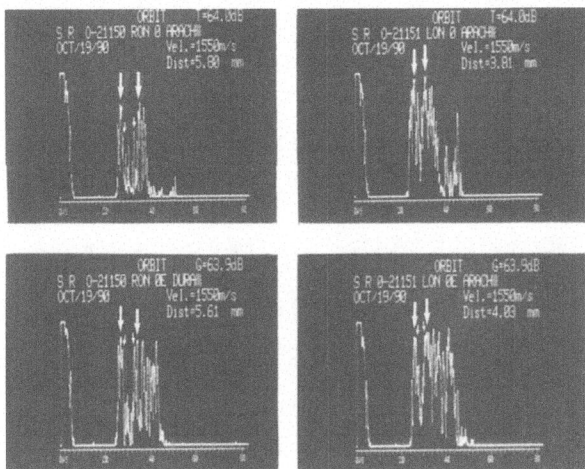

Fig. 37B. Optic neuritis with CON (same patient as decribed in Figure 37A). A-scans: measurements of the anterior right inflamed optic nerve (left echograms) in comparison with the left normal optic nerve (right echograms) of this patient. The top left echogram shows the markedly increased arachnoidal diameter measured in straight gaze direction during initial examination: 5.80 mm) of the right retrobulbar optic nerve caused by swelling of the nerve and by overlying subarachnoidal fluid. This fluid disappears entirely with exercise (bottom left echogram), while the optic nerve swelling (maximal pial diameter of 4.3 mm) and the thickening of the dural sheaths (dural thickness of about 1.3 mm) remain. In this case, no maximal dural measurements were taken before the exercise. Note, however, that the maximal dural diameter measured after the exercise (5.61 mm) is smaller than the maximal arachnoidal diameter measured initially, proving the CON even without direct comparison of arachnoidal or dural diameters before and after the exercise and on top of the fact that the optic nerve is wet before, but dry after the exercise. Also the marked sheathing sign still visible in the top left echogram has decreased after the exercise (bottom left echogram), yet another sign of the CON in this case. The right echograms demonstrate, that in the left normal optic nerve without the CON the fluid not only returned promptly into the orbit after the exercise but exceeded slightly (and temporarily) the original amount: normal maximal arachnoidal diameter of 3.81 mm initially (top right echogram) and of 4.03 mm after the exercise (bottom right echogram). The small arrows point at the peaks of the pial spikes (swollen optic nerve in left echograms, normal optic nerve in right bottom echogram), while the large arrows mark the peaks of the arachnoidal spikes in the left top echogram and in both right echograms, and the peaks of the dural spikes (thick dural sheaths) in the left bottom echogram.

mented. Obviously the swelling extended into the optic canal where the limited space did not allow even a minor expansion of the nerve tissues without causing compression.

3.2.6 *Anterior/posterior ischemic optic neuropathy (AION/PION)*

Acute stages of AION or PION are characterized by mild to moderate swelling of the optic nerve in its anterior or posterior orbital portion accompanied by mild but relatively accentuated thickening of the optic nerve

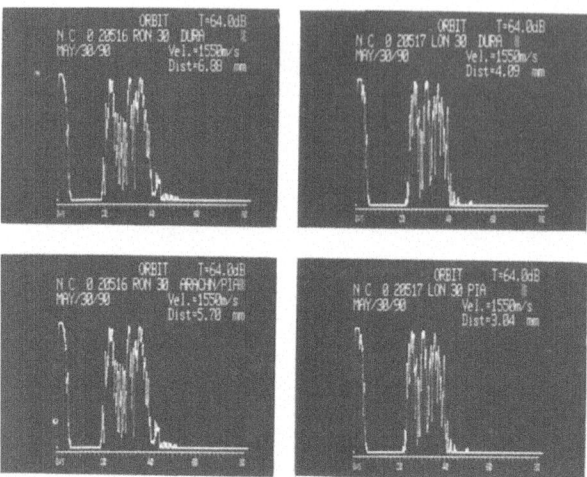

Fig. 38. Severe anterior optic neuritis without CON: maximal dural (top echograms) and pial (bottom echograms) diameters in a 27-year-old male patient with severe right optic neuritis. While the right optic nerve is markedly swollen (left bottom echogram, pial diameter of 5.70 mm) to almost twice the normal thickness of the left optic nerve (right bottom echogram, normal pial diameter of 3.04 mm), the thickness of the right dural sheaths (half the difference between the maximal dural and pial diameters or about 0.6 mm) is not much more than in the normal left optic nerve (about 0.5 mm). Arrows point at the electronic gates as they were placed over the peaks of the dural spikes (top echograms) and the pial spikes (bottom echograms). Because the swelling of the optic nerve affected mostly the anterior orbital portion of the optic nerve including its retrobulbar segment, no signs of CON developed in this case. Note that the reflectivity of the inflamed optic nerve is similar (low) to that of the normal nerve, but that the medium high septa signals, which are dispersed throughout the optic nerve pattern, are enhanced.

sheaths. The affected optic nerve has low reflectivity with enhancement of the medium high septa signals. In addition, the morphological signs of CON may be present. Thus the echographic picture of AION/PION resembles that of mild optic neuritis except for a more regular and more pronounced participation of the optic nerve sheaths. Of course, the very different age group and the absence of pain set these patients clearly apart from those with optic neuritis.

Figure 40A demonstrates optic disk swelling in the right eye (left echograms) of a patient with ischemic optic neuropathy. Such disk swelling may either be part of a very anterior ischemic optic nerve swelling, in which case no subarachnoidal fluid will be detected echographically behind the globe (in addition to a mild optic nerve swelling). Or the optic disk swelling is the consequence of CON, which is proven echographically by the initial presence of subarachnoidal fluid which disappears during exercise and stays away from the orbit following the exercise (as was the case in the patient depicted in Figure 40A).

Figure 40B presents the A-scan measurements in yet another elderly patient with severe right AION and CON. The top echogram was recorded

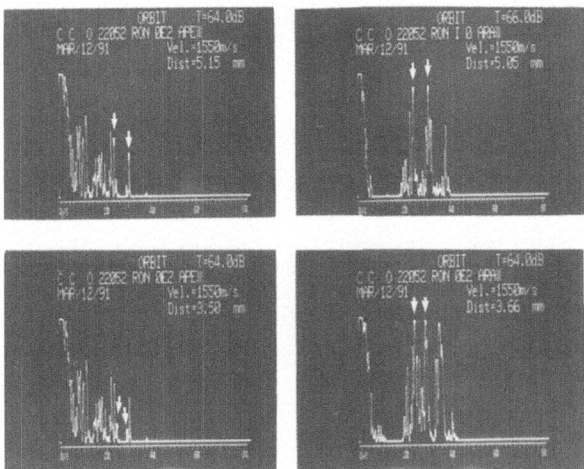

Fig. 39. Mild apical optic neuritis with CON: maximal dural (top left echogram, 5.15 mm) and pial (bottom left echogram, 3.50 mm) diameters of a slightly swollen optic nerve in the right orbital apex of a 44-year-old female patient. The right echograms were obtained in straight gaze direction from the anterior retrobulbar portion of the same optic nerve initially (top right echogram, maximal arachnoidal diameter of 5.05 mm) and following two courses of exercise (bottom right echogram, maximal arachnoidal diameter of 3.66 mm) proving CON. The arrows point at the electronic gates as they were set over the peaks of the dural spikes (top left), pial spikes (bottom left) and arachnoidal spikes (right echograms). Note the extremely oblique beam direction through the globe periphery (hardly any vitreous line left) needed to display the apical optic nerve patterns in the left echograms. This beam obliqueness at the ocular wall together with the consequent dense acoustic shadow cast by the ocular wall on the orbital tissues explains the very low maximal height of the dural and pial spikes as obtained at Tissue Sensitivity of the instrument (compare with the maximal height of the anterior optic nerve sheath signals in the right echograms recorded with a much more favorable sound beam path through the globe (long vitreous lines). See also discussion on p. 21 and Figure 12.

during the initial straight gaze examination of the RON of this patient. It illustrates marked anterior optic nerve sheath distension caused by the CON. The center echogram shows the mild swelling (maximal pial diameter of 3.84 mm measured during 30 degree gaze) of the optic nerve after it was dried out through a prolonged exercise. This echogram also indicates the fairly substantial thickening of the dural sheaths (dural thickness of about 1.60 mm). The bottom echogram demonstrates that the optic nerve stays dry after the exercise proving the CON caused intrinsically by the swelling of the optic nerve and its sheaths.

Late stages of AION or PION may still show minimal thickening of the optic nerve sheaths, while the optic nerve swelling has disappeared and the nerve may even be thinned by atrophy.

3.2.7 *Orbital congestion/hyperemia*

Any type of orbital congestion or hyperemia, be it caused by an intracranial A-V fistula (most pronounced when complicated and aggravated by

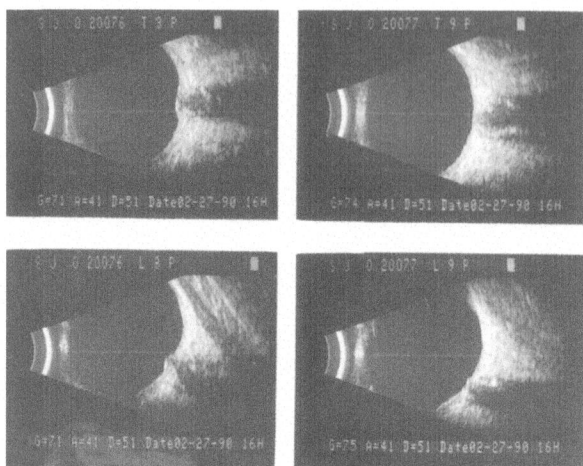

Fig. 40A. Ischemic optic neuropathy with CON: transverse (top) and longitudinal (bottom) B-scans through the right swollen optic disk (left echograms) and the normal left optic disk (right echograms) in a 52-year-old male patient with acute right AION and CON.

thrombosis), an orbital A-V malformation, or by acute inflammatory disease such as orbital cellulitis or severe orbital myositis, will also congest the numerous vessels of the arachnoidal and pial optic nerve sheaths. This sheath hyperemia may produce an echographic picture similar to BIH (i.e., low-reflective widened subarachnoidal spaces displaying a marked sheathing sign). The big difference from a BIH-caused fluid sheath distension is that the blood cannot be pushed out of the orbit by exercise. During the 30 degree test, the sheathing sign as well as the distension of the optic nerve sheaths remain largely unchanged, become slightly aggravated (similar to solid sheath thickening, see p. 21), or decrease only minimally (less than 5%), all depending on the severity of the optic nerve sheath congestion. In acute inflammatory processes, the hyperemia of the optic nerve sheaths is often limited to the anterior optic nerve portion and then often also affects the posterior episcleral tissues surrounding the optic nerve. This results in echographic patterns similar to those in severe posterior scleritis/episcleritis: 'T-sign' in B-scans; low-reflective shell-like episcleral patterns in A-scans.

In addition to revealing the typical optic nerve patterns and results of the 30 degree test, Standardized Echography also confirms optic nerve congestion and hyperemia by detecting other orbital consequences and signs of the underlying conditions: (a) congestion and hyperemia of the extraocular muscles (maximally thickened, low- to medium-reflective mid-portions of the extraocular muscles, especially of the medial and superior rectus as well as superior oblique muscles); or (b) dilated orbital vessels, i.e., the superior and inferior ophthalmic veins, the vertical veins, and other anastomosing

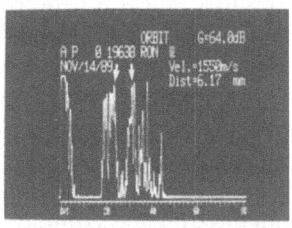

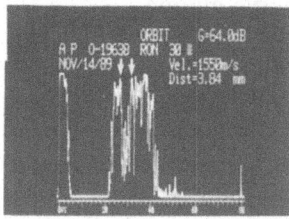

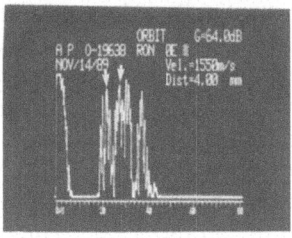

Fig. 40B. Ischemic optic neuropathy with CON: A-scan measurements of the right optic nerve in a 72-year-old female patient with acute severe right AION and CON. Top: maximal anterior arachnoidal diameter (6.17 mm) measured during initial straight gaze examination. Center: maximal pial diameter (3.84 mm) measured in prolonged 30 degree examination during exercise. Note the thickening of the dural sheaths to about 1.6 mm. Bottom: maximal arachnoidal diameter (4.00 mm) measured after a rest period following the exercise, proving CON. Considering the increased pial diameter of this optic nerve, its post-exercise maximal arachnoidal diameter indicates a practically dry nerve. The arrows mark the electronic gates as they were set over the peaks of the arachnoidal spikes (top and bottom echograms) and pial spikes (center echogram), respectively.

vessels; besides being dilated, these veins show only slow, or entirely lack, significant blood flow as evidenced by A-scan and Doppler examinations.

In addition, Standardized Echography helps to clarify the underlying causes of such congestion and hyperemia themselves by diagnosing A-V fistulas, orbital aneurysms, orbital varices, inflammatory sinus disease and orbital cellulitis or abscesses, etc.

3.2.8 *Optic nerve neoplasms*

Optic nerve gliomas
Optic nerve gliomas are low-reflective and therefore easy to diagnose; as a

matter of fact, they are the lesions that after increased intracranial pressure are the easiest ones to identify by Standardized Echography. In addition they are often much larger than other optic nerve lesions. It is therefore not surprising, that historically, optic nerve gliomas were the first of all the optic nerve disorders to be detected and differentiated with Standardized Echography (Ossoinig et al. [17]). Also, when the author for the first time succeeded to display and measure a normal optic nerve with the A-scan method in 1972, it was through a routine comparison of the normal fellow orbit in a case of an optic nerve glioma.

Apart from the young age of the patients, which already should make the examiner think of the possibility of an optic nerve swelling to be an optic nerve glioma, the echographic findings in this tumor are typical:

a) Quantitative criteria are a regular heterogeneous structure with low reflectivity (low spikes representing the cellular structures, and interspersed medium high spikes from the connective tissue septa), and a mild but distinct sound attenuation (small angle kappa). This typical quantitative appearance may change drastically if larger cystic spaces form within the tumor, especially in later stages of glioma. These cystic spaces by themselves produce typical echographic patterns and thus do not distract from the reliability and accuracy of echographic diagnoses. Rather, the echographic detection of cystic spaces in these tumors enhance their diagnosis.

b) Topographic criteria include an axial location within the muscle cone, frequently a fusiform shape, a sharp delineation by the thickened optic nerve sheaths (cyst wall appearance), and sometimes a thin optic nerve pattern detectable within the tumor.

c) Kinetic criteria are an absence of significant vascularity, a slight concomitant movement with changes in gaze direction, a solid consistency (no decrease in pial diameter during 30 degree testing), and a significant variation in size (in both directions) over long follow-up periods (changing fluid contents). Only when excessive amounts of cerebrospinal fluid, caught anteriorly by the CON, surround an optic nerve glioma (see Figure 43), a partially soft consistency is established with kinetic echography.

Figures 41A and B illustrate the typical A-scan and B-scan patterns of an optic nerve glioma with increased subarachnoidal fluid anteriorly as caused by CON. Figures 42A and B represent the typical echograms of particularly large optic nerve gliomas filling the muscle cone from globe to orbital apex. Figure 43 shows the echograms of a small optic nerve glioma being surrounded by large amounts of subarachnoidal fluid as a consequence of CON caused by posterior nerve swelling.

Figures 44A and B depict another huge optic nerve glioma with a 10-year follow-up showing increasing tumor volumes as well as fluid amounts within the tumor caused by cystic degeneration. During the course of this follow-up it was noted that the measured maximal diameters fluctuated markedly together with the amount of fluid within the tumor boundaries as well as the thickness of the solid tumor portions.

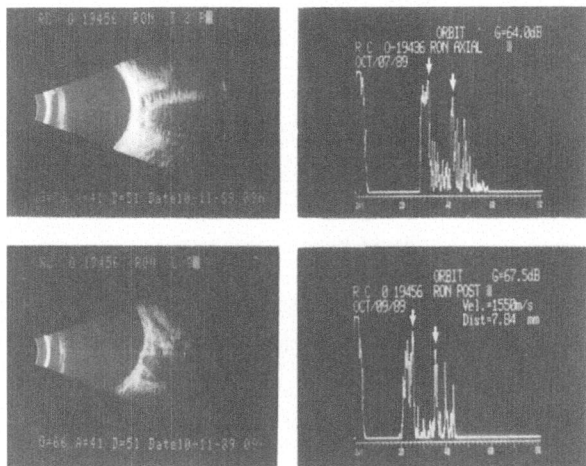

Fig. 41A. Optic nerve glioma of the posterior orbit in a 14-year-old male patient with slowly progressive painless proptosis OD. The top echograms show long-sections through this large tumor. The separation of the optic nerve sheaths as seen in the transverse (top) B-scan anteriorly is caused by great amounts of cerebrospinal fluid caught in the subarachnoidal space anterior to the tumor because of CON. For the same reason a flying bat configuration can be seen in the longitudinal B-scan echogram at the bottom left. The A-scan patterns on the right represent a long-section (top) and a cross-section (bottom) of the tumor. Note the typical low reflectivity and connective tissue septa (single medium high spikes outgrowing the very low tumor spikes) as well as the clear-cut angle kappa (decline of the tumor spike height from left to right as a consequence of sound absorption in the tumor tissue). The bottom A-scan was recorded from the posterior optic nerve portion indicating an overall thickness of the optic nerve of 7.84 mm (maximal pial diameter). Note the sharp delineation of the A-scan echograms by the much higher optic nerve sheath signals in both A-scans. The arrows point at the electronic gates which were placed over the peaks of the pial spikes.

Optic nerve sheath meningiomas

Optic nerve sheath meningiomas are acoustically characterized by thickened high-reflective optic nerve sheaths, and frequently by severe optic atrophy. In addition the morphological signs of CON are usually noted from the fluid distension of the retrobulbar optic nerve sheaths and the decrease or disappearance of the subarachnoidal fluid after exercise. The psammoma bodies imbedded in the tumor cause high, irregularly arranged spikes in the A-scan echograms; they are better appreciated as drusen-like, bright dot signals in the B-scan echograms.

These calcium deposits together with other characteristics of the affected optic nerve and the absence of any of several signs of Graves' orbitopathy let the echographic appearance of optic nerve sheath meningiomas differ clearly from that of Graves' orbitopathy. In Graves' orbitopathy, other orbital tissues than the optic nerves are primarily involved: often marked, usually asymmetric thickening primarily of the posterior segments of the

84

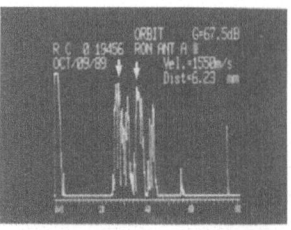

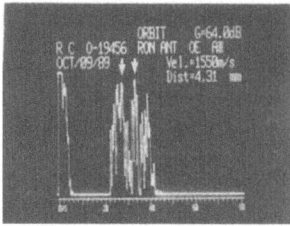

Fig. 41B. CON signs in same case as illustrated in Figure 41A: A-scan measurements of the maximal arachnoidal diameters of the retrobulbar portion of the right optic nerve during the initial examination (top echogram, 6.23 mm) and following a rest period after exercise (bottom echogram, 4.31 mm), both obtained in straight gaze directions, indicating CON. The arrows point at the electronic gates which were placed over the peaks of the arachnoidal spikes.

extraocular muscles in both orbits; bumpy thickening of the periorbitae OU; and frequently swollen lacrimal glands. Even the thickening of the optic nerve sheaths, which at a first glance appears to be a finding common to both diseases, differs markedly: in Graves' orbitopathy the thickening of the optic nerve sheaths is minor, always diffuse and similar in extent throughout the entire orbit, and is usually bilateral. The thickened nerve sheaths have a tendency toward low reflectivity. In contrast, the sheath thickening is usually unilateral, often localized, asymmetric, bumpy, irregular, tumor-like and mostly high-reflective in optic nerve sheath meningiomas.

Thus the echographic differential diagnosis between Graves' orbitopathy and optic nerve meningiomas is fairly easy and clear-cut. Nevertheless, it should be pointed out that in a patient with severe Graves' orbitopathy the early diagnosis of a coexisting optic nerve sheath meningioma may be difficult or impossible to achieve. In the thousands of Graves' patients seen in our institution over the past two and a half decades, not a single such co-existing optic nerve meningioma occurred, however. Also, the early echographic diagnosis of optic nerve sheath meningiomas is more difficult than that of optic nerve gliomas, mainly for two reasons: (a) their high reflectivity, and (b) their relatively small sizes when the first clinical signs and symptoms arise.

All other tumors of the optic nerve sheaths, e.g., inflammatory pseudotumors and sarcoidosis, produce low reflectivity of the thickend sheaths very much in contrast to the high reflectivity seen in optic nerve sheath meningi-

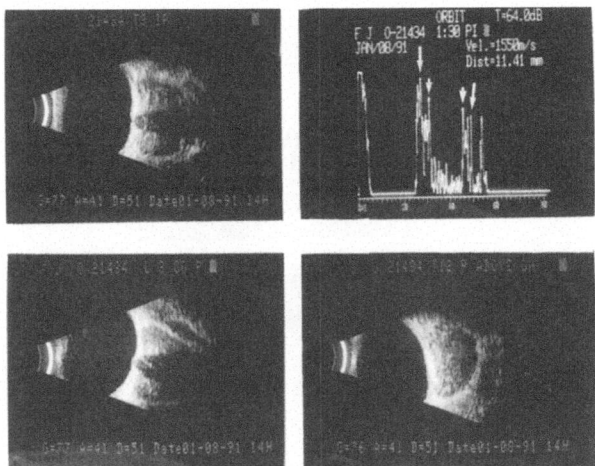

Fig. 42A. Huge glioma affecting the entire orbital portion of the right optic nerve in a 40-year-old female patient: anteriorly the tumor is still confined within the optic nerve sheaths assuming the flying bat configuration as seen in the transverse (top left) and the longitudinal (bottom left) B-scans. This phenomenon, so typical for fluid distension of the retrobulbar arachnoidal sheaths, however, by far exceeds in size everything sofar seen in fluid distension. No decrease in the size and no change in the shape of these flying bat patterns were noted during 30 degree examination (clearly solid consistency; also confirmed by A-scan). This optic nerve tumor is so huge (maximal pial diameter of 11.41 mm) that even in the cross-sectional view represented by the A-scan the angle kappa is clearly visible (top right). Note the enormous thickening of the optic nerve sheaths as marked by the pairs of arrows (the larger arrows pointing out the dural surface spikes, while the smaller arrows point at the electronic gates which were set over the peaks of the pial spikes). The anterior transverse B-scan section through the optic nerve as seen at the bottom right also demonstrates the huge size of this glioma.

omas. Also, those other optic nerve sheath tumors usually occur together with several other abnormal structures within an orbit, i.e., enlarged and infiltrated lacrimal glands, low-reflective tumors of the extraocular muscles, etc.

CT scans are well suited to diagnose larger optic nerve sheath meningiomas, mostly because of the high vascularity and dense calcifications in these tumors. A CT scan should therefore always be obtained when the diagnosis of an optic nerve meningioma is entertained echographically. In our experience, however, the early diagnosis of small optic nerve sheath meningiomas has been achieved more successfully with Standardized Echography than with radiological imaging procedures.

Figures 45A and B illustrate the typical A-scan and B-scan patterns of a diffuse ring-meningioma of the optic nerve with the signs of psammoma bodies, severe optic atrophy, and CON. Figures 46A–D present the echograms of another ring-like optic nerve sheath meningioma affecting mostly the mid-orbit, but extending posteriorly into the optic canal on the left side of a male patient. Standardized Echography was the first test clearly diagnos-

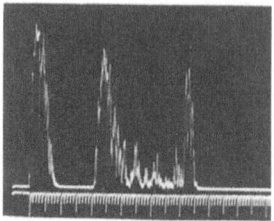

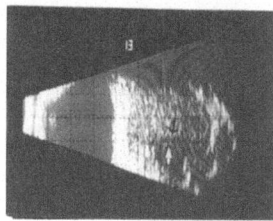

Fig. 42B. Another very large optic nerve glioma in a 17-year-old male patient: the A-scan, indicating the heterogenous internal structure and low reflectivity as well as weak sound absorption of the tumor, represents the tumor's antero-posterior axis (long-section). The B-scan, also a cut along the entire orbit from anterior to posterior, demonstrates a thin intact portion of the optic nerve imbedded along the axis of the tumor (between the two arrows) and several small cystic spaces within the posterior portion of the glioma near the right end of the echogram. The B-scan showed clearly more such details of the tumor than did the radiological imaging procedures which were also performed in this patient.

ing optic nerve sheath meningioma in this fairly young patient. Again, the tumor has caused atrophy of the left nerve, and signs of psammoma bodies and CON are noted. The extension of the tumor into the optic nerve canal was also documented by A-scan in this patient (see Figure 46D). Months later it was noted on CT that the tumor extended into the intracranial space and a combined orbital/intracranial surgical procedure was performed.

Figures 47A and B illustrate the echograms of an optic nerve sheath meningioma affecting the apical portion of a right optic nerve only. Careful A-scanning of the entire optic nerve from globe to apex is paramount to make the diagnosis and not simply state CON with unknown cause. It is the typical mistake of a beginner in Standardized Echography, to readily recognize the increased anterior subarachnoidal fluid caused by CON in such a case but to fail the pursuit of a thorough investigation of the more posterior portions of the optic nerve. Figure 48 finally illustrates a rare case of long-standing optic nerve meningioma with such a tremendous amount of calcification that it was difficult to echographically visualize the posterior portion of the tumor due to the very dense shadows cast by the calcium plaques beneath the anterior surface of the tumor.

Other optic nerve neoplasms: Thickening of the optic nerve and/or its sheaths has been documented also in cases of orbital 'pseudotumor' and sarcoidosis.

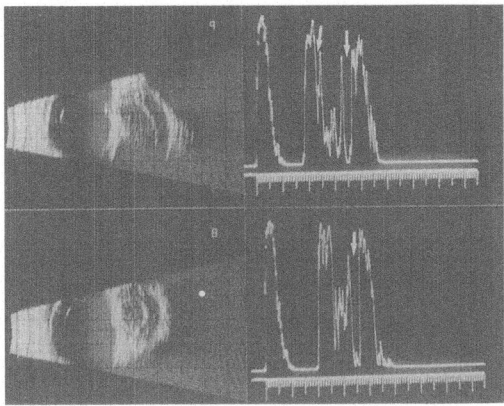

Fig. 43. Small optic nerve glioma with large amounts of surrounding subarachnoidal fluid in the left orbit of a 3-year-old male patient: Standardized Echography performed intraoperatively made the correct diagnosis which had not been made by radiological imaging in this patient. *Top left:* longitudinal B-scan showing a long-section of anterior slightly thickened optic nerve with wide optic nerve sheaths distended greatly by fluid surrounding the tumor (CON). *Bottom left:* anterior cross-section of the same area showing the slightly enlarged optic nerve surrounded by the increased amount of subarachnoidal fluid. *Right:* Maximal anterior (top) and intermediate (bottom) cross diameters of the left thickened optic nerve demonstrating the marked sheathing sign as caused by the large amount of subarachnoidal fluid (non-reflective zone as indicated by the arrows on each side of the thickened optic nerve). By pressure with the A-scan probe on the globe the fluid-filled space clearly diminished in width (a 30-degree test was not possible, since the examination was performed in the operating room under general anesthesia).

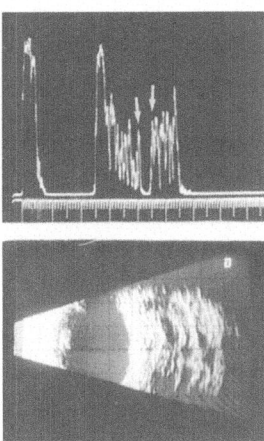

Fig. 44A. Large cystic optic nerve glioma in the left orbit of an 11-year-old female patient: the A-scan shows a long-section of the tumor in an antero-posterior direction demonstrating its typical heterogenous internal structure as well as a larger, cystic, fluid-filled space (non-reflective, well delineated) in the tumor's mid-portion (between the arrows). The numerous dark roundish areas in the retrobulbar B-scan section also indicate cystic spaces within this large tumor.

88

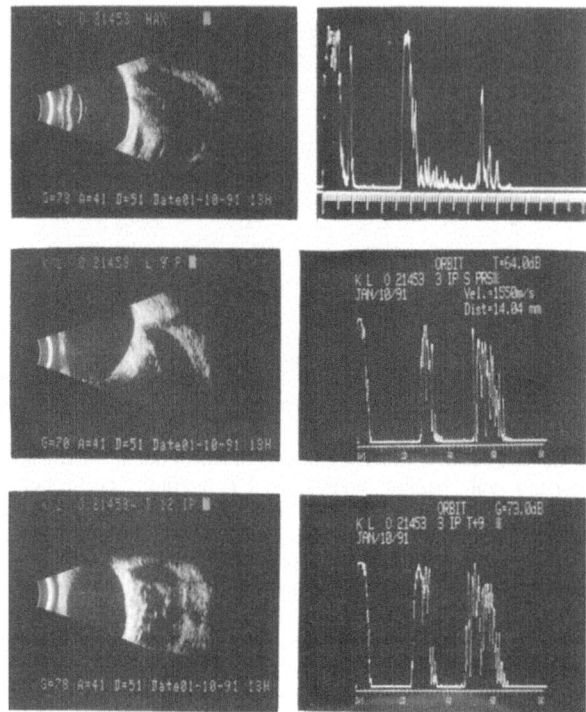

Fig. 44B. Large cystic glioma as shown in Figure 44A, ten years later. The B-scans (a horizontal axial scan through the optic disk and most anterior tumor, on top; a longitudinal scan showing an anterior long-section of the tumor, in the center; and a transverse section from below displaying an anterior cross-section of the thickened nerve, at the bottom) all show extensive fluid-filled (dark appearing) spaces surrounding the optic nerve tumor and being confined by the markedly distended optic nerve sheaths. The top A-scan (Kretztechnik 7200 MA) was obtained along the axis of the eye (note the posterior lens spike) and along the glioma in an antero-posterior direction (note the low reflectivity of the tumor and its sound absorption as expressed by the small angle kappa). The center and bottom A-scans represent cross-sectional views of the fluid-filled bag surrounding the optic nerve and confined by the markedly distended optic nerve sheaths. The optic nerve glioma itself was by-passed by the beam and is not shown in these two echograms. The center echogram was recorded at Tissue Sensitivity, whereas the bottom echogram was obtained with a 9 db higher system sensitivity still displaying only minimal blips from the very homogenus fluid.

The term 'pseudotumor' nowadays excludes all those inflammatory lesions that can be classified by Standardized Echography, and in part, especially when more severe, also by radiological imaging procedures, but often enough not on clinical grounds, as 'acute' (idiopathic) orbital myositis, dacryoadenitis, dacryocystitis, posterior scleritis and episcleritis, optic neuritis, periorbititis, orbital cellulitis, or abscesses. Only a combination of several of these conditions and the finding of tumor-like circumscribed masses in the orbital fat tissues, within the sheaths of extraocular muscles or the optic nerve, or

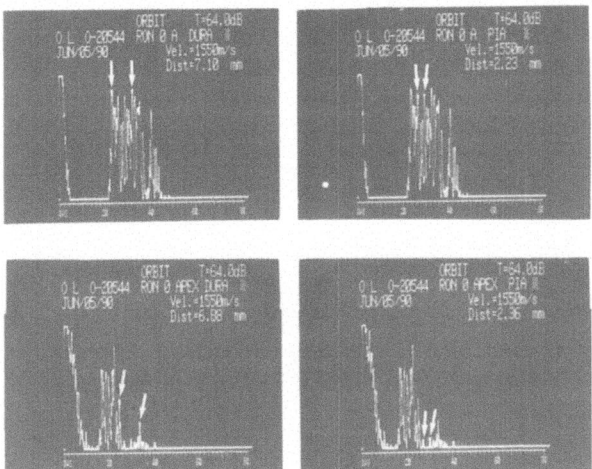

Fig. 45A. Ring-meningioma of the optic nerve sheaths in the right orbit of a 72-year-old female patient with mild proptosis and count fingers vision OD: the A-scan measurements of the anterior optic nerve (top echograms) show a maximal dural diameter of 7.10 mm (left) and a maximal pial diameter of 2.23 mm (right), and measurements within the orbital apex (bottom echograms) reveal a dural diameter of 6.88 mm (left) and a pial diameter of 2.36 mm, indicating an average dural thickening of 2.5 mm anteriorly and of 2.3 mm posteriorly in the orbit as well as severe optic atrophy. The arrows mark the electronic gates as they were placed over the peaks of the dural spikes in the left echograms, and the pial spikes in the right echograms. Note the high reflectivity (high spikes) of the dural tumor in the anterior echograms (top) as delineated by the dural and pial spikes. High reflectivity of the dural tissues may also be concluded from the fact that the tumor spikes are still visible in the apex echograms (bottom echograms) although all the orbital soft tissue signals in these echograms are very low (shadows from the ocular wall reached by oblique sound beam, see p. 21). The single towering spike in the middle of the orbital pattern in the bottom echograms represents a psammoma body (better recognizable as such in the B-scan echograms of Figure 45B).

spreading diffusely along the bony orbital wall (sclerosing pseudotumor), is still called 'orbital pseudotumor'.

In both disorders, orbital pseudotumor and sarcoidosis, other orbital structures are usually involved to such an extent as to allow their echographic differentiation from other lesions. However, the echographic features of low reflectivity, hard consistency, poor or lacking vascularity and multiple locations within an orbit are common to both conditions and histological differentiation through a biopsy is always required to separate these two conditions from each other.

Metastatic carcinomas and leucemic cells have been noted to spread from the brain into the orbit along the subarachnoidal space distending the optic nerve sheaths in the way fluid does but sometimes also infiltrating and thickening the optic nerve and its sheaths. Acoustically such optic nerve sheath distension is similar to hyperemia of the arachnoidal and pial sheaths (e.g., in A-V fistulas). Like hyperemia (and unlike simple fluid distension),

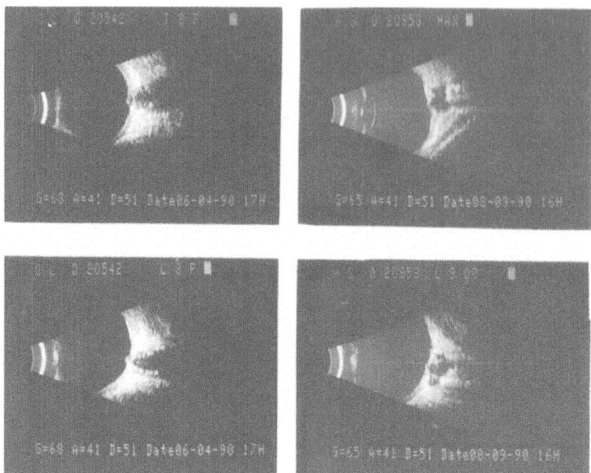

Fig. 45B. Optic nerve sheath meningiomas of the patient depicted in Figure 45A (left echograms) and of another patient described in Figures 46A–D (right echograms): the B-scans indicate slight elevation of the optic disks and show psammoma bodies to be imbedded in the thickened optic nerve sheaths (more pronounced in the echograms on the right). The B-scans on the right also suggest CON in this case (flying bat patterns).

the subarachnoidal space is slightly higher reflective than in simple fluid distension and the optic nerve sheath diameter does not decrease more than 5% (if that much), during a 30 degree test. Unlike hyperemia, no other signs of orbital congestion such as hyperemic, swollen extraocular muscles and dilated orbital veins are seen with those neoplastic metastases. In both conditions, which usually also affect the intracanalicular portion of the optic nerve, CON may be present. On the other hand, metastases of carcinomas and leukemia to other orbital structures which may co-exist with those to the optic nerve, are acoustically very different from hyperemia and congestion and thus support rather than confuse the diagnosis of optic nerve involvement by metastatic carcinoma or leukemia.

Figure 49 presents a case of acute promyelocytic leukemia with involvement of both optic disks and nerves. B-scan imaging confirmed the bilateral elevation of the optic disks (noted ophthalmoscopically) and surrounding retinochoroidal layer, which in contrast to papilledema appeared irregular and "bumpy" in the B-scan sections. The B-scans also suggested enhanced optic nerve sheath distension. The A-scan examination indicated low reflectivity of the disk and adjacent choroidal tissues confirming cellular infiltration. The A-scans also proved marked distension of the arachnoidal/dural sheaths by increased cerebrospinal fluid, which upon exercise decreased and following the exercise stayed away from the orbits, thus confirming CON. This compression probably took place within the optic canals where the sheath infiltration prevented the free fluid exchange between brain and orbits.

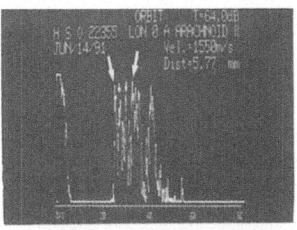

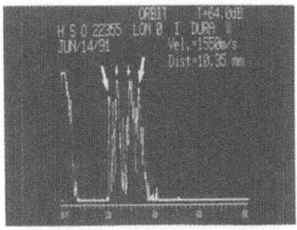

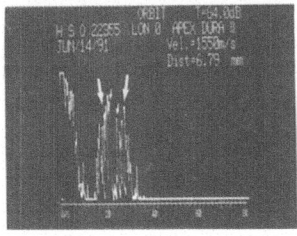

Fig. 46A. Optic nerve sheath **meningioma** with **CON** in the left orbit of a 41-year-old male patient with counting fingers vision in OS (same patient as in Figures 45B, right echograms, and 46B, C and D): these initial A-scan echograms were obtained in straight gaze direction from the most anterior portion (top), the mid-portion (center) and the apical portion (bottom) of the left optic nerve. Increased subarachnoidal fluid retrobulbarly caused the arachnoidal diameter there to measure 5.77 mm (CON; see also right B-scans in Figure 45B). The marked dural thickening (of up to 3.7 mm in the mid-orbit as measured indirectly − 1/2 of the difference between the maximal dural and pial diameters) caused the dural diameter to measure 10.35 mm there (center echogram) and 6.79 mm in the apex (bottom echogram). The small arrows mark the peaks of the pial spikes, while the large arrows point at the electronic gates as they were set over the peaks of the arachnoidal (top echogram) and dural spikes (center and bottom echograms), respectively. Note that the subarachnoidal space filled with fluid (between the pial and arachnoidal spikes in top echogram) presents with a much lower reflectivity than the dural tumor tissue in the center echogram (area between the pial and dural spikes, especially on the right end of the echogram) inspite of the fact that all orbital spikes are lower in this center echogram due to the more oblique beam incidence at the posterior ocular wall (note also the shorter vitreous line in the central echogram as compared to the top echogram). In the bottom echogram the dural tumor spikes as seen between the dural and pial signals are still relatively high inspite of the extremely oblique sound beam incidence at the lateral ocular wall required to reach the orbital apex (almost no vitreous line left).

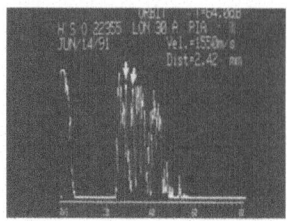

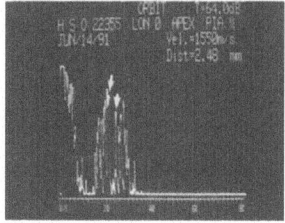

Fig. 46B. Severe optic atrophy in the same case of optic nerve sheath meningioma as depicted in Figures 46A, C and D: the maximal pial diameters as measured anteriorly (top echogram: 2.42 mm) and in the orbital apex (bottom echogram: 2.48 mm) indicate severe optic atrophy. Arrows point at the electronic gates as they were placed over the peaks of the pial spikes.

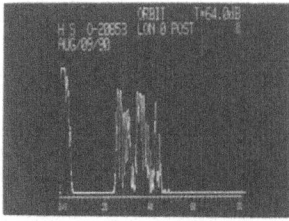

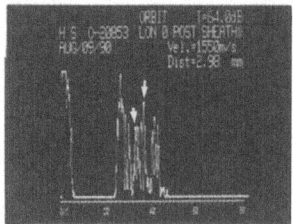

Fig. 46C. Optic nerve sheath ring-meningioma (same case as described in Figures 46A, B and D): A-scan echograms from the posterior portion of the optic nerve demonstrate the marked, high-reflective thickening of the dural sheaths. This time the dural thickness is measured directly as 2.98 mm (arrows point at the electronic gates as they were placed over the peaks of the nasal pial and dural spikes in the bottom echogram). The inner dural signals are almost as strong as the maximized large surface signals indicating the presence of psammoma bodies.

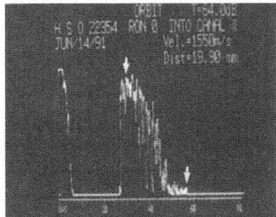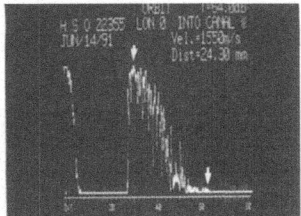

Fig. 46D. Extension of optic nerve sheath meningioma into the optic canal (same case as depicted in Figures 46A, B, and C): A-scan echograms of the right normal orbit and optic canal (left echogram) and of the left orbit and optic canal with the optic nerve sheath meningioma extending into the optic canal (right echogram). The acoustic beam was aimed along the axis of the orbit into the optic canal in each orbit; the electronic gates (arrows) were placed over the peaks of the scleral spike and the last spike of the chain of orbital signals on the right. Note that the right abnormal orbital echogram (left orbit) is 4.4 mm longer than the left normal one (right orbit). Even when considering the left proptosis of 2 mm in this patient and a shortening of the left globe by 0.2 mm (as determined with immersion axial eye length measurement), a surplus of 2.2 mm remains: this is the distance the acoustic beam was able to follow the optic nerve into the optic canal as it was slightly widened by the expanding tumor.

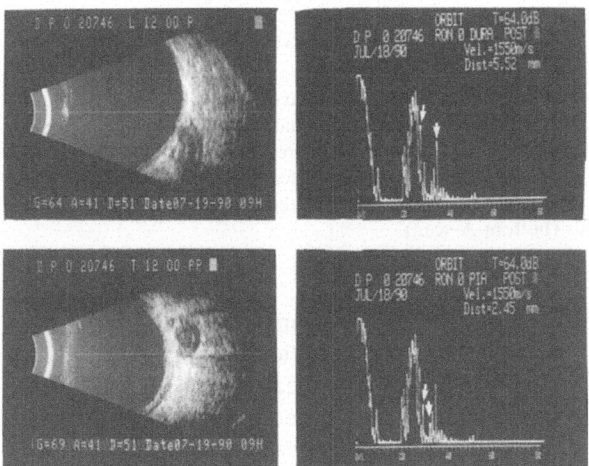

Fig. 47A. Small ring-meningioma of the right optic nerve in the posterior orbit of a 55-year-old female patient with minimal proptosis and moderate decrease in her vision OD: the longitudinal long-section (top B-scan) and the transverse cross-section (bottom B-scan) show the increased subarachnoidal fluid surrounding the anterior portion of the affected nerve (caused by CON). The A-scans were obtained from the most posterior orbital portion of the optic nerve measuring the dural diameter as 5.52 mm (top A-scan) and the pial diameter as only 2.45 mm (bottom A-scan) thus indicating optic atrophy and a dural sheath thickening of slightly more than 1.5 mm. The arrows point at the electronic gates as they were placed over the peaks of the dural spikes (top A-scan) and the pial spikes (bottom A-scan) for the measurements.

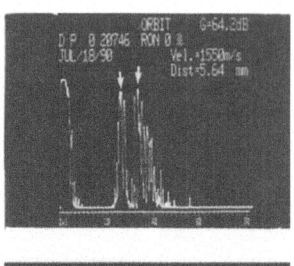

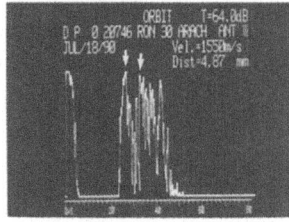

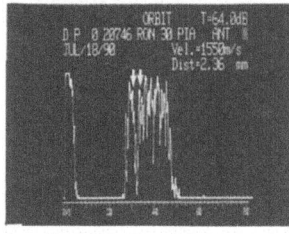

Fig. 47B. CON caused by small ring-meningioma of the optic nerve in the right posterior orbit of the patient depicted in Figure 47A: the maximal anterior arachnoidal diameter measures 5.64 mm during the initial straight gaze examination (top A-scan), and decreases to 4.87 mm (by 14%, enough to prove fluid) during 30 degree examination (center A-scan). The maximal pial diameter is reduced to 2.36 mm (bottom A-scan) indicating optic atrophy. The arrows point at the electronic gates placed over the peaks of the arachnoidal spikes (top and center A-scans) and the pial spikes (bottom A-scan).

In addition the A-scan examination revealed diffuse thickening of the arachnoidal/dural sheaths of both optic nerves throughout the orbits. The thickness of these sheaths, normally measuring between 0.3 and 0.8 mm, was locally increased to 2.3 mm. A low reflectivity of the sheaths suggested dense cellular infiltration. When the optic nerves were stretched during a 30 degree test, the thickness of the sheaths decreased minimally (clearly less than 5%) indicating firm consistency of the sheath infiltrates. All these echographic findings were well consistent with leucemic infiltration of the optic disks and nerves. Treatment with oral trans-retinoic acid was undertaken and resulted in the resolution of these leucemic infiltrations, as evidenced by clinical improvement and confirmed by Standardized Echography.

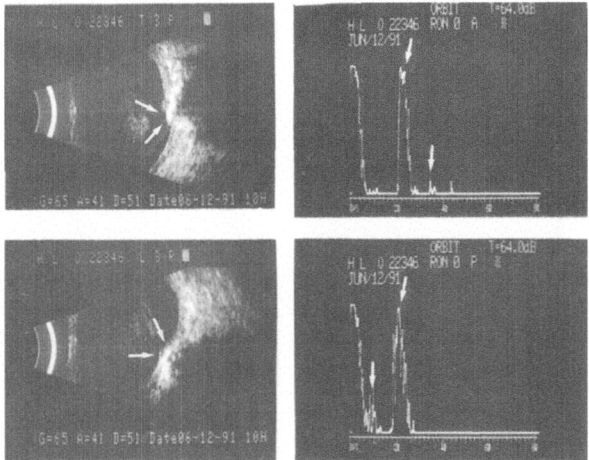

Fig. 48. Heavily calcified optic nerve meningioma in the right orbit of an 83-year-old female patient with long-standing right optic nerve sheath meningioma, 2 mm proptosis and no light perception of the right eye: this meningioma is so heavily calcified, that only a few weak signals (from strongly reflective calcium deposits) were obtained from behind the most anterior heavy calcification (arrows) of this meningioma in the B-scans. The top A-scan was obtained from the anterior portion of the optic nerve and shows mostly the temporal calcified (high spikes as marked by left arrow; dense shadowing) optic nerve sheaths. Very weak signals are still obtained from the nasal heavily calcified sheaths of the nerve as indicated by the right arrow in this echogram. The bottom A-scan was recorded from the posterior orbit. Inspite of the fact of dense shadowing by the obliquely traversed ocular wall (left arrow; hardly any vitreous baseline is visible and virtually no orbital soft tissue signals are displayed at tissue sensitivity), the dense calcification of the temporal tumor surface can still be appreciated from the almost 100% high spikes representing that posterior temporal surface of the tumor (right arrow). By comparison, non-calcified posterior surface signals of the optic nerve are much lower under these circumstances (see left A-scans in Figure 39).

4. CONCLUSIONS

Standardized Echography plays an indispensable role in the diagnosis and management of disorders of the optic disk and of the optic nerve, or of other diseases which indirectly affect the optic nerve. This method provides a wealth of clinically important information including real-time kinetic data and precise measurements, clearly surpassing the resolution and accuracy of radiological neuro-imaging procedures. Standardized Echography is both a reliable front-line screening method and an important secondary test by offering highly accurate differential diagnoses and precise measurements, and is optimally suited for frequent follow-up examinations because of its time-proven safety. It thus effectively complements the radiological tests which on the other hand provide a more comprehensive topographic over-view of the region and also crucial information about intracranial structures not available from echographic imaging. Fine topographic details, precise

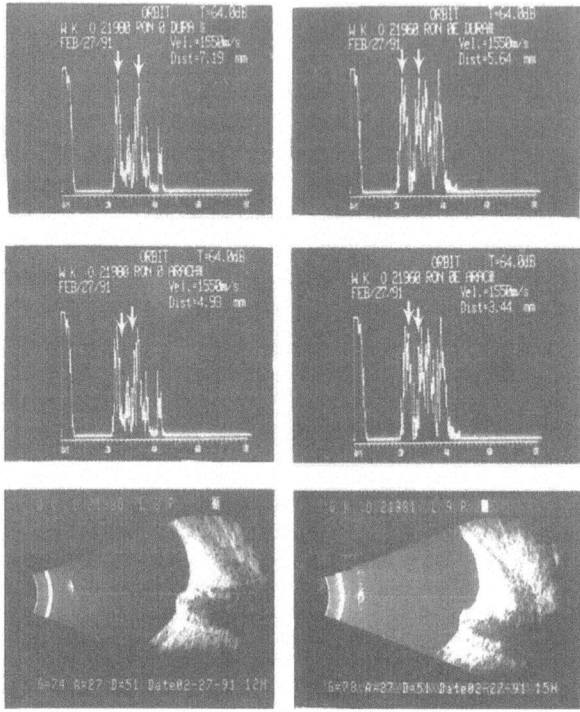

Fig. 49. Acute promyelocytic infiltration of both optic disks and nerves in a 37-year-old female patient. The left A-scans represent the display and measurements of the maximal dural (top: 7.19 mm) and arachnoidal (center: 4.93 mm) diameters of the right optic nerve during initial 0 degree gaze. The difference between the dural and arachnoidal diameters, divided by 2, indicates the thickness of the arachnoidal/dural sheaths (1.13 mm). The right A-scans show the maximal diameters measured in straight gaze after an exercise, indicating (a) CON as evidenced by a clear decrease of subarachnoidal fluid (by 30%) and (b) firm consistency of the sheath infiltrates (only minimal decrease in sheath thickness by 0.03 mm). Note the fairly substantial drop in reflectivity between the dural and arachnoidal spikes suggesting low reflectivity of the thickened sheaths. The arrows point at the placement of the electronic gates over the peaks of the dural spikes (top A-scans) and the arachnoidal spikes (center A-scans). The B-scans show horizontal longitudinal sections through the right optic disk aimed from temporal (left B-scan) and through the left optic disc (right B-scan). Note the bumpiness of the elevated disk tissues as well as the marked sheathing sign of the optic nerve.

measurements and the great differential diagnostic capabilities of Standardized Echography make this method indispensable for the evaluation of the orbital portion of the optic nerve, however.

Further progress in the echographic imaging of the optic disk and the optic nerve may be expected from the development of new, improved technology ranging from three-dimensional displays and color flow mapping to advanced computerization of digitized echographic signals and data. However, artefacts are both frequent and significant in the echographic scanning of the eye and orbit, particularly in the area of the optic nerve. In order to avoid them and to prevent them from rendering the echographic data invalid, the signals from the large optic nerve interfaces, i.e., the dural, arachnoidal and pial surfaces, must be maximized. This is accomplished through a meticulous adjustment of beam position and direction. It is totally unrealistic to expect that some day this may be achieved through the design of a both effective and economic, automated, signal-guided mechanical probe movement device. The elimination of detrimental artefacts and the extraction of valid and correct information from the echograms will always require the trained and skillful hand of an experienced and knowledgeable echographer who guides the ultrasonic beam effectively and safely through what is called visual pattern recognition. The echographer does this in a reflex-like reaction to the dynamic changes of the signals as observed on the screen during the scanning procedure. Technological advances will unquestionably facilitate Standardized Echography in the foreseeable future. The success of this method will, however, remain a major function of the human operator, because Standardized Echography is not only a matter of science and technology, but also represents – to a considerable degree – a skill.

References

1. Atta, H.R. 1988. Imaging of the optic nerve with Standardized Echography. Eye 2(4): 358–366.
2. Baum. G. 1960. Ultrasonography – an aid in orbital tumor diagnosis. Arch. Ophthal. 64: 180–194.
3. Byrne, S.F. 1987. The echographic measurement and differential diagnosis of optic nerve lesions. In: Ophthalmic Echography (K.C. Ossoinig, ed.), Docum. Ophthal. Proc. Series 48: 571–585. Martinus Nijhoff/Dr. W. Junk Publishers, Dordrecht/Boston/Lancaster.
4. Cennamo, G., Sorrentino, A., Scanni, E., & Rosa, N. 1985. Echographic study of the optic nerve during anesthesia. Orbit 4(4): 231–234.
5. Cennamo, G., Gangemi, M., & Stella, L. 1987. The correlation between endocranial pressure and optic nerve diameter: an ultrasonographic study. In: Ophthalmic Echography (K.C. Ossoinig, ed.), Docum. Ophthal. Proc. Series 48:603–606. Martinus Nijhoff/Dr. W. Junk Publishers, Dordrecht/Boston/Lancaster.
6. Darnley-Fisch, D.A., Byrne, S.F., Hughes, J.R., Parrish, R.K., & Feuer, W.J. 1990. Contact B-scan echography in the assessment of optic nerve cupping. Am. J. Ophthalmol. 109: 55–61.
7. Doro, D., Perrone, S., Fiore, D., & Moro, F. 1987. Optic nerve evaluation by echography and computerized tomography in patients with optic disk drusen. In: Ophthalmic Echography (K.C. Ossoinig, ed.), Docum. Ophthal. Proc. Series 48: 615–618. Martinus Nijhoff/Dr. W. Junk Publishers, Dordrecht/Boston/Lancaster.
8. Galetta, S., Byrne, S.F., & Smith, J.L. 1989. Echographic correlation of optic nerve sheath size and cerebrospinal fluid pressure. J. Clin. Neuro-Ophthalmol. 9(2): 79–82.
9. Gerstner, R. & Ossoinig, K.C. 1971. A new Instrument (Kretz 7200 MA, Prototype) for the diagnosis and differential diagnosis of tissues (Ger.). In: Ultrasonographia Medica (Proc. 1st World Congress on Ultrasonic Diagnosis in Medicine and SIDUO III, Vienna 1969; J. Boeck and K. Ossoinig, eds.), Vol. I: 55–60, Verlag Wiener Med. Akad., Vienna.
10. Hasenfratz, G. 1987. Experimental studies on the display of the optic nerve. In: Ophthalmic

Echography (K.C. Ossoinig, ed.), Docum. Ophthal. Proc. Series 48: 587–602. Martinus Nijhoff/Dr. W. Junk Publishers, Dordrecht/Boston/Lancaster.

11. Hodes, B.L. 1978. Ultrasonographic demonstration of glaucomatous optic nerve excavation. J. Clin. Ultrasound 6(4): 223–225.

12. Jackson, W.E. & Freed, S. 1985. Ocular and systemic abnormalities associated with morning glory syndrome. Ophthalmic.-Paediatr.-Genet. 5(1–2): 111–115.

13. Levine, R.A. 1987. Orbital ultrasonography. Radiol. Clin. North. Am. 25(3): 447–469.

14. Magli, A., Cennamo, G., Corvino, C., & Mele, A. 1985. Genetic and ultrasound study of abnormalities of the optic nerve head. Ophthalmic-Paedriatr.-Genet. 5(1–2): 71–78.

15. Ossoinig, K.C. 1971. Clinical Echo-Ophthalmography of orbital lesions (Ger). In: Ultrasonographia Medica (Proc. of 1st World Congress on Ultrasonic Diagnosis in Medicine and SIDUO III, Vienna 1969; J. Boeck and K.C. Ossoinig, eds.), Vol. II: 423–435, Verlag Wiener Med. Akad., Vienna.

16. Ossoinig, K.C. 1971. Basics of Clinical Echo-Ophthalmography (Ger). Verlag Wien. Med. Akad., Vienna.

17. Ossoinig, K.C. & Blodi, F.C. 1974. Preoperative differential diagnosis of tumors with echography. IV. Diagnosis of orbital tumors. In: Current Concepts in Ophthalmology 4:313–343.

18. Ossoinig, K.C. 1975. A-scan echography and orbital disease. In: Mod. Probl. Ophthal. 14: 203–235. Karger, Basel.

19. Ossoinig, K.C., Kaefring, S.L., McNutt, L., & Weinstock, S.J. 1977. Echographic measurement of the optic nerve. In: Ultrasound in Medicine, Vol. 3A (D. White and R.E. Brown, eds.), pp. 1065–1066, Plenum Press, New York.

20. Ossoinig, K.C. 1977. Echography of the eye, orbit and periorbital region. In: Orbit Roentgenology (P.H. Arger, ed.), John Wiley & Sons Publishers, New York.

21. Ossoinig, K.C. 1979. Standardized Echography: basic principles, clinical applications and results. In: Ophthalmic Ultrasonography: comparative techniques (R.L. Dallow, ed.), Internat. Ophthal. Clinics 19: 127–210. Little, Brown and Co., Boston.

22. Ossoinig, K.C., Cennamo, G., & Frazier-Byrne, S. 1981. Echographic differential diagnosis of optic nerve lesions. In: Ultrasonography in Ophthalmology (J.M. Thijssen and A.M. Verbeek, eds.), Docum. Ophthal. Proc. Series 29: 327–332. Dr. W. Junk Publishers, The Hague/Boston/London.

23. Ossoinig, K.C. 1982. Diagnostic ultrasound. In: Neuro-Ophthalmology, Vol. 2: 373–388 (S. Lessell and J.T.W. van Dalen, eds.). Excerpta Medica, Amsterdam/Oxford/-Princeton.

24. Ossoinig, K.C. 1984. Ultrasonic diagnosis of Graves' ophthalmopathy, In: The Eye and Orbit in Thyroid Disease (C.A. Gorman, R.R. Waller, and J.A. Dyer, eds.), pp. 185–211. Raven Press, New York.

25. Ossoinig, K.C., Reshef, D.S., Weingeist, T.A., Folk, J.C., & Packer, A.J. 1987. Echographic findings in Terson's syndrome. In: Ophthalmic Echography (K.C. Ossoinig, ed.), Docum. Ophthalmol. Proc. Series 48: 247–256, Martinus Nijhoff/Dr. W. Junk Publishers, Dordrecht/Boston/Lancaster.

26. Ossoinig, K.C. 1989. The role of standardized opthalmic echography in the management of Graves' orbitopathy. Dev.-Ophthalmol. 20: 28–37.

27. Sampaolesi R. 1990. Echometry in congenital glaucoma: long-term results after 10 to 17 years of surgery. In: Ultrasonography in Ophthalmology 12 (R. Sampaolesi, ed.), Docum. Ophthal. Proc. Series 53:181–191. Kluwer Academic Publishers, Dordrecht/Boston/London.

28. Singh, J., Ghose, S., Vashisht, S., & Goulatia R.K. 1985. Optic nerve hypoplasia: clinical and ultrasonographic study. Can. J. Ophthalmol. 20(6): 205–210.

29. Singh, J. & Ghose, S. 1987. Isolated coloboma of the optic nerve head: an echographic evaluation. Ann. Ophthalmol. 19(5): 184–186.

30. Skalka, H.W. 1978. Ultrasonographic demonstration of glaucomatous optic nerve excavation. J. Clin. Ultrasound 6(6): 23.

31. Skalka, H.W. 1978. Neural and dural optic nerve measurements with A-scan ultrasonography. South Med. J. 71(4): 399–400.
32. Spector, R.H. 1991. Echographic diagnosis of dural carotid-cavernous sinus fistulas. Am. J. Ophthalmol. 111 (1): 77–83.
33. Spencer, W.H. 1979. Diagnostic modalities and natural behavior of optic nerve gliomas. Ophthalmology 86(5): 881–885.
34. Stanowsky, A. & Kreissig, I. 1987. Echographic examination of the optic nerve and its meninges in the diagnosis of pseudotumor cerebri. In: Ophthalmic Echography (K.C. Ossoinig, ed.), Docum. Ophthal. Proc. Series 48: 607–613. Martinus Nijhoff/Dr. W. Junk Publishers, Dordrecht/Boston/Lancaster.
35. Stanowsky, A. 1988. Echographically determined changes of the optic nerve in hypertensive retinopathy (Stage IV). In: Ultrasonography in Ophthalmology 11 (J.M. Thijssen, J.S. Hillman, P.E. Gallenga, and G. Cennamo, eds.), Docum. Ophthal. Proc. Series 51: 291–295. Kluwer Academic Publishers, Dordrecht/Boston/London.
36. Till, P. 1976. Solid tissue model for the standardization of the echo-ophthalmograph 7200 MA (Kretz-Technik). Docum. Ophthal. Proc. Series 41: 205–240.

Address for correspondence: Department of Ophthalmology, University of Iowa Hospitals, Iowa City, IA 52242, USA.

2. CSF dynamic parameters and changes of optic nerve diameters measured by standardized echography

C. TAMBURRELLI, C. ANILE, A. MANGIOLA,
B. FALSINI & P. PALMA

(Rome, Italy)

Abstract. By means of infusion of Ringer lactate in the subarachnoidal spaces, different CSF intracranial dynamic parameters have been studied in 20 subjects. During the infusion, optic nerve diameters were evaluated with Standardized A-Scan. Anterior, posterior and intermediate transverse optic nerve diameters were obtained during the infusion test. The correlation between intracranial CSF dynamic parameters and optic nerve diameters showed: (a) a direct, biphasic, positive relation between diastolic intracranial pressure and optic nerve diameters, (b) a direct relation with the intracranial absorptive reserve, (c) rapid changes of optic nerve diameters in response to variation of intracranial pressure, (d) based on normal intracranial pressure values, we could define an echographic biometric range of normal optic nerve diameters, (e) the echographic investigation of increased intracranial pressure showed a high level of sensitivity and specificity of the Standardized A-Scan for detection of increased CSF pressure.

Introduction

Standardized A-scan echography can be used to evaluate variations in the thickness of the optic nerve between the bulb and the beginning of the optic canal. Increases in the transverse diameter of the optic nerve may be caused by various pathological processes. Solid enlargements can be ultrasonically distinguished from those due to increases in the volume of the cerebro-spinal fluid (CSF) in the subarachnoid space [4–6]. Correlation between ultrasound findings in the latter cases and increases in intracranial pressure (ICP) has now been firmly established: the distance between the lateral and nasal arachnoid surfaces of the nerve shows proportional increases or decreases with those of intracranial pressure [4, 5, 7]. Standardized A-scans show increases in the transverse diameters of both optic nerves in cases of benign intracranial hypertension.

The objective of the present study was to identify those CSF parameters (systolic and diastolic ICP, intracranial elasticity, CSF absorption) that cause variations in the thickness of the optic nerve. In addition, we wanted to determine the degree to which each of these parameters influences the increase or decrease of the perioptic subarachnoid CSF. Finally, we hoped to obtain data that would allow us to identify normal values for optic nerve thickness in relation to CSF dynamics. There is still, in fact, disagreement over this last point in spite of the large volume of literature dealing with ultrasonic examination of the optic nerve. Twenty patients were thus exam-

P. Till (ed.), Ophthalmic Echography 13, pp. 101–109.
© 1993 *Kluwer Academic Publishers.*

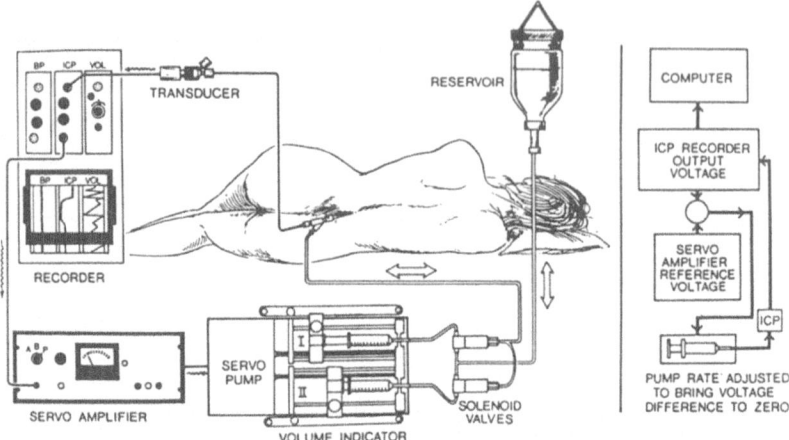

Fig. 1. A needle is inserted into the subarachnoid lumbar space and connected to a servocontrolled pump and pressure transducer. The infusion liquid can be introduced or removed according to the intracranial conditions found. The patient lies on his right side and the ultrasound evaluation of the transverse diameter of the left optic nerve is performed (from Sklar et al.).

ined using standardized A-scan of the optic nerve during variations in ICP induced by Ringer's lactate infusions into the spinal and endocranial subarachnoid spaces.

Materials and methods

The study group was composed of 20 patients (14 females and 6 males). Neurosurgical consultations had been requested for all patients because of suspected alterations in CSF dynamics. In order to evaluate the production and absorption of CSF these patients were subjected to the infusion test described by Katzmann and Hussey. This test is used to study patients with altered CSF absorption, those with tumors of the choroid plexus and those with presumed disorders involving CSF dynamics.

Ringer's lactate was introduced into the spinal subarachnoid space via lumbar puncture. The volume of liquid introduced was controlled by a perfusion pump based on continuous measurements of ICP by means of a special pressure transducer (Fig. 1).

The test lasts approximately 30 min and involves three phases. During the first phase the baseline ICP was measured prior to initiation of the infusion. At this point, the Ringer's lactate was introduced. In response to this infusion, the ICP will show a variable increase depending on the endocranial condition of the individual; in a few cases there is no increase at all. During the final phase the pressure increase induced by the infusion was eliminated.

Table 1. The table shows the type of data collected for each patient. The figures shown, as examples, are those found in case no. 9

Diam. ON			T.	ICP diast.	ICP puls.	AR	IV	IE
ant.	mid.	post.						
4.2	4.3	4.6	0	16	6	0.1	0.5	0.7
4.4	4.5	4.8	10	19	5			
4.5	4.7	4.9	20	20	4			
4.8	5.0	5.3	30	25	4			
4.3	4.4	4.6	−10	12	3			

ON Diam.: arachnoidal optic nerve diameter measured by standardized A-Scan immediately behind the bulb (ant.) in the mid-orbital segment (mid.) and near the orbital apex (post.).
T: Time of measurement expressed in minutes after initiation of the infusion.
Diast. ICP: Minimum intracranial pressure.
Puls. ICP: Pulsatile intracranial pressure, i.e. difference between systolic and diastolic ICPs.
AR: CSF absorptive reserve. For each ICP value, the arithmetic difference between CSF absorption and formation.
IV: Volume infused.
IE: Intracranial elasticity: capacity of the system to absorb sudden increases in volume; the more rigid the system, the lower the elasticity value.

This step is not necessary unless the ICP remains above 15 mm Hg after the infusion has been completed. In this case, liquid must be removed from the system until the pressure falls below this level [1–3].

The lumbar puncture was performed while the patient was lying on his right side with head and legs flexed. In this position, the optic nerve of the left eye is accessible for the ultrasound study. The transverse diameters were measured at three points along the intraorbital portion of the nerve: right behind the bulb, at the mid-orbital portion and near the orbital apex. Measurements were made before the infusion was begun and at 10-minute intervals thereafter during the infusion for a total of four measurements in each patient.

Standardized A-scan was performed with Ophthascan S and Mini A using techniques already described in the literature [4]. With the eye in the primary gaze position, these scans show peaks corresponding to the lateral and nasal subarachnoid surfaces of the optic nerve. When the ICP increases, these surfaces can be visualized even more clearly because of the volume of liquid separating them from the underlying nerve tissue. Diastolic and pulsatile ICP, volume of liquid infused, intracranial elasticity and velocity of diastolic ICP variations were recorded with each ultrasound measurement of the nerve. Table 1 shows the figures obtained for one of the patients studied.

Results

On the basis of baseline diastolic ICP values, the patients could be divided into three categories: those with baseline values between 1 and 7 mm Hg,

Table 2. Diastolic ICP and mean mid-orbital O.N. diameters (ϕ)

	I	II	III
Patients	5	9	6
ICP baseline	1–7 mm Hg	8–15 mm Hg	16–30 mm Hg
O.N. ϕ mid.	3.0–3.7 mm	3.2–4.5 mm	4.7–6.2 mm
	(3.6)	(3.95)	(5.25)

Table 3. Ranges of diastolic ICP and corresponding optic nerve diameters observed during infusion test. The patients have been divided into three groups based on ICP values

	I	II	III
Patients	4	9	7
Diastolic ICP	0–5 mm Hg	8–14 mm Hg	15–35 mm Hg
O.N. ϕ	3.0–3.9 mm	3.6–4.5 mm	4.4–6.5 mm

Table 4. Increase in diastolic ICP (in mm Hg) with respect to baseline ICP are shown with corresponding increases in transverse diameters of the mid-orbital portion of the optic nerve. Group A is composed of patients with baseline ICPs of less than 15 mm Hg; Group B contains patients with baseline ICPs of 15 mm Hg or more. Three subgroups (I, II and III) have been distinguished within group A on the basis of the degree of ICP increase during infusion

Group A	I	II	III	Group B	
Patients	3	6	7	Patients	4
D ICP					
(ICP max – ICP base)	0–5 mm Hg	6–10 mm Hg	10–16 mm Hg	D. ICP	10–25 mm Hg
ϕ O.N.					
(Diameter max – base)	0.0–0.6 mm	0.7–0.9 mm	0.2–0.8 mm	D. ϕ O.N.	0.2–0.9 mm
	(0.3)	(0.83)	(0.82)		(0.47)

those with values ranging from 8 to 15 mm Hg and those whose baseline diastolic pressure exceeded 15 mm Hg (in one case as high as 30 mm Hg). In the first category of patients, the diameters measured at the mid-orbital portion of the optic nerve ranged from 3.0 to 3.7 mm (mean 3.6). The same diameters for the second group were between 3.2 and 4.5 mm (mean 3.95 mm) and, for the third group, from 4.7 to 6.2 mm (mean 5.25 mm) (Table 2).

If we examine variations in the diastolic ICP during the test three categories of patients can also be distinguished (Table 3). In the first group of patients, diastolic ICP never exceeded 5 mm Hg during the infusion test (range 0–5 mm Hg). Maximum values in the second group ranged from 8 to 14 mm Hg and in the third group from 15 to 35 mm Hg. The variations in the diameter of the optic nerve were closely correlated with those of the ICP. Maximum diameters of 3.0 to 3.9 mm were observed in the first group, from 3.6 to 4.5 in the second and from 4.4 to 6.5 in the third.

The variations in diastolic ICP correlated with those of the mean optic nerve diameters observed during the infusion are shown in Table 4. Variations are expressed as differences (in mm Hg for ICP; in mm for optic nerve diameter) between initial baseline figures and the highest figure observed during the infusion. It is important to keep in mind that the response of the optic nerve in patients with initial diastolic ICPs of 15 mm Hg or more differs from that seen in patients with lower baseline pressures. For this reason, patients with baseline pressures less than 15 mm Hg (Group A) will be considered separately from those with higher baseline readings (Group B) (Table 4).

Within the first group (A) we could distinguish three subgroups based on the ICP response to the infusion: those with pressure increases of 0–5 mm Hg, those with increases of 6–10 mm Hg and those whose ICP increased from 10 to 16 mm Hg over baseline values. These increases were accompanied by increases in optic nerve diameters measured midway between the nerve's insertion at the bulb and its passage through the orbital apex which ranged from 0.0 to 0.6 mm (mean 0.3 mm) for the first subgroup, from 0.7 to 0.9 mm (mean 0.83 mm) for the second subgroup and from 0.2 to 0.8 mm (mean 0.82 mm) for the third.

The patients with baseline diastolic ICPs greater than 15 mm Hg (Group B) experienced increases during the infusion that ranged from 10 to 25 mm Hg. These increases were associated with increases in optic nerve diameter that ranged from 0.2 to 0.9 mm (mean 0.47 mm).

In Fig. 2 the diastolic ICPs observed during the infusion are plotted against the corresponding diameters of the optic nerve segments (anterior, intermediate and posterior) measured ultrasonographically. The resulting curves clearly show that the responses of the optic nerve to these increases in pressure are biphasic. In the first phase of the response in which ICP values are 12 or 13 mm Hg or less, there is no increase in the transverse diameter of the optic nerve which ranges from 3.4 to 3.9 mm. When the diastolic ICP exceeds 13–14 mm Hg, however, the optic nerve begins to expand and a linear correlation can be observed between its enlargement and simultaneous increases in the ICP. This correlation can be observed in the curves for all three diameters measured although it is most evident in those based on the intermediate and posterior segment measurements. The correlation coefficients are 0.78 for the anterior segment diameters, 0.79 for the intermediate and 0.79 for the posterior. There were no significant correlations between the pulsatile ICP or intracranial elasticity and optic nerve diameter.

The relationship observed between optic nerve diameter and CSF absorptive reserve (AR) was similar to that observed between the latter and ICP. Abnormal AR values (less than 0.1 ml/min per mm Hg) were recorded whenever the optic nerve diameter exceeded (in baseline readings or in those made during the test) 4.6 mm (intermediate segment) or 4.7 mm (posterior segment). This finding indicates that an optic nerve diameter of 4.6 mm or more is an index of AR alteration. However, lower values prior to the initiation of the infusion test cannot be considered proof of normal AR. During the test diameters of less than 4.6 mm can increase. The relation

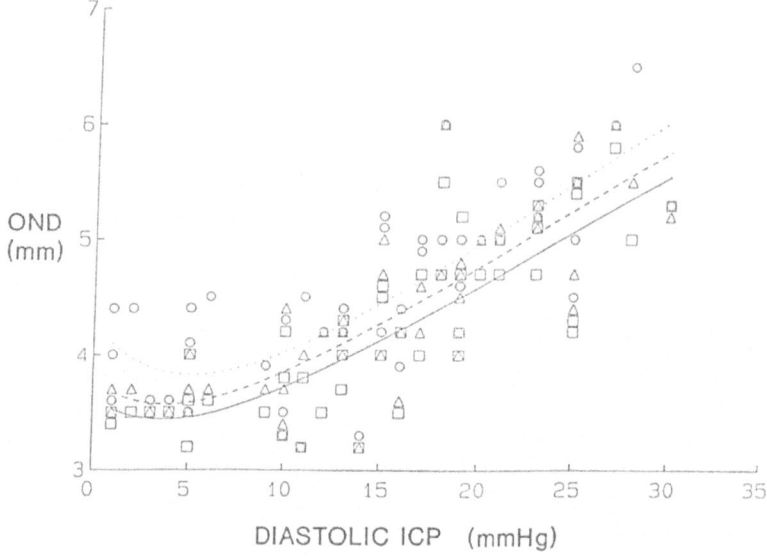

Fig. 2. Diastolic ICP readings are plotted along the abscissa and corresponding measurements of the transverse diameter of the left optic nerve are shown on the ordinate. Measurements were made during the infusion test of Katzmann and Hussey. □: anterior diameter of optic nerve; △: mid-orbital diameter; ○: posterior diameter. The response curve is biphasic with an initial phase in which increases in diastolic ICP are not associated with any increase in the diameter of the optic nerve. During the second phase the nerve expands as diastolic ICP increases.

between ICP and AR is similar in that while an abnormal baseline ICP value is a certain index of altered AR, normal baseline ICPs can reach pathologically high levels during the test and reveal AR alteration.

No correlation could be found between the volume of liquid infused and the transverse diameter of the optic nerve. The rapidity with which the ICP responded to the introduction or removal of a given volume depended on the characteristics of the individual system. Variations in the ICP were continuously monitored while corresponding changes in the diameter of the optic nerve were evaluated every 10 minutes. In spite of this limitation rapid variations in the nerve diameter could be documented: the shortest interval observed between a change in the ICP and a corresponding change in the nerve diameter was 3 minutes; the longest was 8 minutes.

Discussion and conclusions

Katzmann and Hussey's infusion test is a useful model for the in vivo study of CSF dynamics. The method used here allowed us to evaluate within a very short period of time the repercussions on the optic nerve of changes in certain hydrodynamic parameters of the CSF system. The constant monitoring of the ICP allowed us to correlate these data with those of optic nerve diameters. Our findings confirm that there is a definite correlation ($R = 0.81$) between baseline diastolic ICP and the diameter of the optic nerve (Table 1). This correlation persists when the pressure is increased artificially during the infusion test ($R = 0.79$).

It is, therefore, reasonable to assume that the optic nerve responds dynamically to changes in intracranial pressure transmitted to its structures through the optic canal. The increase in the diameter of the nerve differs depending on whether the baseline ICP is normal or already elevated prior to initiation of the infusion. In fact, (Table 4), the same increase in ICP produces less expansion of the optic nerve sheath in cases in which the baseline ICP is greater than 15 mm Hg (0.43 versus 0.82). It may be that the expansive capacity of the arachnoidal and dural sheaths has already been partially exhausted in an attempt to accomodate the baseline elevation. The same mechanism may be responsible for an interesting finding that emerges from Table 4: the variations in the diameter of the optic nerve for subgroups II and III (0.83 mm and 0.82 mm respectively) were almost identical in spite of the differences between the two groups as far as ICP increases were concerned. This finding would seem to refute the existence of a direct correlation between increases in the ICP and those of the diameter of the optic nerve. It is possible that a sudden increase in the ICP does, indeed, cause a proportional increase in the diameter of the nerve which is, however, limited by factors such as the elasticity of the nerve sheath and intraorbital pressure, on the one hand, and on the ICP itself, on the other.

The validity of this interpretation is, in any case, limited in situations in which there is a rapid increase in the ICP. Persistent increases in the ICP and the consequent distensions of the optic nerve may possibly lead to changes that are more significant than those that could be observed with the infusion test, as, for example, occurs in patients with benign intracranial hypertension in which the ICP is persistently elevated.

It should be noted that the optic sheath maintains a certain degree of elasticity even after it has been distended for long periods of time as demonstrated by the fact that ventriculo-peritoneal shunts created in patients with benign intracranial hypertension produce decreases not only in ICP but also in the transverse diameter of the optic nerve.

The response curve of the optic nerve to progressive increases in the diastolic ICP reveals an interesting aspect, i.e. the two phenomena are fairly independent up to a certain point. In fact, after the ICP has exceeded 13 or 14 mm Hg, the optic nerve diameter begins to show a response that parallels further pressure increases. It is reasonable to assume that a certain pressure balance exists between the intracranial and intraorbital subarachnoid spaces and that when the ICP exceeds the forces of elastic resistence in the nerve sheath and intraorbital pressure caused by fat, extraocular muscles, vascular structures and endobulbar pressure, the subarachnoid liquid is forced toward the orbit.

When the ICP is close to 0, as occurs in cases of patent CSF fistulas, the gradient that results pushes the CSF in the opposite direction, i.e. from the intraorbital to the intracranial compartment and the optic nerve diameters in these patients are, in fact, markedly reduced (3.0–3.2 mm). A state of relative equilibrium between the two compartments is maintained at ICPs ranging from 4 to 14 mm Hg, and within this range there is greater variability in the responses of the optic nerve (3.2–4.5 mm). This may explain why the slope of the initial portion of the curve shown in Fig. 2, correlating diastolic ICP and optic nerve diameter, is less steep than that of the second part of the curve.

We did not find any correlation between pulsatile ICP and the diameter of the optic nerve. The former has only instantaneous effects on intracranial conditions. Any effects transmitted to the optic nerve could only have been revealed by means of continuous monitoring of nerve diameter changes which was not used in this study. This approach would also have proved useful in determining the relative influences of intracranial elasticity and velocity of ICP variations on the changes in optic nerve diameters. Even though the findings of the present study do not suggest any correlation between intracranial elasticity and optic nerve diameter, it is not unreasonable to imagine that the instantaneous changes in nerve diameter would be greater and more immediate in a system characterized by inelastic intracranial structures with respect to one more capable of more effectively absorbing rapid changes in ICP.

Absorptive reserve was altered whenever the diastolic ICP (baseline or infusion-induced) exceeded 14–15 mm Hg. Additional confirmation of the close correlation between ICP and optic nerve diameter is provided by our observation that AR was also altered whenever the nerve diameter exceeded 4.6 mm indicating that this figure, like 15 mm Hg of ICP, is a cut-off value after which AR alteration invariably occurs.

Based on the findings of this study the upper limits of normal values for optic nerve diameters can be considered 4.4 mm for the anterior portion, 4.5 mm for the mid-orbital portion and 4.6 mm for the segment near the orbital apex. We believe that the mid-orbital diameter is the most important. If we consider 15 mm Hg to be the upper limit of the normal range of ICPs, the figure of 4.5 mm can reliably be assumed to be the upper limit for a normal optic nerve diameter.

Ultrasonographic studies can be used to obtain an indirect diagnosis of elevated ICP or, more precisely, an ICP that has exceeded 15 mm Hg. The accuracy of this method based on the cut-off values reported here is over 90% with circa 88% sensitivity and 90% specificity.

References

1. Hussey, F., Schanzer, B. & Katzman, R. A simple constant infusion manometric test for measurement of CSF absorption. II Clinical studies. Neurology (Minneapolis) 20: 665–680 (1970).

2. Katzman, R. & Hussey, F. A simple constant infusion manometric test for measurement of CSF absorption. I Rationale and method. Neurology (Minneapolis) 20: 534–544 (1970).
3. Sklar, F.H., Beyer, C.W., Jr., Ramanathan, M., Elashvili, I., Cooper, P.R. & Clark, W.K. Servocontrolled lumbar infusions: a clinical tool for the determination of CSF dynamics as function of pressure. Neurosurgery 3: 170–175 (1978).
4. Ossoinig, K.C., Cennamo, G. & Byrne, S.F. Echographic differential diagnosis of optic nerve lesions. Doc. Ophthalmol. Proc. Ser. 29: 327–31 (1981).
5. Ossoinig, K.C. & Tamburrelli, C. Otticopatia compressiva studio ecografico nella ipertensione endocranica benigna. Atti del congresso Giornate di Ecografia Oftalmica Standardizzata.: 62–3 Roma Ott. (1986).
6. Byrne, SF. The echographic measurement and differential diagnosis of optic nerve lesions (review). Doc. Ophthalmol. Proc. Ser. 48: 571–85 (1987).
7. Cennamo, G., Gangemi, M. & Stella, L. The correlation between endocranial pressure and optic nerve diameter: an ultrasonographic study. Doc. Ophthalmol. Proc. Ser. 48: 603–606 (1987).

Address for correspondence: Department of Ophthalmology, Catholic University of Rome, Largo F. Vito 1, I-00168 Rome, Italy.

3. Functional echographic biometry of extraocular muscles

C. TAMBURRELLI
(Rome, Italy)

Abstract. Standardized A-scan echography was used to measure the thickness of the lateral and medial recti in the primary gaze position, abduction and adduction in normal subjects and patients with Graves ophthalmopathy. Graves patients' muscles were significantly thicker in all positions studied. While increases in muscle diameter caused by contraction were similar in controls and patients, the latter showed less thinning during relaxation.

Introduction

Ophthalmic echography is one of the most sophisticated and reliable methods available for studying extraocular muscle disease. The techniques of standardized ophthalmic echography provide the physician with various types of data upon which diagnosis can be reliably based. The information that can be obtained with these techniques include measurements of muscle thickness, location of muscle thickening, acoustic characteristics of internal structures and internal reflectivity. When these data are collected for each muscle, the overall picture that emerges, together with clinical findings, form a solid basis for diagnosing most cases of extraocular muscle pathology [4–6].

As far as the ultrasound parameters are concerned, decisions regarding the order in which subsequent studies will be carried out, will primarily be made on the basis of the presence or absence of changes in muscle thickness revealed through standardized A-scan echography. These changes accompany a number of different pathological conditions, including Graves' disease, metastases, hematoma, lymphoma, hyperemia, all of which cause thickening, and atrophy, paresis and fibrosis, which are associated with thinning of one or more extraocular muscle [4–6]. For this reason, this parameter is extremely important.

However, the definition of normal thickness values for each of the extraocular muscles is crucial to the ability to individuate such alterations, and, despite the fact that this question has received a fair amount of attention, there are still questions that should be further clarified. Based on their study of a large number of normal subjects, McNutt & Ossoinig [2, 3] have elaborated tables which illustrate the percentage probability that a given measurement is normal or pathological. However, a number of other authors have pointed out that numerous individual factors, including height, weight,

P. Till (ed.), Ophthalmic Echography 13, pp. 111–115.

sex and type of work, must be considered when defining normal extraocular muscle thickness [1, 7–10]. In order to overcome this difficulty, Ossoinig [6] suggests comparing the measurements with those of the corresponding muscle in the contralateral eye. Abnormal findings are suggested when the transverse diameters of the two muscles differ by 0.15 mm (at the insertion tendon) or by 0.3 mm (in the muscle belly).

Biometric evaluations of the extraocular muscles are generally carried out with the eye in the primary gaze position so that the muscles are studied under static conditions. We recently used standardized A-scan to evaluate changes in muscle thickness during contraction and relaxation in a group composed of normal subjects and patients suffering from Graves' ophthalmo-pathy. We hoped to determine whether the thickness changes that occur with contraction or relaxation (during contraction of the antagonist muscle) differed in these two groups of subjects, and, if so, whether they might be used for diagnostic purposes.

Subjects and methods

Thirty-two normal subjects and 38 patients suffering from Graves' ophthal-mopathy (GO) were examined. In the latter group, diplopia was either absent or noted occasionally in certain extreme gaze positions. Standardized A-scan was used to assess the thickness of the muscle belly by measuring the maximum distance between two muscle-sheath spikes of maximum or quasi-maximum height (Fig. 1). Measurements were taken in the primary position (Fig. 1P), with the eye abducted 30 degrees (rotated toward the probe) (Fig. 1R) and in adduction (30 degrees away from the probe) (Fig. 1C). The primary-position measurements were taken as baseline values against which increases (during contraction) or decreases (during relaxation) were evaluated. Only the medial and lateral recti were examined. The only difficulty we encountered in obtaining these measurements arose when we tried to measure the muscles during contraction. In these cases, it was somewhat difficult to keep the probe positioned so that the ultrasound beam passed through the muscle sheath at a 90–degree angle. This problem did not arise when the muscle was relaxed.

Results

In the primary position, both the lateral and medial recti were found to be thicker in patients with GO than in the normal subjects (Table 1). These differences were maintained in the measurements taken during contraction and relaxation.

Analysis of variance showed a significant difference in the primary-position measurements from the two groups ($p = 0.000$). Within each group, the increases and decreases seen during the dynamic studies also proved to be

---

113

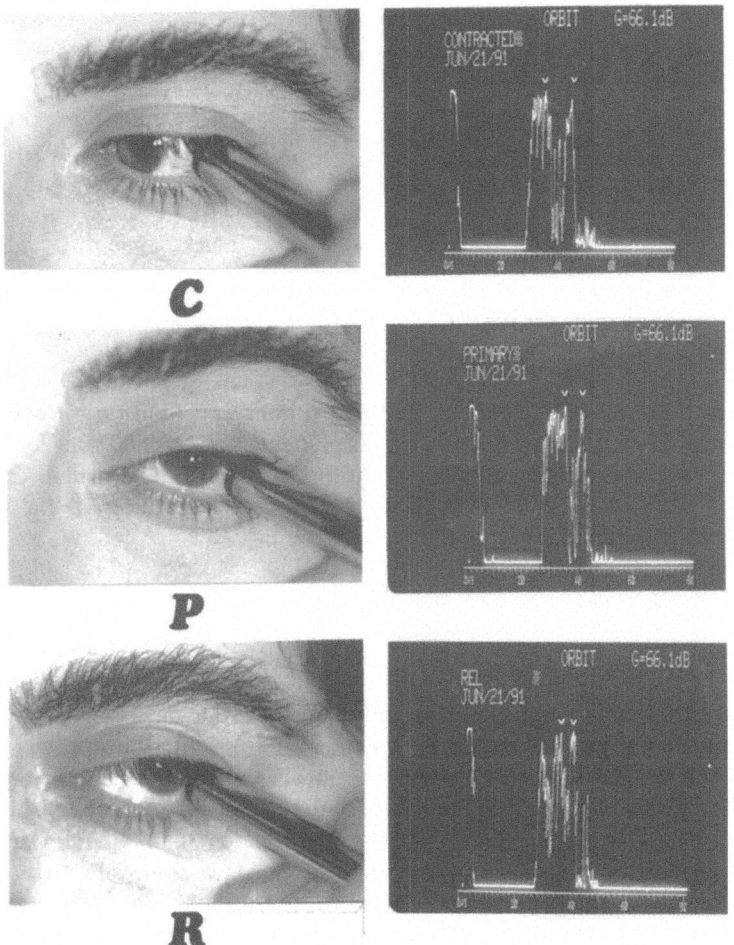

Fig. 1. C = Contracted; P = Primary; R = Relaxed.

Table 1.

	Primary Position	Contracted	Relaxed
Medial rectus			
Normals	4.72 (0.72 sd)	5.36 (0.74 sd)	3.75 (0.54 sd)
GO	5.75 (0.79 sd)	6.46 (0.83 sd)	5.15 (0.79 sd)
Lateral rectus			
Normals	4.06 (0.61 sd)	4.67 (0.60 sd)	3.35 (0.54 sd)
GO	4.72 (0.53 sd)	5.16 (0.49 sd)	4.20 (0.50 sd)

114

muscle thickness (mm)

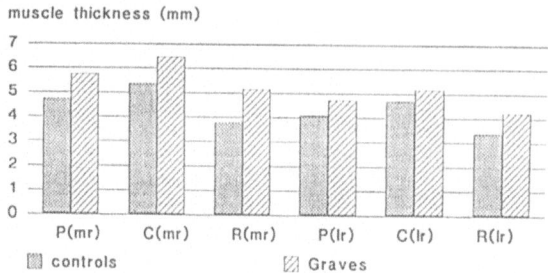

Fig. 2. P = Primary; C = Contracted; R = Relaxed.

significantly different from those of the primary position ($p = 0.000$). The two groups of subjects also differed significantly ($p = 0.002$) as far as the degree of thinning of both muscles during relaxation is concerned. Contraction was, in contrast, similar in the two groups regardless of the muscle considered ($p = 0.356$) (Fig. 2).

Discussion

Echographic measurement of extraocular muscle thickness is a sensitive and accurate method for distinguishing normal subjects from those with GO. As our experience shows, the extraocular muscle enlargment characteristic of GO is apparent even when the ultrasound studies are performed during contraction or relaxation. Both the lateral and medial recti undergo the same proportional increase in thickness during contraction. The proportional increases in thickness caused by contraction are almost identical ($p = 0.326$) in the two groups of subjects. In contrast, the decrease in thickness observed during relaxation in the patient group was not as great as that seen in the normal subjects.

It is important to remember that none of the patients we examined showed signs of overt diplopia or restrictive strabismus which rules out the possiblility of severe interstitial muscle fibrosis. The fact that the muscles of the Graves patients behave differently from those of normal subjects only during relaxation and not contraction is probably related to the type of involvement that characterizes the early phases of this disease. Interstitial swelling is accompanied by accumulation of lymphocytes and progressive deposition of collagen fibers that reduce elasticity and flexibility [2, 6, 11]. The muscle's ability to shorten and contract is less compromised by this process at least until the disease is fairly advanced.

Functional biometry is useful for studying the dynamic changes that occur in the extraocular muscles. However, because of the wide variation in measurements with high standard deviation, it is less applicable for clinical purposes.

References

1. Avitbile, T. & Uva, M.G., Fiordalisi, F. Inostri valori ecobiometrici normali per la misurazione dei muscoli retti. I Congr. S.I.E.O., Ferrara (1985).
2. McNutt, L.C. Ultrasound of Graves' orbitopathy. Seminar Department of Ophthalmology. Iowa City: University of Iowa (1975).
3. McNutt, L.C., Kaefring, S.L. & Ossoinig, K.C. Echographic measurement of extraocular muscles. In: White, D.N. and Brown, R.E. (eds.), Ultrasound in Medicine, Vol. 3A, pp. 927–932. New York: Plenum (1977).
4. Ossoinig, K.C. Preoperative differential diagnosis of tumors with echography, I: Physical principles and morphologic backgound of tissue echograms. In: Blodi, F.C. (ed.), Current Concepts in Ophthalmology, Vol. 4, pp. 264–280. St. Louis: Mosby (1974).
5. Ossoinig, K.C. Standardized echography: basic principles, clinical applications and results. Int. Ophthalmol. Clinics, 19–127 (1979).
6. Ossoinig, K.C. Ultrasonic diagnosis of Graves' ophthalmopathy. In: Gorman, C.A. et al. (eds.), The eye and orbit in thyroid disease. New York: Raven Press (1984).
7. Reibaldi, A., Scuderi, G.L. & Avitabile, T. Attuali possibilità diagnostiche ecografiche nella oftalmopatia di Graves. Atti VIII Conv. Soc. Oftalmol. Siciliana, Taormina-Giardini Naxos, 303 (1983).
8. Reibaldi, A., Avitabile, T., Uva, M.G. & Tritto, M. Utility of ultrasounds in monolateral endocrine exophthalmos. 5th International Symposium on Orbital Disorders. Amsterdam (1985).
9. Reibaldi, A., Assennato, G., Avitabile, T. & Uva, M.G. The echobiometric measurements of the extraocular muscles in normal subjects. In: Thijssen, J.M. (ed.), Ultrasonography in Ophthalmology. Dordrecht: Kluwer Acad. Publ. (1988).
10. Tane, S. & Komatsu, A. Echographic measurement of extraocular muscles in normal person and in patients with thyroid orbitopathy. Acta XXIV Int. Congress of Ophthalmology, San Francisco, 120 (1982).
11. Tamburrelli, C., Focosi, F., Savino, G., Dickmann, A. & Buratto, E. Criteri ecografici nella diagnosi differenziale degli esoftalmi e delle diplopie da interessamento muscolare. Clinica Oculistica e Patologia Oculare, 10(5): 347–353 (1989).

Address for correspondence: Department of Ophthalmology, Catholic University of Rome, Largo F. Vito 1, I-00168 Roma, Italy.

4. Standardized A-scan echography of the optic nerve in a patient with leukemic meningeosis and papilledema

A. STANOWSKY

(*Augsburg, Germany*)

Abstract. A 21-year-old patient with acute lymphatic leukemia and leukemic meningeosis had unilateral papilledema and extracranial enlargement of the optic nerve. Standardized A-scan echography played a decisive role in differentiating the optic nerve disease and in planning a lumbar tap.

Introduction

Standardized echography is particularly suitable for examining the extracranial part of the optic nerve [1–8, 10, 11]. Increases and reductions in the total diameter become especially apparent in the left-right comparison [9], and the optic nerve sheats (dura, arachnoid, pia) can be demonstrated separately as an additional means of analyzing highly complicated problem situations [1, 6].

A further factor of fundamental importance is that echography is a kinetic examination method with high resolution capacity. This permits distinction of solid from fluid-induced enlargements of the subarachnoidal space within the optic fascicle during the abduction test [1, 6, 11].

We were asked whether complications were to be expected from a lumbar tap planned for a patient with pronounced, unilateral papilledema and CT-confirmed leukemic meningeosis.

Case history

The patient, born in 1968 and admitted to our outpatient clinic in March, 1990, had been diagnosed 3 years earlier as having lymphatic leukemia. The disease had been treated with cytostatics (COP protocol) but without skull irradiation. After 6 asymptomatic months, an isolated meningeal recurrence appeared in March of 1990. Clinically, no pathological changes were found in the peripheral blood count or the bone marrow. However, computed tomography (Fig. 1) showed leukemic meningeosis and infiltration of the sphenoid bone with enlargement of the right optic nerve. The left optic fascicle appeared normal.

At the time of examination, visual acuity was hand movements at 50 cm

P. Till (ed.), Ophthalmic Echography 13, pp. 117–121.

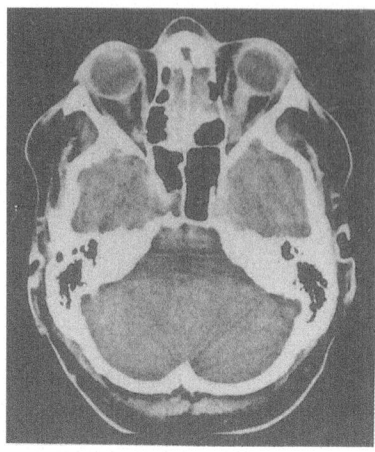

Fig. 1. Distension of the right optic nerve shown by computed tomography.

in the right eye, 20/20 in the left. Visual field examination with the Goldman perimeter showed only a residual island located in the temporal periphery of the right eye and a normal visual field in the left eye.

The anterior segments were normal. The posterior pole of the right eye showed a severe, chronic papilledema (Fig. 2), the disc of the left eye was normal in appearance.

An echographic examination was performed to clarify whether the papilledema of the right eye was caused by infiltrative opticoneuropathy with or without increased intracranial pressure.

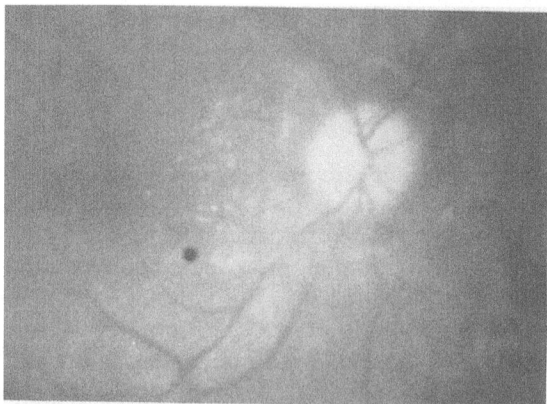

Fig. 2. Fundus photo of the right eye with chronic papilledema.

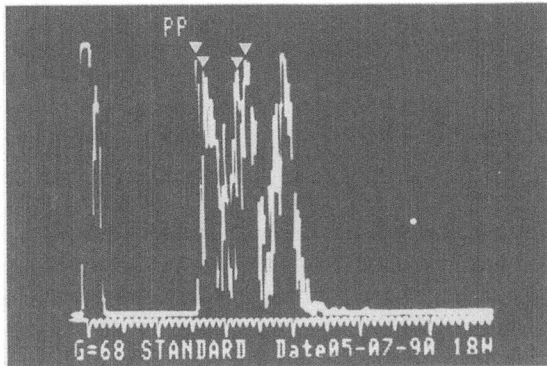

Fig. 3a. A-scan echogram of the right optic nerve in primary position (arrows, Fig. 3b).

Material and method

Echographic examination was carried out with the Ophthascan S unit, starting with both optic nerves in primary position in both the A-scan and B-scan procedures. In each instance, the transducer was positioned temporally at the level of the insertion of the lateral rectus muscle. The optic fascicle was then examined by swinging the transducer along its whole extracranial part. This yielded the best pictures and centration in the B-scan and the highest vertically rising dura spikes in the A-scan. Examination was then repeated with maximum abduction, starting with the right eye.

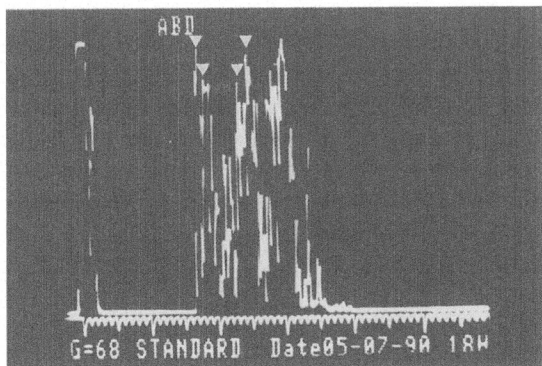

Fig. 3b. Even after 5-minute abduction, there was practically no change in total diameter (distance between outer arrows) or the subarachnoidal space on both sides of the nerval tissue (distance between neighboring outer and inner arrows).

Results

The right optic nerve was distended to 7.5 mm in primary position (Fig. 3a). Both the outer and inner surfaces of the dura were clearly shown. The diameter of the subarachnoidal space was a consistent 1.1 mm on both sides of the optic nerve.

The total diameter of the left optic nerve was 4.5 mm, and the subarachnoidal space was barely discernable on both sides of the optic nerve.

Upon gaze to the right, total diameter and the width of the subarachnoidal space at the right optic fascicle remained practically unchanged even after 5 minutes abduction (Fig. 3b).

There were likewise no changes in the left optic fascicle upon gaze to the left.

Discussion

Clinically, the question prior to planned lumbar tap was whether intracranial pressure was abnormally high. Computed tomography was incapable of answering this question.

The possibility of increased intracranial pressure appeared clinically remote, even though unilateral papilledema occurs in ca. 5% of these patients [12].

Standardized A-scan echography at first permitted exclusion of a fluid-caused distension of the left fasciculus opticus. This provided an additional argument against increased intracranial pressure.

The decisive factor, however, was that standardized A-scan echography pinpointed the cause of the distension of the right fasciculus opticus (and so of the unilateral papilledema).

The total diameter and the width of the subarachnoidal space remained practically unchanged after 5-minute abduction, in contrast to their behaviour in compressive opticoneuropathy [1, 6, 8, 11]. This unequivocally contradicted an additional fluid-caused distension of the right optic nerve, i.e. compressive opticoneuropathy or increased intracranial pressure, and proved a solid tumorous process along the lines of infiltrative (leukemic) opticoneuropathy.

The lumbar tap was subsequently performed without complications.

References

1. Byrne, S.F. The echographic measurement and differential diagnosis of optic-nerve lesions. In: Ossoinig, K. C. (ed.) Ophthalmic Echography. Proceedings of the 10th SIDUO Congress Doc. Ophthalmol. Proc. Ser. 48: 571–585 (1987).
2. Cennamo, G., Gangemi, M. & Stella, L. The correlation between endocranial pressure and optic nerve diameter: an ultrasonographic study. Ophthalmic Echography. Proceedings of the 10th SIDUO Congress, pp. 603–606 (1987).

3. Hasenfratz, G. Experimental studies on the display of the optic nerve. In: Ossoinig, K. C. (ed.), Ophthalmic Echography. Proceedings of the 10th SIDUO Congress, pp. 587–602 (1987).
4. Ossoinig, K.C. Echography of the eye, orbit and periorbital region. In: Arger, P.H. (ed.), Orbit Roentgenology, pp. 224–269. New York: Wiley (1977).
5. Ossoinig, K.C. Standardized echography. Basic principles, clinical applications and results. In: Dallow, P.L. (ed.), Ophthalmic ultrasonography: Comparative techniques (Int Ophthalmol Clin) Boston: Little, Brown (1979).
6. Ossoinig, K.C., Cennamo, G. & Frazier-Byrne, S. Echographic differential diagnosis of optic nerve lesions. Doc. Opthalmol. Proc. Ser. 29: 327–335 (1981).
7. Ossoinig, K.C. Die Bedeutung der standardisierten Echographie in der Neuro-Ophthalmologie. In: Aktuelle ophthalmologische Probleme. Stuttgart: Enke Verlag, pp. 61–75 (1981).
8. Rochels, R. Ultraschalldiagnostik in der Augenheilkunde. Lehrbuch und Atlas. Landsberg a.L.: Ecomed (1986).
9. Schroeder, W. Ergebnisse der A-Bildechographie bei einseitigen Sehnervenerkrankungen. Klin. Mbl. Augenheilk. 169: 30–38 (1976).
10. Skalka, H.W. Ultrasonography of the optic nerve. Neuro-ophthalmol. 1: 109–116 (1980).
11. Stanowsky, A. & Kreissig, I. Hat die echographische Untersuchung des Nervus opticus und seiner Meningen eine Bedeutung in der Diagnostik eines Pseudotumor cerebri? Fortschr. Ophthalmol. 81: 604–607 (1984).
12. Walsh, F.B. & Hoyt, W.F. Clinical Neuroophthalmology. Baltimore: Williams and Wilkins Co., 3rd ed. (1969).

Address for correspondence: Zentralklinikum, Augenklinik, Stenglinstrasse 2, W-8900 Augsburg, Germany

5. Optic nerve anomalies in childhood

Á. SZABÓ, Zs. PELLE, J. NÉMETH & M. JANÁKY

(Szeged and Budapest, Hungary)

Abstract. Contact real-time B-scan echography was used to examine the optic nerve in 17 children with optic nerve anomalies. The examinations took place between August 1988 and September 1989. The following developmental abnormalities were present: (1) Megalopapilla, (2) Coloboma of the optic nerve, (3) Optic disc pit, (4) Hypoplasia of the optic nerve, and (5) Glioma of the optic nerve. We found decreased echographic diameters of the optic nerve in 16 eyes, normal diameters in 11 eyes and increased diameters in 5 eyes in comparison to our control group. Our results suggest that echography is a very important adjunct to other methods of diagnosing optic nerve anomalies.

Introduction

Developmental abnormalities of the bulb may result in developmental anomalies of the optic nerve. It is very important to diagnose the developmental abnormalities of the optic nerve from both ophthalmological and neurological points of view.

The following symptoms call attention to these pathological changes: decreased visual acuity, nystagmus and strabismus.

Materials and methods

We examined 17 children with optic nerve anomalies from August 1988 to September 1989.

Five types of optic nerve abnormalities were diagnosed (Table 1). Seven of the 17 patients were female, and 10 were male. Their age varied between 3 months to 13 years, the average age was 5 years.

The examinations were conducted with CooperVision contact real-time A/B-scan instrument (10 MHz). We measured the optic nerve diameter using the method of Schroeder [4]. The children were examined without using general anaesthesia, after topical anaesthesia they were instructed to look in the required direction.

Our control group included healthy children of the same average age.

We completed our studies by using ophthalmoscopic, electrophysiologic, neurologic and computed tomographic examinations.

P. Till (ed.), Ophthalmic Echography 13, pp. 123–125.
© 1993 *Kluwer Academic Publishers*.

Table 1. The number of eyes with developmental abnormalities

Megalopapilla	2
Coloboma of the optic nerve	5
Optic disc pit	1
Hypoplasia of the optic nerve	20
Glioma of the optic nerve	2

The children underwent the following electrophysiological examinations: VEP, ERG and PERG.

Results and discussion

The optic nerve anomalies are considered uncommon pathological changes [2].

In comparison to our normal control group we found decreased optic nerve diameters in 16 eyes, normal in 13 eyes and increased in 5 eyes (Table 2). In the control group we obtained values in the range 3.2–4.3 mm for the optic nerve diameter. We did not observe a significant correlation between the age and the optic nerve diameter.

Our echographical examinations confirmed the diagnosis in all cases of our patients with the above mentioned optic nerve abnormalities. The smallest optic nerve diameter measured by us was 2.0 mm in the case of a severe form of optic nerve hypoplasia (Fig. 1). The largest optic nerve diameter, 6.0 mm, was detected in the case of a megalopapilla (Fig. 2). We found normal optic nerve diameter in the cases of mild optic nerve hypoplasia, optic disc pit and optic nerve colobomas except the cystic form.

We found abnormal echographic patterns in 21 eyes, e.g. high internal echoes of the optic nerve, uncommon shapes of the optic nerve cross sections, abnormal axial lengths, drusen, epipapillary echoes and remnants of hyaloid artery.

Boynton et al. [1] reported the measurements with B-scan ultrasonography in a longitudinal section of a case of bilateral optic nerve hypoplasia. Guthoff [3] considers the contact B-scan method very suitable for the measurement of the optic nerve diameter.

We claim that the echographic examination is essential in diagnosis of patients suspected of having developmental abnormalities of the optic nerve.

Table 2. Echographic results

Diameter of the optic nerve	No. of eyes
– Decreased	16
– Normal	13
– Increased	5

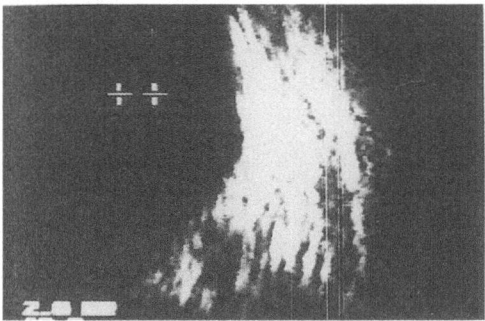

Fig. 1. The optic nerve diameter is 2.0 mm in a case of severe form of optic nerve hypoplasia.

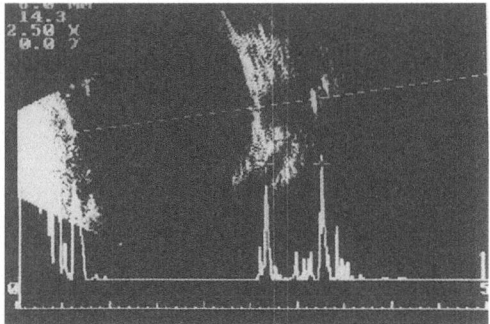

Fig. 2. The optic nerve diameter is 6.0 mm in a case of megalopapilla.

Measurements using ultrasound can confirm initial diagnoses, and the echographical results can call attention to the anomalies of the central nerve system.

References

1. Boynton, JR et al. Hypoplastic optic nerve studied with B-scan ultrasonography and axial tomography of the optic canals. Can J Ophthal 10: 473 (1975).
2. Duke-Elder, S. Embryology. In: System of Ophthalmology, Vol 3, pt 2, p. 668. London: Kimpton (1964).
3. Guthoff, R. Ultraschall in der ophthalmologischen Diagnostik, p. 109. Stuttgart: Enke Verlag (1988).
4. Schroeder, W. Ergebnisse der A-Bild-Echographie bei einseitigen Sehnervenerkrankungen. Klin Mbl Augenheilk 169: 30 (1976).

Address for correspondence: A. Szent-Györgyi Med. Univ. of Ophthalmology, P.O. Box 407, H-6701 Szeged, Hungary.

6. A case of bilateral chronic myositis with compressive optic neuropathy

V. JUVAN

(*Varaždin, Croatia*)

Muscular changes comprise, according to literature (Ossoinig & Hermsen 1984), a considerable percentage of orbital pathology, about 40%, this number being mainly due to endocrine myopathy. Myositis of EOM is far less frequent, about 4–5%, bilateral and especially oligosymptomatic forms, as in our case, being rather rare.

Extraocular myositis can be considered as a specific form of idiopathic inflammatory orbital pseudotumour (Jakobiec & Jones,1979; Walsh & Hoyt 1985) involving predominantly the muscles. Within this myositic group of orbital pseudotumour, depending on the onset, duration and symptoms acute and chronic, exophthalmic and nonexophthalmic oligosymptomatic forms can be distinguished (Schulze 1972).

Pathohistologically there is small cell infiltration of the muscle, followed by hyalinisation and disintegration of the fibers in the advanced stages of the disease (Shibhata et al. 1981). Echographic characteristics consist of low reflectivity, increased homogeneity of the internal structure and enlargement particulary of the anterior portions of the muscle that can be demonstrated both on A and B scan (Ossoinig & Hermsen 1984).

Case report

The patient was a male, aged 56, otherwise healthy. During the last 3 years he complained of transitory migratory pain in both eyes and diplopia on several occasions but he didn't visit an ophthalmologist until April 1989 when he noticed a slight ptosis and complained of headache and reduced vision on the left eye.

The clinical examination revealed a slight bilateral ptosis, the eyes almost completely fixed in the primary position with small remnants of vertical excursions on the right eye, sluggish pupillar reactions with a relative afferent defect on the left eye. There were no inflammatory signs apart from a chronic conjunctival injection, no proptosis. The vision was normal in the right and reduced to 0.4 with severe damage of the visual field on the left eye. Ophthalmoscopy of the left eye showed a swollen hyperemic disc. The echography established the diagnosis of a bilateral myositis with compressive

P. Till (ed.), Ophthalmic Echography 13, pp. 127–131.

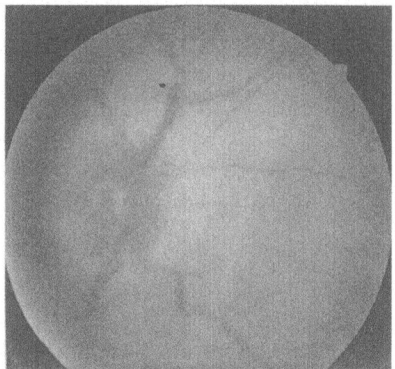

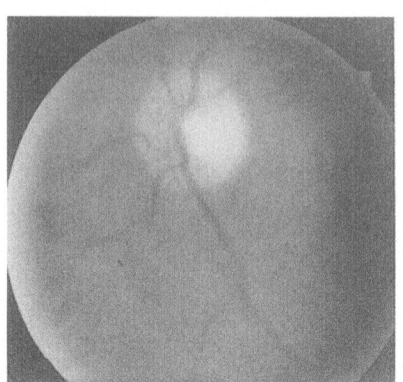

Fig. 1. Fundus-right eye.   *Fig. 2.* Fundus-left eye.

neuropathy on the left and the CT scan also showed an inflammatory process in both orbits.

A high dosage steroid treatment led to the normalisation of the visual acuity and to a considerable improvement of the visual field. Fundus changes disappeared. Motility improved slightly.

A whole battery of laboratory tests and other examinations was performed. To sum up, there was a highly elevated SR, slight anaemia and hypergammaglobulinaemia, particulary of IgA and IgG fractions. The same finding was in the CS fluid. LDH was elevated but CPK normal. All other tests and examinations including thyreoid tests and Tensilon test revealed no abnormalities.

The patient didn't turn up for 8 months. Now he complained of an occasional orbital pain and slight visual disturbance in the right eye.

On examination no visual reduction was found, the visual field didn't show any significant changes but the ophthalmoscopy of the right eye showed a picture similar to that of the left eye 8 months ago, with swollen hyperemic disc and choroidal folds because of the compression (Fig. 1). The left eye had a sectorial atrophy of the disc (Fig. 2). No proptosis was noted. Motility (Fig. 3) was severely restricted in both eyes, on this occasion somewhat more on the right. Echography performed on Ophthascan S showed again a typical low reflective pattern of the muscles (Figs. 4 and 5). A considerable enlargement of virtually all muscles could be demonstrated (Figs. 5 and 6). The inf. rectus muscles were difficult to obtain because of the orbital rim, the measurements were not precise enough and therefore excluded from the list (Table 1). The measurements were made both at tissue and reduced sensitivity (McNutt et al. 1977; Ossoinig 1979) and showed no significant differences. A high dosage corticosteroid treatment was induced again and the fundus changes on the right eye regressed completely, but the motility improved only slightly.

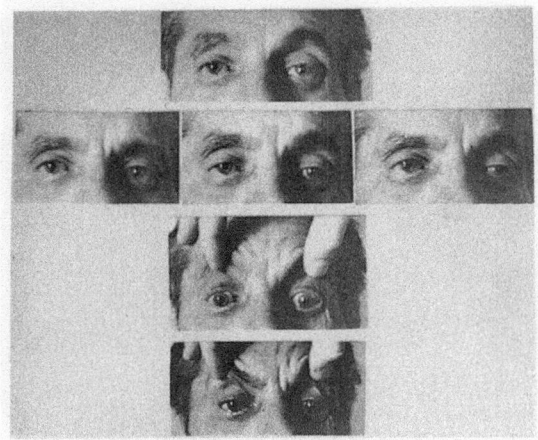

Fig. 3. Motility (secondary directions and convergence).

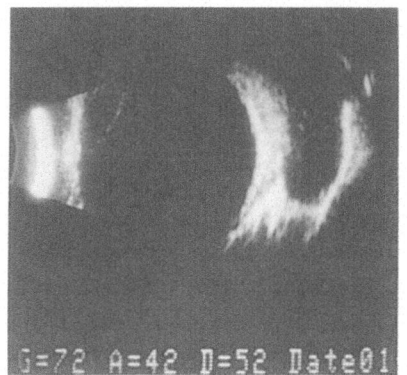
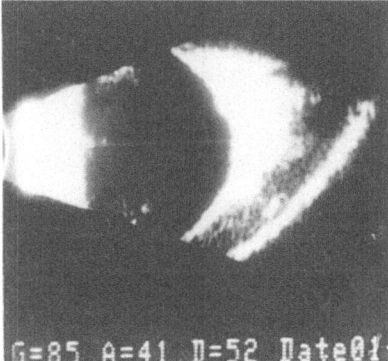

Fig. 4. Typical B scans of the diseased muscles.

Discussion

In conclusion I would like to present a short survey of possible causes of bilateral motility disorders (Table 2). Although some of the entities listed here can be excluded on the basis of clinical examination only, echography is of paramount importance in setting up and confirming the diagnosis of extraocular myositis. Nevertheless, in certain cases CT scan (Trokel & Hilal 1978), biopsy of the muscles and EMG (Esslen & Papst 1961) are valuable in confirming the diagnosis. In the majority of cases these more invasive procedures can be avoided.

130

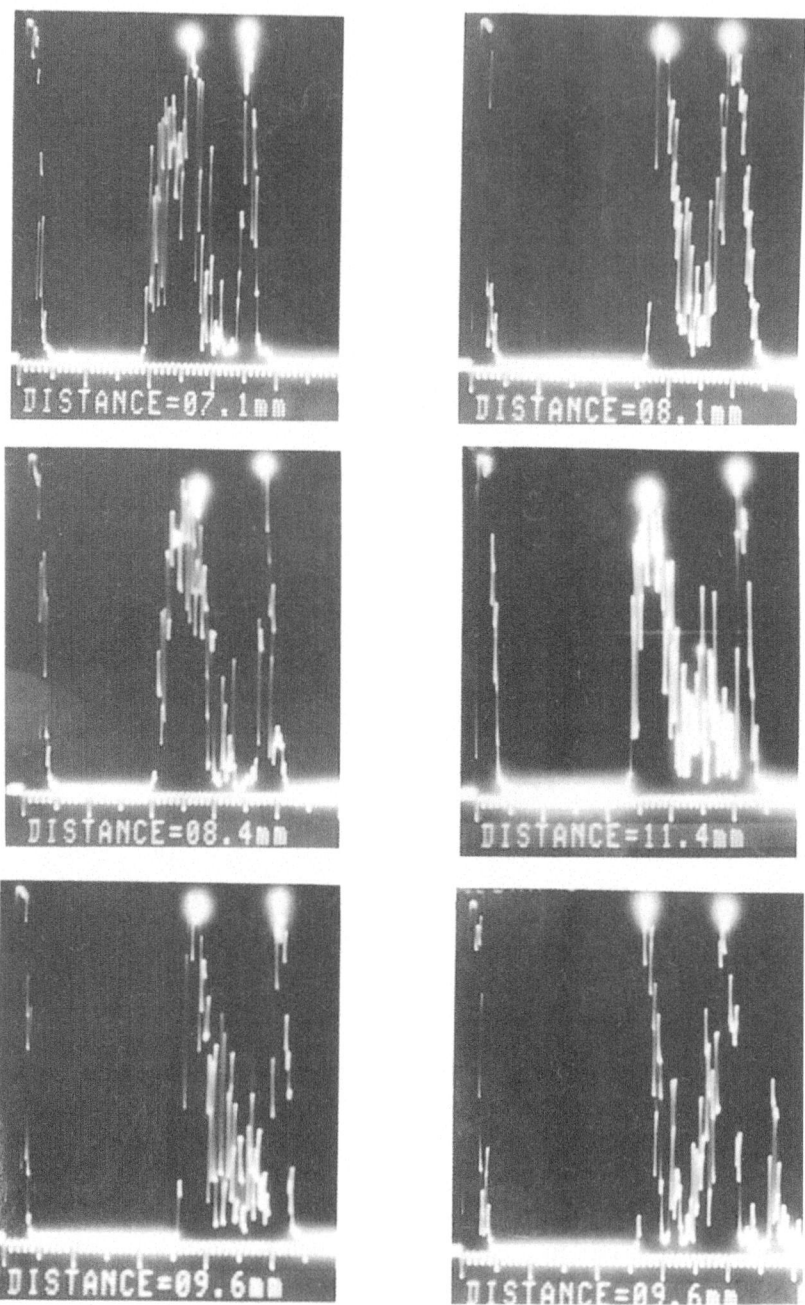

Fig. 5. A scan of lat., sup. and med. rectus m.-right eye (from top to bottom).

Fig. 6. A scan of lat., sup. and med. rectus m.-left eye (from top to bottom).

Table 1. Measurement values of the muscles (mm)

	O.dex.	O.sin.
M. rectus sup.	11.4	9.6
M. rectus med.	9.6	8.1
M. rectus lat.	7.1	8.4
M. obliquus sup.	6.4	6.6

Table 2. Differential diagnosis of bilateral motility disorders

– Cong. fibrotic changes or adhesions of the muscles
– Extraocular myositis: acute and chronic forms
– Myopathies:
Endocrine
Chronic progressive ext. ophthalmoplegia v. Graefe
Oculopharyngeal myodystrophy
– Neuromuscular disturbances: myasthenia sy.
– Neurogenic lesions: nuclear, internuclear or supranuclear
– Nonmyositic form of the orbital pseudotumour
– Bilat. orbital tumours

References

1. Esseen, E. & Papst, W. Die Bedeutung der Elektromyografie fuer die Analyse von Motilitaetsstoerungen der Augen. Bibl. Ophthal. Fasc. 57. Basel: S. Karger (1961).
2. Guthoff, R.F. & Schroeder, W. Swollen extraocular muscles: Ultrasonographic findings and clinical appearance. Doc. Ophthalmol. Proc. Ser. 29: 337. The Hague: Dr. W. Junk (1981).
3. Jakobiec, F.A. & Jones, I.S. Orbital inflammation. Clinical Ophthalmology 2: 35. New York: Harper & Row (1979).
4. McNutt, L.C., Kaefring, S.L. & Ossoinig, K.C. Echographic measurement of extraocular muscles. In: White D. and Brown R.E. (eds.), Ultrasound in Medicines, pp. 927–932. New York: Plenum Press (1977).
5. Ossoinig, K.C. The technique of measuring extraocular muscles. In: Gernet H. (ed.), Diag. Ultrasonica in Ophthalmol. pp. 166–172. Münster: Remy (1979).
6. Ossoinig, K.C. & Hermsen, V.M. Myositis of extraocular muscles diagnosed with standardized echography. Doc. Ophthalmol. Proc. Ser. 38: 381. The Hague: Dr. W. Junk (1984).
7. Schulze, F. Die Ophthalmo-Elektromyographie. pp. 120–134. Leipzig: VEB G. Thieme (1972).
8. Shibhata, H., Masuyama, Y., Nishimoto, Y. & Sawada, A. Echography in orbital myositis. Doc. Ophthalmol. Proc. Ser. 29: 343. The Hague: Dr. W. Junk (1981).
9. Trokel, S.L. & Hilal, S.K. Thin section computerized tomography: Analysis of 600 orbit studies, Proc. 3rd Int. Symp. Orbital Disorders. 107. The Hague: Dr. W. Junk (1978).
10. Walsh and Hoyt's Clinical Neuro-Ophthalmology, 4th ed., 2: pp. 826–830. Baltimore: Williams & Wilkins (1985).

Address for correspondence: Department of Ophthalmology, HR 42000 Varazdin, Mestroviceva bb, Croatia.

PART TWO

Orbital and periorbital lesions

7. Results of standardized echography in orbital diseases
A review of 311 cases

G. HASENFRATZ & U. LEWAN
(Munich, Germany)

Introduction

Clinical echography, particularly the method of standardized echography, is the method of choice for the clinical examination and evaluation, differential diagnosis and follow-up of patients with suspected or proven orbital and periorbital diseases. This is true also if one considers the rapid developing examination-techniques in radiology such as CT-scan and NMR.

Echography offers the advantages of a non-invasive, easy and rapidly performable examination technique which can be performed by the ophthalmologist himself. Together with the possibility to examine the patient and simultaneously approach the differential diagnosis or the definite diagnosis (what can be done in a wide spectrum of diseases), the knowledge of the examiner about orbital and periorbital conditions can be involved immediately into the considerations [6, 12, 13].

Material and method

In this study we report on our results of orbital and periorbital echography. We reviewed 407 patients – excluded were all patients with Graves' disease. In all these patients echography revealed pathology in the orbit or in the periorbit. The study covers six years. All together in these six years over 5,000 orbital examinations were done in the echography-department at the University Eye Hospital in Munich. Thus in approximately 8%, we had pathologic findings. (Patients with Graves' disease were a larger group with about 25% of all orbital examinations.) The majority of examinations were performed to exclude orbital and periorbital pathology in patients with symptoms suspicious for orbital lesions. This demonstrates that echography – with a correct negative result – is a very important clinical examination technique. We had no case were echography failed to detect an orbital lesion, but we had about 40 cases where other examination techniques, particularly CT, showed orbital lesions which could not be verified either by echography, NMR nor by the clinical course. All these cases were Graves disease where CT shows a mass-lesion in the apex, but echography detects the real cause: thickened muscles. On the other hand particularly in cases with vascular

P. Till (ed.), Ophthalmic Echography 13, pp. 135–144.
© 1993 *Kluwer Academic Publishers.*

Table 1.

Standardized Echography/Orbital Diseases/University Munich	
Retrospective study:	1983–1989
Examined cases with	
pathologic echographic findings:	407
(excl. Graves)	
Cases with follow-up data	311 (76%)
Examiners:	9

Table 2.

Correlations	
Echography:	Diagnosis
	First diff. diagnosis
	Second diff. diagnosis
	Follow-up examination
To:	Histopathology
	Clinical data and role of echography
	CT
	NMR
	Follow-up data

changes, thus as A-V-fistulas for instance, CT (and in quite a few cases NMR) fails to make the diagnosis.

In 311 cases we were able to achieve follow-up datas and thus could compare our results with clinical, histopathologic, surgical datas or with the findings in other examination-techniques such as NMR and CT. Additionally we tried to find correlations between the echographic findings and the clinical decisions made by the general ophthalmologist. This was to find out how the echographic results influenced these clinical decisions and what the value of echography was for the patient. The echographic examinations over the six-year period were performed by a total of nine different examiners with a very wide spectrum of echographic experience from beginners (in their first year in echography) to more experienced colleagues with up to 10 years of clinical work in echography. The study includes all kinds of orbital and periorbital conditions where we were able to establish a final diagnosis.

The echographic examinations at the University Eye Hospital in Munich were strictly performed according to the method of standardized echography. We rely very much on all the possibilities of standardized echography: the examination techniques and the evaluation of the different echographic criteria. It has to be underlined again that performing all techniques with the standardized A-scan, the contcat B-scan and the Doppler-sonography during each examination are a conditio-sine-qua-non to achieve good results and to enable the examiner to contribute to the clinical decisions. It also has to be stressed that a thorough examination of the orbit and the periorbit – and this is particularly true in cases where the examiner wants to be sure not to overlook pathology – takes time and demands an examiner who has to know as much as possible about orbital and periorbital diseases as well as he has to be aware of all the clinical and anamnestic datas of the patient. It is very regretable that in many hospitals echography still plays the role of a wall-flower and is performed in a haste by residents who do this in-between their other duties. It should be the task of all ophthalmologists who are really interested in this field to make efforts to change this and thus to achieve more credit for echography.

Results

1. *Inflammatory diseases*

Table 3.

		Histo	Clinic	NV	NF-U
Orbital cellulitis	$n = 2$	–	2	–	–
Pseudotumor	$n = 31$	7	16	2	6
Posterior scleritis	$n = 11$	–	10	–	1
Myositis	$n = 40$	–	37	–	3

(NV = Not-verified; NF-U = No-Follow-Up Datas)

The majority of inflammatory cases evaluated were cases of orbital myositis and of idiopathic inflammatory pseudotumor of the orbit. Besides in seven cases where we had a histopathology (biopsy was done in our hospital in 3 cases, elsewhere in 4 cases) the diagnoses were verified by the clinical courses. Particularly in inflammatory diseases the clinical picture, the symptoms and the course of the conditions is typical in most of the cases. In two cases the diagnosis of an orbital pseudotumor was not verified, both patient suffered from orbital lymphoma. In nine cases no follow-up data could be achieved. The echographic diagnosis was most valuable in cases of extraocular myositis and posterior scleritis. In these cases, besides the primary diagnosis which is the decisive finding in the clinical work-up, follow-up examinations to monitor the course of the disease during and after therapy is of crucial importance. In orbital pseudotumors we very often had the problem of distinguishing the orbital lesion (tumor) from orbital lymphomas and sarcomas. But since orbital idiopathic inflammatory pseudotumors seldomly have a very low reflectivity in the standardized A-scan as, e.g. lymphomas and sarcomas, and are less homogeneous together with the clinical datas the diagnosis could be made correctly in the majority of cases [3–5, 14].

Table 4.

Standardized Echography/Inflammatory Diseases

Summary:

Very good results:	Myositis and post. scleritis
Good results:	Orbital pseudotumor

Clinical value/Influence on clinical decisions: +++

2. *Cellular tumors*

Table 5.

Cellular tumors		Histo	Clinic	NV	NF-U
Lymphoma	$n = 29$	17	3	2	7
Carcinoma/metast./sec.	$n = 48$	17	16	10	5
Rhabdomyosarcoma	$n = 5$	4	–	–	1

In this category there are basically two groups: one with a low to a very low reflectivity of the tumor tissue in standardized A-scan (lymphomas and sarcomas) and the group with a medium to high reflectivity and an often very extensive irregularity of the internal structure (carcinomas). In the cases of intraorbital lymphomas the echographic diagnoses were correct in over 2/3 of the cases. Regarding the remarks made about pseudotumors (see above) it has to be stressed that in these cases very often the examination 'only' may give a differential diagnostic list and to verify the echographic diagnosis follow-up examinations have to be done within a period of days or a few weeks. Thus these very good results can be achieved. Two cases turned out to be clinically classified as orbital pseudotumors, general work-up of the patient showed no basic disease and the tumors disappeared after intensive steroid-therapy. For the clinical work-up of children with a fast growing orbital lesion/tumor echography is very important. CT and NMR to our knowledge (as it also was in our cases) are not capable of making the differential diagnosis. We found that in standardized A-scan the low to very low reflective and not very well outlined lesion, sometimes shows a slight decrease of the echospikes from left to right (angle kappa). In case of suspected rhabdomyosarcoma, follow-up examinations are of crucial importance and show a rapid growth within days. This point – the easily repeatable examinations in children – again underlines the value of clinical standardized echography. In metastatic carcinomas the echographic diagnoses were correct also in about 2/3 of the cases. When looking at the not-verified echographic diagnoses, 2 cases were orbital hemangiomas, 4 cases were idiopathic inflammatory pseudotumors, 1 case was a neurofibroma, 1 case was a schwannoma and 2 cases turned out to be intraorbital, spontaneous hemorrhages (78 and 83 year-old patients with general arteriosclerosis) [8, 14].

Table 6.

Standardized Echography/Cellular tumors	
Summary:	
Very good results:	Lymphoma/Rhabdomyosarcoma
Good results:	Metastatic carcinoma
Clinical value/Influence on clinical decisions:	+++ (Lymph./rhabdomyos.)
	+(+) (Metast.ca.)

3. Vascular tumors

Table 7.

Vascular tumors		Histo	Clinic	NV	NF-U
Orbital varix	$n = 14$	–	10	–	(4)
A-V-fistula	$n = 13$	–	8	–	(5)
Hemangioma	$n = 44$	5	23	3	(11)2
	($n = 29$ adult type; $n = 15$ infant type)				
Lymphangioma	$n = 21$	5	6	5	5

For the diagnosis of vascular tumors and malformations standardized echography proved to be particularly helpful and we found very good results and a decisive influence of echography on the clinical diagnosis. In fact for, e.g. intraorbital varices and for intraorbital A-V-fistulas, it is the method of choice. For these lesions there are echographic key-criteria which enables the examiner to make a very safe diagnosis. In the cases classified here with no follow-up data we found out for the varices by asking the patient or the referring ophthalmologist that no further examinations or therapy had been made and that the patients – though still presenting the symptoms – tolerated the disease without the need or demand for therapy. The 5 cases where we diagnosed an A-V-fistula and had no follow-up data were so-called 'low-pressure/slow-drainage'-fistulas in older patients. These patients too had no further explorations nor therapy and the diagnosis made by standardized echography was not disproved. Intraorbital hemangiomas in adult patients are also among those lesions where echography is usually used in making the diagnosis. In spite of this and the very typical echographic criteria the value of echography in our study was somehow diminished since CT as well as NMR (with correct diagnoses) was already done in 12 of our 29 patients. In 3 cases the lesions turned out to be a pleomorphic adenoma of the lacrimal gland. For the diagnosis of hemangiomas in children, again standardized echography is the method of choice, and 'makes' the diagnosis or proves the clinical suspected diagnosis. As it is true for the vascular malformations (see

Table 8.

Standardized Echography/Vascular tumors

Summary:

Very good results:	Orbital varix/A-V-fistula
	Hemangioma in children
	Hemangioma
Good results:	Lymphangioma

Clinical value/influence on clinical decisions: +++

above) Doppler-sonography gives the pathognomonic echographic criteria by demonstrating the extensive vascularization in these lesions. In cases with intraorbital lymphangiomas we had good diagnostic results except in 5 cases (25%) where the diagnosis was not correct, the tumors turned out to be 1 hemangioma (adult type), 2 lymphomas, 1 orbital varix (a diagnosis close to an orbital lymphangioma) and 1 pseudotumor [9, 14].

4. *Orbital cysts/Hematoma*

Table 9.

Cysts/Hematoma		Histo	Clinic	NV	NF-U
Dermoid	$n = 39$	14	10	3	12
Muco (pyo) cele	$n = 29$	5	14	3	7
Serous cyst	$n = 6$	2	2	–	2
Prolaps/orbital fat	$n = 11$	2	5	–	4
Hematoma	$n = 24$	1	22	–	1

Intraorbital and periorbital cysts turned out to be lesions which can be diagnosed with a very high percentage of accuracy. The echographic criteria in standardized echography correlate very well to the histopathologic features of such cysts and – if present and correctly evaluated – enable the examiner to be sure with the diagnosis, e.g. the proof of the big bony defect in the orbital wall in mucoceles is a pathognomonic finding. Generally cysts show a very sharp outlining with the typical double or triple-peaked surface spikes in standardized A-scan (for most of the cysts this has to be displayed in a paraocular examination technique). For the diagnosis of dermoid-cysts, particularly in children, though the diagnosis often appears to be clear-cut, follow-up examinations, made in all the cases of our study, are important to exclude a rhabdomyosarcoma. The 3 cases, which could not be verified, luckily were not serious tumors, but were all diagnosed as orbital fat prolaps by biopsy. For the post-traumatic orbital hematomas we considered the influence of echography only as good, the clinical findings including the history of these patients were clear in the majority of cases. But in 4 patients who had surgery in the ENT department and in 3 patients who suffered

Table 10.

Standardized Echography/Orbital cysts/Posttraumatic cond.

Summary:

Very good results:	Dermoid/Mucocele
Good results:	Hematoma

Clinical value/influence on clinical decisions:	++ Cysts
	+ Posttraumatic cond.
	++ Postoperative cond.

from motility disturbances after only bland trauma of the periorbital region, echography revealed hematoma of one or more extraocular muscles [1, 7].

5. *Optic nerve*

Table 11.

Optic nerve		Histo	Clinic	NV	NF-U
Meningeoma	*n* = 13	1	1	2	9
Glioma	*n* = 6	–	1	2	3

The results of our study in cases with tumors of the optic nerve diagnosed by echography were giving less evidence. This is because in most of the cases we were not able to achieve follow-up data. In 6 out of the 9 patients with a diagnosed meningeoma and in all 3 cases (children) where we diagnosed a glioma, we discovered, by asking the patient or the referring ophthalmologist, that no further examinations had been made and that the patients still suffered from the clinical symptoms. In the additional cases we could not get any information. On the other hand the method of standardized echography allows to diagnose lesions of the optic nerve by clear and repeatable examination techniques and thus usually other intraorbital conditions and tumors can be ruled out. Though there is a lack of follow-up information, in none of these cases other diagnoses were established. In 4 cases by CT and/or NMR the optic nerve was found to be normal, but other intraorbital lesions could not be found [2].

Table 12.

Standardized Echography/Optic nerve

Summary:

Fair results (due to low case-no.):	Glioma/meningeoma
Clinical value/influence on clinical decisions:	+

Table 13.

Lacrimal sac/gland		Histo	Clinical	NV	NF-U
Dacryoadenitis	$n = 7$	4	2	–	1
Dacryocystitis	$n = 4$	1	–	–	3
Pleomorphic adenoma	$n = 5$	2	2	–	1
Dacryocele	$n = 2$	–	2	–	–
Carcinoma lacr. gland	$n = 2$	1	–	1	–

6. *Lacrimal sac/Lacrimal gland*

Lesions and tumors of the lacrimal sac and the lacrimal gland could be diagnosed correctly in all cases besides 1. One patient had no carcinoma of the lacrimal gland but a pleomorphic adenoma according to histopathology. Inflammatory changes of the lacrimal sac and the gland were followed-up closely under therapy, one lacrimal sac was removed and showed granulomatous changes. In the 4 cases where we had no follow-up data out of our charts the information we could achieve (patient/ophthalmologist) revealed complete disappearence of the symptoms respectively of the tumorous swelling of the lacrimal gland. In case of a suspected carcinoma of the lacrimal gland (high to very high reflectivity, diffus borders, irregularity of the internal structure), though we had only 2 cases, a biopsy within a short time period should be performed [14].

Table 14.

Standardized Echography/Lacrimal sac/gland	
Summary:	
Good results:	Inflammations
Good/fair results:	Adenoma/Carcinoma
Clinical value/influence on clinical decisions:	++ Inflammations
	+ Tumors

Summary/Discussion

When overlooking the variety of diagnoses in our study it correlates in general to other major surveys of orbital tumors [10, 11, 15–19]. The accuracy of the echographic diagnoses made by the method of standardized echography turned out to be in the range of almost 90% which underlines the great importance of this clinical method and is still superior to all other examination techniques. Even when considering that in all the cases where

Table 15.

Summary		
Examined cases	$n = 407$	
Cases with follow-up	$n = 311$	
Verified echographic diagnosis	$n = 279$	(89, 8%)
by histopathology	$n = 88$	(29%)
by clinic/NMR/CT	$n = 191$	(61%)
Non-verified cases	$n = 32$	(10, 2%)
(From all cases ($n = 407$):	$n = 279$	(69%)

we could not achieve follow-up data for our study, the overall accuracy would still be 69% of correct diagnoses.

When we looked at the factors that influenced the echographic diagnoses – as far as this was possible by evaluating the remarks in the written echographic findings and in the charts and by considering which examiner did the echography and how the examinations were performed – we felt that the two major points were how careful and exact the examination was performed (also in terms of time needed for the examination) and how careful the examiner looked for echographic key criteria. Better results were achieved in the cases with lesions of a higher clinical incidence and where the clinical data were known to the echographer (incl. CT and NMR). The echographic experience of the examiner (provided that the examiner did the complete examination exactly according to the method of standardized echography, which was assumed for this study, though we could not check to verify this in detail), in our opinion, was less important for a correct diagnosis or differential diagnostic considerations than the general clinical knowledge and experience, particularly about the histopatholgy of orbital lesions/tumors.

Table 16.

Influence on echographic diagnosis: (orbital diseases)	Duration of examination (evaluation of criteria)
	Presence of key criteria
	Incidence of condition
	Follow-up examination
	Clinical data
	CT/NMR
	Experience of echographer (echography/clinic/histo)

References

1. Byrne, S.F. Orbital dermoid cysts. Doc. Ophthalmol. Proc. Ser. 48: 465–475. Dordrecht: M. Nijhoff/Dr. W. Junk (1987).
2. Byrne, S.F. The echographic measurement and differential diagnosis of optic nerve lesions (review). Doc. Ophthalmol. Proc. Ser. 48: 571–585. Dordrecht: M. Nijhoff/Dr. W. Junk (1987).
3. Green, R.L. Echographic diagnosis of posterior scleritis. Doc. Ophthalmol. Proc. Ser. 48: 515–519. Dordrecht: M. Nijhoff/Dr. W. Junk (1987).
4. Goes, F. Ultrasonographic and clinical characteristics of orbital pseudotumors. Doc. Ophthalmol. Proc. Ser. 48: 499–507. Dordrecht: M. Nijhoff/Dr. W. Junk (1987).
5. Guthoff, R.F. & Singh, G. Posterior scleritis – the role of ultrasonography in the follow-up of the disease. Doc. Ophthalmol. Proc. Ser. 38: 169–174. The Hague: Dr. W. Junk (1984).
6. Harrie, R.P. Standardized echography of the orbit (review). Doc. Ophthalmol. Proc. Ser. 48: 445–451. Dordrecht: M. Nijhoff/Dr. W. Junk (1987).
7. Hasenfratz, G. & Ossoinig, K.C. The diagnosis of orbital mucoceles and pyoceles with standardized echography. Doc. Ophthalmol. Proc. Ser. 38: 407–415. The Hague: Dr. W. Junk (1984).
8. Hasenfratz, G. Diagnosis of orbital metastases with standardized echography. In: Thijssen, J.M., Hillman, J.S., Gallenga, P.E., & Cennamo, G. (eds.), Ultrasonography in Ophthalmology. Proc. of the 11th SIDUO Congress. Doc. Ophtalmol. Proc. Ser. 51: 243–258. Dordrecht: Kluwer Acad. Publ. (1988).
9. Hauff, W. & Till, P. Echography in carotid-cavernous fistulas. Doc. Ophthalmol. Proc. Ser. 38: 399–405. The Hague: Dr. W. Junk (1984).
10. Henderson, J.W. Orbital tumors, 2nd ed. New York: B.C. Decker/Stuttgart, New York: G. Thieme (1980).
11. Moss, H.M. Expanding lesions of the orbit. Am. J. Ophthalmol. 54: 761–770 (1962).
12. Ossoinig, K. Basics, methods, and results of ultrasonography used in diagnosis of intraorbital tumors. In: Gitter K.A., Keeney A.H., Sarin L.K. and Meyer D. (eds.), Opthalmic ultrasound. Proc. of the 4th Int. Congr. of ultrasonography in ophthalmology. pp. 282–293. St. Louis: C.V. Mosby (1969).
13. Ossoinig, K.C. The role of clinical echography in modern diagnosis of periorbital and orbital lesions. In: Orbital Centre of the Amsterdam University Eye Hospital et al. (eds.), Proc. of the 3rd Int. Symposium on orbital disorders. pp. 496–540. The Hague: Dr. W. Junk (1978).
14. Ossoinig, K.C. Standardized echography: Basic principles, clinical applications, and results. In: Dallow, R.L. (ed.), Ophthalmic ultrasonography: Comparative techniques. Int. Ophthal. Clin. 19/IV: 127–210. Boston: Little, Brown & Co. (1979).
15. Reese, A.B. Tumors of the eye. 3rd ed. Hagerstown: Harper & Row (1976).
16. Reibaldi, A., Lorusso, V.V. & Delle Noci, N. Eight years of A- and B-scan ultrasonography in tumoural diagnostics of the globe and orbit. In: Thijssen, J.M. & Verbeek, A.M. (eds.), Ultrasonography in Ophthalmology. Doc. Ophthalmol. Proc. Ser. 29: 323–326. The Hague: Dr. W. Junk (1981).
17. Silva, D. Orbital tumors. Am. J. Ophthalmol. 65: 318–339 (1968).
18. Skalka, H.W. Ultrasound diagnoses of orbital masses and intraocular tumors. In: Ossoinig, K.C. (ed.), Ophthalmic echography. Proc. of the 10th SIDUO Congr. Doc. Ophthalmol. Proc. Ser. 48: 463–464. Dordrecht: M. Nijhoff/Dr. W. Junk (1987).
19. Till, P. & Hauff, W. Differential diagnostic results of clinical echography in orbital tumors. In: Thijssen, J.M. & Verbeek, A.M. (eds.), Ultrasonography in Ophthalmology. Doc. Ophthalmol. Proc. Ser. 29: 277–282. The Hague: Dr. W. Junk (1981).

Address for correspondence: University Eye Clinic, Josef-Schneider-Str. 11 W-8700 Würzburg, Germany

8. Lacrimal gland amyloidosis
Characteristics in standardized A-scan echography

A. STANOWSKY

(*Augsburg, Germany*)

Abstract. Lacrimal gland tumors are rare and have therefore been only partially studied with standardized A-scan. We had the opportunity to examine an isolated amyloid tumor of both lacrimal glands prior to histological confirmation. The tumor's echographic characteristics are described and an attempt is made to differentiate it from other lacrimal gland tumors.

Introduction

Lacrimal gland tumors are classified according to WHO criteria [7, 15] into epithelial tumors (adenomas, mucoepidermoid tumors, carcinomas), tumors of hematopoietic and lymphatic origin, metastatic and inflammatory (pseudo-) tumors. The clinical determinants for distinguishing among these tumors are changes in blood count, fever, swelling, reddening, pain (carcinoma!) and bone erosion. Even though enlargement of the lacrimal gland can be ascertained by computed tomography, diagnosis according to the histological type is not possible in most of the patients [6, 8].

Standardized A-scan echography, on the other hand, nearly always permits a reliable differential diagnosis [1–5, 9–12]. For example, epithelial tumors (high reflectivity), can be distinguished [13, 14] from tumors of hematopoietic and lymphatic origin (low reflectivity). It is also possible to differentiate within the group of epithelial tumors between pleomorphic adenomas and adenoid cystic carcinomas [5, 12].

Isolated amyloid tumors, on the other hand, constitute a very rare form. We report in the following on their A-scan characteristics.

Case history

A female patient (Fig. 1), born in 1913, first came to our out-patient clinic in November, 1988. She had noticed an increasing sensation of pressure with slight pain, primarily in the right eye. Clinically, a clearly defined, firm, mobile, only moderately pressure-sensitive tumor was bilaterally diagnosed in the anterosuperior temporal orbit. When ectropionating the upper lid a subconjunctival growth in the temporal upper fornix was visible. Except for bilateral incipient cataract and a slight exophthalmus of both eyes (Hertel

P. Till (ed.), Ophtalmic Echography 13, pp. 145–149.

146

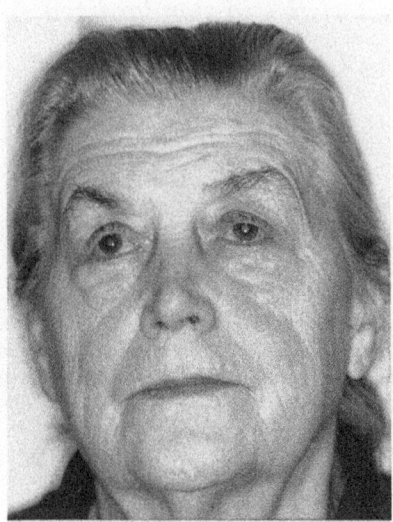

Fig. 1. Patient with amyloidosis of the lacrimal gland showing slight bilateral exophthalmus.

basis 110; right eye 20 mm, left eye 21 mm), no other pathological changes were confirmed on both sides. Motility was free.

Computed tomography showed an enlargement of both lacrimal glands, a differential diagnosis however could not be performed though intravenous injection of contrast medium. There were no signs of bone erosion.

Material and method

Both orbits were subjected to parabulbar and transocular echography with an Ophthascan S unit. Since the tumor was mobile, a light pressure with the finger-tip on the medial eyelid during echography kept the tumor in place.

Results

Standardized A-scan of both eyes showed a clearly defined, plum-shaped process originating in the fossa lacrimalis and extending into the temporal orbit. The tumor showed a maximum depht of 23 mm (right side)/18 mm (left side), with a maximum width of 8/6 mm and a maximum height of 9/6 mm. It was solidly configurated, mobile, showed no signs of increased vascularization and was encapsulated. Bilateral reflectivity was very high, the structure was heterogeneously regular, and absorption ranged from low

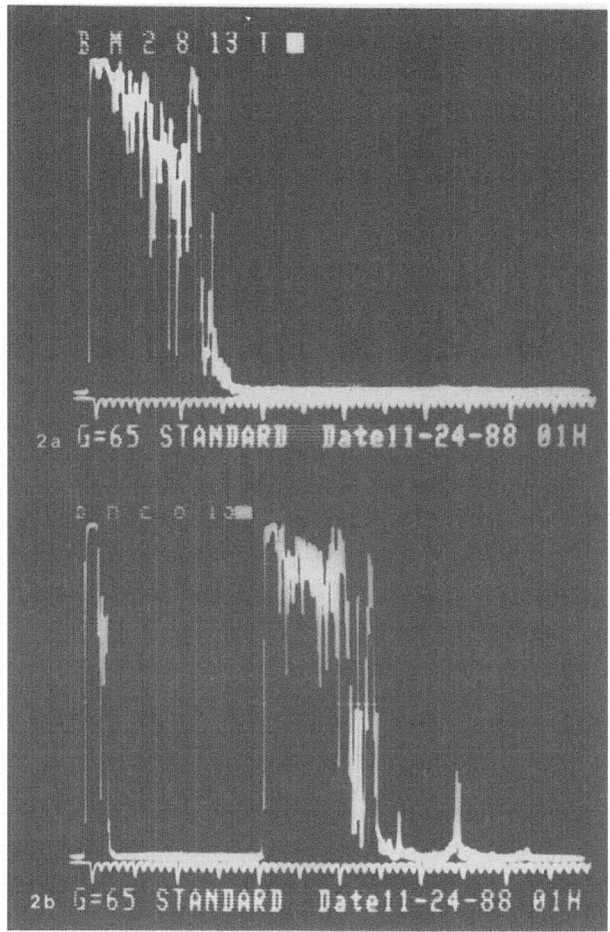

Fig. 2. Standardized A-scan echograms of the right lacrimal gland by parabulbar (Fig. 2a) and transocular (Fig. 2b) examination technique.

to medium (Fig. 2). Histological examination of a tissue sample acquired from the right orbit by excisional biopsy showed an amyloid tumor of the lacrimal gland (Fig. 3).

Discussion

Even though amyloid tumors of the lacrimal gland are very rare, they must be kept in mind for differential diagnosis even in the absence of clinical signs of amyloidosis. Distinguishing such tumors clinically from acute dacryoadenitis is usually unproblematic unless they should be located strictly unilaterally

148

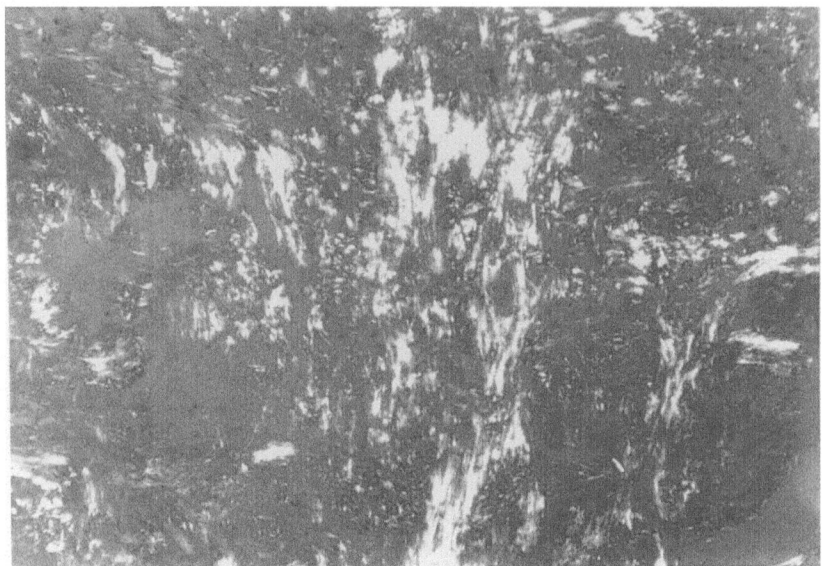

Fig. 3. Biopsy material of the right lacrimal gland shows amorphous eosinophilic material lightening up in polarized light (Kongo-red staining).

and be inflamed. They are clearly distinguished from lacrimal gland tumors of hematopoietic or lymphatic nature by characteristics such as inner structure, good delineability and reflectivity. Distinguishing them from tumors of a primarily epithelial nature will be more difficult. In general, pleomorphic adenoma can be highly reflective, showing a heterogenous regular internal structure and strong to medium absorption. It therefore can make a differentiation very difficult. Adenoid cystic carcinoma, on the other hand, can make the differential diagnosis difficult too, though showing a lower degree of reflectivity with regular internal structure. In such cases, one should determine whether the lacrimal gland tumor is mobile or immobile, uni- or bilateral, painful, and whether signs of bone erosion are visible by roentgenology.

References

1. Baker, S. & Ossoinig, K.C. Ultrasonic evaluation of salivary glands. Trans. Amer. Acad. Ophthalmol. Otolaryngol. 84: 750–762 (1977).
2. Bellone, G. & Gallenga, P.E. Echography of mixed tumors of the lacrimal gland. Ophthalmologica 166: 156–160 (1973).
3. Dagher, G., Anderson, R.L., Ossoinig, K.C. & Baker, J.D. Adenoid cystic carcinoma of the lacrimal gland in a child. Arch. Ophthalmol. 98: 1098–1100 (1980).
4. Divine, R.D., Anderson, R.L. & Ossoinig, K.C. Metastatic carcinoid unresponsive to radiation therapy presenting as a lacrimal fossa mass. Ophthalmology 89: 516–520 (1982).

5. Hackelbusch, R., Rochels, R. & Knieper, P. Korrelation echographischer und histologischer Befunde bei Erkrankungen der Tränendrüse. Opthalmologica 186: 113–124 (1983).
6. Hammerschlag, S.B., Hesselink, J.R. & Weber, A.L. Computed tomography of the eye and orbit. pp. 74–75 and 105–111. (1983).
7. Jakobiec, F.A. Tumors of the lacrimal gland and lacrimal sac. In: Anderson, R.L. (ed.), Symposium on diseases and surgery of the lids, lacrimal apparatus, and orbit. pp. 190–202. Saint Louis: Mosby (1982).
8. Kazner, E., Wende, S., Grumme, Th., Lanksch, W. & Stochdorph, O. Computertomographie intrakranieller Tumoren aus klinischer Sicht. pp. 475–475. Berlin: Springer (1981).
9. Ossoinig, K.C. & Blodi, F.C. Preoperative differential diagnosis of tumors with echography. Part IV: Diagnosis of orbital tumors. In: Blodi, F.C., (ed.), Current concepts in opthalmology. pp. 313–342. Saint Louis: Mosby (1974).
10. Ossoinig, K.C. Echography of the eye, orbit and periorbital region. In: Arger, P.H. (ed.), Orbit roentgenology. pp. 224–269. New York: Wiley (1977).
11. Ossoinig, K.C. Orbital disorders. In: de Vlieger, M. (ed.), Handbook of Clinical ultrasound. pp. 881–904. Philadelphia: Wiley (1978).
12. Rochels, R. Ultraschalldiagnostik in der Augenheilkunde: Lehrbuch und Atlas. Landsberg a.L.: Ecomed (1986).
13. Till, P. & Hauff, W. Differential diagnostic results of clinical echography in orbital tumors. Doc. Opthalmol. Proc. Ser. 8, 29: 277–282. The Hague: Dr. W. Junk (1981).
14. Till, P., Steinkogler, F.J. & Hauff, W. Die Bedeutung der echographischen Gewebsdifferenzierung für die Orbitachirurgie. Klin. Mbl. Augenheilk. 186: 296–299 (1985).
15. Zimmerman, L.E. & Sobin, L.H. Histological typing of tumors of the eye and its adnexa. No. 24. pp. 35–36. Geneva: World Health Organization (1980).

Address for correspondence: Zentralklinikum, Augenklinik, Stenglinstrasse 2, W-8900 Augsburg, Germany.

9. Standardized echography in adenoid-cystic carcinomas of the orbit

P. TILL

(*Vienna, Austria*)

Introduction

Epithelial tumors of the orbit commonly arise from the lacrimal glands as primary tumors and are located in the temporal upper orbit (pleomorphic adenomas, adenocarcinomas, adenoid-cystic carcinomas etc.). Otherwise the same epithelial tumors arise from the minor salivary glands of the submucosa of parasinuses, lacrimal sac or epiglottis and reach the orbit by engrowth or metastases as secondary tumors in any location of the orbit.

Standardized Echography can differentiate these high reflective epithelial tumors preoperative from other high reflective tumors as cavernous hemangiomas, an important fact for managment of epithelial tumors by excisional biopsies [1, 2].

Case report

Case 1. An 80-year-old female with a 10-year history of progressive lacrimal sac swelling with epiphora was diagnosed clinical as chronic dacryocystitis (Fig. 1); before the planned dacryorhinostomy the lesion was examined with Standardized Echography. MINI-Ascan echograms paraocular demonstrated at tissue sensitivity a high reflective lacrimal sac tumor with a medium high angle k (Fig. 2) with extraorbital echos into the direction to the nasal cavity and maxillary sinus (Fig. 2 bottom). These echograms were very similar to the echographic pattern of cavernous hemangiomas, but with a 10% lower reflectivity and a 10% higher angle k. The prolonged pressure test was negative. Delayed continuous compressibility is a specific criterion for cavernous hemangiomas (Fig. 3). Blood is squeezed out by continuous pressure with the probe and only cavernous hemangiomas became smaller in diameter, when compressed over a period of time. No other orbital lesion can be squeezed out [3, 4]. NMR showed a large lacrimal sac tumor with engrowth into the nasal cavity and maxillary sinus (Fig. 4). Total tumor excision was performed (Fig. 5) and histology diagnosed an adenoid-cystic carcinoma of the lacrimal sac (Fig. 6); postoperative local radiotherapy followed and the patient has been without recurrence for more than two years.

P. Till (ed.), Ophtalmic Echography 13, pp. 151–159.

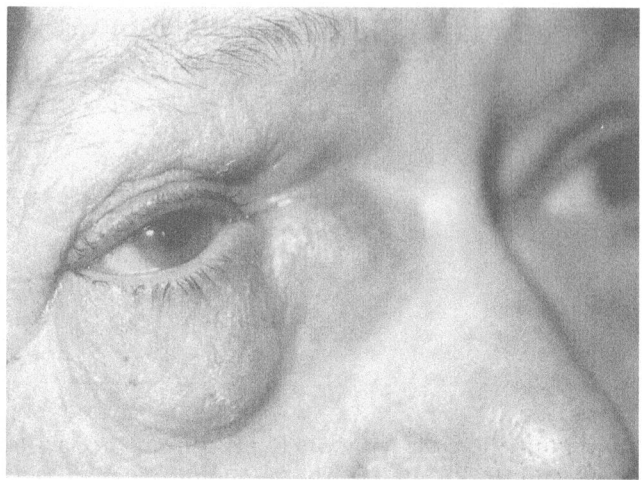

Fig. 1. 80-year-old female with a lacrimal sac swelling for more than 10 years.

Case 2. A 61-year-old male complained of progressive proptosis and diplopia of 14 days duration. Standardized A-scan echograms demonstrated a large, high reflective lesion in the muscle cone (Fig. 7) with negative prolonged pressure test; reflectivity was 10% lower and angle k 10% higher than in cavernous hemangiomas and echographic diagnosis of an adenoid-cystic carcinoma was made. Two years ago an epiglottis tumor with enlarged lymph nodes was operated (Fig. 8). Histology diagnosed an adenoid-cystic carcinoma of the epiglottis (Fig. 9) originated from the minor salivary glands of the epiglottis (Fig. 10). The patient died 1 year later with distant metastases also in the skin (histologically varified).

Case 3. A 33-year-old male with minimal displacement of his right eye nasally downwards was examined with Standardized A-scan. MINI-Ascan echograms (Fig. 11) showed at tissue sensitivity in the temporal upper orbit a solid lesion with high reflectivity and medium high angle k like in cavernous hemangioma but with negative delayed compression test. Echographic diagnosis was pleomorphic adenoma of the lacrimal gland and excision in the capsule was therefore indicated and performed. Histology confirmed the echographic diagnosis of pleomorphic adenoma of the lacrimal gland (Fig. 12).

Conclusion

Preoperative differential diagnosis of epithelial tumors of the orbit is possible with Standardized A-scan echography. These tumors can arise primary from the lacrimal gland or secondary from the minor salivary glands of the submu-

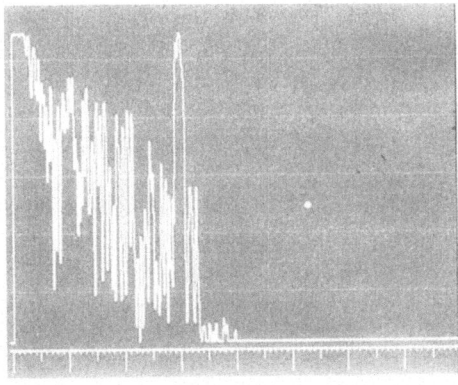

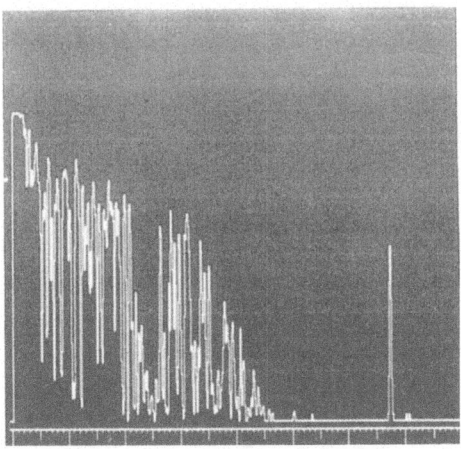

Fig. 2. Paraocular MINI-Ascan echograms with a reflectivity 10% lower and 10% higher angle k than in pleomorphic adenomas and cavernous hemangiomas. The echogram below demonstrate extraorbital echos from the maxillary sinus engrowth (both echograms at tissue sensitivity).

cosa of the parasinuses and involve the orbit by ingrowth in the orbit with destruction of the orbital bone or originate from the lacrimal sac. A secondary epithelial tumor can envolve the orbit as distant metastasis in case of a primary epiglottis tumor. Echographically the important criterion of a pleomorphic adenoma is the high reflectivity and the medium high angle k of the tumor echogram identical with the echogram of cavernous hemangiomas. In adenoid-cystic carcinomas reflectivity is 10% lower and angle k 10% higher than in pleomorphic adenomas and cavernous hemangiomas. The prolonged pressure test is negative in epithelial tumors; this is the key criterion to differentiate epithelial tumors from cavernous hemangiomas; only cavernous hemangiomas can be squeezed out und shortened by the delayed compression test.

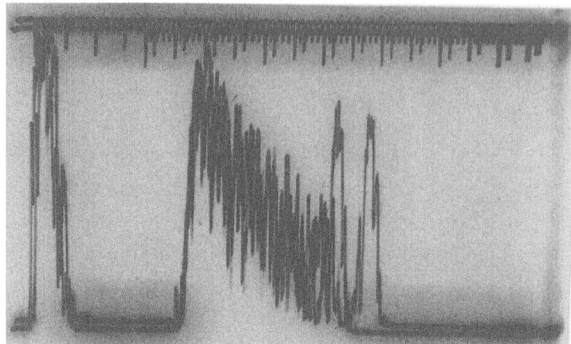

Fig. 3. A-scan echograms at tissue sensitivity (7200 MA Kretztechnik) of a cavernous hemangioma in the muscle cone before and after the delayed compression test (demonstrated as sandwich from both echograms); the tumor is squeezed out and the tumor length shortened.

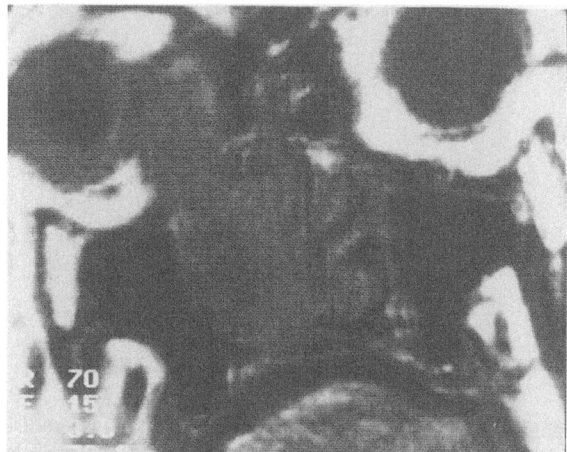

Fig. 4. NMR of the lacrimal sac tumor with engrowth in the nasal cavity and maxillary sinus.

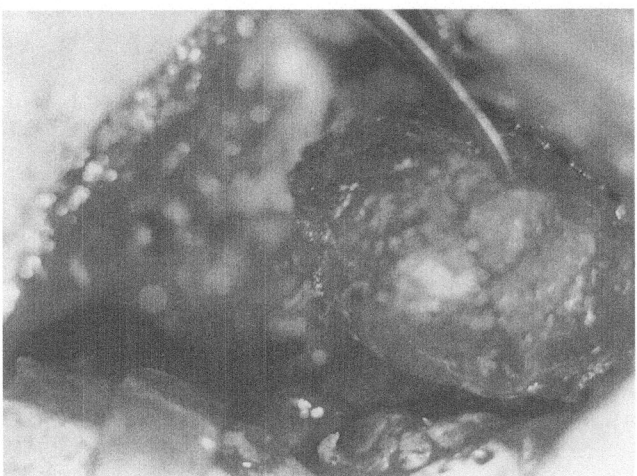

Fig. 5. Complete surgical tumor excision.

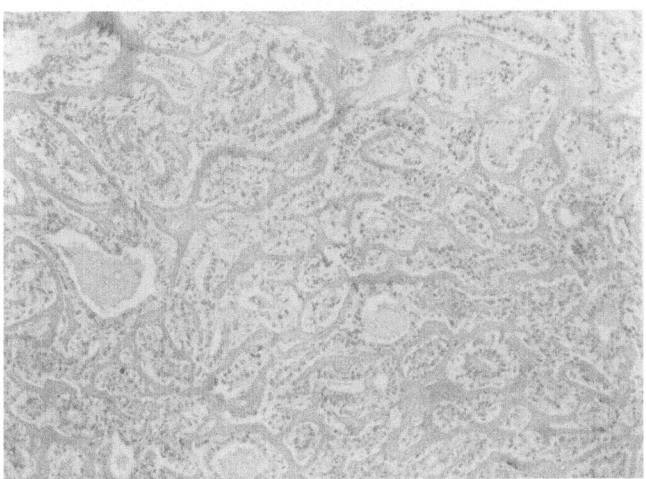

Fig. 6. Histology diagnosed an adenoid-cystic carcinoma.

156

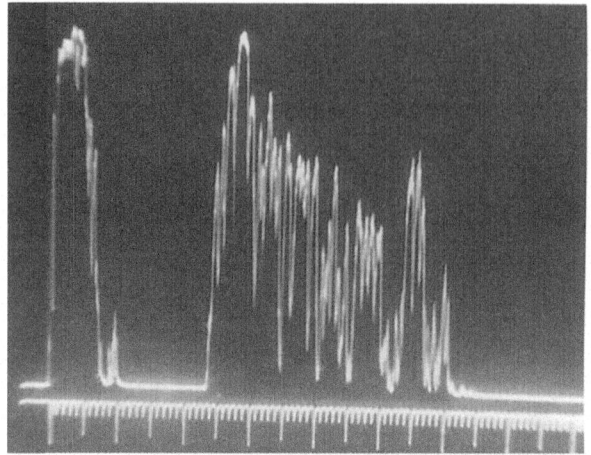

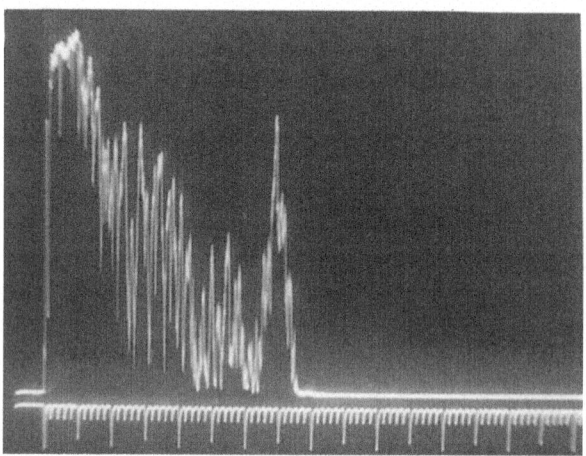

Fig. 7. Metastatic adenoid-cystic carcinoma of the orbit in the muscle cone. Transocular (top) and paraocular (bottom) A-scan echograms at tissue sensitivity (7200 MA Kretztechnik) show a 10% lower reflectivity and a 10% higher angle k than in pleomorhic adenomas and cavernous hemangiomas. The prolonged pressure test was negative.

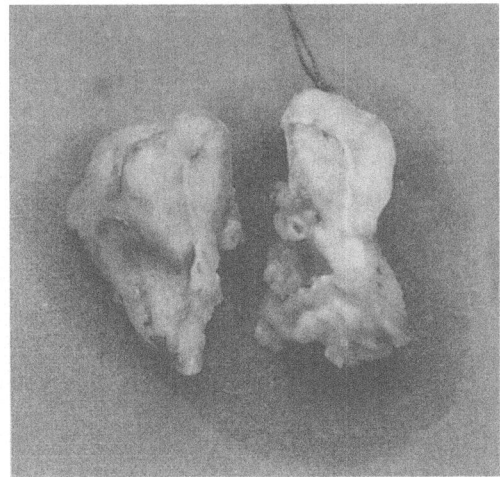

Fig. 8. Primary epiglottis tumor excised two years ago.

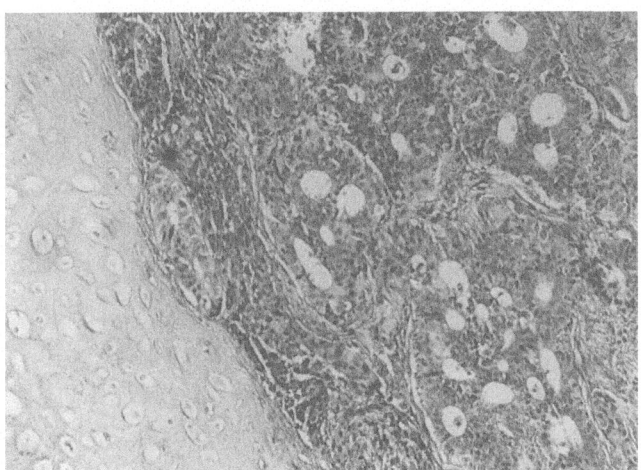

Fig. 9. Histology of the adenoid-cystic carcinoma of the epiglottis.

158

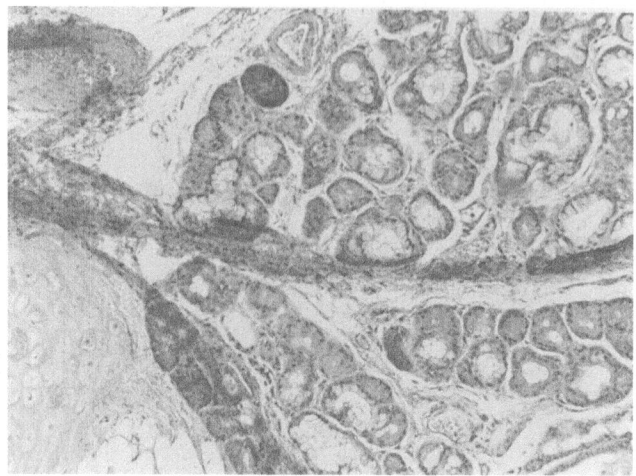

Fig. 10. Histology of a minor salivary gland of the epiglottis.

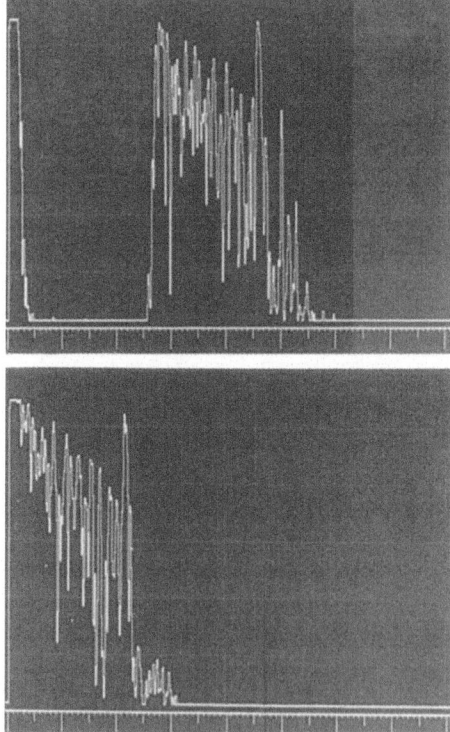

Fig. 11. MINI-Ascan echograms of a pleomorphic adenoma of the lacrimal gland at tissue sensitivity: transocular and paraocular echograms show high reflectivity and medium high angle k like in cavernous hemangiomas. Sharp delineation is seen in the paraocular echogram: a high posterior surface echospike.

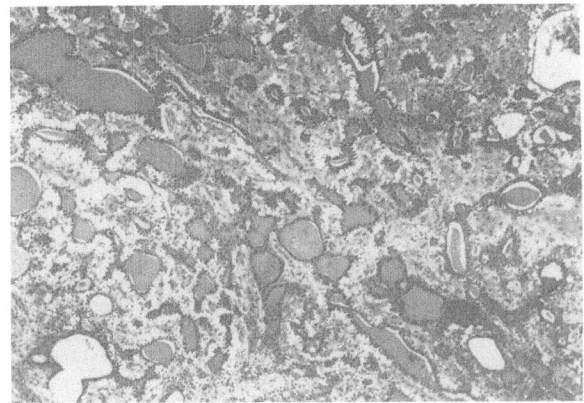

Fig. 12. Histology of the pleomorphic adenoma of the lacrimal gland.

References

1. Dagher, G., Anderson, R.L., Ossoinig, K.C. & Baker, J.D. Adenoid cystic carcinoma of the lacrimal gland in a child. Arch. Ophthalmol. 98: 1098–1100 (1980).
2. Cennamo, G., Franfa, F. & Bonavolonta, G. Lesions of the lacrimal fossa: a retrospective echographic study. Doc. Ophthalmol. Proc. Ser. 53: 63–78. Dordrecht: Kluwer Acad. Publ. (1990).
3. Ossoinig, K.C. Standardized Ophthalmic Echography of the Eye, Orbit and periorbital Region. A Comprehensive Slide Set and Study Guide. Iowa City: Goodfellow, Inc. (1985).
4. Ossoinig, K.C. Echographic differentiation of vascular tumors in the orbit. Doc. Ophthalmol. Proc. Ser. 29: 283–291. The Hague: Dr. W. Junk (1981).

Address for correspondence: 2nd University Eye Clinic, Alserstrasse 4, A-1090 Vienna, Austria.

10. Two cases of benign lacrimal gland tumors
Correlation between echographic and histopathologic findings

J. FUKIYAMA, N. NAO-I, F. MARUIWA & A. SAWADA

(Miyazaki, Japan)

Abstract. Two cases of benign lacrimal gland tumors are described. Preoperative CT and MRI showed a well-circumscribed oval lesion in the superotemporal orbit in both cases. Standardized echography revealed that both tumors had pseudocapsules and different internal reflectivity patterns. The patients underwent lateral orbitotmy and the tumors were excised in their pseudocapsules without performing incisional biopsy. During the operations the tumors proved to be enlarged lacrimal glands themselves. Histopathologically, the first case was a benign mixed tumor (pleomorphic adenoma) and the second case was a benign lymphoepithelial lesion (Mikulicz's disease).

Introduction

Lacrimal gland tumors are relatively rare among orbital tumors. We recently had the opportunity to treat two middle-aged women with lacrimal gland tumors. Preoperative radiologic and echographic assessment indicated that these tumors were solid and encapsulated. So in both cases, we did not perform incisional biopsy, and selected lateral orbitotmy as a surgical intervention. The excised tumors were examined histopathologically, with which preoperative echographic findings were compared.

Case report

Case 1. A 57-year-old woman was referred to us on May 9, 1989 with a complaint of left proptosis of 3 years' duration. She also complained of pain, blurred vision, and dryness in the left eye. Past medical history was unremarkable. Best-corrected visual acuity was R.E.: 24/20 and L.E.: 20/20. The patient had full range of ocular motility except slight limitation of elevation in the left eye and right hypertropia was present. A nontender, firm, immobile mass was present in the superior lateral lid. The globe was displaced inferonasally. Hertel exophthalmometer readings disclosed 12 mm for the right eye and 20 mm for the left eye. Results of slit-lamp examination of the anterior segment was normal but funduscopic examination disclosed choroidal folds in the superotemporal quadrant extending to the macula (Fig.

P. Till (ed.), Ophthalmic Echography 13, pp. 161–177.
© 1993 *Kluwer Academic Publishers.*

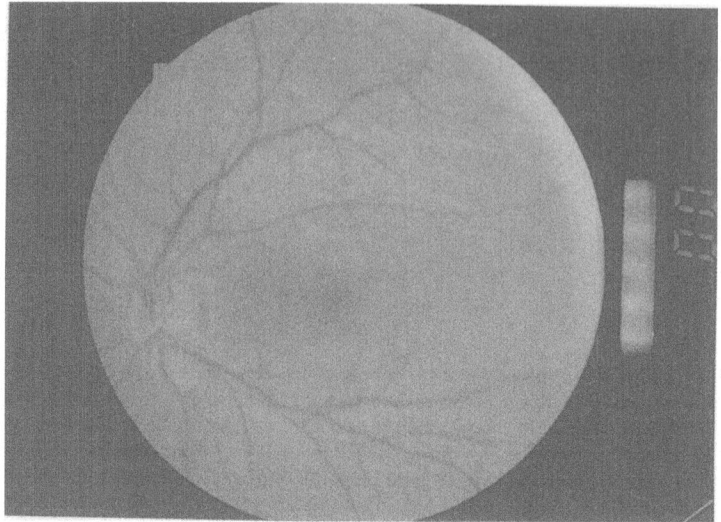

Fig. 1. Fundus photograph of the left eye showing the presence of choroidal folds in the superotemporal quadrant extending to the macula.

1). The results of the laboratory investigations disclosed normal values for the following: complete blood cell count, urinalysis, electrolytes, liver, renal and thyroid function studies. Orbital CT with axial section showed an enhancing mass in the lacrimal gland region with relatively well-defined margins. No bony destruction was evident. On MRI, the mass appeared as a well-circumscribed oval lesion that was enhanced with Gd-DTPA (Fig. 2). Standardized echography was performed disclosing a rounded mass with moderate internal reflectivity and a high reflective posterior surface suggestive of encapsulation (Fig 3).

First, we suspected orbital pseudotumor on CT because of rectus muscle involvement. So steroid was administered orally for two weeks but it made no change in proptosis then discontinued. Another differential diagnosis included benign lacrimal gland tumor, hemangioma, meningioma and epithelial cyst. On July 3, 1989, the tumor was excised by lateral orbitotomy. We utilized the curved L-incision of the anterolateral orbitotomy (Henderson 1976, Wright 1983). During the operation, the tumor was found to be encapsulated and enlarged lacrimal gland itself. The tumor was excised in its pseudocapsule using silk and retinal cryoprobe. It measured 15 × 15 × 30 mm and was light pink, firm and encapsulated. Grossly, the outer aspect of the entire circumference was delimited by a hyaline fibrous capsule. On its cut surface, multiple small cysts were discerned in otherwise firm and solid lesion. Some cysts contained secretory products (Fig. 4). The tumor was dominated by spindle-shaped and cuboidal duct-forming cells. The ductular component varied from large cystic spaces to small compressed lumens. The ducts were

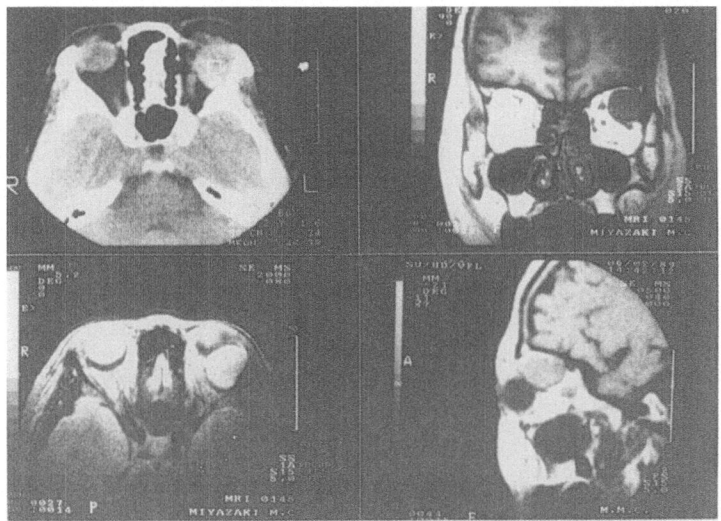

Fig. 2. Top left: Axial CT scan showing the orbital tumor in the lacrimal gland region. It reveals as an enhancing mass which is relatively well defined. No overlying bony destruction is found. Top right: T-1-weighted coronal MR scan showing a round shaped, well-circumscribed tumor with low signal intensity. It makes distortion of the muscle cone and inferonasal displacement of the optic nerve. Thickening of the rectus muscles is observed. Bottom left: T-2-weighted axial MR scan showing an oval-shaped, well-circumscribed tumor with high signal intensity. Bottom right: parasagittal MR scan showing the tumor which is enhanced with Gd-DTPA. It indents the left globe.

formed by a double row of cuboidal to columnar cells (Fig. 5). Small foci of squamous metaplasia were in evidence, and in some areas there was a hyalinized and myxomatous stroma (Fig. 6). Results of histopathologic examination were diagnostic for a benign mixed tumor of the lacrimal gland. After the surgery, the left proptosis and choroidal folds disappeared entirely.

Case 2. A 59-year-old woman with bilateral parotid gland swelling and multiple nuckal lymphnodes swelling was referred to us on August 3, 1989 with a complaint of slowly growing painless right upper lid swelling of approximately one year duration (Fig. 7). She also noted tearing of the right eye for recent two months. Previous treatment included an oral steroid administration three years previously for parotid gland and nuckal lymphnodes swelling by otorhinolaryngologist. Sjögren syndrome was suspected at that time. So a biopsy of the left parotid gland was performed which showed no sign of inflammation. The patient's medical history was otherwise unremarkable, and the family history was noncontributory. On examination, the best-corrected visual acuity was R.E.: 20/25 and L.E.: 20/20. Her right upper lid was swollen and Hertel exophthalmometer readings disclosed 18 mm for

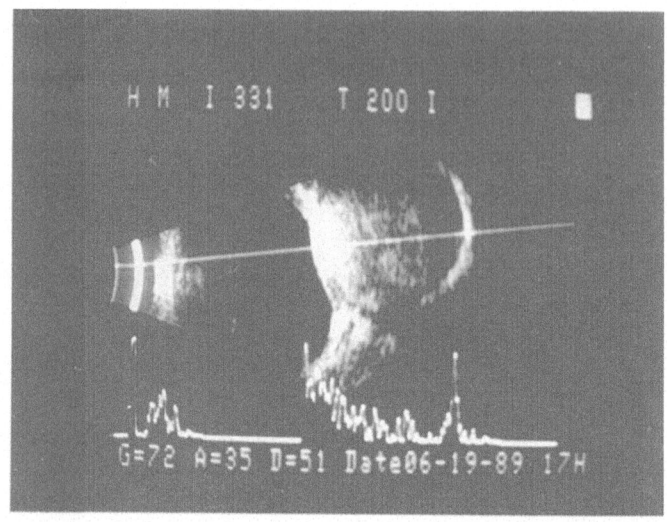

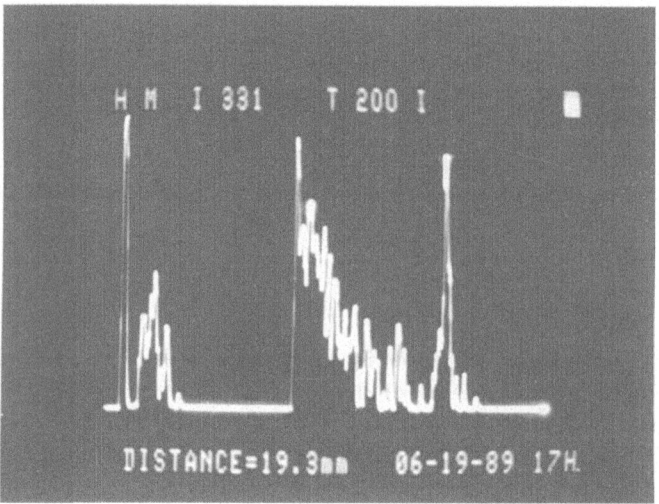

Fig. 3. Echograms of the tumor. Top: B and CV-A (cross vector-A) mode echogram showing a round-shaped tumor which has an heterogeneous internal structure. The high reflective posterior wall suggesting the presence of a pseudocapsule. Bottom: A mode echogram showing the low to medium internal reflectivity with great sound attenuation and high reflective spike from the posterior surface of the tumor.

the right eye and 13 mm for the left eye. The elevation was restricted in the right eye and the patient noted diplopia at right and upward gaze. An elastic hard immobile mass was palpable in the lateral aspect of the right upper lid. Results of the slit-lamp examination of the anterior segment was normal

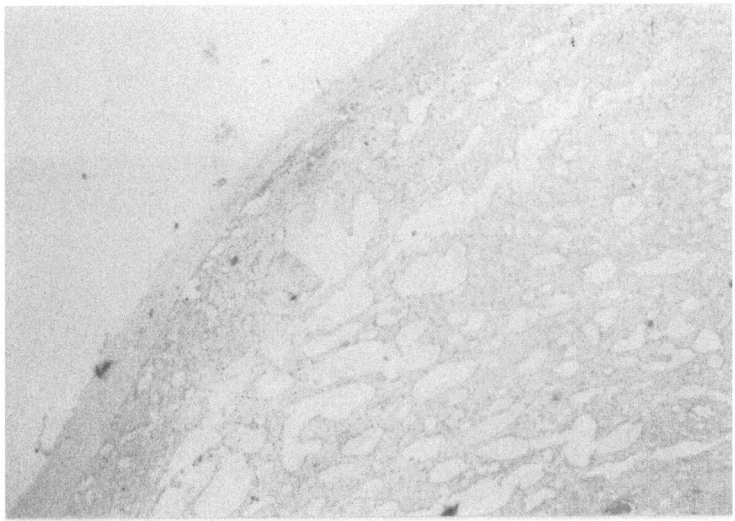

Fig. 4. Top: The pathologic specimen of the excised tumor. The tumor is solid. There are numerous cystic spaces, some of which have secretory products (hematoxylin-eosin; original magnification, ×5). Bottom: A fibrous pseudocapsule is seen and many cystic spaces adjacent to it are shown (hematoxylin-eosin; original magnification, ×20).

except chemosis of bulbar conjunctiva of the right eye. Funduscopic examination of the right eye disclosed superotemporal retinal degeneration. Schirmer testing showed decreased lacrimal secretion in both eyes (right eye 3 mm of Schirmer test strip wetting; left eye 4 mm). The results of laboratory

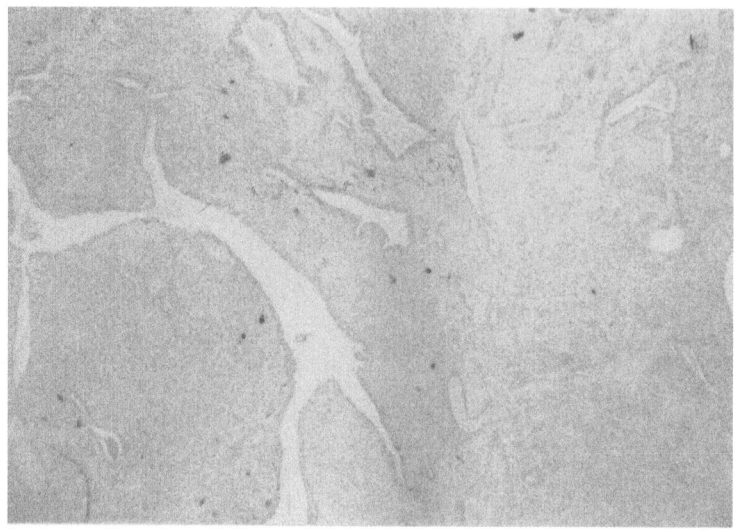

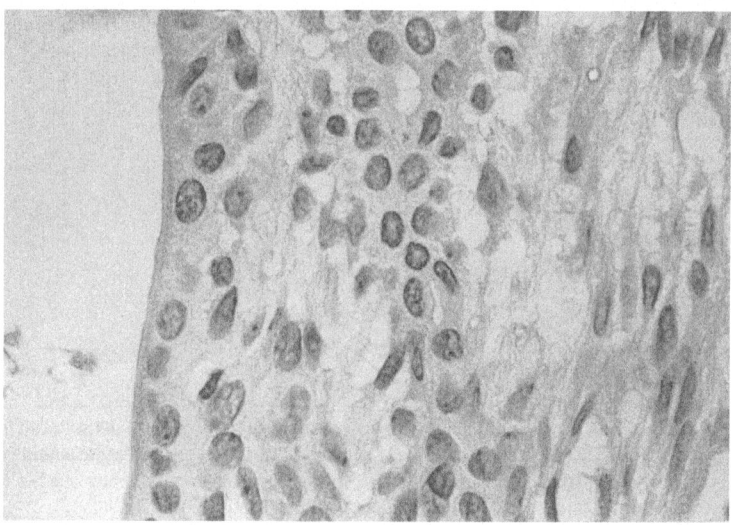

Fig. 5. Top: Higher magnification of the tumor parenchyma. Ductular components are compressed by stromal cell proliferations. The walls of them are made up of double-layered epithelial cells (hematoxylin-eosin; original magnification, ×20). Bottom: The layer of the ductular wall consists of cuboidal to columnar epithelial cells which are also found in the stroma. Spindle-shaped myoepithelial cells are also present in the stroma (hematoxylin-eosin; original magnification, ×400).

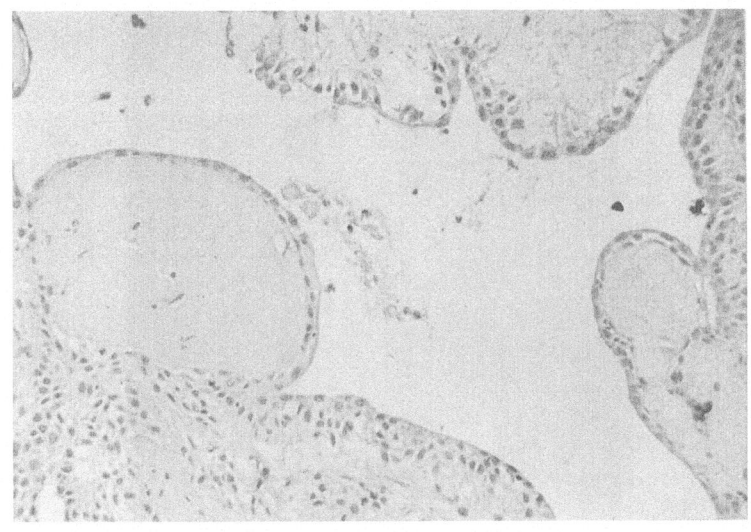

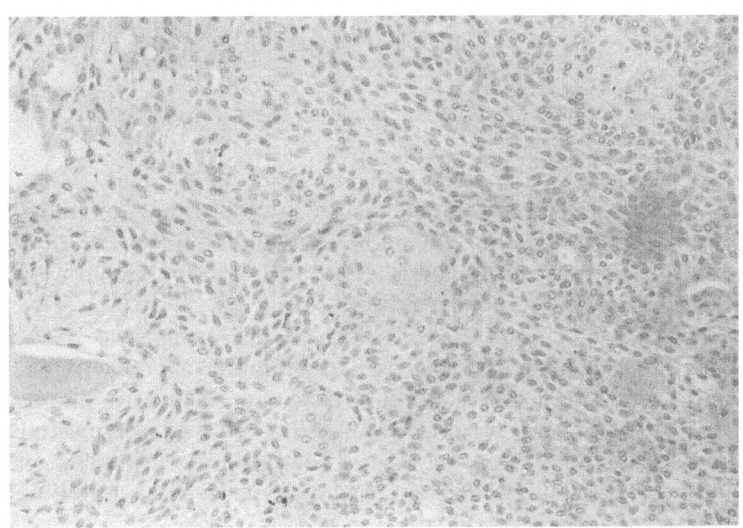

Fig. 6. Top: Hyalinization is observed adjacent to the lumen of the ductular component (hematoxylin-eosin; original magnification, ×100). Bottom: Squamous metaplasia is observed in the stroma (hematoxylin-eosin; original magnification, ×200).

168

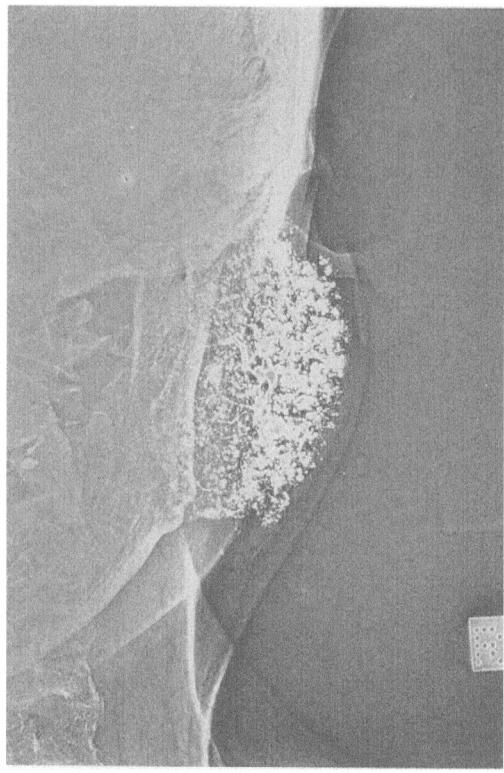

Fig. 7. Sialography of the left parotid gland showing its swelling and typical 'apple tree sign'.

investigations disclosed normal values for the following: complete blood cell count, urinalysis, electrolytes, liver and renal function studies, tumor markers (AFP, CEA), and immunogloblins. Neither RA factor nor antibody for anti-SS A and anti-SS B antigen were positive.

Standardized echography was performed disclosing an oval-shaped mass in the lacrimal gland region which had low internal reflectivity. Scattered sonodense areas were observed within the tumor and the tumor was well-defined at the high gain setting (Fig. 8). But the low internal reflectivity of the tumor and the presence of the pseudocapsule revealed on standard gain setting (Fig. 9). Echodense tail was observed by repeated echographic examination.

Orbital CT and MRI disclosed a well-circumscribed oval lesion in the right lacrimal gland region. Bony erosion (enlargement of the bony lacrimal fossa) was evident but no bony destruction was found (Fig. 10). The preoperative differential diagnosis included benign lacrimal gland tumor, epithelial cyst, and meningioma. On September 13, 1989, the tumor was excised in its pseudocapsule by the same procedure as the case 1 (Fig. 11). The tumor measured 30 × 25 × 20 mm and was yellow, firm and encapsulated. Besides

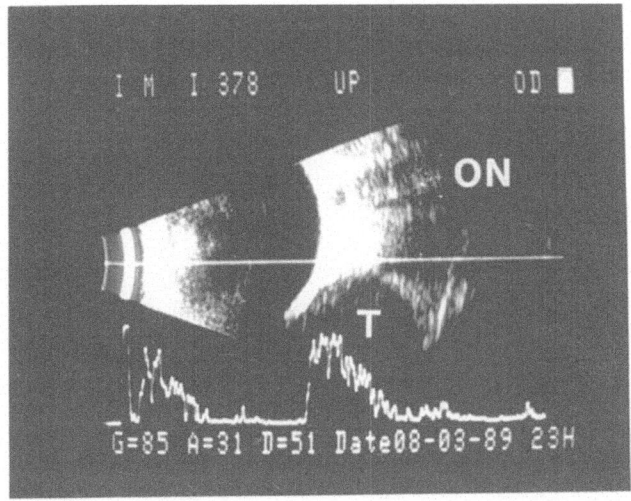

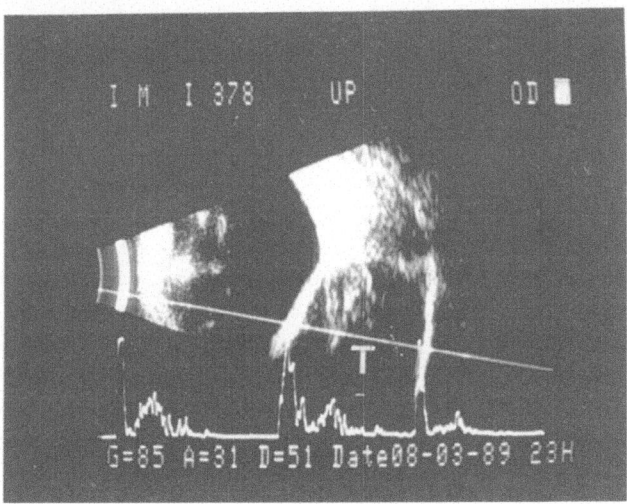

Fig. 8. Echograms of the tumor. Top: Transocular echogram showing the tumor lateral to the optic nerve (T: Tumor, ON: Optic nerve). Bottom: The tumor is well-circumscribed and the low internal reflectivity is shown on CV-A mode. High reflectivity of the posterior wall is also shown.

having fibrous capsule, this tumor had multiple internal fibrous septae (Fig. 12). The whole tumor was infiltrated by lymphocytes and the structure of acini and ducts had disappeared. Well-developed germinal centers were observed (Fig. 13). Several 'epimyoepithelial island' were found by the careful observation of the specimen. Cholesterin clefts were observed in some areas.

Histopathological diagnosis was a benign lymphoepithelial lesion. Postop-

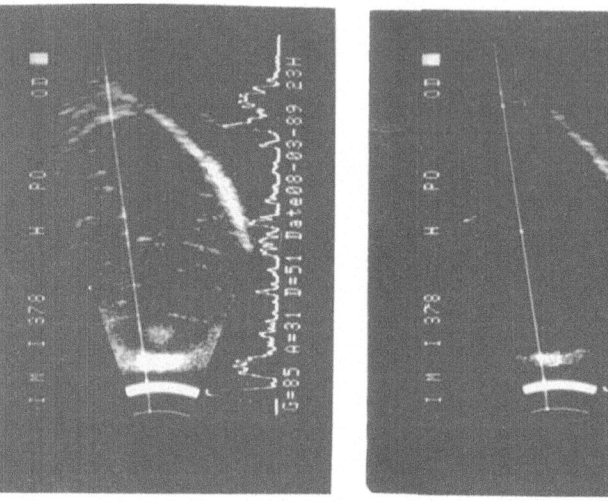
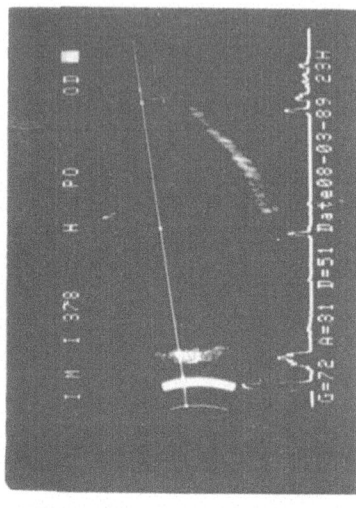
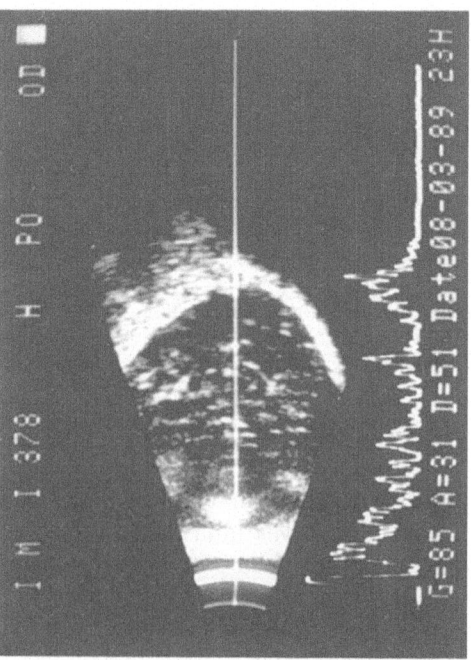

Fig. 9. Echograms obtained with direct contact to the tumor by the probe. Left: Many scattered sonodense areas are seen in the tumor. The tumor has smooth outline at its margin. Top right: Encapsulation of the tumor is evident in this echogram. Bottom right: Low internal reflectivity of the tumor reveals on B and CV-A mode at standard gain setting.

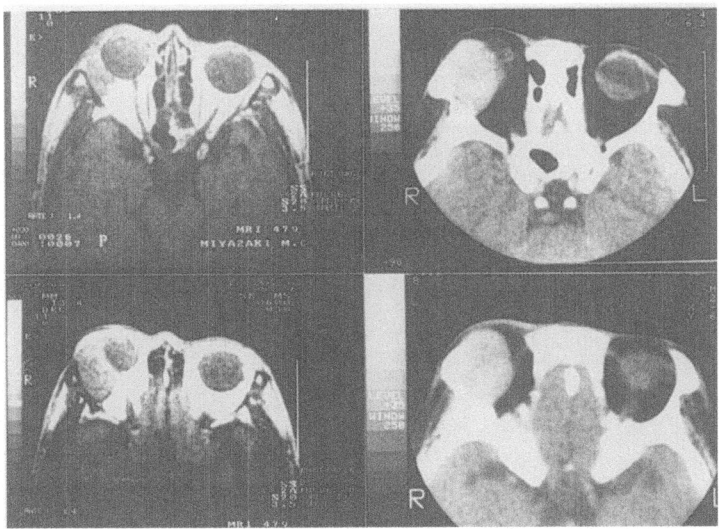

Fig. 10. Top left: T-1-weighted axial MR scan showing right proptosis and inferonasal displacement of the right globe by the tumor. Top right: Axial CT scan showing oval-shaped, well-cicumscribed, enhancing tumor. No bony destruction was found. Bottom left: A higher horizontal MR section (T-1-weighted) showing the oval-shaped tumor. Bottom right: A higher horizontal CT section showing overlying bony erosion (enlargement of the bony lacrimal fossa).

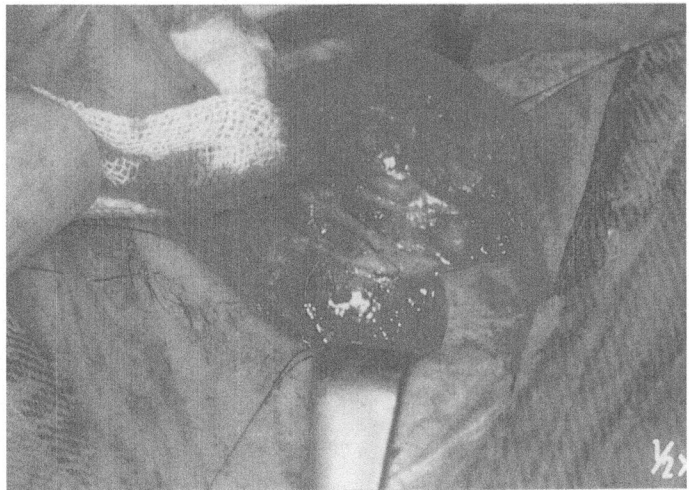

Fig. 11. The exposed lacrimal gland tumor after removal of the lateral bony orbit and the periorbita.

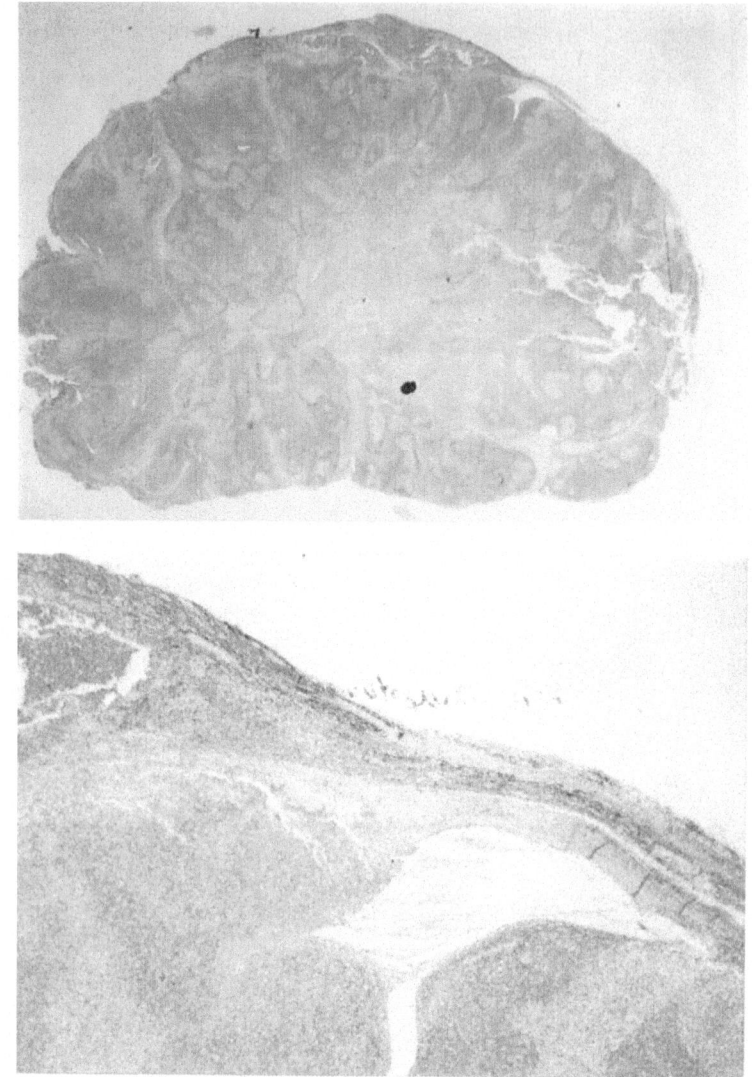

Fig. 12. Top: The pathologic specimen of the excised tissue. The lacrimal gland is replaced by lymphocytes and the structure of the acini and ducts can not be seen. Fibrous pseudocapsule and internal septae are noted (hematoxylin-eosin; original magnificaton, ×5). Bottom: A fibrous pseudocapsule with lymphocytic infiltration (hematoxylin-eosin; original magnification, ×10).

Fig. 13. Top: At higher magnification, germinal centers and fibrous internal septae are noted (hematoxylin-eosin; original magnification, ×10). Middle: So called 'epimyoepithelial island' is observed in the 'lymphocytic sea' (hematoxylin-eosin; original magnification, ×200). Bottom: Cholesterin clefts are present which may be the cause of the radiodense tail (hematoxylin-eosin; original magnification, ×10).

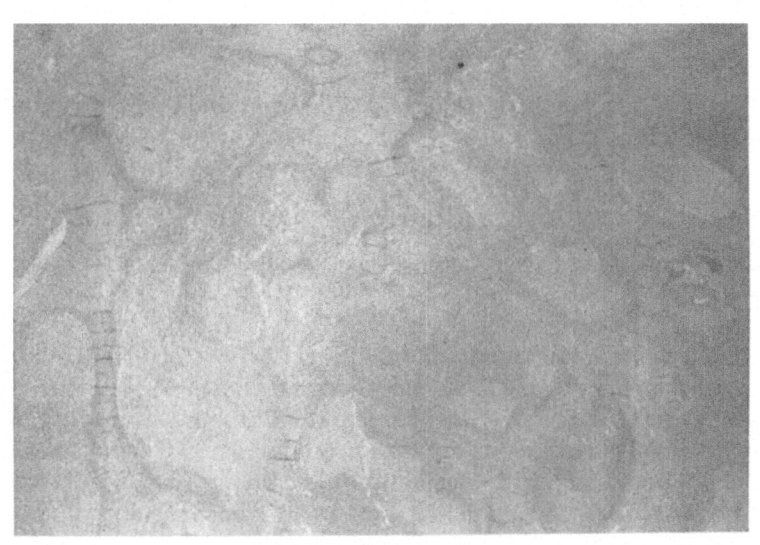

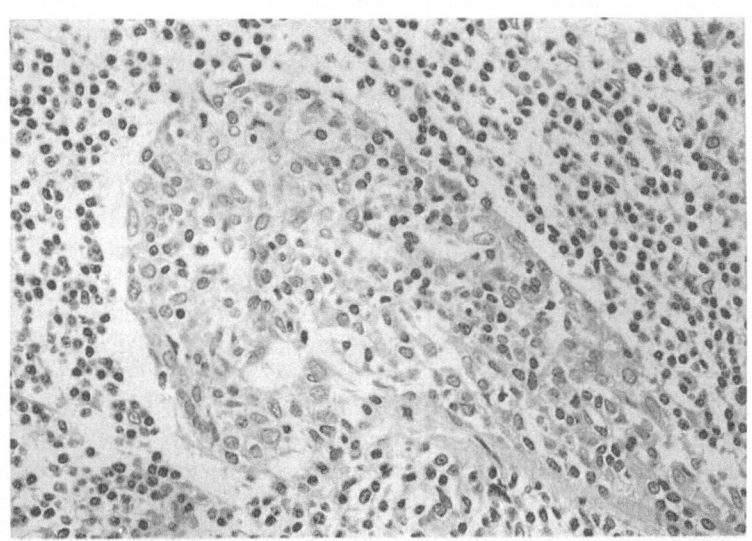

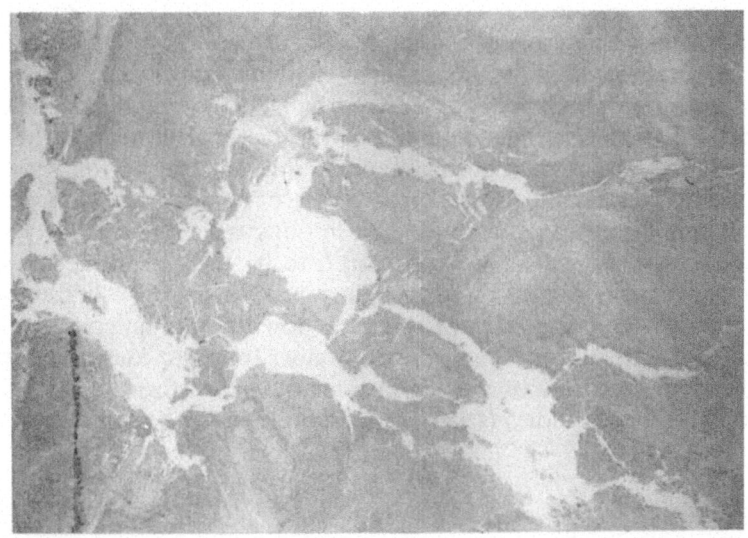

eratively, the right upper lid swelling disappeared and the eye returned to its normal position.

Discussion

Lacrimal gland tumors are mainly devided into epithelial and nonepithelial ones, and most authors state that approximately 50% of lacrimal fossa tumors are of epithelial origin and 50% are of nonepithelial origin. But Shields recently analysed 142 cases of lacrimal gland lesions and reported that non-epithelial lacrimal gland lesions are more common and epithelial malignancies of the lacrimal gland are considerably less common than generally believed (1989). Among the epithelial tumors, the benign mixed tumors are the most common intrinsic lacrimal gland tumors, accounting for approximately 50% of the epithelial tumors (Auran 1988). Cheng reported 56% incidence of benign mixed tumor in 160 cases of primary epithelial tumors (1982). It usually arises from the orbital lobe of the lacrimal gland but the one from the palpebral lobe has been reported by many authors (Murphy & Rodrigues 1974, Auran et al. 1988, Parks & Glover 1990), and the one from ectopic lacrimal gland tissue in the orbit (Mindlin 1977), and aberrant lacrimal gland ploemorphic adenoma within the muscle cone (Mueller 1979) were also reported. It usually occurs in adults but a case in a seven-year-old boy was reported (McPherson 1966). While most of the patients with malignant lacrimal gland tumors experience pain but usually few patients with benign mixed tumor do. Our patient was the exception. On CT, it appears as an oval-shaped, well-circumscribed enhancing mass. Jakobiec (1982) stated that the benign tumors had smooth encapsulated outlines at their margins, whereas the malignant tumors displayed microserrations indicative of infiltration. Enlargement of the lacrimal gland fossa due to pressure erosion of the overlying bone is sometimes observed (Wright et al. 1979). Hornblass et al. reported a case of benign mixed tumor of long standing duration which caused complete erosion of the orbital roof and dura (1981). Echographically, this tumor showed heterogeneous internal structure with pseudocapsule on B-mode (Auran et al. 1988) and low to medium internal reflectivity with sound attenuation on CV-A mode. According to the criteria published by Ossoinig (1974), benign mixed tumor of the lacrimal gland has the echographic characteristics of high to medium internal reflectivity with great sound attenuation. Byrne also reported a case of benign mixed tumor of the same echographic characteristics (1983). In our case, more cellular proliferation and less cystic spaces are considered to be the reason of the low to medium reflectivity. Auran stated benign mixed tumor with a homogeneous matrix without cystic spaces have relatively low internal reflectivity (1988). Concerning the origin for benign mixed tumor, Iwamoto considered a close relationship to the ducts of the lacrimal gland rather than to the acini on electron microscopic studies (1982). A ductal origin for benign mixed tumor has also been suggested in a ultrastructual study of a tumor arising from the palpebral lobe of the lacrimal gland (Auran 1988). The benign mixed tumors, if totally excised, have a good prognosis (Wright 1982, Shields 1987).

The second case was a benign lymphoepithelial lesion. This tumor is a relatively rare non-epithelial lacrimal gland tumor. Meyer et al. reported four cases of Mikulicz's syndrome in their literature entitled 'Differential diagnosis in Mikulicz's syndrome, Mikulicz's disease and similar disease entities' (1971). Considering the clinical findings and laboratory investigations, this patient was suspected of so called 'Mikulicz's disease'. Meyer et al. stated that Mikulicz's disease is a disorder of unknown etiology following benign course, while Mikulicz's syndrome is a symptom complex caused by a variety of systemic disorders and the term 'benign lymphoepithelial lesion' should replace the confusing term Mikulicz's disease. (Meyer, Yanoff & Hanoo 1971; Yanoff & Fine 1982). On echographic examination, this tumor had scattered sonodense spots within the tumor with pseudocapsule on B-mode echogram which may corresponded the internal fibrous septae. But this tumor showed the low internal reflectivity at normal gain setting. This may be due to the homogeneous internal structure of densely packed lymphocytes. Echodense tail was observed which may derived from the secondary dacryoadenitis or cholesterin clefts.

These two tumors showed similar configurations both on CT and MRI and enhancing patterns did not help us to differentiate these tumors, while standardized echography was very useful to differentiate these tumors by internal reflectivity patterns. Balchunas et al. reported CT is of proved value in determining the size, location, and extent of orbital masses, but their appearances are often similar making differentiation between various pathological entities difficult. Further, they found enhancing patterns were generally not helpful in arriving at a diagnosis (1983). Hesselink et al. stated ultrasonography and CT was remarkably complementary, together giving a 97% accuracy in the evaluation of orbital diseases (1979). However there exists malignant tumors which have pseudocapsule and heterogenous internal structure such as an adenoid cystic carcinoma (Byers 1975). Dagher et al. reported a case of adenoid cystic carcinoma which could not be distinguished on echography from a benign mixed tumor (1980). Char (1982) stated no clinical parameters reliably differentiate benign from malignant epithelial lacrimal gland tumors. We also believe it is difficult to predict the malignancy of a tumor by even echography but it is at least possible to know the tissue type diagnosis. Because it is apparent that the tumors were encapsulated on the echogram, we did not perform prior incisional biopy and selected lateral orbitotomy as a surgical procedure (Stewart, Krohel & Wright 1979). Histopathological investigation of two cases of malignant transformation of benign mixed tumors after incomplete excision have been reported by Perzin (1980). If recurrence is suspected, early reoperation is nessesary (Forrest 1971). We are following up the patients carefully for recurrence, especially case 1, because a part of the pseudocapsule had been damaged maybe during the operation.

176

Acknowledgments

The authors would like to acknowlege gratefully to Dr. Inoue who provided the pathologic evaluation and Mr. Kazunori Maeda who took the photographs.

References

Auran, J., Jakobiec, F.A. & Krebs, W. Benign mixed tumor of the palpebral lobe of the lacrimal gland. Ophthalmology 95: 90–99 (1988).

Balchunas, W.R., Quencer, R.M. & Byrne, S.F. Lacrimal gland and fossa masses: Evaluation by computed tomography and A-mode echography. Radiology 149: 751–58 (1983).

Byers, R.M., Berkeley, R.G., Luna, M. & Jesse, R.H. Combined therapeutic approach to malignant lacrimal gland tumors. Am. J. Ophthalmol. 79: 53–55 (1975).

Byrne, S.F. Standardized echography in the differentiation of orbital lesions. Surv. Ophthalmol. 29: 226–28 (1984).

Char, D.H. & Norman, A.D. The use of computed tomography and ultrasonography in the evaluation of orbital masses. Surv. Ophthalmol. 27: 49–63 (1982).

Cheng, C.N., Cheng, S.C., Dryja, T.P. & Cheng, T.Y. Lacrimal gland tumors: A clinico-pathological analysis of 160 cases. Int. Ophthalmol. Clin. 22: 99–120 (1982).

Dagher, G., Anderson, R.L., Ossoinig, K.C. & Baker, J.D. Adenoid cystic carcinoma of the lacrimal gland in a child. Arch. Ophthalmol. 98: 1098–1100 (1980).

Forrest, A.W. Pathological criteria for effective management of epithelial lacrimal gland tumors. Am. J. Ophthalmol. 71: 178–92 (1971).

Henderson, J.W. & Neault, R.W. En bloc removal of intrinsic neoplasms of the lacrimal gland. Am. J. Ophthalmol. 82: 905–910 (1976).

Henderson, J.W. & Farrow, G.M. Primary malignant mixed tumors of the lacrimal gland. Ophthalmology 131: 143–7 (1980).

Hesselink, J.R., Davis, K.R., Dallow, R.L., Roberson, G.H. & Taveras, J.M. Computed tomography of masses in the lacrimal gland region. Radiology 131: 143–7 (1979).

Hornblass, A., Friedman, A.H. & Yogoda, A. Erosion of the orbital plate (frontal bone) by a benign tumor of the lacrimal gland. Ophthalmic Surg. 12: 737–43 (1981).

Iwamoto, T. & Jakobiec, F.A. A comparative ultrastructural study of the normal lacrimal gland and its epithelial tumors. Hum. Pathol. 13: 236–62 (1982).

Jakobiec, F.A., Yeo, J.H., Trokel, S.L., Abbott, G.F. & Anderson, R. Combined clinical and computed tomographic diagnosis of primary lacrimal fossa lesions. Am. J. Ophthalmol. 94: 785–807 (1982).

Marsh, J.L., Wise, D.M., Smith, M. & Schwartz, H. Lacrimal gland adenoid cystic carcinoma: Intracranial and extracranial en bloc resection. Plastic and Reconstructive Surg. 68: 577–85 (1981).

Meyer, D., Yanoff, M. & Hanno, H. Differential diagnosis in Mikulicz's syndrome, Mikulicz's disease, and similar disease entities. Am. J. Ophthalmol. 71: 516–24 (1971).

McPherson, S.D., Jr. Mixed tumor of the lacrimal gland in a seven-year old boy. Am. J. Ophthalmol. 61: 561–3 (1966).

Mindlin, A., Lambeerts, D. & Barsky, D. Mixed lacrimal gland tumor arising from ectopic lacrimal gland tissue in the orbit. J. Ped. Ophthalmol. 14: 44–7 (1979).

Mueller, E.C. & Borit, A. Aberrant lacrimal gland and pleomorphic adenoma within the muscle cone. Ann. Ophthalmol. 11: 661–3 (1979).

Murphy, M.B. & Rodrigues, M.M. Benign mixed tumor of the (palpebral) lacrimal gland presenting as a nodular eyelid lesion. Am. J. Ophthalmol. 77: 108–111 (1974).

Ossoinig, K.C., Blodi, F.C. Preoperative differential diagnosis of tumors with echography, Part

IV: Diagnosis of orbital tumors. In: Blodi, F.C. (ed): Current Concepts of Ophthalmology. St Louis: CV Mosby: 313–41 (1974).

Parks, S.L. & Glover, A.T. Benign mixed tumors arising in the palpebral lobe of the lacrimal gland. Ophthalmology 97: 526–30 (1990).

Perzin, K.H., Jakobiec, F.A., Livolsi, V.A. & Desjardins, A.L. Lacrimal gland malignant mixed tumors. (Carcinomas arising in benign mixed tumors): A clinico-pathologic study. Cancer 45: 2593–2606 (1980).

Shields, J.A., Shields, C.L., Eagle, P.C. & Rizzo, J. Pleomorphic adenoma ('Benign mixed tumor') of the lacrimal gland. Arch. Ophthalmol. 105: 560–1 (1987).

Shields, C.L., Shield, J.A., Eagle, R.C. & Rathmell, J.P. Clinicopathologic review of 142 cases of lacrimal gland lesions. Ophthalmology 96: 431–5 (1989).

Stewart, W.B., Krohel, G.B. & Wright, J.E. Lacrimal gland and fossa lesions: An approach to diagnosis and management. Ophthalmology 86: 886–95 (1979).

Wright, J.E., Stewart, W.B. & Krohel, G.B. Clinical presentation and management of lacrimal gland tumours. Br. J. Ophthalmol. 63: 600–606 (1979).

Wright, J.E. Factors affecting the survival of patients with lacrimal gland tumours. Can. J. Ophthalmol. 17: 3–9 (1982).

Wright, J.E. Lacrimal gland tumours. Trans. Ophthal. Soc. N.Z. 35: 101–6 (1983).

Yanoff, M. & Fine, B.S. Ocular Pathology (2nd ed). p. 605. Philadelphia: Harper & Row (1982).

Address for correspondence: Dept of Ophthalmology, Miyazaki Medical College, 5200 Kihara, Kiyotake, Miyazaki 889-16, Japan.

11. Bilateral orbital and adnexal lymphoma

L. HENČ-PETRINOVIĆ
(*Zagreb, Croatia*)

Introduction

Being of either extranodal presentation of non-Hodgkin's lymphoma or primary orbital lymphoma, lymphoid tumours account for 10 to 15% of space occupying orbital lesions (Shields 1986; Flanders 1987).

An extranodal presentation occurs in about 40% of patients with non-Hodgkin's lymphoma, and orbital location in 5–14% of all extranodal presentations (Bessell et al. 1988; McNally 1987).

The clinic features of slowly enlarging, painless hard resistance is in the majority of cases unilateral, but bilateral lymphoma do occur or become over time, only if we wait long enough (Vogiatzis 1984).

Bilateral lesions are representatives of the same tumor with similar morphologic features and identical immunophenotypic profiles. The patients with bilateral orbital lymphoma do not appear to have an increased incidence of malignant monoclonal disease (McNally 1987).

Computed tomography and magnetic resonance imaging characteristics of orbital lymphoma are relatively nonspecific (Krahe et al. 1987; Atlas et al. 1987).

Standardized echography provides data about exact location, extent and tissue differentiation of orbital tumors (Till et al. 1985). Well circumscribed orbital mass with acoustic hollowness and good sound transmission with oval contours molding to the surface of the eyeball and orbital bone is a typical echographic picture of orbital lymphoma.

To determine the nature of the orbital lesion, surgical biopsy specimen analysis is indispensable. Histopathologic criteria supported by immunophenotypic analysis provide diagnostic and prognostic data (Knowles et al. 1979; Bennett et al. 1985).

The location of previous nonocular non Hodgkin's lymphoma is mostly to the lymph nodes but extranodal location also occurs as is the case in the first of the patients to be presented.

P. Till (ed.), Ophthalmic Echography 13, pp. 179–183.
© 1993 *Kluwer Academic Publishers*.

180

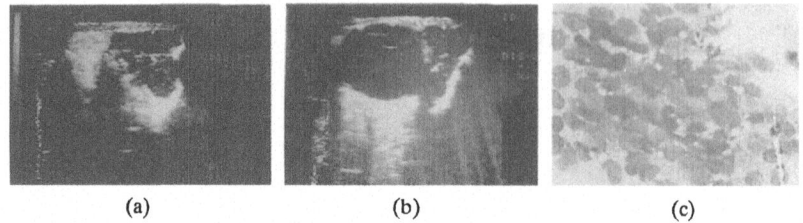

Fig. 1. Non-Hodgkin's lymphoma; a) echographic picture with parabulbar presentation of low reflective, well outlined orbital echo defect, right orbit; b) similar picture in the left orbit; c) biopsy specimen histopathologic picture was also the same for both orbits as well as for previous lung tumor-immunocytoma.

Patients and methods

In December 1986 a 35-year-old patient had thoracotomy and lobectomy due to the lung tumor identified as immunocytoma. Follow-up in the next year disclosed no pathology other than higher IgM.

Twenty months later CT scanning without pathologic finding but bone marrow biopsy specimen was positive with nodular infiltration of lymphoplasmocytoid cells. Immunoelectrophoresis with IgM still higher.

At the same time bilateral eyelid swelling occured causing diplopia, positive Lancaster test and low reflective orbital echo defects indicating bilateral orbital infiltration.

The defects were well outlined, non compressable tumors in the superotemporal aspects of both orbits with no signs of bone destruction (Fig. 1a,b).

Biopsy of both orbits with cytology and histopathology results being the same as for previous lung tumor-immunocytoma. Immunophenotypic analysis was performed by immunoperoxidase staining. Monotonous picture of lymphoplasmocytoid cells (Fig. 1c). Immunohistochemistry: PAP method positivity to kappa light chains of immunoglobulin, consistent with monoclonal proliferation. The patient was treated with steroid and cytostatic therapy without further changes in the three years' follow-up period.

The other patient, a 60-year-old man, was referred to the ophthalmologist due to bilateral upper eyelid swelling. A general survey revealed cervical adenopathy.

Surgical biopsy specimen analysis of lymph nodes and palpebral infiltrates gave the same result as bone marrow biopsy: non-Hodgkin's lymphoma.

Orbital echography revealed bilateral palpebral low reflective hard, well outlined masses, while the picture of biopsy specimen consisted of monotonous lymphoplasmocytoid infiltration and immunoperoxidase studies suggested that it was a monoclonal lesion (Fig. 2a,b). Corticosteroid and cytostatic treatment resulted in regression of the palpebral infiltrations.

The problem of clinical, radiographic and echographic methods in discerning lymphoma among other low reflective orbital lesions will be illustrated by another two cases.

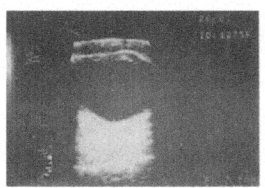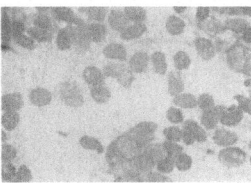

Fig. 2. Non-Hodgkin's lymphoma; a) echographic picture with low reflective infiltrates in both upper eyelids; b) biopsy specimen analysis with the same result for both eyelids as well as for cervical lymph nodes – monotonous lymphoplasmocytoid infiltration.

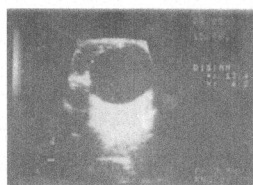

Fig. 3. Epibulbar amyloidosis: a) bilateral epibulbar hard mass showing low reflectivity, sharp contours, molding to the surface of the eyeball; b) surgical biopsy specimen analysis showing extracellular accumulation of amyloid (congo-rot staining).

The first one is a 57-year-old woman with bilateral low reflective epibulbar and orbital hard masses. Unilateral biopsy was done and histopathology confirmed amyloidosis. Congo rot staining revealed extracellular accumulation of amyloid. Further clinical work-up disclosed liver involvement with amyloid accumulation in the portal region. Echographic pictures with low reflective, well outlined epibulbar masses and histopathologic findings are presented in Fig. 3a,b. Two years of follow-up discovered no further changes in clinical as well as in echographic studies.

The other patient, with parabulbar low reflective well-outlined orbital echo defect in the upper temporal quadrant of the right orbit and indolent low reflective infiltration of the left lower lid, was subjected to clinical examination and biopsy analysis of both infiltrations. The histopathologic result was plasmocytoma on both sites (Fig. 4a,b,c). The distribution of lymphoma infiltrations was similar, orbital on one side and palpebral on the other as described by Mamalis (1988).

Immunohistochemistry showed that the lesion specifically expressed immunoglobulin lambda light chain and immunoglobulin A-chain. The patient remained well almost three years with the process localized to the right orbit and left lower eyelid.

182

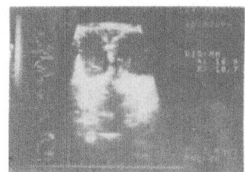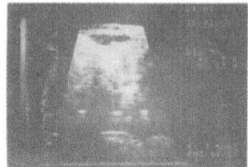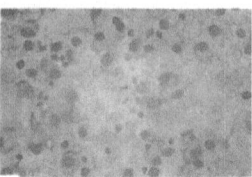

Fig. 4. Orbital plasmocytoma: a) low reflective, well outlined echo defect in the upper temporal quadrant of the right orbit; b) similar low reflective infiltration of the left lower eyelid; c) surgical biopsy specimen analysis disclosed plasma cell infiltration, the same on both sides.

Discussion and conclusion

The presented bilateral orbital and adnexal immunocytoma is histo- and cyto-morphologically as well as immunologically identical to the previous tumor, extranodal lung tumor in the first patient, and nodal in the second – representing separate deposits of the same neoplasm.

In spite of its monoclonality-indicating malignancy, the clinical course in our patients is, up to now, slow and indolent. Diagnostic value of clinical, radiologic, echographic and magnetic resonance imaging techniques are limited in discerning lymphoid orbital neoplasms concerning their benign or malignant nature because orbital pseudotumors as well as some other tumorous lesions such as presented plasmocytoma and orbital amylidosis fullfil almost the same criteria.

However echography is the easiest method of detecting of orbital and adnexal lymphoid infiltration indicating further clinical work-up.

Histo- and cyto-morphologic as well as immunohistologic techniques are being used in hope of discerning benign and malignant lesions, but classification and predictability of clinical behaviour of orbital lymphomas continue to be a problem.

References

1. Atlas, S.W., Bilaniuk L.T., Zimmerman, R.A., Hackney, D.B., Goldberg, H.I. & Grossman, R.I. Orbit: Initial experience with surface coil spin-echo MR Imaging at 1,5 T. Radiology 510–509 (1987).
2. Bennett, C.L., Petterman, A., Bitran, J.D., Recant, W., Shapiro, C.M., Karesh, J. & Kalokhe, U. Staging and therapy of orbital lymphomas. Cancer 1204–1208 (1986).
3. Bessel E.M., Henk, J.M., Wright, J.E. & Whitelocke, R.A.F. Orbital and conjunctival lymphoma treatment and prognosis. Radiotherapy and Oncology 237–244 (1988).
4. Flanders, A.E., Espinosa, G.A., Markiewicz, D.A. & Howll, D.D. Orbital lymphoma, Role of CT and MRI. Radiologic Clinics of North America. 601–613 (1987).
5. Krahe, Th., Koster, O., Trier, H.G., Lackner, K. & Flatten, M. Computertomograpie primärer and sekundärer Tumoren des Auges and der Orbit. Fortschr. Rontgenstr. 599–606 (1987).
6. Mamalis, N., Mackman, G., Holds, J.B., Anderson, R.L., Apple, D.J. & Scholes, G.

Simultaneous bilateral conjunctival and orbital lymphoma presenting as a conjunctival lesion. Ophthalmic Surgery 662–663 (1988).

7. McNally, L., Jakobiec, F.A. & Knowles, D.M. Clinical, morphologic, immunophenitypic and molecular genetic analysis of bilateral ocular adnexal lymophoid neoplasms in 17 patients. Am. J. Ophthalmol. 555–568 (1987).
8. Shields, J.A., Cooper, H., Donoso, L.A., Augsburger, J.J. & Arbizo, V. Immunohistochemical and ultrastructural study of unusual IgM lambda lymphoplasmocytic tumor of the lacrimal gland. Am. J. Ophthalmol. 451–457 (1986).
9. Till, P., Steinkogler, F.J. & Hauff, W. Die Bedeutung der echographischen Gewebsdifferenzierung für die Orbitachirurgie. Klin. Mbl. Augenheilk. 296–299 (1985).
10. Vogiatzis, K.V. Lymphoid tumors of the orbit and ocular adnexa. A long-term follow-up. Ann. Ophthalmol. 1036–1055 (1984).

Address for correspondence: Ophthalmology Department, General Hospital 'Sueti Duh', Sueti Duh 64, 41000 Zagreb, Croatia.

12. Unusual orbital mucocele

J. McADAM, W.A.J. VAN HEUVEN & K.S. HELD
(San Antonio, USA)

Abstract. An orbital muco(pyo)cele is described as a cystic lesion that has invaded the orbit by eroding the bony wall. Based on acoustic characteristics typical for mucocele, the sensitivity of Standardized Echography in correctly diagnosing this lesion reaches 97.6% [1]. Ultrasound, being noninvasive and of relatively low cost, should usually be the first choice in diagnostic tools. However, in atypical cases, such as the one presented here, the typical echographic diagnostic features may be altered or absent, and other diagnostic modalities must be combined with ultrasound in order to make the correct diagnosis.

Introduction

Mucoceles represent 2–15% [1–3] of all invasive orbital masses. Adults in the 4th to 7th decades are most often affected [2], and a unilateral exophthalmos is usually the first ophthalmic sign. Although a history of chronic sinus inflammation or past trauma is often present, other formation factors include metastasis (especially squamous cell carcinoma of the ethmoid), surgery of the sinuses, sinus polyps, and allergies. The average duration of symptoms (proptosis, headache, visual disturbances) is ten months.

Mucocele formation is usually thought to be due to the entrapment of secretory epithelium [2] and subsequent filling of the sinus cavity, most often the ethmoid. The progressively increasing pressure of the retained mucus on the bony structures causes thinning, erosion of the bony wall and extension of the cyst into the orbit, with displacement of orbital soft tissues. The majority of mucoceles contain a clear sterile fluid (mucoid) [2], leading to the characteristic acoustic pattern. Secondary infection of the cyst is termed pyocele which cannot be reliably differentiated from the sterile condition by ultrasound. Spontaneous fluid drainage with air replacement or air entrapment during progressive formation (aerocele) [5] can occur that can compromise the echographic examination. Hemorrhage within mucoceles is rare [2] and can be associated with cholesterol crystals.

Standardized echographic diagnosis of orbital muco(pyo)celes consists of ten acoustic criteria [1]: low internal reflectivity, regular internal structure, weak sound attenuation, supero-nasal location (most often), sharply defined borders, rounded shape, lack of mobility, no vascularity, hard consistency (orbital portion can be soft), and presence of a bony defect. Nasr [5] lists four characteristics as being sufficient for pathognomonic diagnosis: regular

P. Till (ed.), Ophthalmic Echography 13, pp. 185–191.

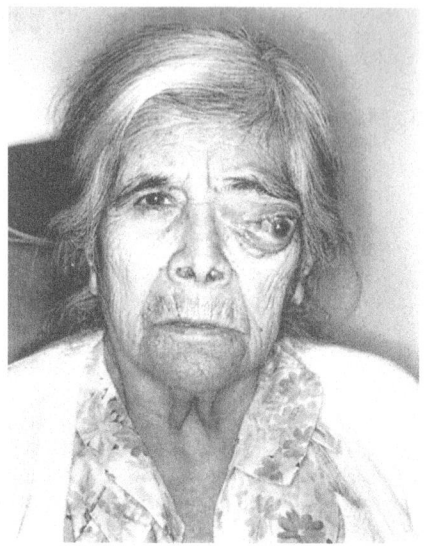

Fig. 1. A 20-year history of slowly progressive proptosis resulted in massive inferior and temporal displacement of the left eye with 19 mm of exophtholmos.

internal structure, low reflectivity, sharply-outlined shape with cyst walls, and a typical (supero-nasal orbit/ethmoid) location. Rootman [2] describes mucoceles as having few internal echoes, good sound transmission, good definition of the far wall, and a smooth rounded outline. Other cyst-like masses which may be included in the differential diagnosis are dermoid cyst, aneurysmal bone cyst, eosinophilic granuloma, and cholesteatoma. Lesions with debris may show internal echoes and appear as solid lesions. When ultrasound shows an internal structure with irregularity, a solid tumor (such as carcinoma) should be suspected [1].

Case report

On 10/17/89, a 72-year-old Hispanic female was referred with severe left exophthalmos, poor vision, and occasional pain. The patient had a 20-year history of slowly progressive proptosis and decreasing vision; she stated that recent gall bladder surgery seemed to worsen her eye condition. She was taking medication for hypertension and congestive heart failure, but denied any history of cancer, other systemic illnesses, or trauma.

External examination revealed a slightly obese Hispanic female with massive disfiguring proptosis of the left eye (19 mm by Hertel exophthalmometry), causing exposure keratitis (Fig. 1). Globe displacement was inferior and temporal by a large, palpable, superior medial orbital mass. The mass was without bruit or pulsation, and ocular motility was only mildly restricted.

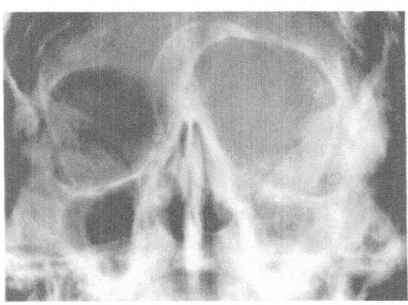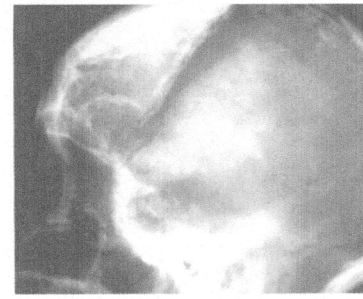

a
b

Fig. 2. (a) Frontal (Caldwell) X-ray projection shows enlargement of left orbit and opacification of left sinuses. (b) Lateral X-ray projection shows the roof of the lesion expanding into the cranial fossa.

Best corrected visual acuity was 20/50+ in the right eye and hand motion at one foot in the left eye. Pressures were 10 and 15 mm Hg. The left visual field showed generalized constriction, and fundoscopic exam showed some optic atrophy, but no choroidal folds. There was a left 2+ afferent pupillary defect, as well as a preauricular node. Laboratory tests were consistent with her congestive heart failure. Plain x-ray films, orbital echography, CAT scan, MRI scan, and angiography were obtained in addition to neurosurgical and otolaryngological consultation.

X-ray films showed enlargement and extensive remodeling of the left orbit with erosion of the normal bony structures and opacification of the adjacent sinuses (Fig. 2). Normal orbital landmarks were obliterated on the left, indicating extensive tumor growth.

Standardized echography was done using the Biophysic Ophthascan S and the Kretztechnik 7200MA equipment. A very large, firm mass with irregular internal structure and low- to- medium internal reflectivity was detected in the supero-nasal quadrant of the left orbit. The lesion extended from the anterior orbit to beyond machine resolution posteriorly with globe indentation and either nerve displacement or compression (Fig. 3). The sound attenuation was medium to strong (Fig. 4), and at least two small areas of increased echo intensity with posterior shadowing were detected in the posterior portion of the mass (suggestive for calcium). Due to the large size of the lesion, its borders as well as the demonstration of a discrete bony defect, i.e. the 'see-saw' effect [1], were difficult to assess. Doppler testing was negative, although A-scan detected a very anterior area of possible vascularity.

Based on the internal irregularity, medium to strong sound attenuation, and low to medium internal reflectivity, a suspicion was present for a solid tumor (Fig. 5). The recent history of a sudden increase in symptoms suggested hemorrhage or malignancy. Included in the differential diagnosis were dermoid cyst, lymphangioma, meningioma, and muco(pyo)cele.

A CAT scan of the head and orbits (Fig. 6), with and without contrast,

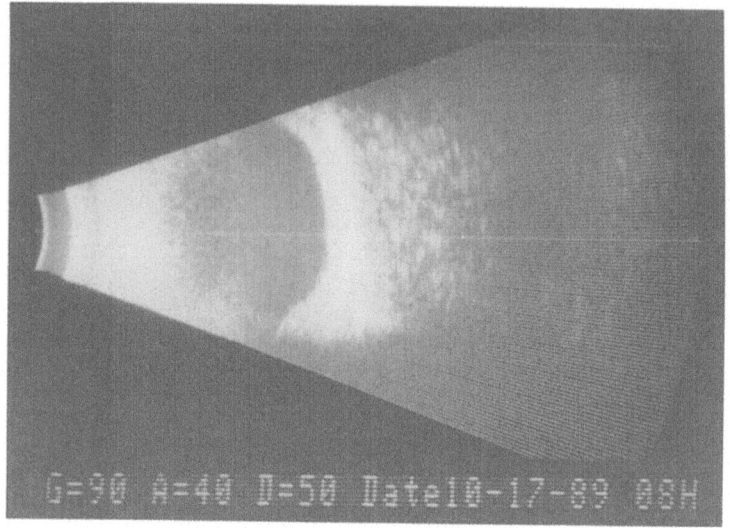

Fig. 3. B-scan shows a very large mass indenting the posterior nasal globe.

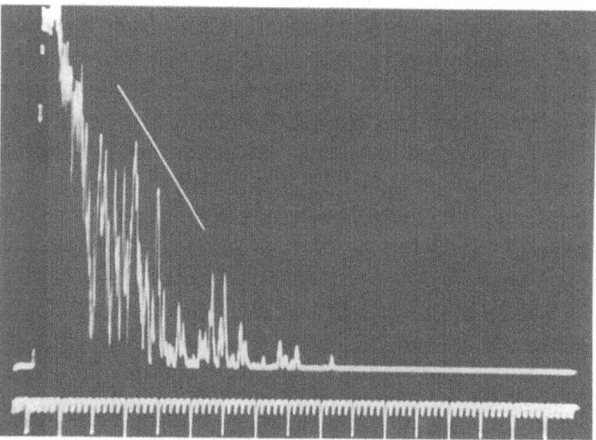

Fig. 4. A-scan demonstrates medium to high sound attenuation (slope of slanted line).

revealed a cystic lesion with ring calcification in the nasal cavity and superior intracranial extension with associated calcium. The cribiform plate was under apparent compression. The differential diagnosis was mucocele from the ethmoid sinus, benign intracranial tumor, and cribiform neuroblastoma.

The MRI scan showed one large mixed-signal intensity mass with ring calcification and areas of hemorrhage involving the paranasal sinus, with intracranial extension. It was suspicious for mucocele. Strong signal intensity

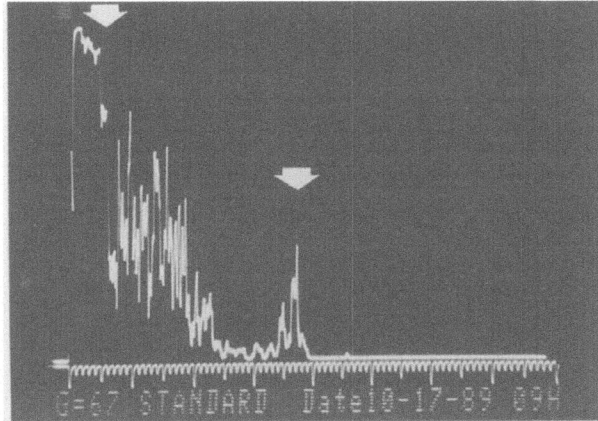

Fig. 5. The Standardized A-scan shows low to medium internal reflectivity and variable irregularity of the internal structure. Arrow indicates posterior tumor border.

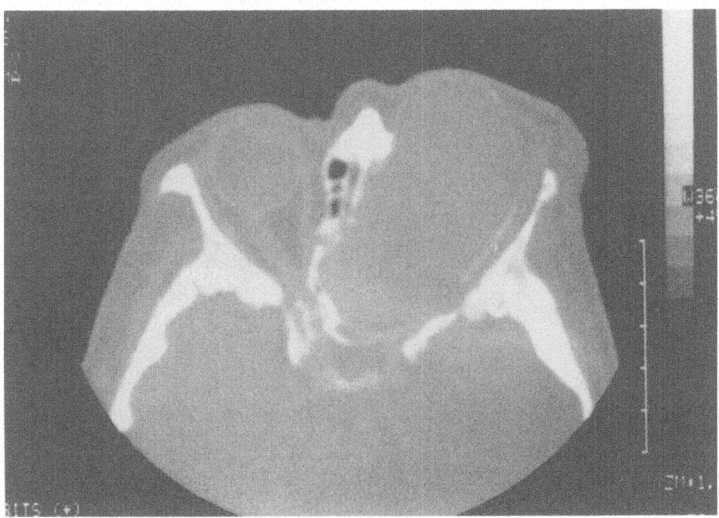

Fig. 6. The axial CAT scan displays an expansile lesion on the left, with globe displacement and obliteration of the ethmoid sinus.

and enhancement, compatible with fat, raised the possibility of a dermoid (Fig. 7).

Differential diagnosis at that time included mucocele (most likely), giant thrombosed aneurysm, cavernous hemangioma, dermoid, meningioma, neuroasthesioma, and lymphangioma. Subsequent angiography showed no tumor vascularity or vascular encasement and displacement of the anterior cerebral artery and left ophthalmic artery.

190

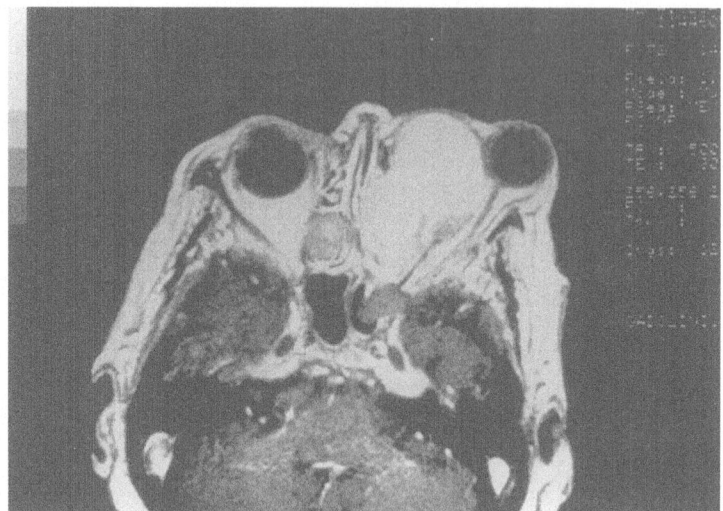

Fig. 7. The axial MRI through the middle of the orbit shows strong signal intensity of the lesion. Note the long stretched optic nerve (black).

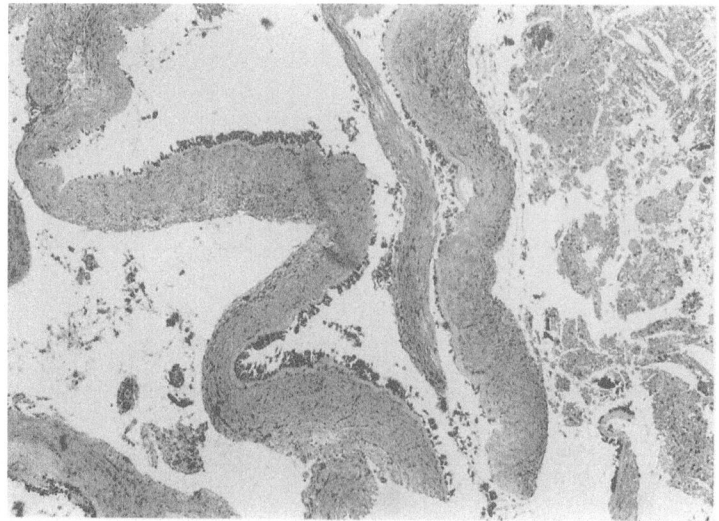

Fig. 8. Pathologic specimen shows a cystic structure lined with respiratory mucosa.

The patient underwent a left frontal osteoplastic craniotomy and exenteration of the cystic mass, a dural patch graft, and placement of a spinal epidural drain. The pathology specimens were consistent with mucocele and were notable for inflammatory and fibrotic tissue (Fig. 8). Areas of old hemorrhage with cholesterol formation were interspersed with thick, yellow-ish-brown, jelly-like mucoid secretions.

Discussion

We have described an atypical mucocele. Both it's longstanding presence and the hemorrhage within it probably contributed to it's unusual history, appearance, and echographic characteristics. These varied significantly from most mucoceles which can usually be diagnosed by echography alone. Thus, ophthalmic B-scan and Standardized A-scan, which are quick, low cost, and portable, are sufficient to make the correct diagnosis in most cases and should always be utilized first. Only in complex cases, such as the one presented here, are x-ray, CAT scan, and MRI also needed in order to reach the correct diagnosis.

Acknowledgement

Supported by a unrestricted research grant from Research to Prevent Blindness, Inc., NY.

References

1. Hasenfratz, G. & Ossoinig, K.C. The diagnosis of orbital mucoceles and pyoceles with standardized echography. In: Hillman, J.S. & LeMay, M.M. (eds.), Doc. Ophthalmol. Proc. Ser. 38: 407–415. The Hague: Dr. W. Junk (1983).
2. Rootman, J. Diseases of the Orbit, A Multidisciplinary Approach. pp. 496–502. Philadelphia: J.B. Lippincott Co. (1988).
3. Shields, J.A. Diagnosis and Management of Orbital Tumors. pp. 113–15. Philadelphia: W.B. Saunders Co. (1989).
4. Kaltreider, S.A. & Dortzbach, R.K. Destructive cysts of the maxillary sinus affecting the orbit. Arch. Opthalmol. 106: 1398–1402 (1988).
5. Nasr, A.M. & Ipektchi, A. The diagnosis of an aerocele with standardized echography. orbit (Amsterdam) 3: 275–280 (1984).
6. Johnson, L.N., Krohel, G.B., Yeon, E.B. & Parnes, S.M. Sinus tumors invading the Orbit. Ophthalmology 91: 209–217 (1984).

Address for correspondence: The University of Texas, Health Science Center at San Antonio, 7703 Floyd Curl Drive, San Antonio TX 78284-6230, USA.

13. Importance of ultrasound diagnostics in lacrimal sac disease

M. VÉGH & J. NÉMETH

(Szeged and Budapest, Hungary)

Abstract. Ultrasound examination can be used routinely in the diagnostics of diseases of the lacrimal sac, to indicate operation and to control the condition after the operation, in most cases without other expensive and more complex diagnostic methods. A new examination method has been devised, in which a rubber tube filled with fluid is placed between the transducer and the skin surface. This technique can be carried out as easily as the direct contact method, and the quality of the echograms is as good as in the water bath method. Special advantages are that the examinations are very easy, especially in cases of children, and infection of the patient with the ultrasound probe can be avoided.

Introduction

As concerns the lacrimal apparatus, a number of works are known about the ultrasound diagnosis of lacrimal gland patholgy, but it is not often used in the diagnostics of the lacrimal drainage system (Oksala 1959; Ossoinig 1966; Scott et al. 1979; Mazzeo 1981; Montanara et al. 1981; Rochels et al. 1982; Weinstein et al. 1982; Reibaldi 1987; Végh et al. 1988b; Buschmann 1989; Dutton 1989). Most ophthalmologic ultrasound equipment is suitable in the diagnostics of the lacrimal sac diseases.

In our department, ultrasound examinations have been used in everyday practice for 4 years. We have devised a new examination method (Végh and Németh 1988a; Végh and Németh 1988b). This paper presents the results of our examinations of the lacrimal sac by means of echography.

Material and methods

The ages of the patients varied in a wide range. The examinations were made with an Ultrascan Digital B™ System IV (Cooper Vision), at 10 MHz. We used our own new examination method (Végh and Németh 1988a; Végh and Németh 1988b) in which a water-filled sterilized rubber tube 30–40 mm wide, 30–40 mm high and 80 mm long was applied between the transducer and the skin surface. The examinations were performed on patients lying on their back with their eyes closed. The upper part of the rubber tube and the medial lid region of the skin were coated with 2% methylcellulose solution to attain a better contact. The ultrasound probe was fixed on the upper part

P. Till (ed.), Ophthalmic Echography 13, pp. 193–197.
© 1993 *Kluwer Academic Publishers.*

of the rubber tube, adjusted in the correct direction for the examination. For differential diagnosis the following methods have been used:

a) pressure test;

b) a repeat examination on the filling up and rinsing out of the cavity of the lacrimal sac.

A- and B-scan echograms were recorded on video-tape and pictures were copied by a Mitsubishi Video Copy Processor, Model P60B.

Results

Anatomical disorders were detected in 2 cases (diverticulum and congenital absence of lacrimal sac), mucocele in 3 cases, inflammation in 72 cases, and tumor (histology: adenocarcinoma) in 1 case; in the surrounding tissue dermoid cyst in 2 cases, hemangioma in 1 case, granuloma (histology: pyogenic granuloma) in 1 case, and inflammation with abscess in 2 cases.

Discussion

The ophthalmologic ultrasound equipment can be used in the diagnostics of the diseases of the lacrimal sac and the upper part of the nasolacrimal duct (Végh et al. 1988a; Végh et al. 1988b). Our results indicate that ultrasound diagnostics is very informative in the diagnostics of the lacrimal sac, in most cases without to need for other expensive diagnostic methods. It gives the possibility to differentiate an inflammation from a tumor (Rochels et al. 1987). In complicated cases, for differential diagnosis dacryocystography (Radnót and Gáll 1966; Denffer et al. 1981; Montanara et al. 1983; Steinkogler et al. 1987) and computed tomography (Nishimoto et al. 1981) or computed tomographic dacryocystography (Zinreich et al. 1990) examinations are very important before the surgical treatment. Furthermore echography helps in the clinical follow-up of surgery of the lacrimal drainage system (Mazzeo 1981; Rochels et al. 1984; Reibaldi 1987; Végh et al. 1988a; Végh et al. 1988b; Dutton 1989). After Toti operations, the bone window is well detectable, and in cases of failed operations the membrane-like obstruction is also detectable.

In ultrasound diagnostics of the lacrimal sac diseases, the following methods were earlier used: direct contact (Oksala 1959; Rochels 1984), water bath (Coleman et al. 1969; Okamoto 1983) and transocular contact (Ossoinig 1966; Rochels et al. 1984). The examinations with the direct method are easy: the probe is placed directly on the medial lid region, but the echograms of the wall closer to the skin surface are not clear in most cases (Fig. 1). The water bath method is not so easy to carry out as the direct contact method, especially in examinations of children, but the wall closer to the skin surface can be seen well. The distance from the skin can also readily be measured. Use of this method is more difficult after the operation, when

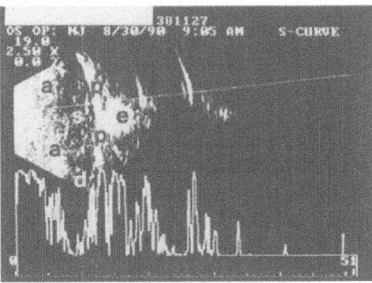

Fig. 1. A- and B-scans of acute dacryocystitis with fistulization, using the direct contact method. The posterior wall (p) of the lacrimal sac, the discharge within (s), and the initial part of the ductus nasolacrimalis (d) are well visible, but the wall closer to the skin surface (a) is not clearly visible. The phlogistic process in the ethmoidal air cells (e), is also well visible (histology of the ethmoidal pathology: pyogenic granuloma).

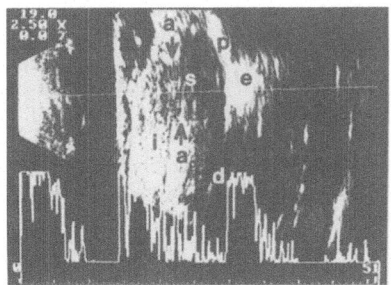

Fig. 2. A- and B-scans of chronic dacryocystitis, using the rubber tube method. The anterior (a) and posterior (p) walls of the lacrimal sac, the discharge within (s), and the initial part of the ductus nasolacrimalis (d) are well visible. The site of fistulization (arrows), and the phlogistic process in the skin (i) and in the ethmoidal cells (e) are also clearly visible (histology of the ethmoidal pathology: pyogenic granuloma). The distance from the skin surface could be measured.

the skin of the wound may become softened by water. In the transocular contact method, the probe is placed on the anesthetized conjunctiva in the lateral palpebral fissure; only the A-scan echogram is available, because of the size of the B probe. For the patient this method is not comfortable, especially in examinations of children. We have devised a new examination method (Végh and Németh 1988a; Végh and Németh 1988b), in which a rubber tube filled with water is placed between the transducer and the skin surface. This method can be carried out as easily as the direct contact method, and the quality of the echograms is as good as in the water bath method (Fig. 2). Special advantages are that the examination is more comfortable, especially in children, and infection of the patient with the ultrasound probe can be avoided.

196

References

1. Buschmann, W. Erkrankungen der ableitenden Tränenwege. In: Buschmann, W. & Trier, H.G. (eds.), Ophthalmologische Ultraschalldiagnostik. pp. 288–289. Berlin: Springer-Verlag (1989).
2. Coleman, D.J., Koenig, W.F. & Katz, L. A hand operated ultrasound scan system for ophthalmic evaluation. Am. J. Ophthalmol. 68: 256–263 (1969).
3. Denffer, H.V., Gullotta, U. & Dressler, J. Dakryozystographie und Radionukliddakryographie. In: Hanselmayer, H. (ed.), Neue Erkenntnise über Erkrankungen der Tränenwege. Bücherei des Augenarztes. Vol. 84. pp. 19–29. Stuttgart: Enke (1981).
4. Dutton, J.J. Standardized echography in the lacrimal drainage dysfunction. Arch. Ophthalmol. 107: 1010–1012 (1989).
5. Mazzeo, V. Some less important use of ultrasound in ophthalmology. In: Thijssen, JM & Verbeek, A.M. (eds.), Ultrasonography in Ophthalmology. Doc. Ophthalmol. Proc. Ser. 29: 399–403. The Hague: Dr. W. Junk (1981).
6. Montanara, A., Mannino, G., Scorcia, G. et al. Studio ecografico del sacco lacrimale. Clin Ocul Patologia Oculare 2: 377–382. (1981). Loc cit: Montanara, A., Mannino, G. & Contestabiles M.T. Macrodacryocystography and echography in diagnosis of disorders of the lacrimal pathways. Surv. Ophthalmol. 28: 33–41 (1983).
7. Montanara, A., Mannino, G. & Contestabile, M.T. Macrodacryocystography and echography in diagnosis of disorders of the lacrimal pathways. Surv. Ophthalmol. 28: 33–41 (1983).
8. Nishimoto, Y., Baba, Y., Shibata, H. & Sawada, A. Combination of echography with coronal CT in the diagnosis of orbital disorders. In: Thijssen, J.M. & Verbeek, A.M. (eds.), Ultrasonography in Ophthalmology. Doc. Ophthalmol. Proc. Ser. 29: 301–316. The Hague: Dr. W. Junk (1981).
9. Okamoto, H. A simplified water immersion method using a thin film. In: Hillmann, J.S. & Le May, M.M. (eds.), Ophthalmic ultrasonography. Doc. Ophthalmol. Proc. Ser. 38: 387–493. The Hague: Dr. W. Junk (1983).
10. Oksala A. Diagnosis by ultrasound in acute dacryocystitis. Acta Ophthalmol. (Kbh) 37: 176–179 (1959).
11. Ossoinig, K. Die Ultraschalldiagnostik der Orbita. Mbl. Augenheilk. 149: 817–839 (1966).
12. Radnót, M. & Gáll, J. Die Röntgendiagnostik der tränenableitenden Wege. Budapest: Akadémiai Kiadó (1966).
13. Reibaldi, A., Avitabile, G.L., Scuderi, G.L. & Lorusso, V.V. Echography in the lacrimal apparatus diagnosis. In: Ossoinig, K.C. (ed.), Ophthalmic echography. Doc. Opthalmol. Proc. Ser. 48: 553–556. Dordrecht: Dr. W. Junk (1987).
14. Rochels, R. & Hackelbusch, R. B-Bild-Echographie bei Erkrankungen der ableitenden Tränenwege. Klin. Mbl. Augenheilk. 181: 181–183 (1982).
15. Rochels, R., Lieb, W., & Nover, A. Echographische Diagnostik bei Erkrankungen der ableitenden Tränenwege. Klin. Mbl. Augenheilk. 185: 243–249 (1984).
16. Rochels, R., Scherer, U., Nover, A. & Lieb, W. Echographical diagnosis of lacrimal sac tumors. In: Ossoinig K.C. (ed.), Ophthalmic echography. Doc. Ophthalmol. Proc. Ser. 48: 545–552. Dordrecht: Dr. W. Junk (1987).
17. Scott, W.E., Fabre, J.A. & Ossoinig, K.C. Congenital mucocele of the lacrimal sac. Arch. Ophthalmol. 97: 1656–1658 (1979).
18. Steinkogler, F.J., Karnel, F. & Canigiani, G. Die digitale Dacryozystographie. Klin. Mbl. Augenheilk. 191: 55–57 (1987).
19. Végh, M., Németh J. & Bordás, P. A könnyelvezetö rendszer ultrahangvizsgálata. Szemészet 125: 90–95 (1988a).
20. Végh, M., Németh, J. & Bordás, P. Dacryocystography or echography. Orbit (Amsterdam) 7: 191–195 (1988b).
21. Végh, M. & Németh, J. A new device in ultrasound diagnostics of the lacrimal sac. Orbit (Amsterdam) 7: 197–200 (1988a).
22. Végh, M. & Németh, J. Új segédeszköz a saccus lacrimalis és ductus nasolacrimalis ultrahanggal való vizsgálatára. Szemészet 125: 116–120 (1988b).

23. Weinstein, G.S., Biglan, A.W. & Patterson, J.H. Congenital lacrimal sac mucoceles. Am. J. Ophthalmol. 94: 106–110 (1982).
24. Zinreich, S.J., Miller, N.R., Freeman, L.N., Glorioso, L.W. & Rosenbaum, A.E. Computed tomographic dacryocystography using topical contrast media for lacrimal system visualization. Orbit (Amsterdam) 9: 79–87 (1990).

Address for correspondence: Department of Opthalmology, Albert Szent-Györgyi Medical University, P.O. Box 407, H-6701 Szeged, Hungary

14. Standardized echography in a case of orbital varix

H.R. Atta
(Aberdeen, UK)

Standardized Echography is a useful imaging technique in the differentiation of orbital vascular lesions. By employing the topographic, quantitative and kinetic methods of examination as described by Ossoinig (Byrne, Glaser 1983) an accurate and reliable 'Tissue Diagnosis' can often be made of these lesions (Ossoinig 1981).

A case of Orbital Varix (Primary Venous Malformation) in a young patient is described and the echographic appearance is presented. The usefulness of Valsalva test in securing the diagnosis is highlighted.

Case presentation

A twenty-nine year-old male, caucasian, presented with a twelve year history of intermittent right proptosis and red subconjunctival mass (Fig. 1). On presentation in 1979 a limited biopsy of the lesion was obtained from its anterior portion. Histologically this was reported as 'Non-specific Vascular

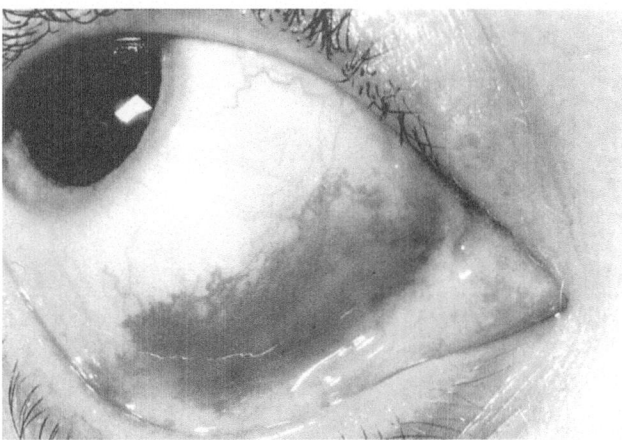

Fig. 1. Clinical appearance of orbital varix. A sheet of tortuous vascular channels and hemorrhage are seen subconjunctivally.

P. Till (ed.), Ophthalmic Echography 13, pp. 199–203.
© 1993 Kluwer Academic Publishers.

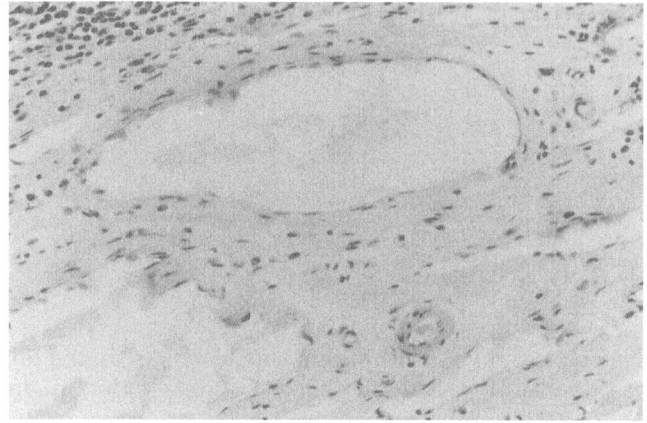

Fig. 2. Histological appearance of a biopsy of the subconjunctival lesion. Large endothelial lined, thin walled, vascular channel is seen. Lumen containing scanty amount of blood. Courtesy of Dr. G. Scott, University of Aberdeen.

Connective Tissue' (Fig. 2). In 1980 the patient received an orbital MRI examination using one of the earliest machines developed in the University of Aberdeen. This clearly demonstrated an abnormal soft tissue mass in the right orbit but tissue diagnosis was not then available (Fig. 3).

Over the ensuing years recurring episodes of proptosis, painful at times was recorded but in between attacks the eyes appeared normal with preservation of normal vision. In 1989 the patient was referred for echographic examination in an attempt to achieve tissue diagnosis.

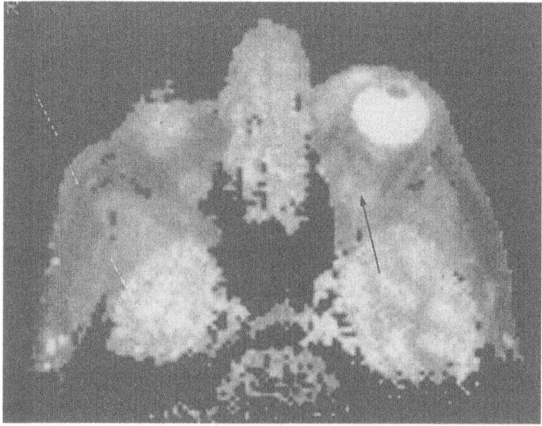

Fig. 3. MRI examination showing an abnormal retrobulbar soft-tissue mass lesion (arrow). Courtesy of Dr. F. Smith, University of Aberdeen.

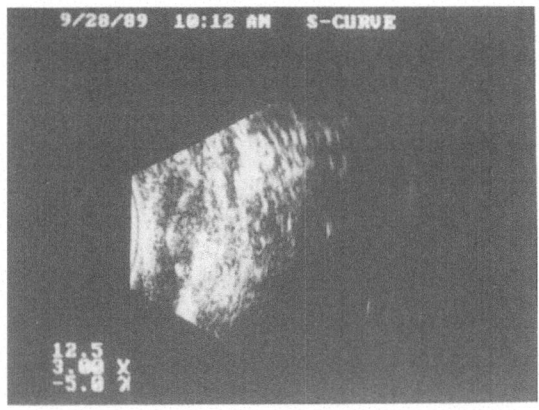

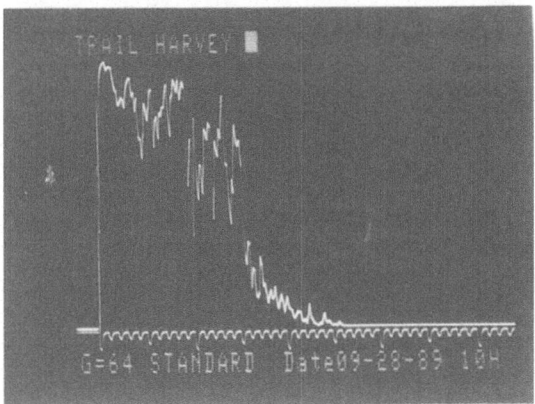

Fig. 4. Paraocular B-Scan (top) and A-Scan (bottom) of the supranasal aspect of right orbit before valsalva manoeuvre. Slight widening of orbital fat pattern was noted but no defect was seen.

Echographic findings

A lesion best seen on 'Para-ocular Examination' was found in the supranasal aspect of the right orbit (Figs. 4 and 5). Compared to the corresponding area in the left orbit there was widening and slight irregularity of the echo-pattern. On valsalva manoeuvre a wide, sharply oulined vascular channel became apparent showing low reflectivity, weak sound attenuation and no detectable blood flow. The lesion was easily compressable and collapsed readily on repeated valsalva manoeuvre. The extra-ocular muscles and optic nerves appeared normal and symmetrical to that on the left side. The echographic findings were consistent with the diagnosis of an Orbital Varix. The histological specimen, obtained in 1979, was revised and was considered compatible with such a diagnosis.

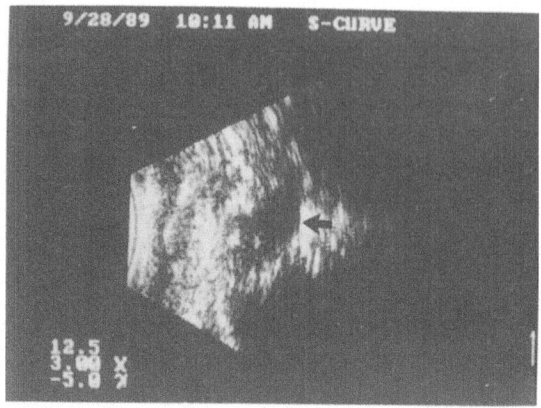

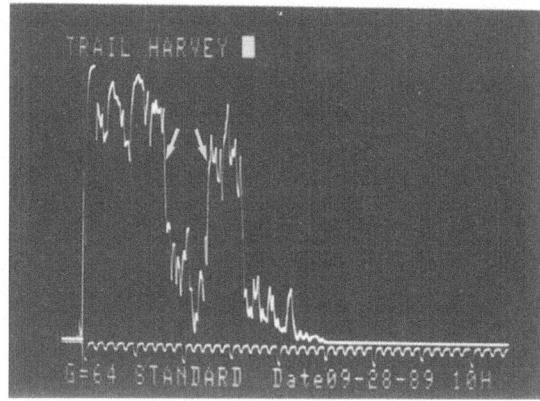

Fig. 5. Same examination as in Figure 4 during valsalva manoeuvre. A large dark 'vascular' channel is apparent on B-Scan (top) (arrow) and a sharply outlined, low reflective defect is seen on A-Scan (bottom) (arrows). No vascularity was noted on kinetic examination.

Table 1. Echographic features of orbital vascular lesions

	Orbital varix	A–V fistula	Lymphangioma
Shape	Enlarged vessel	Enlarged vessel	Irregular channels
Borders	Sharp	Sharp	Irregular
Location	Superior–Nasal orbit	Superior orbit	Retrobulbar
Reflectivity	Low	Low	Irregular
Sound attenuation	Weak	Weak	Weak
Blood flow	Absent	Present	Absent
Valsalva test	Highly positive	Positive (hazardous)	Negative
Orbital congestion	Absent	Present	Absent

Comment

Vascular tumours and abnormalities constitute one of the most common disorders in the orbit with Orbital Varices or primary vascular anomalies as one of its most frequent sub-groups (Wright 1988).

Orbital Varices are typically present in young adults. The clinical course is varied, consisting of intermittent uniocular proptosis with or without a visible sub-conjunctival or lid lesion. When visible the lesion appears as a fleshy red mass usually in the nasal aspect of the orbit. Proptosis can be acute and painful due to hemorrhaging and is usually precipitated by an upper respiratory tract infection or physical exertion. In between attacks the eye may appear normal with no visual disturbance. Surgical removal is usually incomplete and reserved for severe cases.

Other orbital vascular lesions produce sufficiently different clinical and echographic findings making their distinction possible with the exception of arteriovenous fistula affecting the orbit and lymphangioma.

Arteriovenous fistula can produce a similar echographic appearance but have a different clinical course and presentation. On the other hand lymphangioma produces a very similar clinical presentation to that of Orbital Varix making some authors believe that they are one and the same lesion with two different names (Rootman 1986). However the echographic appearance of these two lesions is so distinct thus supporting the view that they are two separate entities.

Table 1 summarizes the main echographic features of the three lesions. In this case the strongly positive valsalva manoeuvre, the absence of detectable blood flow within the lesion and the typical clinical appearance made the diagnosis secure.

References

1. Byrne, S.F. & Glaser, J.S. Orbital Tissue Differentiation with Standardized Echography. Ophthalmology **90**: 1071–1090 (1983).
2. Ossoinig, K.C. Echographic Differentiation of Vascular Tumours in the Orbit. Docum. Ophthalmol. Proc. Ser. **29**: 283–291 (1981).
3. Rootman, J., Hay, E., Graeb, D. and Miller, R. Orbital Adnexal Lymphangiomas. A spectrum of hemodynamically isolated vascular hamartomas. Ophthalmology **93**: 1558–70 (1986).
4. Wright, J.E. Doyne Lecture: Current Concepts in Orbital Disease. Eye **2**: 1–11 (1988).

Address for correspondence: H.R. Atta, Department of Ophthalmology, Aberdeen Royal Hospitals, Foresterhill, Aberdeen AB9 2ZB, Scotland, United Kingdom.

15. A case of orbital phlebectasy

A. CANTALLOUBE & J. POUJOL
(Paris, France)

Introduction

We present one case of orbital phlebectasia, seen in the ultrasound laboratory of the Quinze-Vingts Hospital. Clinical semiology is described, with the results of various complementary investigations.

Material and methods

A 34-year-old woman had a violent pain in her right eye. This severe pain appeared suddenly, and increased with lateral ocular movements and ante-flexion of the head. Visual acuity was not altered. Suffering got worse in the first 24 hours and when she arrived at the Quinze-Vingts Hospital, slit-lamp anterior segment examination, applanation tonometry, and dilated ophthal-moscopy were normal, (except for an isolated conjunctival hemorrhage). No exophthalmos, but little weeping. As local pain was significant, an orbital echographic examination and cerebral nuclear magnetic resonance were rapidly performed.

Results

Contact B-scan ultrasonography found an acoustically silent mass in the right superior orbit (Fig. 1); corresponding to an enormous superior ophthal-mic vein. NMR showed an expansive lesion in the retro-ocular position, in the superior and internal orbit; the brain and ventricules, were normal, as was the internal carotid.

Right carotid arteriography found no arterio-venous shunt in the cavern-ous sinus, but many venous development anomalies were present in various part of the hemisphere and occipital region. The ophthalmic symptoms were then assumed to be due to a spontaneous complication of an orbital varix. However two months later, the dilatation disappeared completely spon-taneously, and the orbit then became echographically normal, except for a small papillar swelling due to oedema which regressed after few weeks of

P. Till (ed.), Ophthalmic Echography 13, pp. 205–207.

206

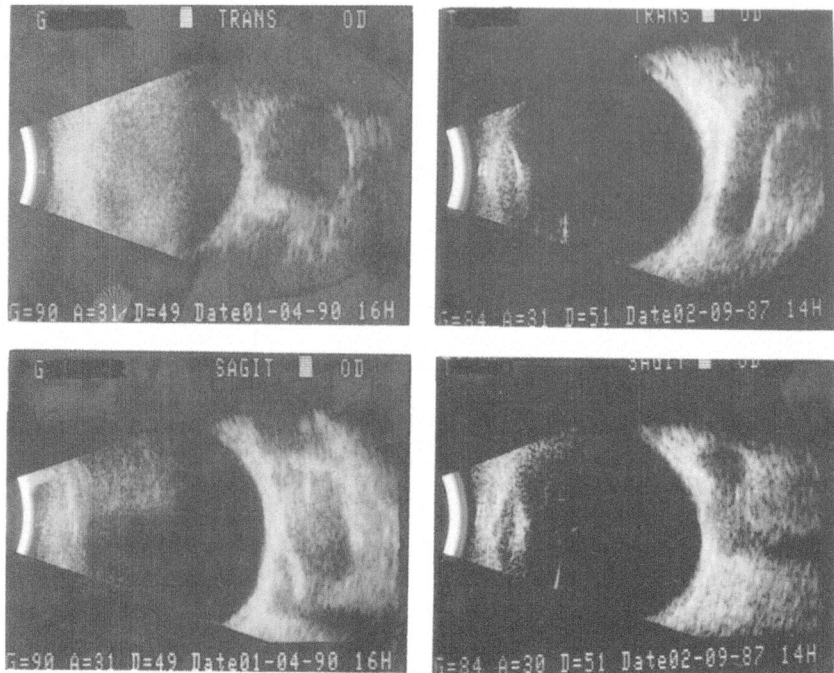

Fig. 1. Upper left and lower left: orbital phlebectasy. Right: transverse (upper) and sagittal (lower) section of a typical dilatation of superior ophthalmic vein.

corticosteroids. So the final diagnosis is that of an isolated and temporary orbital phlebectasy.

Discussion and comments

This image is a little different from the characteristic aspect of a dilated superior ophthalmic vein (Fig. 1) in carotid-cavernous fistulas (Phels 1982). It is a well-known image, amply described over the years (Coleman 1977). The probe is placed horizontally through the lower eyelid, showing a horizontal acoustic section of this dilated and arterialized vein in the superior orbit (from anteronasal to posterotemporal) (Poujol 1984), associated sometimes with thickened sheaths of the optic nerve. A cross section of the dilated vein can also be seen in a vertical acoustic section with the probe placed vertically along the temporal part of the globe.

In our case, the retrobulbar anechoic section is not so clear: the borders are not parallel, the image is not linear but oval. Probe positioning is the same as for carotid-cavernous fistulas. There is no other diagnosis possible when faced with this image: liquid, but no cystic, given its shape, and located at the superior ophthalmic vein.

Conclusion

We were unable to explain the evolution of this lesion. We could only see the ultrasonic image of this aqueous dilatation with echography which is a fast, non-invasive, cheap diagnostic method with no side effects.

References

1. Coleman, D.J., Lizzi, F.L., & Jack, R.L. Ultrasonography of the eye and orbit, pp. 340–342. Philadelphia: Lea & Febiger (1977).
2. Phelps, C.D., Thompson, H.S. & Ossoinig, K.C. The diagnosis and prognosis of atypical carotid-cavernous fistula (red-eyed shunt syndrome) Am. J. Ophtalmol. 93: 423–436 (1984).
3. Poujol, J. Echographie en ophtalmologie. Monographie, 2nd edition, pp. 65–67. Paris: Masson (1984).

Address for correspondence: Centre National d'Ophtalmologie, des Quinze-Vingts, 28 Rue de Charenton, F 75012 Paris, France.

16. The diagnosis of intracranial AV malformation with orbital involvement by B-scan, colour Doppler and CT-scan

ZHONGYAO WU, YANGIONG MO, YOUGIAN PANG,
JIANWEN LIAN, QIXIANG ZENG and JOHN S. KENNERDELL*
(Guangzhou, Peoples Republic of China)
(*Pittsburgh, USA)

Abstract. Eleven patients with intracranial AV malformations with orbital involvement were examined by B-Scan ultrasonography, colour Doppler and CT scan. The imaging features and their role in the diagnosis are discussed.

Introduction

Intracranial arteriovenous malformations (AVM) can involve the orbit causing proptosis and other ocular dysfunctions. The position of carotid-cavernous fistulas (CCF) and cerebral arteriovenous fistulas (CAVF) can be confirmed by carotid angiography or digital subtraction angiography (DSA) [1]. Real-time B-scan, colour Doppler and CT scan can yield valuable diagnostic information.

Method

Between 1985 and 1989, 10 patients with CCF and one patient with CAVF were examined. All of the 11 patients had ultrasound and CT scan at the same time and clinical evidence of vascular malformation. There were 4 men and 7 women with ages ranging from 7 to 65. The main signs and symptoms of these patients are seen in Table 1.

Results

B-scan ultrasonography showed dilatation of the superior ophthalmic vein (SOV) (diameter 2–7 mm) in 11 patients which was sharply outlined, echo-free space and SOV pulsating with synchronized heart beating. The echo-free space changed in shape upon compression with the probe in 5 patients. There were thickened extraocular muscles in 6 patients. Doppler colour ultrasonography in 5 patients showed arterized blood flow and continued frequency in the dilated SOV. Eleven patients were examined by CT scan. A dilated SOV in 9 cases, the enlargement of intraocular muscles in 5 cases and cavernous sinus dilation in 5 cases were seen.

P. Till (ed.), *Ophthalmic Echography 13*, pp. 209–216.

Table 1. Principal symptoms and signs of AVM

Symptoms and signs	No. of cases
Proptosis	11
Dilated epibulbar vessels	9
Noise synchronized with heart beat	9
History of trauma	6
Increased intraocular pressure	6
Intraocular hemorrhage	3
Diplopia	1

Equipment:
Ultrasound – Ophthascan B (Real-Time contact B-Scan)
Doppler – Acuson 128 with colour
CT – GE 8800 and GE 9000

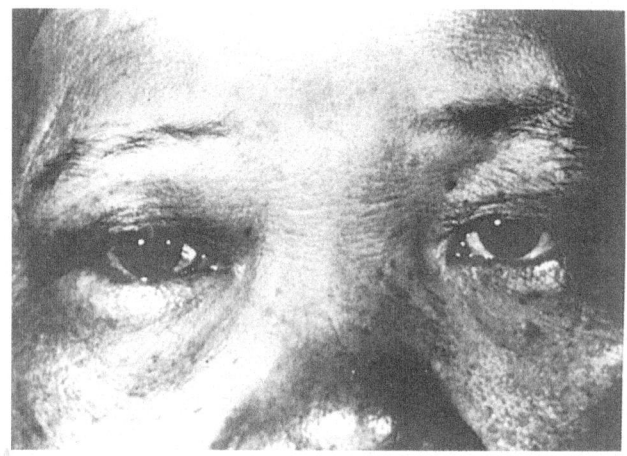

Fig. 1. There was proptosis and swelling in the right eye.

Examples

Case 1. A 49-year-old woman had a red, swollen right eye for 25 days with no history of trauma. Her visual acuity was 0.8 in the right eye and 1.0 in the left eye. Her intraocular pressure (Schiotz) was 24.4 mm Hg in the right eye and 18.9 mm Hg in the left eye. Hertel exophthalmometry showed 3 mm right proptosis (Fig. 1). A noise synchronized with the heart beat could be heard through the right upper lid. There were dilated episcleral veins in the right eye (Fig. 2). B-scan ultrasonography showed an oval shape, echo-free space in the retrobulbar nasal superior orbit, which pulsed with the heart beat (Fig. 3). The echo-free space narrowed in shape upon compression with the probe. CT scan revealed dilation of the right SOV (Fig. 4).

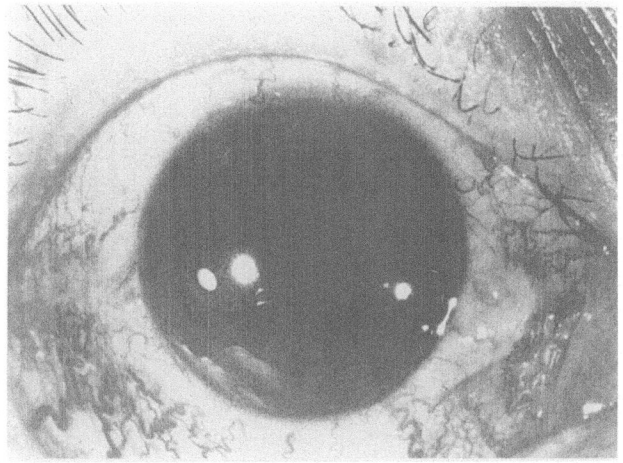

Fig. 2. There were dilated episcleral veins in the right eye.

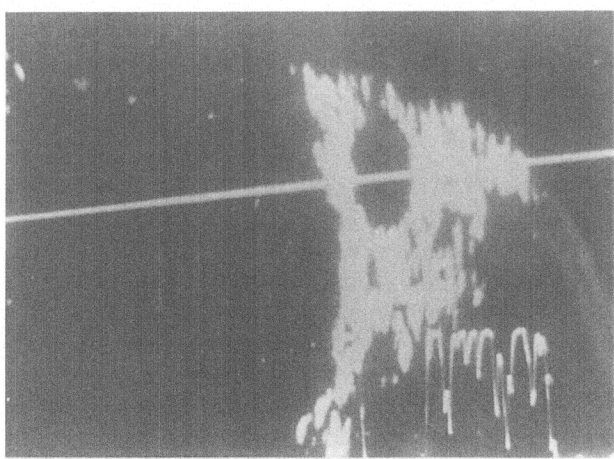

Fig. 3. B-scan showed an oval shape, echo-free space in the right retrobulbar nasal-superior orbit, which pulsed with the heart beat.

Case 2. After suffering trauma (traffic accident) to the head, a 40-year-old man complained of swelling and bulging of his left eye with diplopia for more than a month. His visual acuity was 1.2 in the right eye and 1.0 in the left eye. Both intraocular pressures were normal. Hertel exophthalmometry showed 5.5 mm left proptosis. He had a left pulsatile proptosis, epibulbar injection and an orbital bruit. B-scan showed a dilated left superior ophthalmic vein (3.5 mm diameter), which pulsated synchronous with the heart beat. The echo-free space of SOV changed in shape upon compression with the probe. Doppler showed a dilated and arterialized SOV on a continued fre-

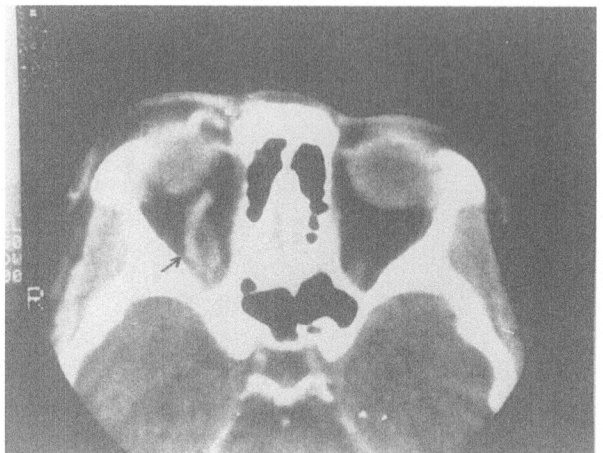

Fig. 4. CT scan showed dilation of the superior ophthalmic vein (SOV) (arrow) in the right eye.

quency chart (Figs. 5 and 6). CT scan showed a dilated SOV and an enlarged cavernous sinus (Fig. 7). The CCF diagnosis was proven by DSA (before and after treatment, Figs. 8 and 9).

Discussion

Intracranial AV malformations present in the orbit in two basic ways, the carotid-cavernous sinus fistulas (high flow type) and dural cavernous sinus fistulas (low flow type). The clinical presentation is often misdiagnosed as dysthyroid orbitopathy, orbital inflammatory disease, conjunctivitis, or an orbital tumor. B-scan, Doppler and CT scan have great value in differential diagnosis.

On ultrasonography, the main acoustic features in orbital involvement of intracranial AVM's are the following: (1) dilatation of SOV in the retrobulbar space, a sharply outlined echo-free space changing with the scan angle (round, oval, and strip shape); (2) SOV pulsation synchronized with the heart beating; (3) the echo-free space changed in shape upon compression with the probe; (4) thickened extraocular muscles; (5) the reverse flowing pulsation of blood stream (arterized SOV) [1–5]. Continued frequency chart showed on colour Doppler. In low flow form, SOV revealed a weak pulsation and there was a spontaneous closure sometimes.

In our series, the above acoustic features all can be seen, especially on lacuson 128, with colour Doppler showing clearly a dilated and arterized SOV and the sound and volume of blood stream. There were two cases with low-flow fistulas that had spontaneous closure within 6–9 months.

Concerning the differential diagnosis, if the dilated SOV can't be com-

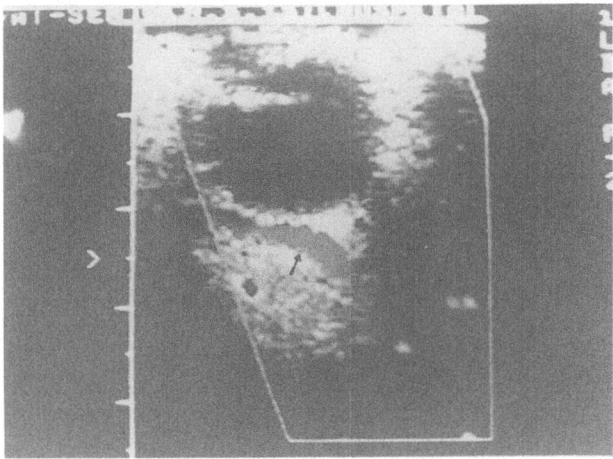

Fig. 5. Colour Doppler revealed a dilated and arterialized SOV, (arrow) which showed the reverse flowing pulsation of blood stream.

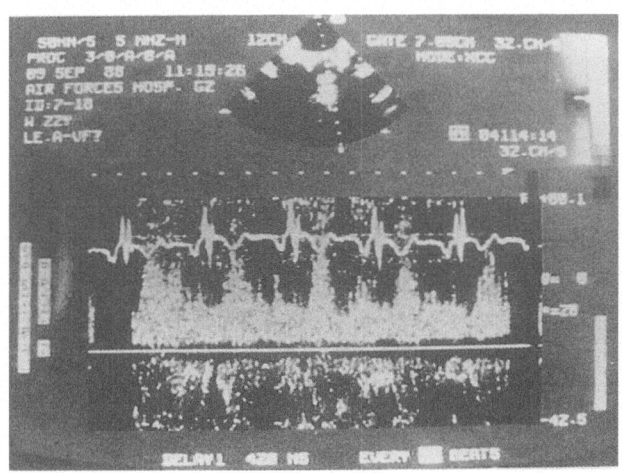

Fig. 6. Colour Doppler showed a SOV pulsation synchronized with heart beat on the continued frequency chart.

pressed, it could be an occlusion of the SOV or the cavernous sinus. If the dilated SOV doesn't pulsate and can't be completely compressed, it could be space-occupying lesions (such as tumor, pseudotumor) or dysthyroid orbitopathy [5]. If it can be compressed with no pulsation, then it is likely a low flow vascular malformation of fistula.

CT scan can show the orbit and intracranial lesions at the same time. In CCF, the CT scan features are the following: Dilated SOV of tube shape from trochlear area to orbital apex; epsilateral cavernous sinus dilation,

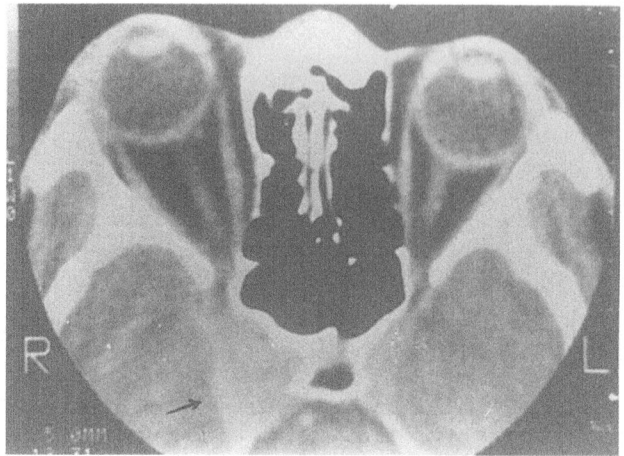

Fig. 7. CT scan showed an enlarged cavernous sinus (arrow).

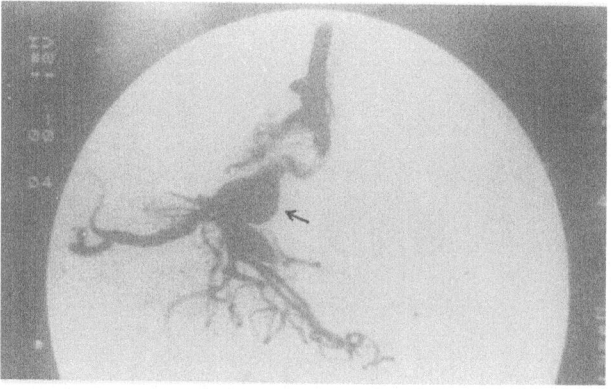

Fig. 8. The position of carotid-cavernous fistulas (arrow) was confirmed by digital subtraction angiography (before treatment).

occasionally, both cavernous sinuses are dilated, thickened extraocular muscles and exophthalmos [6, 7]. After intravenous injection of contrast medium, the dilated SOV and cavernous sinus enhanced and showed the cerebral AVM's. We had one patient whose B-scan revealed dilated SOV which pulsed with the heart beat. CT scan showed the enlarged SOV cavernous sinus and left-sided cerebral AV malformation (Fig. 10). The diagnosis was conformed by the carotid angiography (Fig. 11). Therefore, CT enhanced scan is helpful in the differential diagnosis.

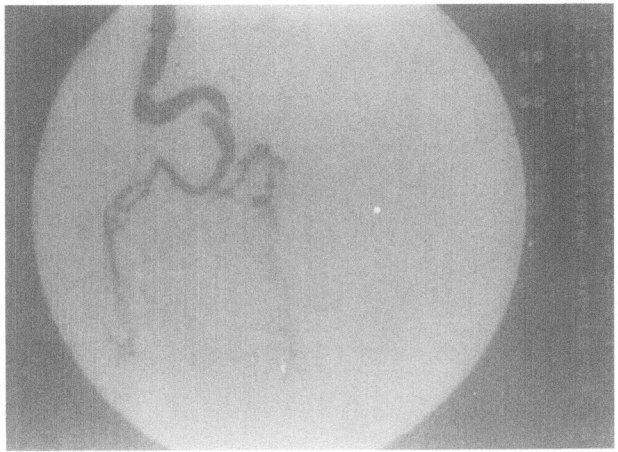

Fig. 9. After treating, the carotid-cavernous fistulas were not revealed by digital subtraction angiography.

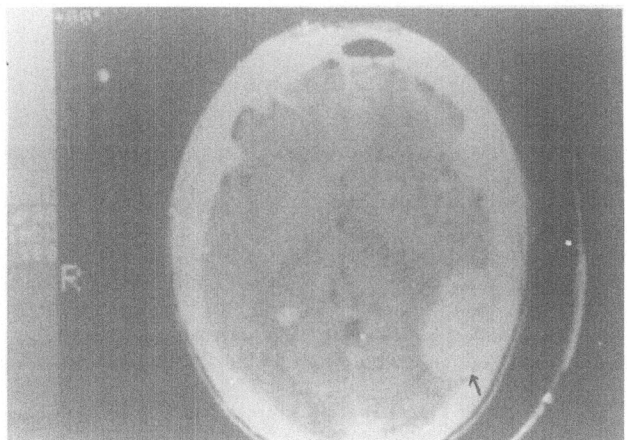

Fig. 10. Contrast-enhanced CT axial view through brain showing left-sided cerebral AV malformations (arrow).

Conclusion

There are many advancements in ultrasound and CT scan. By combining ultrasound and CT scan, we can improve the differential diagnosis of some orbital diseases. For pulsating exophthalmos, we can distinguish AVM's from vascular tumors of the orbit or intracranial area, cavernous sinus thrombosis, mucocoele of ethmoid or sphenoidal sinus and malignant tumor with abundant vessels.

216

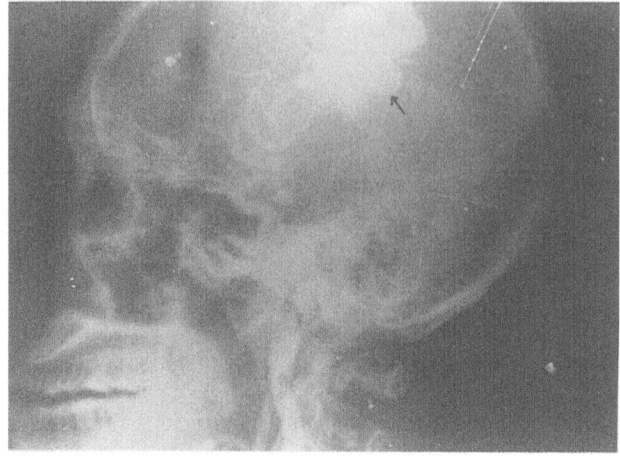

Fig. 11. The cerebral AV malformation was proven by the carotid angiography.

Therefore, B-scan, colour doppler and CT scan are also of value for diagnosing AVM's of the intracranial area.

References

1. Lee Xin-Wei & Song Quo-Xiang. Carotid-cavernous fistula. Ophthalmology of Foreign Country Medicine [China] 1: 42 (1988).
2. MacNeill, J. The diagnosis of intracranial AV malformation with orbital involvement by standardized echogaphy'. Orbit 6(3): 217–222 (1987).
3. Ossoinig, K.C. Echographic differentiation of vascular tumors in the orbit. Thijssen, J.M. & Verbeck, A. M. (ed.), Doc. Ophthalmol. Proc. Ser. 29: 283. The Hague: Dr. W. Junk (1981).
4. Moster, M.R. & Kennerdell, J.S. B-scan ultrasonic evaluation of a dilated superior opthalmic vein in orbital and retro-orbital arteriovenous anomalies. J. Clin. Neuro-Ophthal. 3: 105–108 (1983).
5. Guthoff, R. & Jorgensen, J. Long-term follow up in patients with spontaneous AV-fistulas affecting the orbit. Orbit 6(4): 229–235 (1987).
6. Zilkha, A. & Daiz, A.S. Computed tomography in carotid cavernous fistula. Surg. Neurol. 14: 325–329 (1980).
7. Hemmerschlag, S.B. et al. Computed tomography of the eye and orbit. East Norwalk: Appleton-Century Crafts, 155–157 (1983).

Address for correspondence: Prof. Zhongyao Wu, Zhongshan Ophthalmic Center, 54 Xianlie Road, Guangzhou 51060, P.R. China.

17. Traumatic carotid-cavernous fistula affecting the orbit

K. JANEV, K. SPAHIU, N. SALIHU &
D. PEROVIĆ-STAMENKOVIĆ
(*Pristina, Serbia*)

Abstract. Two cases with carotid-cavernous fistulas have been presented. The general and ocular symptoms were a lot milder in one of them. As the goal was to make cavernous sinus thrombosis, a hypotensive treatment was applied in this particular case. The condition of the fistula was followed by ultrasound during the whole treatment.

Introduction

Traumatic carotid-cavernous fistulas arise during a fracture of the base of the scull mainly because of the break of sphenoid bone. The bone particles rupture either the internal carotid artery, which lies on the side of the body of sphenoid or some of the small meningeal arteries from the internal or external carotid artery touching the sinus (dural communications). That is the very moment when arterial blood flows into the sinus. From here the blood enters the ophthalmic vein expanding it in the orbit. It comes about easily since there are no valves in the ophthalmic veins (Duke-Elder & MacFaul 1974). All ophthalmological symptoms originate from this reflux of arterial blood (Brismar & Brismar 1976).

Materials and methods

We have had two patients who suffered from traumatic fistula of internal carotid artery in cavernous sinus. In one of them the injury was before we introduced echography in our hospital, while the other one was after we started using ultrasound as diagnostic procedure. The first one, 21-year-old male who was injured in a traffic accident, suffered from a terrible noise in the head and had a distinct protrusion of the eye. We diagnosed the case in a classical way: by angiography of internal carotid which showed the dye entering the cavernous sinus. The patient was operated immediately.

The second case was a 25-year-old worker who was hit on the head by a falling plank. He continued working but about fifteen days later he came to the hospital because of some redness of the left eye and an irritating noise in the head. Examinations showed that the conjunctival and episcleral veins were dilated and twisted (Phelps et al. 1982). The blood in them was red

P. Till (ed.), Ophthalmic Echography 13, pp. 217–220.

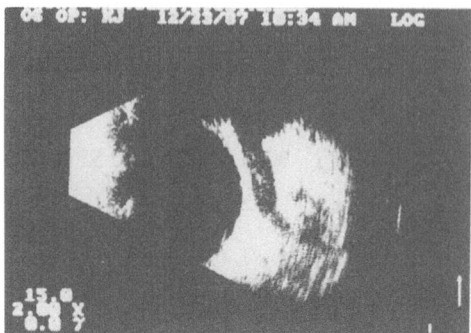

Fig. 1. Upper and nasally large echo free groove demonstrating the upper ophthalmic vein.

due to its arterial origin. The veins of the lower half of conjunctiva did not show the same dilations and twistings since the upper ophthalmic vein is larger and communicates more directly with cavernous sinus than it does with the lower one. The eyeball showed hardly visible pulsations which became evident under slit-lamp.

We did not perform angiography but diagnosis was established by ultrasound. As the general and ophthalmological symptoms of this particular case were a lot milder, an hypotensive treatment was applied. For five months the blood pressure was maintained at the levels from 10 to 15 mm Hg under its normal value with Dexason plus Nimodipin which were administered regularly.

Echographic findings and comments

At the first examination by echography a large echo free groove in the upper and inner part of the orbit could be seen on the B-scan (Fig. 1). This acoustically empty space pulsated synchronously with the systolic beat. Moreover, the surrounding tissues showed some fine motions simultaneous with the pulsations of the groove. Obviously, this groove was the upper ophthalmic vein itself.

Two defects were shown on the A-scan. The first defect, which could be easily compressed, presented the vein while the second one was the medial rectus muscle (Ossoinig & Blody 1974) (Fig. 2). On the horizontal section the defect resembled a hole, size of 4.1 mm, whereas the normal size of this vein is 1 mm (Guthoff & Jørgensen 1987). The echo free space which occupies the upper part of the echogram are contours of the medial rectus (Fig. 3).

The hypotensive treatment was applied during the five-month period. Unfortunately, no reduction of the symptoms was observed. On the contrary, the whole condition was worsening. The defect was growing larger and at that time measured 5.2 mm (Fig. 4). Having realized that these efforts showed no

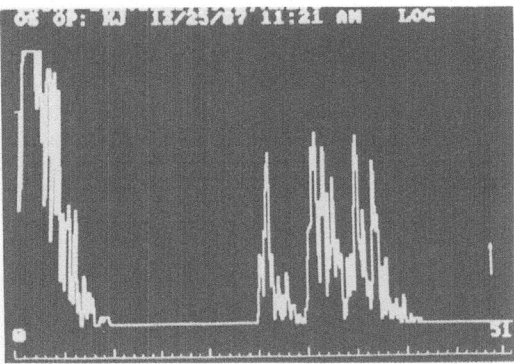

Fig. 2. Two defects could be seen on the A-scan. The first one corresponds to the superior ophthalmic vein and the second one to the medial rectus muscle.

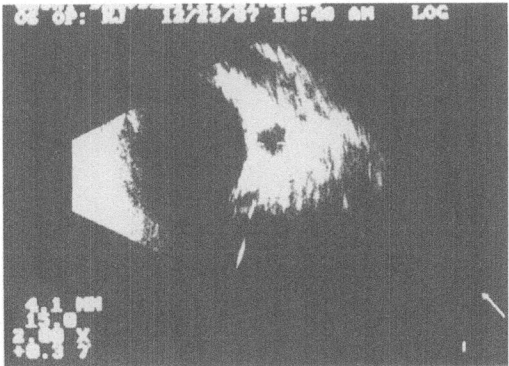

Fig. 3. On the horizontal section the vein resembles a hole, size of 4.1 mm (as indicated in the left lower corner). Upper and posteriorly are the contours of the medial rectus muscle.

results, the patient was sent to Neurosurgery, where the fistula was closed. After the surgery the symptoms disappeared and the defects on the echogram were completely gone. Only some loose edema of retrobulbar space remained (Fig. 5).

Conclusion

Our presentation has once again confirmed that the echographic pattern of carotid-cavernous fistula is rather typical. The echography can be applied instead of an invasive and risky carotid angiography. The hypotensive therapy, at least regarding the traumatic carotid cavernous fistulas, is without any effect.

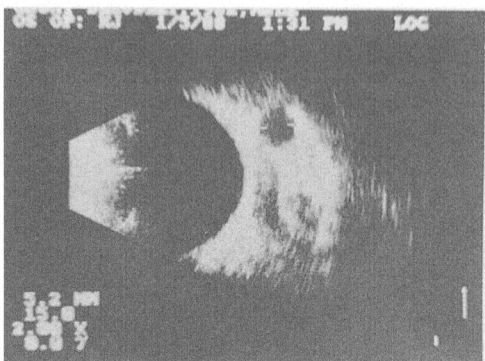

Fig. 4. Horizontal section of the same patient five months later. The defect is larger and measured 5.2 mm. In the lower part of the orbit some echo free spaces can also be seen. They show a dilated lower ophthalmic vein and a swollen lower rectus muscle.

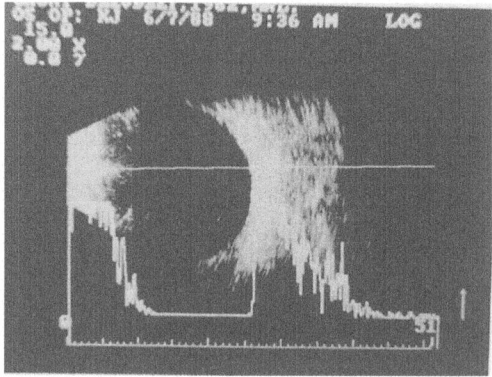

Fig. 5. The echogram after surgery (done on 7 June 1988). The defects in the orbit are completely gone. Only some loose edema of retrobulbar space remained.

References

1. Brismar, G. & Brismar, J. Spontaneous carotid-cavernous fistulas. Clinical symptomatology. Acta Ophthalmol. (Kbh) 54: 542–552 (1976).
2. Duke-Elder, S. & MacFaul, P.A. System of ophthalmology, Vol. 13. London: Kimpton (1974).
3. Guthoff, R. & Jørgensen, J. Long-term follow-up in patients with spontaneous AV-fistulas affecting the orbit. Orbit 4: 229–235 (1987).
4. Ossoinig, K.C. & Blodi, F.C. Preoperative differential diagnosis of tumors with echography. Current Concepts in Ophthalmology 4: 313–341 (1974).
5. Phelps, C.D., Thompson, H.S. & Ossoinig, K.C. The diagnosis and prognosis of atypical carotid cavernous fistula (red eye shunt-syndrome). Am. J. Ophthalmol. 93: 423–436 (1982).

Address for correspondence: Medical Faculty, Eye Clinic, Ulpijana D7/III-8, 38000 Pristina, Serbia.

18. Standardized A-scan examination of the eye and orbit in a newborn child after forceps delivery

E. FRIELING & A. STANOWSKY

(*Augsburg, Germany*)

Abstract. Protrusion of the globe, lid hematoma, dense corneal edema and ocular hypotonia by ultrasound caused considerable difficulties in examining the ocular and adnexal structures of a newborn infant after forceps delivery. Standardized A-scan echography proved to be decisive for diagnosis.

Introduction

Ocular examination of newborn infants with the ultrasonic B-scan probe is possible only through the eyelids, since the palpebral fissure is very small and narrow [2, 3]. In spite of some degree of attenuation and scattering of the ultrasonic beam, this normally causes no diagnostic problems, since the anatomical structures especially in the lids of newborn infants are very fine [4]. Use of the much smaller A-scan probe common to standardized echography (8 mm in diameter), however, permits direct eye examination even in newborn infants. In this case the transducer is placed directly on the conjunctiva. Following there is a report on a newborn infant whose special situation [1] made it difficult to diagnose by means of B-scan examination through the eyelids. The problem was solved by using standardized A-scan echography.

Case history

In December, 1989 we were consulted concerning a newborn baby which had been referred as an emergency case from an outlying area to the Children's Clinic of the Zentralklinikum in Augsburg. The infant incurred a trauma due to a forceps delivery the previous day. In addition to a fracture of the left clavicule and a pronounced cephal-hematoma above the right occiput, x-ray showed a frontotemporal skull fracture with possible involvement of the orbital roof.

CT-scan additionally revealed an epidural hematoma in the left frontal region with a thickness of 2 cm, producing a displacement of the midline structures and a marked subarachnoidal hemorrhage in the area of forceps closure over the right occiput. Emergency neurosurgical intervention was required.

P. Till (ed.), Ophthalmic Echography 13, pp. 221–226.
© 1993 *Kluwer Academic Publishers*.

The first ophthalmological examination took place preoperatively, with the patient already under general anesthesia. There was protrusion of the left globe with pronounced upper and lower lid hematoma. Dense edema of the corneal stroma hid deeper-lying ocular structures from view. The eye was hypotonic, and concealed globe rupture was a possibility. These factors and the question whether Terson's syndrome was present made echographic examination mandatory.

Material and method

Echographic examination was performed with the Ophthascan-S unit, which offers both high resolution B-scan and standardized A-scan echography.

The first echographic examination of the intubated one-day-old patient took place in the operating room. Subsequent examinations were performed on the 4th and 14th day in a heated crib. After topical anesthesia with proparacaine hydrochloride, the eye and orbit were first examined with standardized A-scan (the probe was placed on the conjunctiva) followed by the B-scan procedure through the closed eye lids.

Results

The first examination with standardized A-scan revealed thickening of the retinochoroid layer (1.4 mm) in the circular mid-periphery. However, no sign of vitreous hemorrhage was found even after tissue sensitivity was increased by 6 dB (Fig. 1). Although the intraorbital portion of the optic nerve showed a normal appearance (total diameter: 3.9 mm), a subperiostal hematoma extending to the orbital apex was found below the bony roof of the orbit. It was up to 5.2 mm high and up to 24 mm wide.

In contrast to the undamaged right eye, an adequate representation of the posterior pole of the left eye was obtained only after increasing the system sensitivity by 12 dB during B-scan examination. At this sensitivity echos were obtained from the vitreous space which prompted the suspicion of a vitreous hemorrhage (Fig. 2). Due to the large hematoma and consequent immobility of the globe it was impossible to determine whether these echos changed position with movement of the globe. However, the optic nerve also showed a normal appearance in the B-scan and the subperiostal hematoma was clearly visible (Fig. 2).

At the second examination (4th day after birth), the lid and orbital hematoma had regressed slightly. The extent of the subperiostal hematoma remained practically unchanged (Fig. 3). In B-scan, however, in contrast to standardized A-scan, there were continued indications of vitreous hemorrhage (Fig. 4). Kinetic B-scan examination remained impossible.

At the time of the third examination (14th day after birth), only a slight hematoma of the eyelids and the orbit remained. The retinochoroid layer

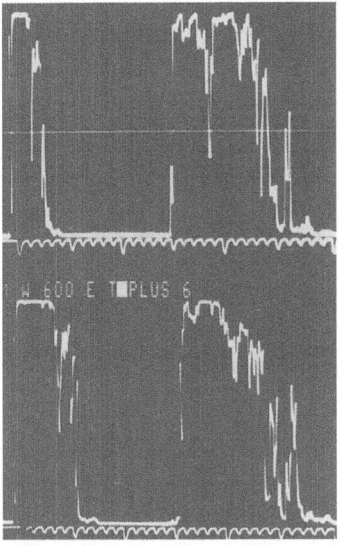

Fig. 1. Free vitreous space at tissue sensitivity (above) and at tissue sensitivity +6 dB (T + 6 dB, below), 2nd day post partum.

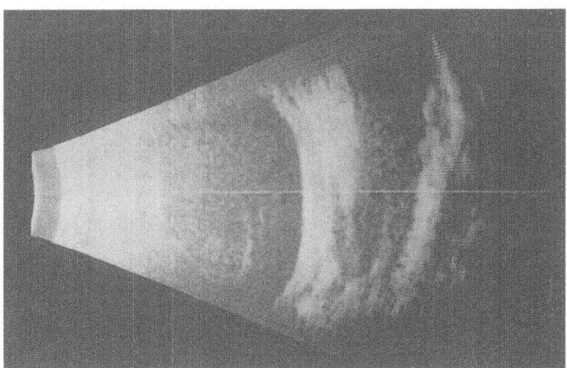

Fig. 2. 'Opacities' in the vitreous space, suspicious for vitreous hemorrhage (system sensitivity increased by 12 dB). Subperiostal hematoma beneath the orbital roof, extending to the orbital apex (2nd day post partum).

had regained a normal thickness of 0.7 mm (mid-periphery) in standardized A-scan examination. The subperiostal hematoma was still 4 mm high and up to 18 mm wide, but did not extend to the orbital apex anymore (Fig 5). The B-scan no longer showed any echographic structures within the vitreous space (Fig. 6).

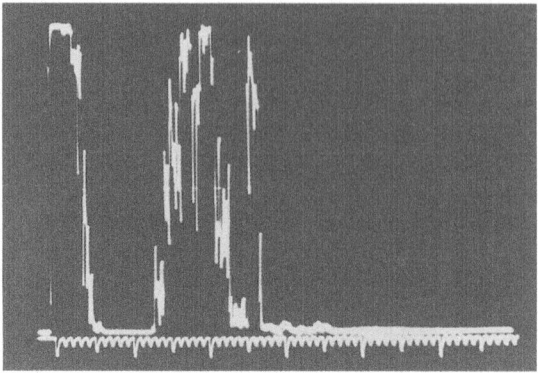

Fig. 3. Subperiostal hematoma (5.2 mm high, 24 mm wide) extending to the the orbital apex (4th day post partum).

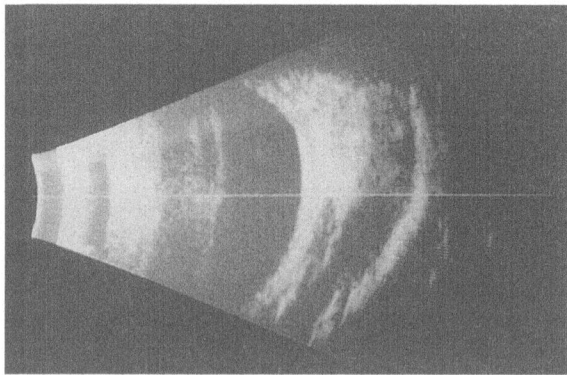

Fig. 4. Vitreous 'opacities', subperiostal hematoma (4th day post partum).

Discussion

Ultrasonic examination of newborn children is restricted by their narrow palpebral fissure. B-scan examination is only possible through the closed lids due to the size of the ultrasonic probe.

This causes few problems when the lids are structured normally. However, when there is pronounced lid hematoma, as in the case of the patient described here, considerable attenuation of the ultrasonic beam results, along with reflection and scattering. In our patient, additionally artefacts appeared after system sensitivity was increased by 12 dB.

Standardized A-scan thus was pivotal for us as a means of answering the question whether this patient actually had vitreous hemorrhage or whether the echos were only artefacts. This was all the more so because of the need

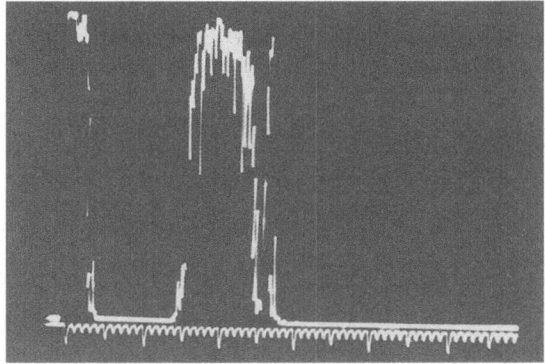

Fig. 5. Remnant of the subperiostal hematoma (4 mm high, 18 mm wide) at the 14th day post partum.

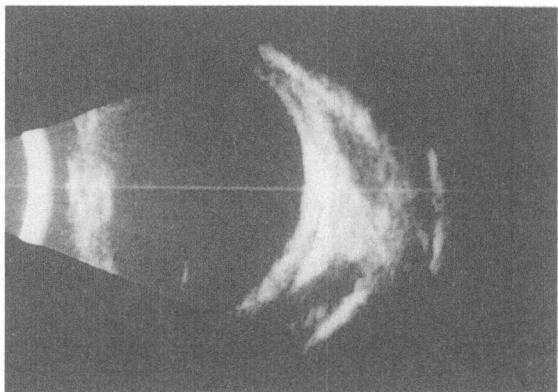

Fig. 6. Free vitreous zone, remnants of the sub-periostal hematoma (14th day post partum).

to determine whether a concealed rupture of the globe or a Terson's syndrome were present.

Standardized A-scan therefore proved to be very reliable, and the findings of the initial examination were subsequently verified.

References

1. Durand, L., Burillon, C. & Normand, F. Obstetrical trauma: an exceptional etiology in corneal edema genesis. Bull. Soc. Ophtalmol. Fr. 88: 1215 (1988).
2. Ossoinig, K.C. Echography of the eye, orbit and periorbital region. In: P.H. Arger (ed.), Orbit roentgenology, pp. 224–269. New York: Wiley (1977).

226

3. Ossoinig, K.C. Standardized echography: Basic principles, clinical applications and results. In: P.L. Dallow (ed.), Ophthalmic ultrasonography: comparative techniques (Int Opthalmol Clin). Boston: Little, Brown (1979).
4. Ossoinig, K.C. Personal communication (1989).

Address for correspondence: Zentralklinikum, Augenklinik, Stenglinstrasse 2, W-8900 Augsburg, Germany.

19. Standardized echography in a case of congenital oculodermal melanocytosis with orbital melanoma

P. TILL

(*Vienna, Austria*)

Introduction

Oculodermal melanocytosis is a benign congenital anomalous pigmentation of deep facial skin and ocular tissues; so-called Nevus Ota is a bluish macula of the skin with an ipsilateral slate-gray patch on the sclera. It may be present at birth or later in childhood or adolescence. The lesion tends to gradually enlarge with age. Malignant degeneration of the skin or epibulbar lesions rarely occur. Oculodermal melancytosis is associated with an increased incidence of melanoma of the choroid, especially in white patients. Seven previously described orbital tumors represent the second most frequent area of presentation. Our case of oculodermal melanocytosis with a melanoma of the orbit is the first in literature, that was diagnosed by Standardized Echography.

Case report

A 48-year-old female with a 3-year history of exophthalmos was presented to our clinic with echographic diagnosis of a low reflective orbital tumor of the group of lymphoma/sarcoma; hematologic systemic work-up was negative. The recommending eye department overlooked the bluish colored skin of the left upper lid, when eyes are closed; three hyperpigmented nodules of the nasal eyebrow (Fig. 1) and the epibulbar melanocytosis with hyperpigmentation of the upper conjunctival fornix during down-gaze and lifted upper lid (Fig. 2). This nevus Ota was present since birth and in childhood the patient was called 'blue-eyed'. Standardized A-scan Echography with the MINI-Ascan demonstrated a large sharply outlined retrobulbar tumor in the upper orbit reaching the orbital apex; reflectivity at tissue sensitivity was low (Fig. 3) and MINI-Bscan showed a large necrosis in tumor center (Fig. 4).

Vascularization of the tumor was, in some soundbeam directions, positive; echographic differential diagnosis of a malignant melanoma was made. Because of the well delineation of this encapsulated tumor an excisional biopsy by temporal osteoplastic orbitotomy was planned. During the skin incision along the superior orbital rim dense melanocytic invasion of the subcutaneous fat was visible (Fig. 5); the orbital melanoma was soft and preparation in

P. Till (ed.), Ophthalmic Echography 13, pp. 227–232.

228

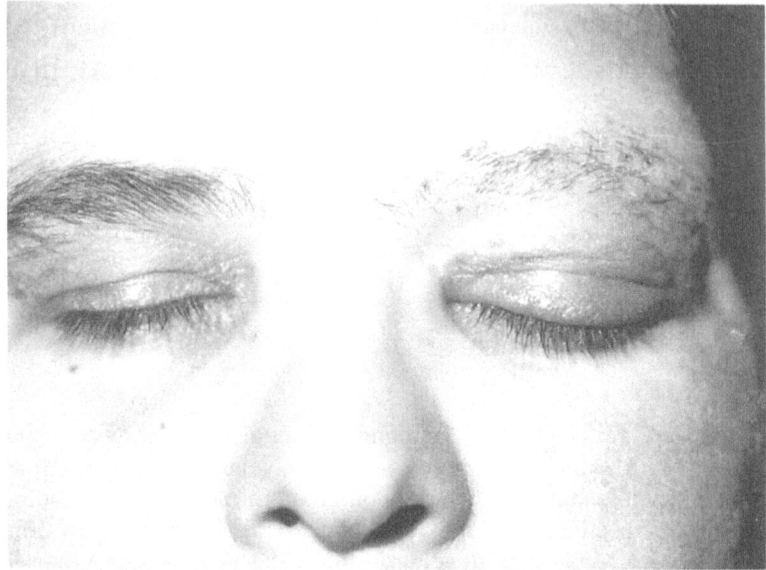

Fig. 1. Only with closed eyes is the bluish colored skin of the left upper lid visible. Three hyperpigmented nodules are in the nasal eyebrow.

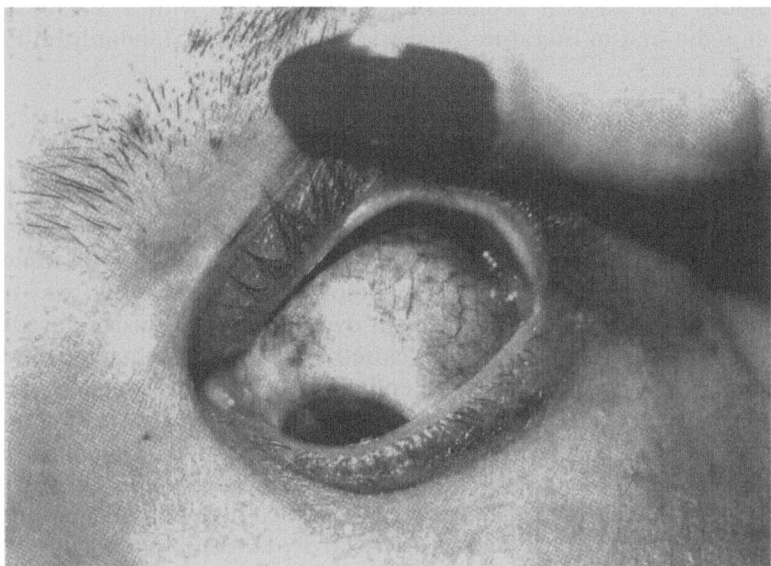

Fig. 2. During lifting upper lid and down-gaze epibulbar melanocytosis and hyperpigmentation of conjunctival fornix is visible.

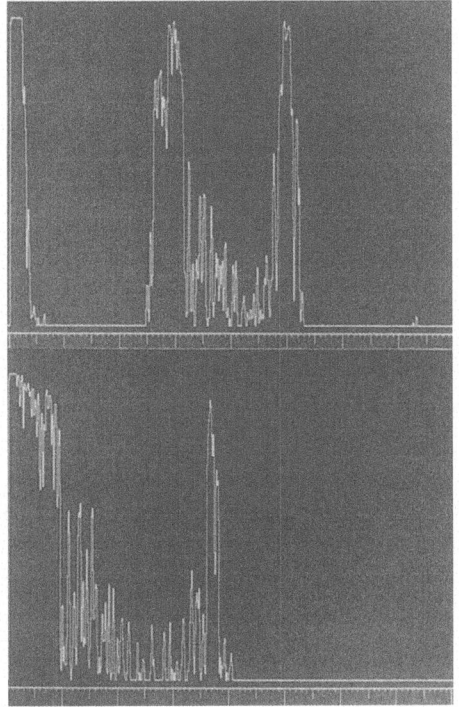

Fig. 3. MINI-A scan echograms of the orbital melanoma demonstrate, at tissue sensitivity, low reflectivity (top and bottom) and sharp delineation (bottom).

the capsule was impossible. Because of diffuse melanocytic infiltration of the sorrounding orbital fat, periorbit and extraocular muscle, an incisional biopsy of the very soft necrotic tumor was made (Fig. 6). Frozen sections of subcutaneous fat and orbital tumor showed malignant melanoma cells; operation was stopped for waiting permanent section-diagnosis: No malignant melanoma cell was found; Ophthalmopathology diagnosed a low grade malignant melanoma (Fig. 7).

Conclusion

The clinical course of primary orbital melanomas in oculodermal melanocytosis is difficult to predict due to tumor rarity and the lack of long-term follow-up. Only two patients in literature have had a follow-up of more than two years. Our patient had exophthalmos for three years before referred to our clinic and has been on follow-up now for more than three years. The unchanged orbital melanoma and the absence of metastasis supports an conservative approach. Aggressive surgery would be unlikely to reduce the risk of future metastasis and would not be indicated in a low grade malignant melanoma in this healthy young patient. Our case also serves as an example

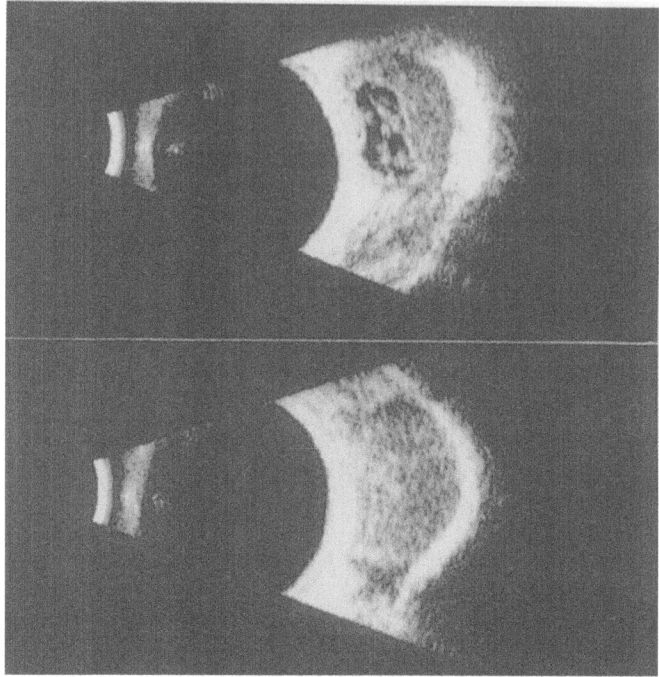

Fig. 4. MINI-B scan echograms of the orbital melanoma in the upper orbit demonstrate tumor necrosis (top) and large horizontal expansion and depth (bottom).

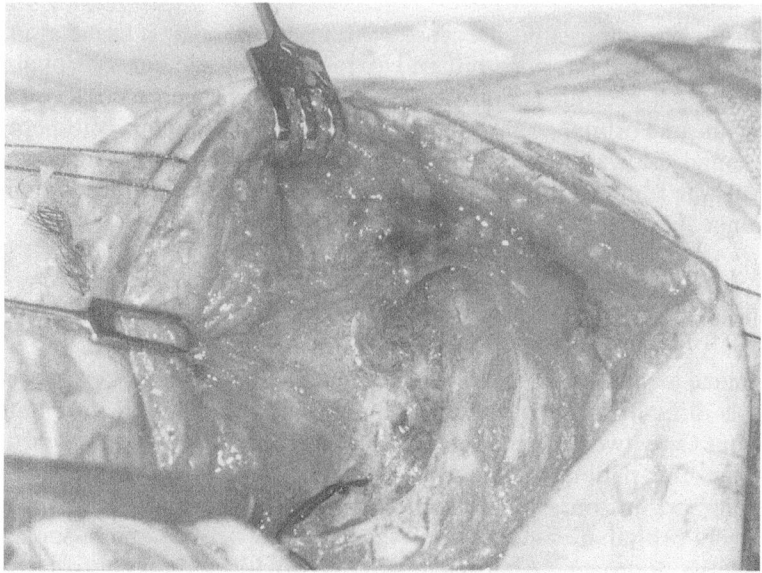

Fig. 5. Skin incision with hyperpigmentation of subcutaneous fat.

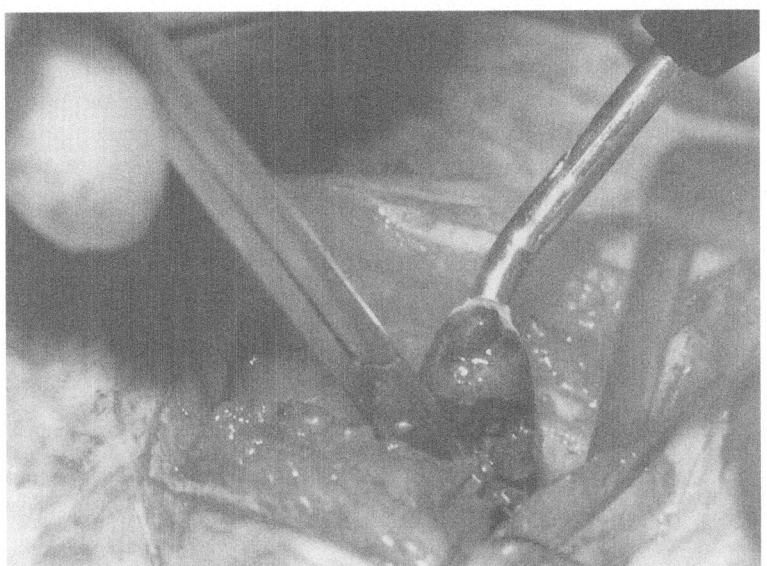

Fig. 6. Part of orbital melanoma during incisional biopsy.

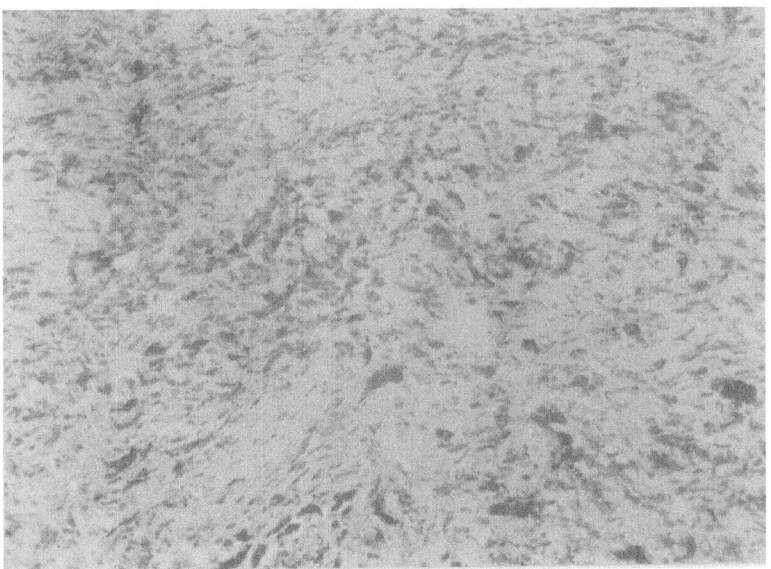

Fig. 7. Ophthalmopathology diagnosed low grade malignant melanoma.

232

of the failure of frozen sections to provide the correct orbital diagnosis dispite a 95% overall accuracy of the technique [1]. In oculodermal melanocytosis pigmentation within the orbit has been reported along extraocular muscles, orbital fat, periorbit, and orbital bones [2]. In most orbital melanomas associated with pigmentary disorders, the ocular or cutaneous pigmentation was visible preoperativly. One case of Rice & Brown [3] is unique since the associated pigmentation was detected only intraorbitally at the time of surgery.

References

1. Howard, G.M. Application of frozen sections to diagnosis of orbital tumors. Am. J. Opthalmol 71: 221–223 (1971).
2. Dutton, J.J., Anderson, R.L., Schelper, R.L., Purcell, J.J. & Tse, D.T. Orbital malignant melanoma and oculodermal melanocytosis: Report of two cases and review of the literature. Ophthalmology 91: 497–507 (1984).
3. Rice, Ch.D. & Brown, H.H. Primary orbital melanoma associated with orbital melanocytosis. Arch. Opthalmol. 108: 1130–1134 (1990).

Address for correspondence: University Eye Clinic, Alserstrasse 4, A-1090 Vienna, Austria.

20. Glomus tumor of the eyelid and anterior orbit
Echographic and histological features

D. DORO, E. MANTOVANI & L. BERGAMO

(Padua, Italy)

Abstract. A roundish slightly mobile mass was found in the superior left eyelid of a 44-year-old man with a two year history of recurrent eyelid edema and frontal headache. Contact B-scan showed an uncompressible roundish eyelid mass extending to the anterior upper nasal orbit with sponge-like internal texture. On standardized A-scan the lesion showed medium to low internal reflectivity with a regular heterogeneous structure and defined borders: no spontaneous vertical movements of the echo spikes were detectable. CT scan evidenced a high density lesion enhanced by contrast. Echo-guided fine needle aspiration twice failed to obtain adequate material. For diagnostic and cosmetic purposes the mass was excised. Histological evaluation evidenced vascular spaces and roundish glomus cells, as confirmed by immunohistochemistry. To our knowledge this is the first pathological echographic correlation of a glomus tumor.

Introduction

Glomus tumor or glomangioma [4, 8] is a rare benign vascular tumor which originates from a normal glomus, a structure with temperature-regulating function [8]. Glomus tumors are usually found in the subungual areas [8], but orbital and eyelid location has also been described [2, 4–6, 9]. The lesion is usually a small solitary reddish-purple nodule which is painful when located in the subungual areas. The differentiation from other orbital vascular masses, such as hemangioma, hemangioendothelioma, hemangiopericytoma and angiosarcoma, is not easy even on histopathological examination [8–10].

To our knowledge the echographic features of an orbital glomus tumor have never been reported.

Case report

On April 1989 a 43-year-old male patient was referred to our clinic. He was under treatment for dilatative myocardiopathy and had been complaining of frontal headache and recurrent right superior eyelid edema for two years. Slow growth of a hard non-compressible mobile mass in the nasal portion of the eyelid and upper nasal anterior orbit was recorded. The lid skin over the mass was reddish, warm and slightly swollen. No pain was evoked by compression of the mass. No proptosis or ocular motility impairment were observed: corrected visual acuity was 20/20 bilaterally, media were clear, fundus and intraocular pressure were normal.

P. Till (ed.), Ophthalmic Echography 13, pp. 233–237.
© 1993 *Kluwer Academic Publishers.*

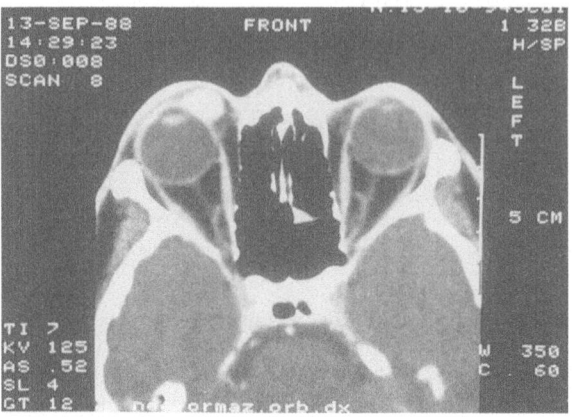

Fig. 1. Glomus tumor. Orbital CT scan evidencing a high density roundish mass lesion enhanced by contrast medium.

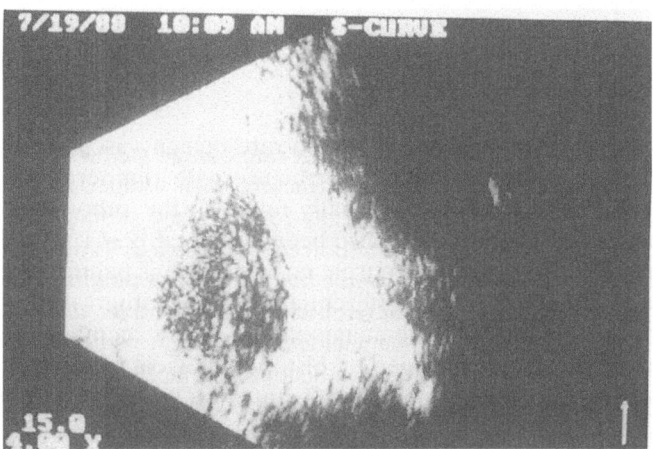

Fig. 2. Glomus tumor. Contact B-scan: extraconal roundish moderately echogenic mass with irregular texture and good sound transmission.

Orbital CT scan evidenced a high density roundish mass lesion in the superior eyelid and upper nasal anterior orbit. The lesion was enhanced by contrast medium (Fig. 1).

Contact B-scan echography evidenced an extraconal roundish moderately echogenic mass with irregular texture and good sound transmission. No bulbus indentation was present (Fig. 2). Standardized A-scan echography showed a (about) 15 microseconds wide, outlined mass lesion with low to medium internal reflectivity and regular heterogeneous structure (Fig. 3);

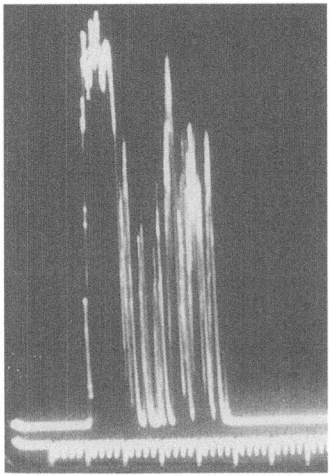

Fig. 3. Glomus tumor. Standardized A-scan: about 15 microseconds wide, outlined mass lesion with low to medium internal reflectivity and regular heterogeneous structure.

there was no evidence of spontaneous vertical movements of the inner echo-spikes; the lesion was not compressible. Rectus muscles were normal.

An aspiration biopsy under B-scan guidance [3, 8] was performed twice, but no adequate material for cytologic diagnosis was obtained.

A definite diagnosis was not reached with standardized echography; cavernous hemangioma was ruled out.

For diagnostic and cosmetic purposes, the mass was excised with its intact capsule. Histopathology showed several round or oval dilated vascular spaces embedded in a densely cellular tissue; each vascular lumen was lined by a single layer of flat endothelial cells and surrounded by multiple rows of round glomus cells with round nuclei and clear cytoplasma, low mitotic ratio and isolated cytonuclear dismetries. Gomori stained material revealed reticulin producing glomus cells (Fig. 4). Immuno-histochemically the cells showed reactivity for factor VIII related antigen (FVIII-RA), Ulex europeaous I lectin, vimentin and myosin; no reactivity was obtained for S-100 antigen and keratin. The pathological report indicated the diagnosis of glomus tumor.

After a one-year follow-up, no recurrence of the orbital mass has been noted.

Discussion

Glomus tumor, hemangioendothelioma and hemangiopericytoma are rare vascular orbital tumors which cannot be differentiated from one another with standardized echography [7]. Actually, in 1983 Byrne [1] reported a case of hemangioendothelioma (diagnosed by several pathologists also as hemangi-

236

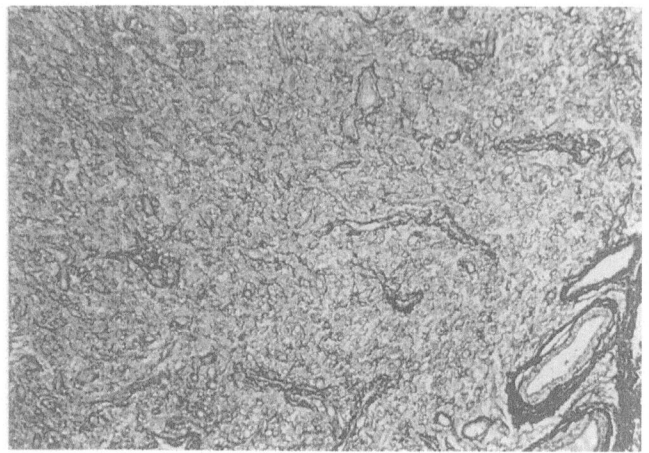

Fig. 4. Glomus tumor. Gomori stained histopathological material revealed reticulin producing glomus cells.

opericytoma), with echographic features very similar to those found in our case. In both cases borders were well outlined (even though the double peak was less clear cut in our case), there was no compressibility or sound attenuation; the reflectivity was slightly higher in our case (low to medium) and structure was regular in both cases but heterogeneous in our patient. Contrary to Byrne's findings [1], we were not able to detect spontaneous vascular movements of the inner echospikes in our case, because probably no fast blood flow was present. Ossoinig, on the other hand, did not report spontaneous vascular movements in different vascular tumors such as capillary hemangioma, hemangioendothelioma, hemangiopericytoma and angiofibroma [7].

The similar histological features of the three above-mentioned vascular tumors make it difficult for the pathologist to reach a sure diagnosis on morphological grounds only. Morphologically, hemangiohendothelioma could not be ruled out in our case, but immunohistochemistry evidenced positive reaction of the tumoral cells not only for FRA-VIII, Ulex europeaus lectin I and vimentin (typical for hemangioendothelioma) but also for myosin (typical for glomus tumor and hemangiopericytoma) [8]. However, the latter vascular tumor could be ruled out because no typical spindle cells were found [8, 10].

The right diagnosis implies different prognosis for the three types of the above-mentioned rare vascular tumors: contrary to reports concerning hemangioendothelioma and hemangiopericytoma, no metastasis has yet been documented from glomus tumor [8].

References

1. Byrne, S.F. Standardized echography in the diagnosis of hemangioendothelioma. In: Hillman, J.S. & Le May, M.M. (eds.), Ultrasonography in Ophthalomology – 8, pp. 347–356. The Hague: Dr. W. Junk (1983).
2. Charles, N.C. Multiple glomus tumors of the face and eyelid. Arch. Ophthalmol. 94: 1283–1285 (1976).
3. Doro, D., Midena, E., Boccato, P., Mantovani, E., Moschini, G.B. & Moro, F. Echography assisted fine needle aspiration biopsy for diagnosing orbital pseudotumor and lymphoma. In: Sampaolesi R. (ed.). Ultrasonography in Ophthalomology-12, pp 27–36. Dordrecht: Kluwer Acad. Publ. (1990).
4. Jensen, O.A. Glomus tumor (glomangioma) of eyelid. Arch. Ophthalmol. 73: 511–513 (1963).
5. Kirby, D.B. Neuromyoarterial glomus tumor in the eyelid. Arch. Ophthalmol. (Chic.) 25: 228–230 (1941).
6. Mortada, A. Glomangioma of the eyelid. Br. J. Ophthalmol. 47: 697–699 (1963).
7. Ossoinig, K.C. Standardized echography: basic principles, clinical applications and results. Intern. Ophthalmol. Clinics 19: 107–210 (1979).
8. Rosai, J. Soft tissue. In: Ackerman's Surgical Pathology, 7th ed., Vol. 2, 1580–1588. St. Louis: The C.V. Mosby Co. (1989).
9. Spoor, T.C., Kennerdell, J.S., Dekker, A., Johnson, B.L. & Rehkopf, P. Orbital fine needle aspiration biopsy with B-scan guidance. Am. J. Ophthalmol. 89: 274–277 (1980).
10. Winter, R. Glomangiom des Augenlides. Klinische und histologische Fallbeschreibung. Klin. Mbl. Augenheilk. 175: 107–109 (1979).
11. Yannof, M. & Fine, B.S. Ocular Pathology. A Text and Atlas, 3rd ed., pp. 519–528. Philadelphia: J.B. Lippincott Co. (1989).

Address for correspondence: Ophthalmology Clinic, University of Padua, Via Giustiniani 2, I-35128 Padua, Italy.

21. Microphthalmus with congenital orbital cyst

M. LOHMEYER & K.B. MELLIN

(*Essen, Germany*)

Abstract. Microphthalmus with orbital cyst is a rare congenital disease. It can present with an exophthalmus and requires extensive investigations in order to exclude other orbital tumors. Standardized echography has proven to be a very helpful diagnostic tool in differentiating this rare disease from other orbital lesions.

Introduction

Microphthalmus with orbital cyst is a rare congenital disease which usually occurs unilaterally and is associated with very poor vision (Makley et al. 1969; Waring et al. 1976). It results from defects in closure of the embryonic fissure and invagination of the optic vesicle (Mann 1957). These abnormalities vary in their clinical picture and are often misdiagnosed. The microphthalmic eye presents a wide spectrum of abnormal development, has anomalous structures such as iridocorneal adhesions and angle defects; the lens is often large, dislocated and cataractous (Waring et al. 1976).

Case report

The following case represents the echographical diagnosis of a microphthalmus with congenital orbital cyst.

A one-month-old baby boy was presented in the Ophthalmology department of the University of Essen for evaluation of an increasing proptosis together with microcornea and cataract of his right eye.

Because of the opaque media an ultrasound examination was performed in order to rule out intraocular pathology, especially a retinoblastoma.

The examination of the globe with standardized A-scan (Ossoinig 1979) and with B-scan revealed no major abnormalities, but unexpectedly a large, very low reflective cystic structure was found in the orbit (Fig. 1). With the A-scan a sharply-outlined orbital cyst could be clearly defined (Fig. 2). In connection with the microphthalmic eye, the syndrome of a congential orbital cyst was diagnosed.

The CT-scan which was performed because of these echographical findings

P. Till (ed.), Ophthalmic Echography 13, pp. 239–243.
© 1993 *Kluwer Academic Publishers.*

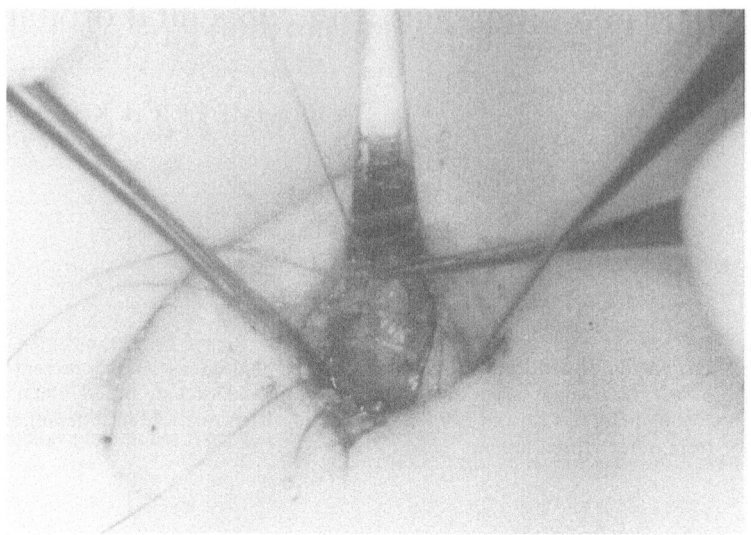

Fig. 1. Cystic bluish tumor during operation.

also demonstrated the orbital lesion on the right side; in contrast to echography, a solid intraorbital tumor with central necrosis was suspected.

Follow-up examinations on the patient were suggested as the proptosis was not painful, but because of the suspicion of a solid tumor on CT-scan, the patient was referred to the reconstructive surgeons who decided to perform an operation on this child.

During the long and extensive operation under general anaesthesia a cystic bluish tumor was found which was removed without complications (Fig. 3).

On histological examination, ectopic neuroepithelial tissue was found in the orbit which had a cystic wall with serous fluid inside. On hyaluronic acid stain degenerated gliotic neuroretinal tissue could be demonstrated confirming the above diagnosis.

Discussion

In our judgement, it was not necessary to take the risk of this operation as the child did not suffer from any pain caused by the proptosis.

Generally speaking, in most cases no intervention is indicated; if the enlarging cyst entails significant pain or proptosis, or if the eye disfigures, surgical treatment may be necessary (Costet et al. 1987; Waring et al. 1976).

Needle aspiration of the cyst is the simplest procedure, but the cyst wall usually recurs. Other therapeutic approaches consist in excision of the cyst alone or of the microphthalmic eye together with the cyst; it should be

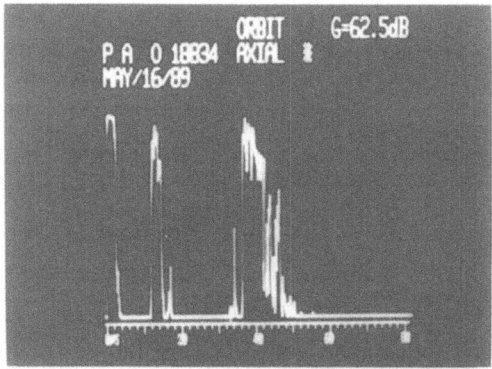

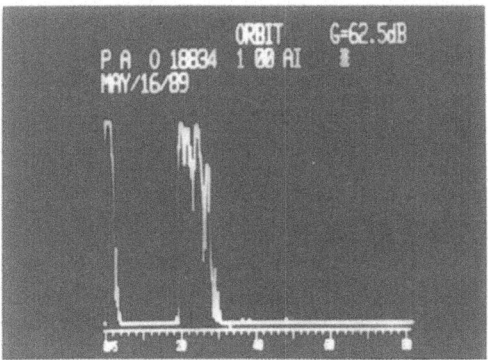

Fig. 2. Transocular (above) and paraocular (below) standardized A-scan echograms showing the sharply outlined extremely low reflective congenital orbital cyst.

intended to remove the whole cyst wall which may be difficult (Waring et al. 1976).

By describing the above case we want to demonstrate that standardized echography is of great value in the diagnosis and differentiation of this disorder; it enables us to show the cystic structure in the orbit which is sharply outlined (representing the double-peaked cyst wall) and has an extremely low interior reflectivity because of the serous fluid. The axial eye length is shortened on the affected side.

On B-scan, the cystic lesion in the orbit can also be demonstrated, a communicating channel between globe and orbital cyst may become obvious (Fisher 1977).

In cases of microphthalmus with congenital cataract an echographical examination should be performed at any rate as a retinoblastoma has to be excluded. Finding this tumor in a microphthalmic eye is rather rare, but some cases have been described in literature.

The differentiation from microphthalmus because of persistent hyperpla-

242

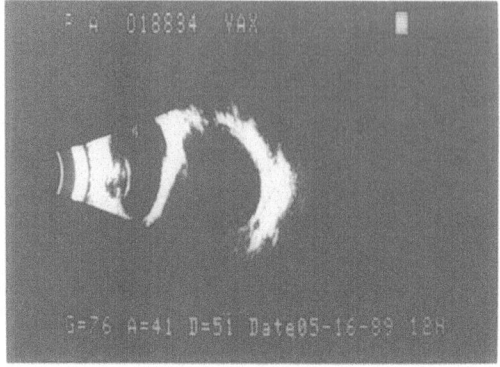

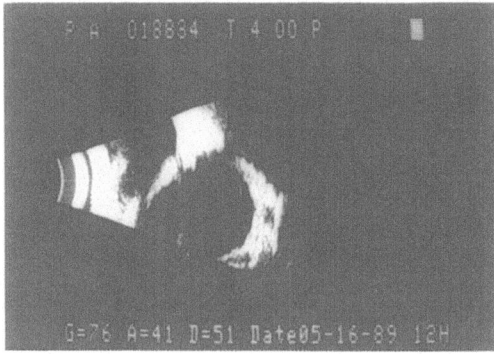

Fig. 3. Contact B-scan echograms demonstrating the microphthalmic globe together with the large congenital orbital cyst.

sia of the primary vitreous or retinopathy of prematurity or isolated microph-thalmus is easily done by echography.

If anterior segment surgery is being considered in a microphthalmic eye with opaque media, preoperative recognition of poor vision implied by the colobomatous cyst may spare the patient an useless procedure.

In our opinion, the differentiation from other orbital lesions by echogra-phy is of great importance. Especially in cases of postnatal enlargement of the cyst, differentiation from a growing malignant tumor may be necessary.

By means of quantitative, topographic and kinetic echography (Ossoinig 1977, 1978), a solid tumor is easily differentiated from the cystic lesion as seen in the syndrome of microphthalmus with congenital orbital cyst.

Other cystic structures as found for example with dermoid cysts and lymph-angiomas are generally not combined with a microphthalmic eye (Weiss et al. 1985) and behave differently on ultrasound examination (Ossoinig 1978). We want to emphasize that an encephalocele should be safely ruled out before performing an operation. On echography, you will find large, regularly outlined bone-defects in the posterior orbit and echo-spikes beyond the extension of the orbit.

Conclusion

Standardized echography has proved to be a very helpful tool in establishing the diagnosis of the above described syndrome and plays a key-role in differentiating it from other intraocular and orbital disorders. It is a safe, not invasive diagnostic test that does not expose the very young patients to radiation. It provides the examining ophthalmologists with clinically related information and allows a very precise follow-up.

References

1. Costet, Ch. Ghenassia, Ch. & Lods, F. Conduite a tenir devant une microphtalmie congenitale à propos de 10 cas. Bull. Soc. Opht. France 87: 485–493 (1987).
2. Fisher, Y.L. Microphthalmus with ocular communicating orbital cyst – ultrasonic diagnosis. Ophthalmology 85: 1208–1211 (1977).
3. Makley, T.A. & Battles, M. Microphthalmus with cyst. Report on two cases in the same family. Survey Ophthalmol. 13: 200–206 (1969).
4. Mann, I. Developmental abnormalities of the eye, 2nd ed. pp. 66–69, Philadelphia: JB Lippincott Co. (1957).
5. Ossoinig, K.C. Echography of the eye, orbit, and periorbital region. In: Arger P.H. (ed.), Orbit roentgenology, pp. 223–269. New York: J Wiley & Sons (1977).
6. Ossoinig, K.C. The role of clinical echography in modern diagnosis of periorbital and orbital lesions. In: Bleeker G.M. (ed.), Proc. of 3rd Int. Symp. on orbital disorders, pp. 496–540. The Hague: Junk. (1978).
7. Ossoinig, K.C. Standardized echography: basic principles, clinical applications and results. In: Dallow R.L. (ed.), Ophthalmic ultrasonography: comparative techniques. Int. Ophthlmol. Clin. 19: 127–210 (1979).
8. Waring, G.O. & Roth, A.M. Clinicopathologic correlation of microphthalmus with cyst. Am. J. Ophthalmol. 82: 714–721 (1976).
9. Weiss, A., Martinez, C. & Greenwald, M. Microphthalmos with cyst: clinical presentations and computed tomographic findings. J. Pedriatr. Ophthalmol. Strabismus 22: 6–12 (1985).

Address for correspondence: University Eye Hospital, Hufelandstrasse 55, W-4300 Essen 1, Germany

PART THREE

Intraocular tumors

22. Choroidal melanoma: Zonal relationship between echographic tracing and cellularity

R. SAMPAOLESI, J.F. CASIRAGHI & J.O. ZARATE

(Buenos Aires, Argentina)

Introduction

At the SIDUO XII conference we presented our conclusions about the relationship existing between the cellular density of intraocular tumours and their reflectivity obtained by means of mode A standardized echography. Intraocular melanomas change their cellular density in relation with their histologic type, as we have shown in the above-mentioned communication. Epithelioid melanomas have a low cellular density, while in the case of the spindle-shaped type, the cellularity per mm^3 is high. Therefore, we have verified a positive linear correlation between cellular density (and consequently, histologic type of melanoma) and reflectivity.

Melanomas of low cellular density (epithelioid) have low reflectivity, while those having high cellular density (spindle-shaped) show high reflectivity.

The aim of this paper is to confirm our findings in a particular case of choroidal melanoma which, due to its morphologic features of zonal distribution, allows an interesting histoechographic correlation.

This case corresponds to a choroidal melanoma in the posterior pole, medium-sized, and of combined histological type, which presents an epithelioid section, a spindle-shaped section and a necrotic area, wholly separated from each other.

Case report

Panoramically, the tumour presents a nodular shape and measures $1.3 \times 1 \times 0.7$ cm (Fig. 1). Four different samples were obtained from this tumour and the cellular density was measured in a total of 270 histologic cuts, according to the study system already mentioned. The eyeball presented retinal detachment and morphologic changes as associated lesions evidencing neovascular glaucoma.

In mode A echography, the tracing presents three distinguishable areas which were called A1, A2 and A3, which correspond with the morphologically numbered sections. Area A1 presents 12 peaks in an extension of 8 useg. (6.2 mm), the average height of which corresponds with a reflectivity of 48.5%. Area A2, also with 12 peaks and 8 useg. (6.2 mm) of extension,

P. Till (ed.), Ophthalmic Echography 13, pp. 247–250.

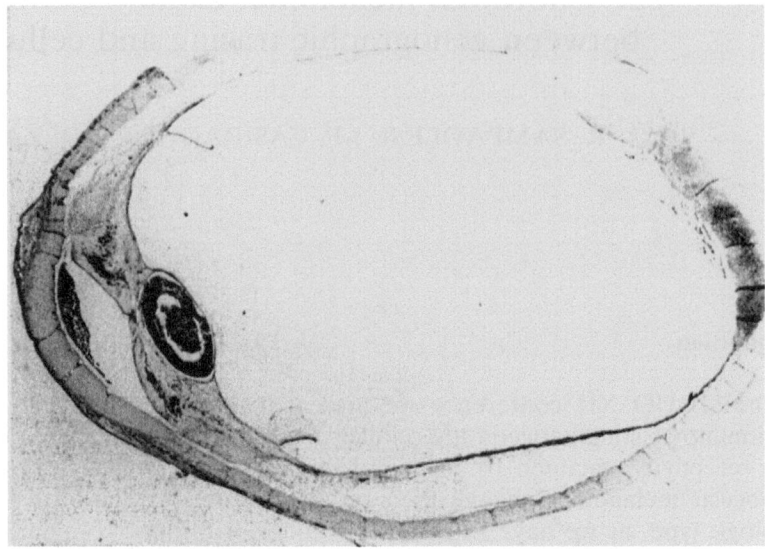

Fig. 1. Panoramic view of one of the histological cuttings of the melanoma located at the posterior pole, which shows 3 different areas: A1, A2 and A3, from the top towards the bottom.

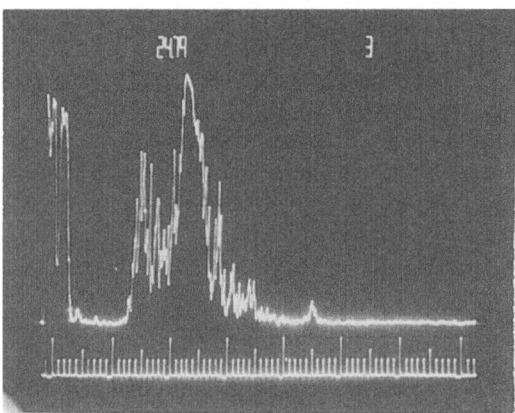

Fig. 2. Mode A echography of the three areas. Area A1 presents 12 peaks in an extension of 8 useg., and an average reflectivity of 48.5%. Area A2 has 12 peaks, 8 useg. of extension and an average reflectivity of 66%, while area A3, with 8 peaks and an extension of 5 useg.; presents an average reflectivity of 14%.

presents an average reflectivity of 66%. Area A3, with 8 peaks and an extension of 5 useg. (3.8 mm), shows an average reflectivity of 14% (Fig. 2).

As regards the cellular density of each of the above-mentioned areas, it has been observed that section A1 relates to an epithelioid melanoma (low cellular density = 175,000 cells/mm^3); section A2 relates to a spindle-shaped

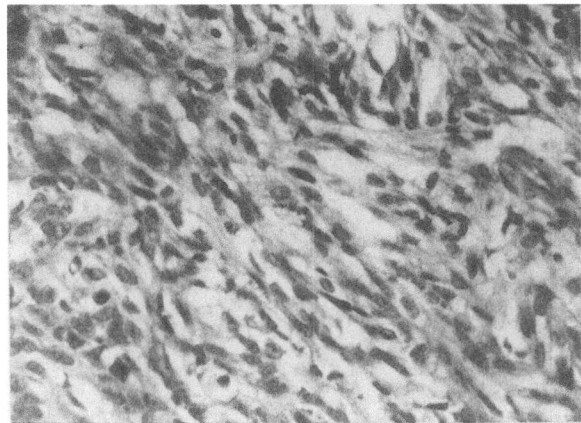

Fig. 3a. Area A1, in which the melanoma belongs to an epithelioid histologic type.

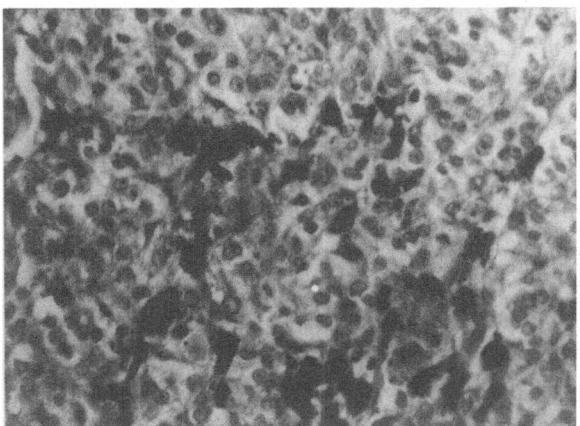

Fig. 3b. At the same size, area A2, of spindle-shaped histologic type.

histologic type (high cellular density = 682,000 cells/mm^3); and section A3, to a necrotic area (very low density = 1,200 cells/mm^3) (Fig. 3a, b and c and Table 1).

Comments

Intraocular melanomas are not distributed zonally in such a distinguishable way very frequently, as in the case we have presented, thus allowing a practical confirmation of our conclusions on the relationship between cellularity – histologic type – and reflectivity.

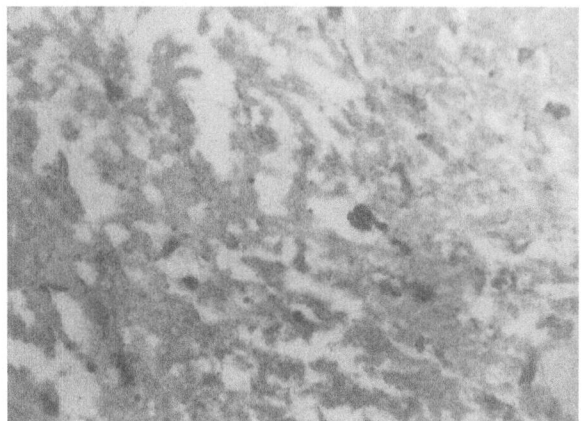

Fig. 3c. Area A3 belonging to the nechrotic histologic type.

Table 1. Correlation among echographic features, cellular density and histologic type of tumour

Echographic area	A1	A2	A3
No. of peaks	12	12	8
Extension	8 useg.	8 useg.	5 useg.
Average height of peaks	1.94	2.65	0.56
Reflectivity (%)	48.5	66	14
Average cellular density (cells/mm^3)	175,000	682,000	1,200
Histologic type	Epithelioid	Spindle-shaped	Necrotic

Reference

Zarate, J.O. & Sampaolesi, R. Morphological parameters of intraocular tumours taking part in echographical tracings. XII Iguazu (Argentina):S.I.D.U.O. Congress. Doc. Ophthalmol. Proc. Ser. 53: 281–292, Dordrecht: Kluwer Acad. Publ. (1990).

Address for correspondence: Parana 1239-1°A, 1018 Buenos Aires, Argentina.

23. The role of echography in small-sized melanomas

P. PERRI, V. MAZZEO, L. RAVALLI,
M. CHIARELLI & P. MONARI
(Ferrara, Italy)

Abstract. Echographic diagnosis of choroidal melanomas is based on well-known criteria. In the following chapter, the authors compare melanomas just large enough to be seen (i.e. smaller than 3 mm) with other small lesions, in order to set differential diagnostic criteria. To this end, all small lesions observed by the authors in the last ten years have been critically re-examined.

Introduction

Solid lesions of the eyeball have been studied by ophthalmological echographers since the introduction of this technique into clinical practice.

The echographic criteria of solid lesions and of other space-occupying pathologies have been codified, [1–4, 6] and nowadays differential diagnosis is possible with an accuracy of between 90 and 100%.

The most important factor is the size of the lesion under examination, since the thicker it is, the easier it is to obtain results in order to formulate a diagnosis.

It is known that to obtain resolution in an echography of a space-occupying lesion, the minimum thickness is 0.5 mm, and for a differential diagnosis a thickness of between 2 and 2.5 mm is required, when this lesion is at the back of the eyeball [2–6].

In the light of these data, we have re-examined all lesions thinner than 3 mm, where an echographic examination was carried out in the last ten years. We evaluated and highlighted the most common echographic criteria which permitted us to give a differential diagnosis between choroidal melanoma and other pathologies (i.e. angioma, metastasis, disciform macular degeneration, hematomas, etc.) (Figs. 1–6).

We have expressly excluded melanomas of the iris and ciliary body, because we believe that in such cases echography can only give an evaluation of the solid characteristics (or cystic) of the lesions under examination.

P. Till (ed.), Ophthalmic Echography 13, pp. 251–256.

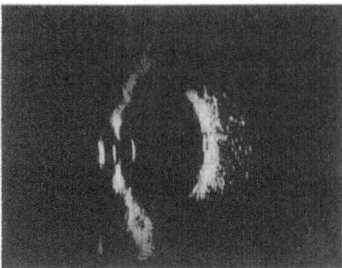

Fig. 1. Very small choroidal melanoma. Choroidal excavation.

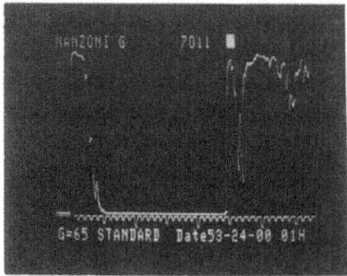

Fig. 2. Small choroidal melanoma. Low internal reflectivity.

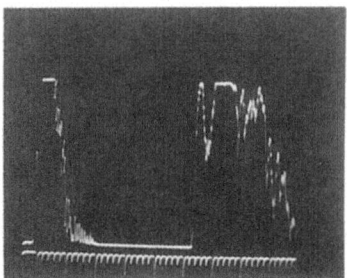

Fig. 3. Small choroidal melanoma. Medium internal reflectivity.

Materials and methods

We have considered and analysed 311 echographic examinations of 250 of our patients, carried out between March 1980 and March 1990 for space-occupying lesions of small dimensions (less than 3 mm).

The echographic examinations carried out by different echographers during the above period were with A-scan and both contact and immersion B-scan.

For the A-scan, a 7200 MA Kretztechnik, and a Biophysic Medical

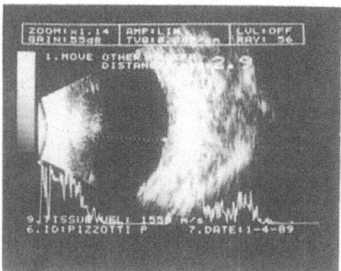

Fig. 4. Small flat lesion. Choroidal metastasis.

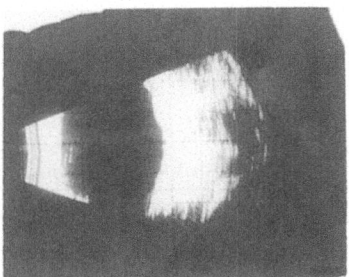

Fig. 5. Small choroidal hemangioma. High internal reflectivity.

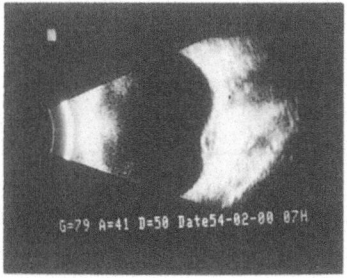

Fig. 6. Solid stratified lesion. Disciform macular degeneration.

Ophthascan S were used; for the B-scan, a Sonometric Inc. Ophthalmoscan 200, a Biophysic Medical Ophthascan S, and a Sonomed 3000 were used.

Results

As can be seen from Table 1, in most lesions (122) the echography provided no clear diagnosis data, both for the thinness, and for the lack of pathogno-monic criteria for well-known pathologies.

Table 1.

Choroidal melanomas	34
Choroidal hemangiomas	16
Choroidal metastases	12
Disciform macular degenerations	26
Hematomas	40
Other unclasified lesions	122

Table 2.

Total choroidal melanomas	34
Histological examination	13
Conservative treatment	9
Only clinic echographic and fluorescein ang. diagnosis	12

Table 3. Pathognomonic echographic findings in 34 cases of choroidal melanomas

Internal reflectivity	Low	20
	Low–medium	6
	medium	8
Shape	Dome-shaped	30
	Mushroom-shaped	2
	Flat-shaped	2
Choroidal excavation		24
Thickness	Minimum	1.5 mm
	Maximum	3 mm
	Medium	2.5 mm

The number of choroidal melanomas diagnosed by us was 34 (Table 2); 13 of these patients were enucleated, and it was therefore possible to verify histologically our diagnosis; 9 were given conservative therapy; the 12 remaining patients were examined echographically and with fluoresceinangiography and clinical tests, but further data are impossible to give, because they subsequently left our area.

In these patients melanomas were found with a thickness of between 1.5 and 3 mm (Table 3). Bearing in mind the pathognomonic criteria, both with A-scan and B-scan, it can be said that the most common form encountered was dome-shaped; in two cases it was flat, and in two cases because of the obvious rupture of Bruch's membrane, it was that of a small mushroom.

In all the above cases, reflectivity was low-medium; the choroidal excavation present in 24 cases indubitable represents a very important criterion for diagnosis.

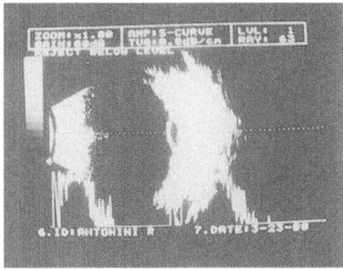

Fig. 7. Small dome-shaped choroidal melanoma. Internal acoustic silence.

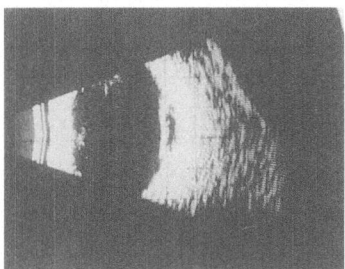

Fig. 8. Small choroidal metastasis from thymoma. Low internal reflectivity. Evident, flat-shaped choroidal excavation.

Because of the small size of the lesions it was impossible to observe the acoustic criteria of absorption or vascularity.

Conclusions

The most up-to-date therapy tends towards conservational treatment of choroidal melanomas, e.g. with Ruthenium or Cobalt-60 plates, proton beams, photocoagulation, etc. To this end, an early diagnosis becomes ever more important, because the thickness of the tumour shows not only the most apt conservative therapy, but is also the most important prognostic criterion.

An analysis of our results shows that a diagnosis was possible in only about 50% of the cases. Of these, melanoma was present in about 25%. Other than reflectivity, the most frequent echographic sign which guided us in differential diagnosis was choroidal excavation, which, as we have seen in our cases, is present in 25 out of 34 (Fig. 7).

From a reading of the literature available, it turns out that especially in small lesions, choroidal excavation is very important. It has never been described in angiomas, while it has been described in one case of tuberculous chorioretinitis, and in some cases of metastases with low reflectivity [2–5] (Fig. 8).

References

1. Coleman, D.J., Lizzi, F.L. and Jack, R.L. Ultrasonography of the eye and orbit. Philadelphia: Lea-Febiger (1977).
2. Mazzeo, V. Ecografia dell'apparato oculare. Testo atlante. Milano: Fogliazza editore (1987).
3. Mazzeo, V. and Scorrano, R. Diagnostica ultrasonica in ophthalmologia. In Gernet H. (ed.), Münster: Augenklink der Westfälischem Wilhelms Universität (1978).
4. Ossoinig, K.C. and Harrie, R.P. Diagnosis of intraocular tumors with standardized echography. In Intraocular tumors. In P.K. Lommatzsch and F.C. Blodi (eds). pp. 154–175. Berlin: Springer-Verlag (1983).
5. Poujol, J. and Le Roy, M. Echographic modifications of the choroid in its tumors and pseudo-tumors. Doc. Ophthalmol. Proc. Ser. 38: 57–62 (1983).
6. Shammas, H. J. Atlas of ophthalmic ultrasonography and biometry. St. Louis/Toronto: The C.V. Mosby Company (1984).

Address for correspondence: Ophthalmology Clinic, Corso Giovecca 203, I-44100 Ferrara, Italy.

24. Ultrasonography in the diagnosis and follow-up of Ruthenium-treated malignant melanomas

F. GOES, J.P. HUYGHE, H. VERBRAEKEN,
P. BRABANT & J.J. DE LAEY

(Antwerp and Ghent, Belgium)

Introduction

There are many unanswered questions regarding the correct treatment of malignant melanoma of the choroid. Is radiation therapy a more effective form than enucleation or local surgical excision? Which form of radiation therapy is most effective? Should adjuvant chemotherapy be used?

Since 1984 Ruthenium treatment was introduced in the Ghent University Eye Clinic as a method of choice for treatment of choroïdal melanomas [1]. Till now 40 eyes were registered in the study.

A- and B-scan ultrasonography was very helpful for the diagnosis and the selection of the cases as well as for the follow-up.

Method

Radiation sources for plaques have included radon seeds, gold 198 seeds, cobalt 60, iridium 192, tantalum 182, iodine 125 seeds, and ruthenium 106.

All of these radioisotopes are photon emitters (gamma rays or x-rays), except ruthenium 106, which is primarily a beta emitter.

The 106 Ruthenium isotope has a half-life time of 366 days and decays to 106 Rodium, with a half-life time of 30 seconds. The decay produces a nearly pure B-ray emission. We chose the 106 Ruthenium isotope because its superior in dose distribution as compared to the 60 Cobalt isotope. The side-effects of the irradiation are also less with 106 Ruthenium [2].

The Ruthenium applicator is formed by a silver shell of 1 mm width. The 106 Ruthenium is equally distributed on the inner concave surface and is covered by a thin film of silver of 0.1 mm. The small film of silver on the inner side has no influence on the B-ray emission, whereas the 1 mm layer on the convex surface absorbs nearly all radiation.

The purpose of this treatment is to get a total dose of 10.000 rad (100 Gy) at the top of the tumor [3, 4]. To obtain this dose in cases of tumors of 5–6 mm height for example, the base of the tumor, and thus also the sclera, will receive between 80.000 and 100.000 rad (800–1000 Gy).

The irradiation time is calculated for each patient individually. This time

P. Till (ed.), Ophthalmic Echography 13, pp. 257–264.
© 1993 *Kluwer Academic Publishers.*

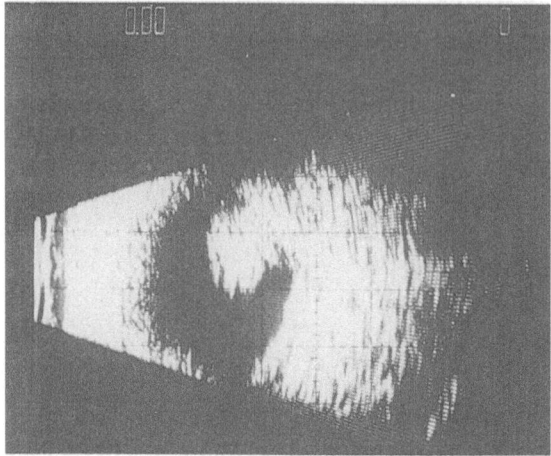

Fig. 1. Tumour height ⩾5 mm in a case that did not fit the criteria.

depends on the prominence of the tumor, measured by A-scan echography, and on the emission power of the applicator.

Recommendations for the case selection for Ruthenium treatment were formulated by Lommatzch [3] (1983) Table 1.

1. First: because of the physical properties of Ruthenium the choroidal melanoma should not exceed 5 mm in height above the scleral surface and 15 mm in diameter at the tumor base. Tumour cells at a distance more than 5 mm away from the applicator will not receive the damaging dose of at least 10.000 rad.
2. Second: the tumour should not involve the ciliary body. Because of the danger of scleral perforation local tumour excision should be preferred if the tumour is too advanced.
3. Third: the distance of the posterior tumour margin should be at least 1 to 2 disc diameters from the optic nerve head.
4. Fourth: there should not be tumour growth outside the eye (Fig. 1).

Table 1. Recommendations for case selection

Ruthenium
1. Maximum 5 mm height
15 mm base
2. No ciliary body
3. 2 d.d. from optic nerve head
4. No growth outside eye

In 1986 Lommatzch [4] reported on the 20 years experience and follow-up of 309 patients with malignant melanoma treated with 106 Ru/106 Rh B-ray applicators with a mean follow-up of 6–7 years after irradiation. This survival

Table 2. Melanoma characteristics

Ultrasound	Reaction
Solid tissue ⩾1.5 mm	
Regular low internal reflectivity	Height reduction
Vascularisation	
Acoustic shadowing	

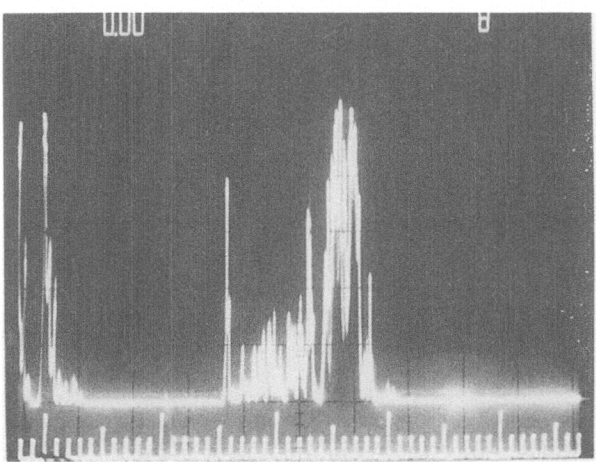

Fig. 2. Tumour height measurement on A-scan.

rate was substantly higher than that for patients whose eyes had primarily been enucleated.

In 17.2% (53 cases) the eye had to be enucleated and 40 patients (12.9%) died from metastasis: 69.9% of the patients were successfully treated. Of the 216 successfully treated patients 49 (22.7%) regained a visual acuity of 1.5–0.5.

Diagnosis – follow-up

Tumour diagnosis and evaluation of regression was based on the fundoscopy, fundus photography, ultrasonography and fluorescein-angiography.

Fluorescein angiography before treatment shows large tumour vessels and mottling during the early phases of the angiogram and dye accumulation within tumour tissue and hyperfluorescence during the late phase.

Tumour regression and cicatrisation of the surrounding tissue causes avascular areas, occlusion of tumour and choroidal vessels within the radiated zone and decreased or no leakage into the tumour remnants.

Successfully treated patients were considered to be those whose tumours

Table 3. Ghent University – treated cases

Ghent University Eye Clinic – Choroidal Melanoma

40 – 26 left – 24 right
  – 18 M – 22 F
  – Follow-up: mean 3.5 (0.5–6y)
  – Localisation: Macular   5
                temporal 22
                nasal   12
                O.N.   1

Table 4. Results of 35 selected cases

Follow-up 35

3+: Liver metastasis
3 Enucleation: glaucoma 1
                vasculitis 2
1 Radionecrosis
1 Add Xenon

Success 27/35: 77%

had either changed to a flat scar or shrunk to a still prominent greyish-black mass with scarification of the tissue on and around the melanoma.

A and B-scan *ultrasound* diagnosis of malignant melanoma was established according to the classical signs:
1. tumour lesion of at least 1.5 mm
2. regular acoustic structure
3. vascularisation
4. low to medium internal reflectivity
5. acoustic shadowing.

Measurement of uveal melanoma thickness is important in the choice of therapy, and monitoring the efficacy of treatment (Table 2).

It has been demonstrated that multiple measurements of the same tumour in the same institutions have a variation of less than 0.5 mm and that there is excellent correlation between ultrasonographic and clinical estimation of tumour height [5] (Fig. 2).

Results

We had the occasion to follow with ultrasound the evolution of 40 treated choroidal malignant melanomas.

The mean follow-up was 3.5 years with a minimum of 6 months and a maximum of 6 years (3 cases). The sex ratio was 18 males, 22 females. The mean age was 57 years (extremes 35–81 years).

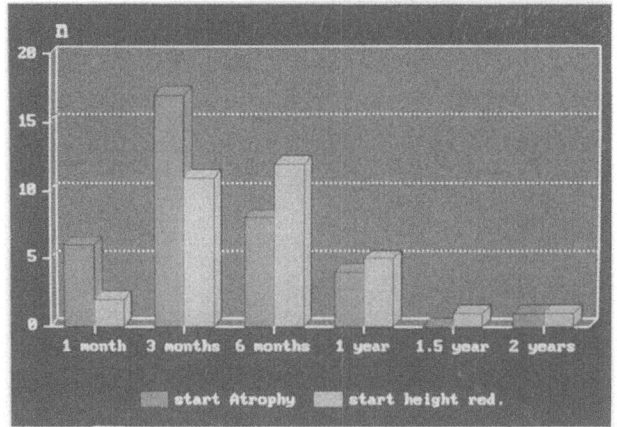

Fig. 3. Start of atrophy, start of height reduction of the treated cases.

The localisation was macular in 5 cases, temporal in 22 cases, nasal in 12 and juxtapapillary in 1 case.

Thirty-five out of the 40 treated cases were suitable for Ruthenium application according to the criteria by Lommatzsch (Table 3).

In our series the regression of the tumour started before 6 months in only one case. In cases of metastatic disease the tumour disappears in 6 to 8 weeks which can be taken as an indication for differential diagnosis. From that time on a gradual regression started. In cases of metastatic, together with the regression of the tumour, some authors found a change of the echographic pattern, increase of internal reflectivity, irregular acoustic structure [6–7]

In the 5 cases that did not correspond to the criteria the thickness of the tumour was always >5.0 mm (5.3 to 10.5 mm, mean 7.5 mm).

All these eyes had to be enucleated because of vitreous hemorrhage without regression of the tumour (2), retinal detachment without tumour reaction (1), radionecrosis (1) and neovascular glaucoma (1). This is a clear indication that one should stick to the selection criteria.

In the 35 cases that fit the criteria, 3 patients died during the follow-up, all of liver metastasis (follow-up 4.5–4.5–3 years, mean age 49, thickness 4–4–5.5 mm). In 3 cases enucleation of the eye had to be performed: (1) neovascular glaucoma; (2) radiovasculitis. In one other case there was mild radionecrosis.

In one case additional Xenon fotocoagulation had to be performed because of lack of reaction to the treatment.

So the success rate in our group was 27/35 = 77% (Table 4)

The visual acuity results of the 35 eligible cases were as follows: in 11 cases decrease in visual acuity, (7 cases macular localisation, 2 radionecrosis,

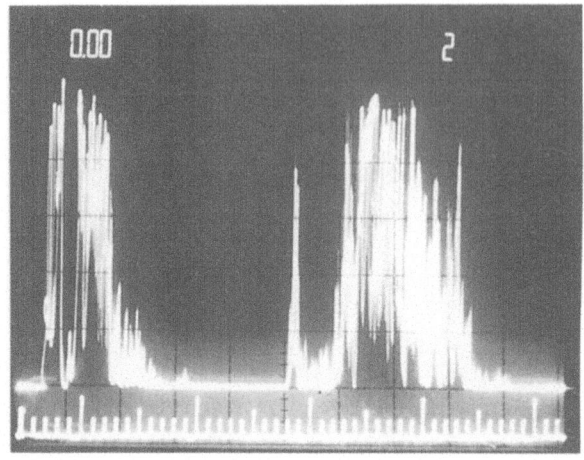

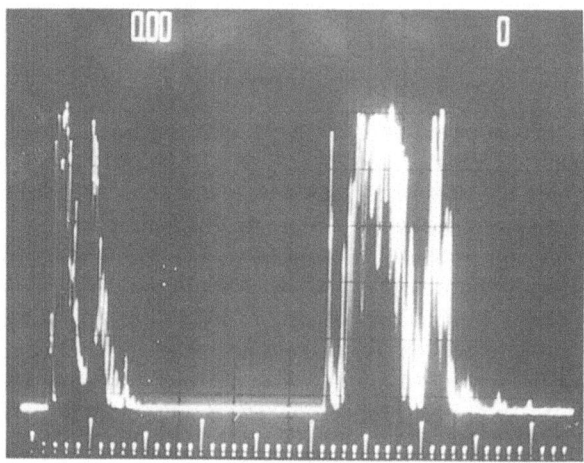

Fig. 4. (a) before, (b) after Ruthenium treatment.

1 Xenon coagulation, 1 keratitis), a status quo in 21 and an amelioration in 3 cases (two cases ameliorated from C.T to 1.0).

Regression of the tumour became usually visible after a mean period of 6 months. The response of the tumour was evaluated by the appearance of atrophic lesions around the tumour and by the ultrasonographically measured shrinkage (Fig. 3–Fig. 4). Both phenomena were not always present at the same moment.

Atrophy was present before echographically measured decrease in 13 cases, both phenomena were present within a 6 months period in 18 cases and echographically measured decrease was present before definite fundoscopic changes of atrophy in only 4 eyes, out of 35 (Fig. 5).

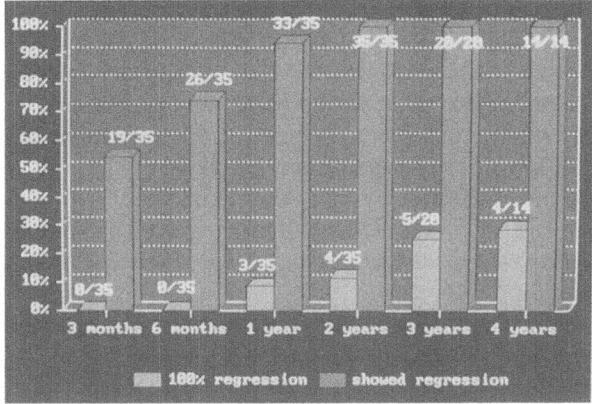

Fig. 5. Start of regression and 100% regression of cases according to the time.

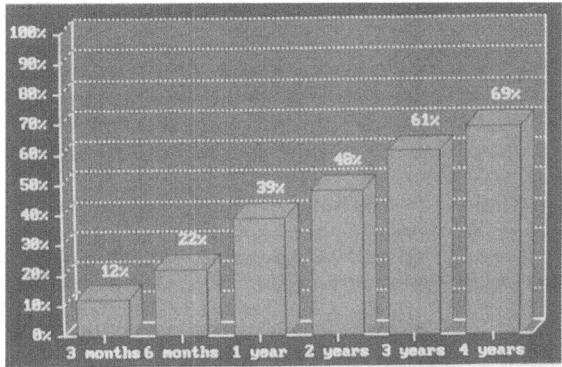

Fig. 6. Mean regression of tumour height according to the time.

We studied echographically the *decrease* of the tumour height in function of time.

At the first control examination after three months 19/35 cases showed no regression and the mean regression of the tumour thickness was 12%.

At the six-month follow-up the mean regression of the tumour was 22%, and still 9 out of 35 cases showing no change.

At the one-year follow-up, still 2 cases out of 35 showed no change of tumour mass, the mean regression being 39% (100% in 3 eyes). At the two-year follow-up all eyes showed some change of volume, the mean change being 48%. In 4 eyes complete regression of the tumour was present.

At the three-year follow-up the mean regression was 61%, and it was 100% in 5/20 cases.

At the four-year follow-up (14 eyes) the mean regression was 69%, and it was 100% in 4/14 eyes (Fig. 6).

Conclusion

Ruthenium application is a valuable mode of therapy for choroïdal malignant melanoma if one adheres strictly to the selection criteria.

A- and B-scan ultrasound was very helpful for the diagnosis of choroïdal melanoma and follow-up of Ruthenium treatment.

With the help of ultrasound we can demonstrate:

1. a reduction in size of the tumour pointing towards a therapeutic success.
2. an eventual growth of the tumour pointing towards a false diagnosis or wrong application.
3. eventual complications as retinal detachment, vitreous hemorrhage or scleral perforation

We presented the follow-up of 35 treated cases. The mean follow-up was 3.5 years and the therapeutic success was 77%.

References

1. Van Hyfte, R., Verbraeken, H. & De Laey, J.J. Ruthenium applications in the treatment of choroidal melanomas. Bull. Soc. Belge. Ophtalmol. 224: 51–58 (1987).
2. Zografos, L. & Gailloud, C. Traitement conservateur des mélanomes de la choroïde avec des applicateurs de Cobalt 60 radioactifs. Kl. Mbl. Augenheilk. 182: 499–501 (1983).
3. Lommatzch, P.K. B-irradiation of choroidal melanoma with 106 Ru/106 Rh applicators 16 years' experience. Arch. Opthalmol. 101: 715 (1983).
4. Lommatzch, P.K. Results after B-irradiation (106 Ru/106 Rh) of choroidal melanomas:20 years' experience. Br. J. Ophthalmol. 70: 844–851 (1986).
5. Char, H., Kroll, S., Stone, D., Harrie, R. & Kerman, B. Ultrasonographic measurement of uveal melanoma thickness: interobserver variability. Br. J. Ophthalmol. 74: 183–185 (1990).
6. Shammas, H.J., Boyer, D.S. & Miller, J.B. Ultrasound characteristics of posterior uveal melanoma treated with cobalt plaque radiotherapy. In K.C. Ossoinig (ed.): Ophthalmic echography, pp. 379–383. The Hague: Dr. W. Junk (1987).
7. Verbeeck, A.M. Uveal melanoma before and after Ruthenium application therapy. In K.C. Ossoinig (ed.): Ophthalmic echography, pp. 385–390. The Hague: Dr. W. Junk (1987).

Address for correspondence: Antwerp Ophthalmic Surgical Centre, Van Eycklei 5 bus 1-2, B-2018 Antwerp, Belgium.

25. Choroidal malignant melanoma masquerading as posterior scleritis

P.G. WOLFF-KORMANN, G. HASENFRATZ,
F. H. STEFANI & K.G. RIEDEL

(*Munich, Germany*)

Abstract. The unusual clinical course and echographic findings of a malignant melanoma simulating posterior scleritis are demonstrated. A forty-year-old man developed epiphora pain and visual loss in his left eye. Biomicroscopy showed sparse exudate in the vitreous. Indirect ophthalmoscopy disclosed left inferior exudative retinal detachment. Ultrasonography revealed a localized subretinal mass. Biopsy was consistent with nodular fasciitis, clinical signs and symptoms however suggested posterior scleritis. Systematic prednisone treatment improved the patient's condition, the retinal detachment resolved and the choroidal elevation decreased. Follow-up examinations showed a recurrent retinal detachment and sonographic signs of a solid tumor with orbital extension two years after initial clinical and histological evaluation. Orbital exenteration was performed as a second orbital biopsy revealed a choroidal malignant melanoma. Light microscopy of the enucleated globe displayed polymorphous amelanotic malignant melanoma of the choroid. The clinical and sonographical features of this case of 'suspected scleritis' are discussed in light of the final diagnosis.

Case report

A forty-year-old white man was admitted to the University Eye Hospital Munich on July 1986 because of a one-week history of left frontal headaches and hazy vision. He complained of pain, tearing and redness of his left eye. Corrected visual acuity was 20/20 on the right and 20/30 on the left eye. The intra-ocular pressure was 16 mm Hg on the right eye and 14 mm Hg on the left eye. The right eye showed no pathological clinical findings. Ocular examination of the left eye revealed eyelid edema and scleral injection in the nasal and upper quadrant. There was evidence of cells in the left anterior chamber as well as in the vitreous. Indirect ophthalmoscopy demonstrated left inferotemporal retinal detachment, thought to be inflammatory in character since no retinal tear could be discovered. A circumscribed fundus mass was noted in the superonasal periphery. By transillumination no shadow could be detected. Ultrasonography (Fig. 1) disclosed a dome-shaped subretinal lesion of 7 mm height. Further criteria were solid consistency, heterogeneous internal structure, medium reflectivity partly with sound attenuation and suspected extraocular growth. No signs of vasculariation could be detected. Ultrasonic evaluation was thought to be consistent with malignant melanoma of the choroid and orbital extension. Biopsy specimens were taken from the sclera within the suspicious area. Histological examination

P. Till (ed.), *Ophthalmic Echography 13*, pp. 265–271.
© 1993 *Kluwer Academic Publishers.*

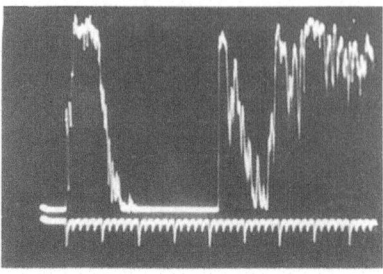

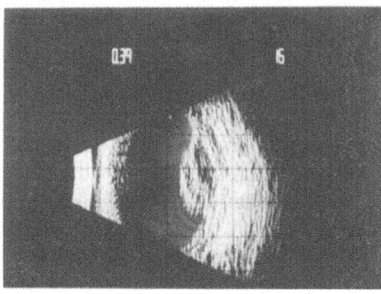

Fig. 1. 7/86 Left eye: A- and B-scan show a dome-shaped subretinal lesion of 7 mm height with solid consistency, medium reflectivity partly with sound attenuation and extraocular growth. No sign of vascularity.

demonstrated collagenous tissue diffusely infiltrated with lymphocytes. plasma cells and some eosinophils, scleral inflammatory changes suspicious of nodular fasciitis. The patient received systemic prednisone, mydriatics and steroid eye drops, which promptly relieved his pain. Clinical follow-up one month later reported cleared scleral injection, normal anterior chamber and vitreous as well as flattened retinal detachment. Ultrasonic workup at this time revealed a significant decrease of the choroidal mass. Further regression of choroidal elevation was noted two months later. A-scan and B-scan echograms (Fig. 2) showed thickening of the posterior sclera and retrobulbar edema suggesting posterior scleritis as the underlying disease [18, 19]. The patient was given gradually tapered doses of corticosteroids. He remained asymptomatic for 17 months. In February, 1988 the condition worsened with the appearence of pain, decreased vision, infection of scleral vessels, anterior chamber and vitreous cells. This exacerbation was accompanied by exudative retinal detachment and recurrent choroidal thickening (Fig. 3). Again remission was achieved by corticosteroid treatment. Ultrasound control on September 1988 more than two years after the initial ocular symptoms, a choroidal tumor of low reflectivity, rather homogenous structure, no signs of vascularity and with large orbital extension (Fig. 4) was detected.

Histological and immunhistological evaluation of a second orbital biopsy finally established the diagnosis of an amelanotic choroidal malignant melanoma. Orbital exenteration was performed. In accordance with the findings

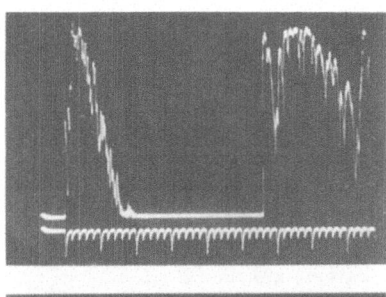

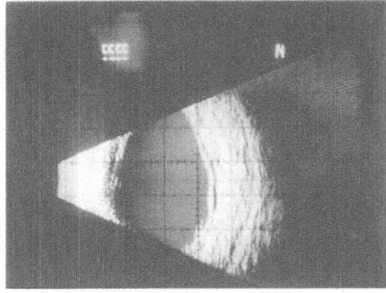

Fig. 2. 10/86 Left eye after corticosteroid treatment: A- and B-scan demonstrate significant decrease of choroidal tumor, scleral thickening and retrobulbar edema.

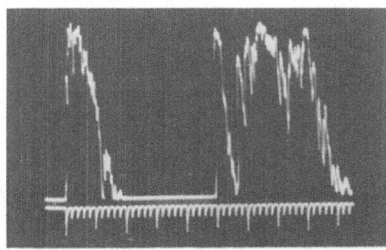

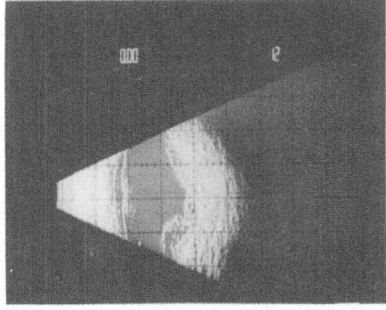

Fig. 3. 02/88 Left eye: A- and B-scan display recurrent choroidal thickening and exudative retinal detachment.

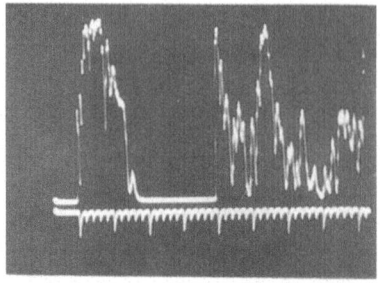

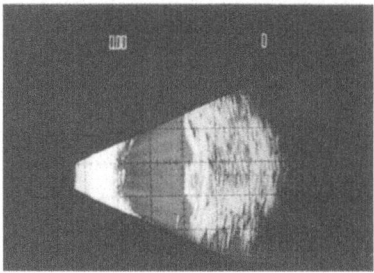

Fig. 4. 09/88 Left eye: A- and B-scan echograms are consistent with malignant choroidal melanoma with orbital extension.

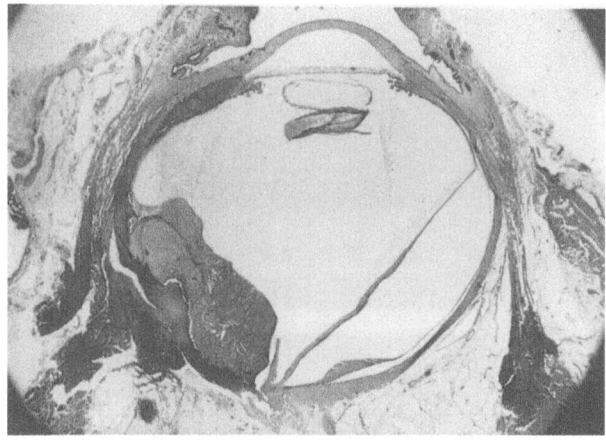

Fig. 5. 09/88 Enucleated globe – Light macroscopy: Amelanotic partially necrotic malignant melanoma of the choroid, measuring 10 × 5.5 mm with extraocular extension of 4 mm.

derived from orbital biopsy, light microscopic examination showed a little pigmented, partly necrotic, polymorphous spindle cell choroidal tumor, measuring 10 × 5.5 mm with an extrascleral extension of 4 mm (Fig. 5). Five months later systemic workup including an abdomen ultrasound study, a computed scan of the abdomen and a radionuclide body scan demonstrated liver, muscle and multiple skeletal metastases. In spite of combination chemotherapy according to the BOLD-regimen (Bleomycin, Vincristine, Lomustine, Dacarbazine), the patient died of metastatic disease in August 1989, ten months after orbital exenteration.

Discussion

In the present case a partially necrotic malignant melanoma of the choroid masqueraded clinically as posterior scleritis attended by exudative retinal detachment. This unusual feature has first been described by Hallden [10] in 1955. In 1979 Fraser [8] reviewed 450 eyes enucleated because of malignant melanoma of the choroid or ciliary body. In 4.9% of the cases ocular inflammation including episcleritis, uveitis, endophthalmitis or panophthalmitis was the initial clinical manifestation of unsuspected malignant melanoma. Posterior scleritis as first harbinger of uveal melanoma was not comprised in his study. Among more than 700 choroidal malignant melanomas this is the only case in our series (1972–1989) simulating posterior scleritis.

Posterior scleritis commonly affects middle-aged individuals (age range from 12 to 77 years); and it occurs more frequently in women than men [2]. The onset of the disease is typically subacute. Pain is the cardinal symptom with which the patient presents and it may be referred to the brow, temple, sinuses or teeth [1]. Recurrences are common. Posterior scleritis can present with uveitis [3], intraocular hemorrhage and vascular occlusion [22]. Further complications include exudative retinal or choroidal detachment [9, 14], choroidal folds [19], a circumscribed fundus mass [2], optic disk edema [22] and angle closure glaucoma [7]. In retrospect several aspects of our patient's history provided clues to the final diagnosis. His sex was atypical for inflammatory scleral disease and he had none of the systemic diseases associated with posterior scleritis such as rheumatoid arthritis [5], lupus erythematode [20], Wegener's granulomatosis [12, 21], Crohn's disease [13], or syphilis [23]. Moreover primary sonographic evaluation indicated malignant melanoma of the choroid.

On the other hand sudden onset of pain, decrease of vision, scleral injection, uveitis and retinal detachment accorded with the clinical picture of posterior scleritis. Severe pain with malignant melanoma is uncommon in the absence of hemorrhage or secondary glaucoma [6]. Initial histological findings were also consistent with inflammatory ocular disease. The immediate and repeated response to systemic corticosteroids seemed to confirm the diagnosis of posterior scleritis. Vascularization is a well established cardinal echographic criterion for malignant uveal melanoma [4, 11, 15–17].

Despite careful screening of different acoustic sections vascularity was missing. Histological findings observed in the enucleated globe (Fig. 6) elucidate the reasons for the lack of spontaneous vertical tumor spike oscillation. The lesion displayed a dense pattern of spindle and polymorphous cells with

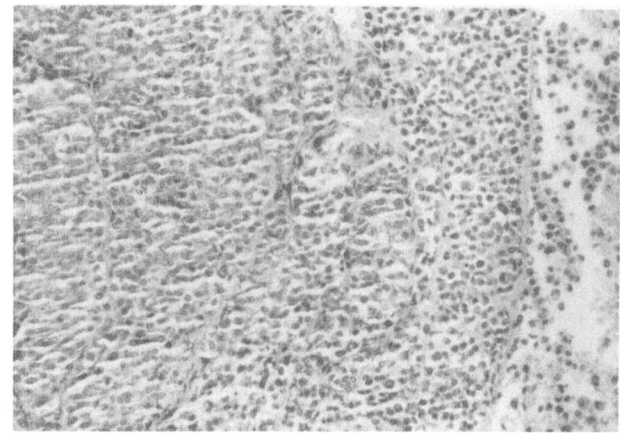

Fig. 6. 09/88 Histological section of malignant melanoma showing a dense pattern of polymorphous spindle cells. Hematoxylin and eosine staining. ×20.

fascicular cell arrangement in part. Only scattered thin-walled blood vessels could be detected suggesting a poor development of tumor capillary network.

We conclude that the sonographic criterion of vasculariation may be absent in highly prominent malignant melanomas of the choroid.

Furthermore this unusual case of malignant melanoma of the choroid lays emphasis on the rare role of posterior scleritis as masquerading syndrome.

References

1. Benson, W.E, Shields, J.A., Tasman, W. & Crandall, A.S. Posterior scleritis – a case of diagnostic confusion. Arch. Ophthalmol. 97: 1482–1486 (1979).
2. Benson, W.E. Posterior Scleritis. Surv. Ophthalmol. 35(2): 297–316 (1988).
3. Calthorpe, C. M., Watson, P.G. & McCartney, A.C.E. Posterior scleritis: a clinical and histological survey. Eye 2: 267–277 (1988).
4. Coleman, D.J., Abramson, D.H., Jacl, R.L. & Franzen, L.A. Ultrasonic diagnosis of tumors of the choroid. Arch. Ophthalmol. 91: 344–354 (1974).
5. Erhardt, C.C., Mumford, P.A., Venables, P.J. & Maini, R.N. Factors predicting a poor life prognosis in rheumatoid arthritis: an eight year prospective study. Ann. Rheum. Dis. 48(1): 7–13 (1989).
6. Feldon. S.E., Sigelman, J., Albert, D.M. & Smith, T.R. Clinical manifestation of browny scleritis. Am. J. Ophthalmol. 85: 781–787 (1978).
7. Fourman, G. Angle-closure glaucoma complicating ciliochoroidal detachment. Ophthalmology 96(5): 646–653 (1989).
8. Fraser, D.J. & Font, R.L. Ocular Inflammation and hemorrhage as initial manifestations of uveal malignant melanoma. Arch. Ophthalmol. 97: 1311–1314 (1979).
9. Fraunfelder, F.T. & Watson, P.G. Evaluation of eyes enucleated for scleritis. Br. J. Ophthalmol. 60: 227–230 (1976).
10. Hallden, U. Malignant melanoma of the choroid clinically simulating posterior scleritis attended by amotio retinae. Acta Ophthalmol. 33: 489–491 (1955).

11. Hodes, B. & Chromokos, E. Standardized A-scan echographic diagnosis of choroidal malignant melanomas. Arch. Ophthalmol. 95: 593–597 (1977).
12. Hodges, E.J., Turner, S. & Doud, R.B. Refractory scleritis due to Wegener's granulomatosis. West. J. Med. 146(3): 361–363 (1987).
13. Knox, D.L., Schachat, A.P. & Mustonen, E. Primary, secondary and coincidental ocular complications of Crohn's disease. Ophthalmology 91: 163–173 (1984).
14. Litwak, A.B. Posterior scleritis with secondary ciliochoroidal effusion. J. Am. Optom. Assoc. 60(4): 300–306 (1989).
15. Ossoinig, K.C. Preoperative differential diagnosis of tumors with echography. In F. C. Blodi (ed.), Current Concepts in Opthalmology 4: 264–343. St Louis: Mosby (1974).
16. Ossoinig, K.C., Bigar, F. & Kaefring, S.L. Malignant melanoma of the choroid and ciliary body: a differential diagnosis in clinical echography. In Ultrasonography in Ophthalmology. Bibl. Ophthalmol. 83: 141–154. Basel: Karger (1975).
17. Ossoinig, K.C. Standardized echography: basic principles. clinical applications and results. In Dallow, R.L. (ed.), Ophthalmic Ultrasonography: Comparative Techniques. Int. Ophthal. Clin. 19/4: 127–210. Boston: Little, Brown & Co. (1979).
18. Rochels, R. & Reis, G. Echographie bei skleritis posterior. Klin. Mbl. Augenheilk. 177: 611–613 (1980).
19. Singh, G., Guthoff, R. & Foster, G.S. Observations on long-term follow-up of posterior scleritis. Am. J. Ophthalmol 101: 570–575 (1986).
20. Turgeon, P.W. & Slamovitz, T.L. Scleritis as the presenting manifestation of procainamide induced lupus. Ophthalmology 96(1): 68–71 (1989).
21. Vogiatzis, K.V. Bilateral blindness due to necrotizing scleritis in a case of Wegener's granulomatosis. Ann. Ophthalmol. 15(2): 185–188 (1983).
22. Watson, P.G. The nature and the treatment of scleral inflammation. Trans. Ophthal. Soc. (U.K.) 102: 257–277 (1982).
23. Wilhelmus, K.R. & Yokoyama, CM. Syphilitic episcleritis and scleritis. Am. J. Ophthalmol. 104(6): 595–597 (1987).

Address for correspondence: Eye Clinic, University of Munich, Mathilden Strasse 8, 8000 Munich 2, Germany.

26. Standardized A-scan diagnosis of bilateral choroidal osteoma in a $4\frac{1}{2}$-year-old girl

A. STANOWSKY

(*Augsburg, Germany*)

Abstract. Choroidal osteoma is a rare eye disease which usually entails meticulous differential diagnosis for final identification. The diagnosis can be made very easily, however, with the aid of standardized A-scan echography. This was reconfirmed in the case of a $4\frac{1}{2}$-year-old girl, where retinoblastoma had to be ruled out especially with regard to the unusual age of the patient. To our knowledge this is the youngest patient with bilateral choroidal osteoma reported in the literature to date.

Introduction

Choroidal osteoma or osseous choristoma of the choroid is a rare tumor [5, 6]. It occurs unilaterally or bilaterally, usually in young adult females [1, 5, 6]. Clinically it appears as an amelanotic placoid choroidal mass, most commonly in the posterior pole. Histologically it is composed of mature bone [3–6]. Hereditary factors [2] as well as antecedent intraocular inflammations [7, 10] are discussed in its etiology. Computed tomography and echographical examination have proved to be the most important examination techniques in establishing the diagnosis. We had the opportunity to see this disease in a $4\frac{1}{2}$-year-old girl involved in the question of whether computed tomography [8] should be performed for final diagnosis as generally recommended in the literature so far.

Case history

The female patient, born in 1983, first presented in our outpatient clinic at the beginning of 1988. Ophthalmoscopically, a placoid choroidal mass was found which extended over the entire posterior pole in both eyes. Although surrounded by a slightly prominent choroidal process, the macular area of the right posterior pole appeared normal for the most part (Fig. 1).

The macular region of the left eye showed additional, pronounced shifts of pigmentation. No intra- or extraocular inflammatory reaction was found. Visual acuity was 20/30 in the right eye, 20/100 in the left.

P. Till (ed.), Ophthalmic Echography 13, pp. 273–276.

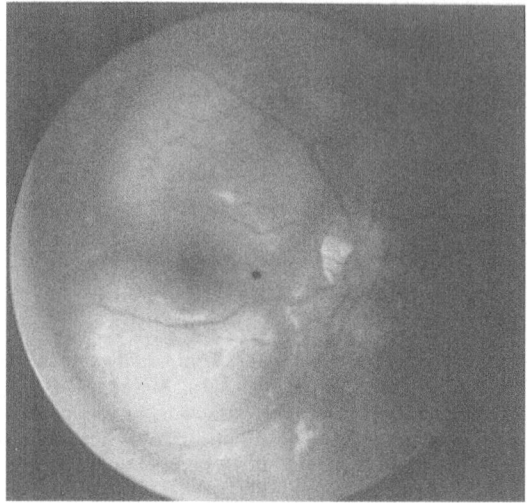

Fig. 1. Both fundi showed a placoid choroidal mass, the macular area of the right eye having a normal configuration for the most part.

Material and method

B-scan and standardized A-scan examinations were carried out with an Ophthascan S unit. Neither sedation nor narcosis were required.

Results

B-Scan. A large, flat, bilateral area of high reflectivity was found stretching from the temporal equator to the disc (Fig. 2a,b). Multiple reverberation echos appeared preferably at the margins. The center of the lesion completely absorbed the ultrasonic sound waves, causing echo-shadowing in the orbital area behind.

Standardized A-scan. An overloaded, 100% highly reflecting echo signal was received from the lesion area (Fig. 3). Here, too, were multiple reverberation echos, especially at the borders of the lesion. An echo-free area behind the lesion was caused by scattering, absorption, and high reflectivity at the level of the lesion. The echo signal had 100% reflectivity [9] even when the ultrasonic beam was oblique (so-called foreign body echo at oblique sound beam).

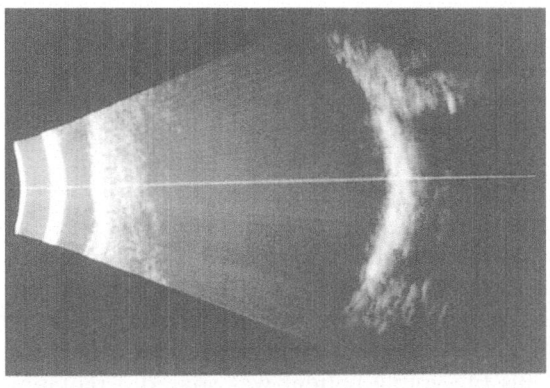

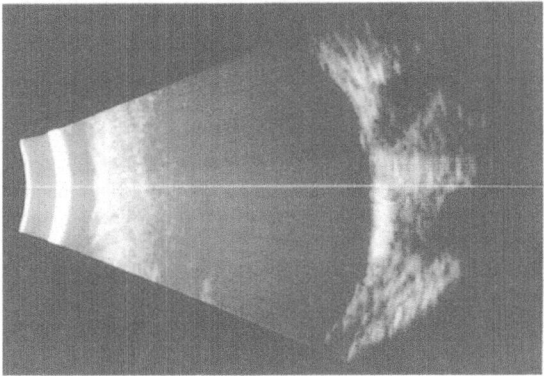

Fig. 2. B-scan of the right (top) and left (bottom) eye shows a flat, hardly prominent area of highly increased reflectivity with marked sound attenuation. The lesion in the left eye extends to the optic nerve showing multiple reverberation echos at its borders.

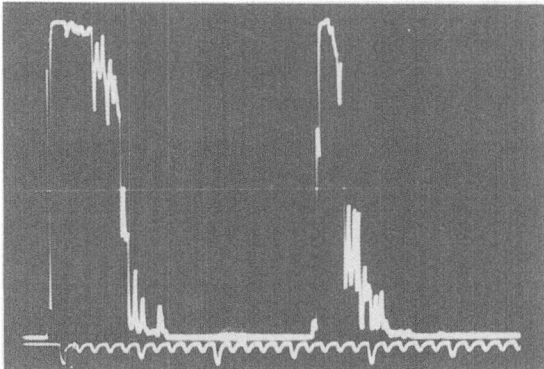

Fig. 3. Standardized A-scan echogram of the right eye. There is an overloaded, 100% high echo signal at the level of the choroidal osteoma with marked sound attenuation behind it.

Discussion

Thanks to prominent characteristics, echographic diagnosis of choroidal osteoma is usually uncomplicated, in conformity with previous examination reports. This makes echographic examination indispensable for this clinical syndrome, and as a consequence further examination techniques such as computed tomography can usually be dispensed with. This was also true of the patient described here, who is to our knowledge the youngest patient with bilateral choroidal osteoma described in the literature to date. On the basis of age, the differential diagnosis of retinoblastoma, in particular had to be considered. Although retinoblastoma causes highly reflecting signals too, these never occur with the standardized A-scan characteristics mentioned above. Thus the young patient was spared a radiation exposure and a narcosis examination for purposes of computed tomography.

References

1. Avila, M.P., El-Markabi, H., Azzolini, C., Jalkh, A.E., Burns, D. & Weiter, J.J. Bilateral choroidal osteoma with subretinal neovascularization. Ann. Ophthalmol. 16: 381 (1984).
2. Cunha, S.L. Osseous choristoma of the choroid: a familial disease. Arch. Ophthalmol. 102: 1052 (1984).
3. Duane, T.D. & Jaeger, E.A. Clinical ophthalmology. Philadelphia: J.B. Lippincott Company Vol. 4: 67, pp. 11–12 (1988).
4. Gass, J.D.M., Guerry, R.K., Jack, R.L. & Harris, G. Choroidal osteoma. Arch. Ophthalmol. 96: 428 (1978).
5. Gass, J.D.M. New observations concerning choroidal osteomas. Int. Ophthalmology 1: 71 (1979).
6. Joffe, L., Shields, J.A. & Fitzgerald, J. Osseous choristoma of the choroid. Arch. Ophthalmol. 96: 1809 (1978).
7. Katz, R.S. & Gass, J.D.M. Multiple choroidal osteomas developing in association with recurrent orbital inflammatory pseudotumor. Arch. Ophthalmol. 101: 1724 (1983).
8. Ogata, T., Hayashi, H., Hashimoto, Y. & Nishimura, Y. Clinical feature and the analysis of choroidal osteoma. Folia Ophthalmol. Jap. 32: 243 (1981).
9. Ossoinig, K.C. Standardized echography: basic principles, clinical applications and results. In Dallow, P.L. (ed.), Ophthalmic ultrasonography: Comparative techniques (Int Opthalmol Clin). Boston: Little, Brown (1979).
10. Trimble, S.N. & Schatz, H. Choroidal osteoma after intraocular inflammation. Am. J. Ophthalmol. 96: 759 (1983).

Address for correspondence:.Zentralklinikum, Augenklinik, Stenglinstrasse 2, W-8900 Augsburg, Germany.

27. Metastatic choroidal lesions
A retrospective study

G. CENNAMO, N. ROSA, T. FOÀ & A. MELE
(*Naples, Italy*)

Abstract. In this retrospective study the authors report their cases of metastatic choroidal lesions. The examinations were performed utilizing Standardized Echography. The authors discuss their findings in some atypical cases, such as low reflectivity that can be related to a fast growth of the lesion with a worst prognosis for the patient.

Introduction

Choroidal metastatic tumors were first described by Horner in 1864 and Perl in 1872. In autoptic series they are the most common malignant intraocular tumors, while they follow malignant melanoma in clinical series [3–8]. In most cases the diagnosis is made in patients suffering from a known neoplastic disease. When a metastatic lesion in the eye is the first clinical sign of a neoplasia, it is very important to differentiate from primary intraocular tumors, such as malignant melanoma, and non neoplastic diseases, such as choroidal hematoma and choroidal detachment [4].

Material and methods

We performed a retrospective study of the choroidal metastatic lesions (Fig. 1) observed in the Echographic Service of our Department in Naples, from 1974 to date. During this period 24 choroidal metastatic tumors were diagnosed. Metastatic leukemia infiltrations were excluded from our study. In all the patients a complete echographic examination with the technique of Standardized Echography was performed. The following machines were used: Kretz 7200 MA, Ophthascan S and Mini A of the Biophysic Medical [9–12].

In our series there were 15 females, aging from 36 to 74 (mean age 54), and 9 males, aging from 57 to 81 (mean age 72). Our echographic diagnoses were supported by history, clinical examination, indirect ophthalmoscopy and, in some cases, by fluorescein angiography and visual field.

P. Till (ed.), *Ophthalmic Echography 13*, pp. 277–283.

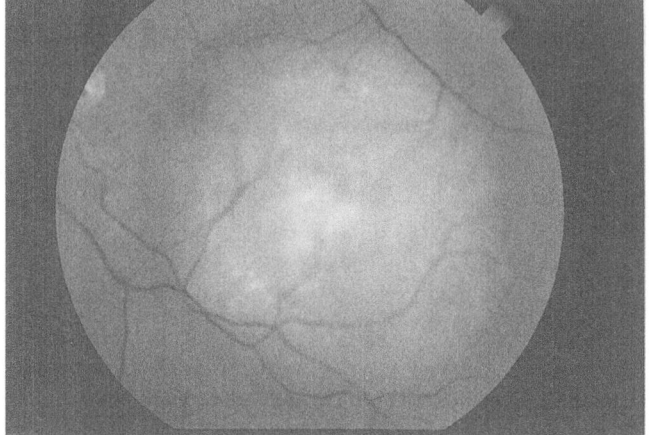

Fig. 1. Ophthalmoscopic aspect in one case of metastatic choroidal lesion.

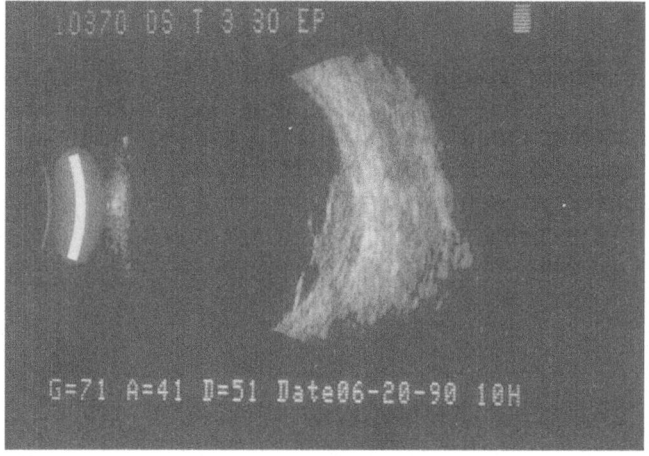

Fig. 2. B-Scan showing a wax flow lesion with an associated retinal detachment.

Results

Our echographic diagnoses were correct in 23 choroidal metastatic tumors. Two cases were false-positive diagnosed, one was a choroidal malignant melanoma, the other one a disciform like lesion. Only one case, with the echographic diagnosis of choroidal hematoma, at the histological examination turned out to be a metastatic tumor from a cutaneous malignant melanoma. The left eye was involved in 11 patients, the right eye in 8. In 5 cases both

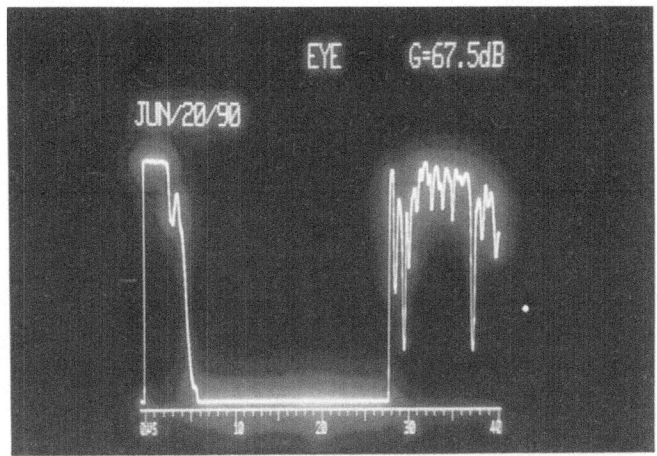

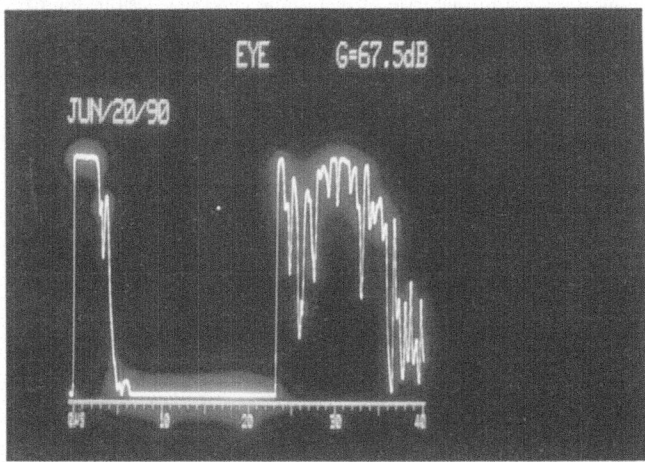

Fig. 3. Typical A-Scan patterns in a case of metastatic choroidal lesion, showing a solid lesion with irregular internal reflectivity.

eyes were affected, in 5 cases there were multiple focuses in a single eye, and in one case, multiple and bilateral focuses. The most common location was the posterior pole, and this is related to the most abundant supply of the posterior ciliary artery in the macular area. An exudative retinal detachment is frequently associated (8 cases) (Fig. 2). Ten cases were metastatic carcinoma from the breast, 6 from the lung, 1 from the prostate gland, 1 from the thyroid gland, 1 from the stomach, 2 from cutaneous malignant melanoma, 1 from the testicle, and in 1 case the primary site was unknown. In 6 cases the ocular metastasis was the first clinical sign of the neoplastic disease.

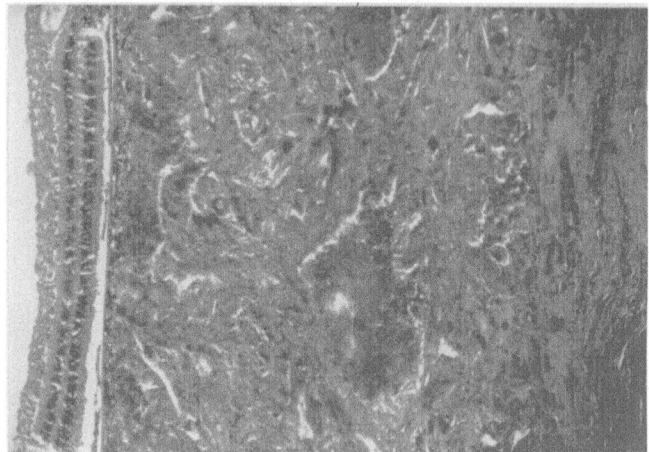

Fig. 4. Histological section in one case of metastatic choroidal lesion, the irregular interfaces of this lesion explain the irregular A-Scan pattern.

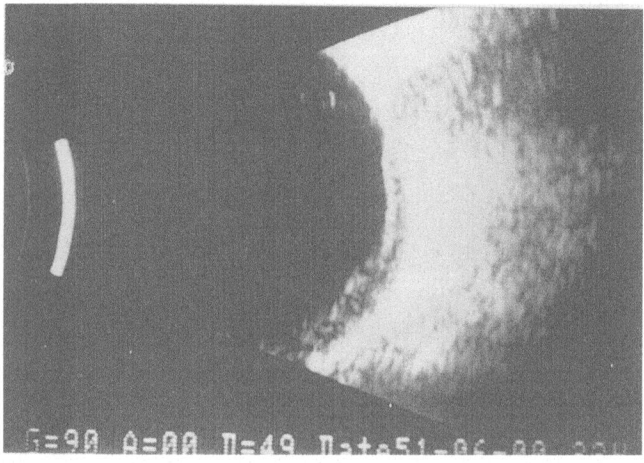

Fig. 5. B-Scan showing a diffuse, flat metastatic lesion.

Discussion

The typical echographic pattern of a choroidal metastatic tumor shows a solid lesion with irregular structure, high-to-medium reflectivity (Fig. 3). In some cases the echographic pattern has a V shape [1]. These echographic features were found in 21 patients, related to the macroscopic structure of the tumor, consisting of connective tissue which irregularly separates different wide zones of neoplastic cells (Fig. 4). In 3 cases we found a lesion with a regular structure, low-to-medium reflectivity, and in 2 cases, there were

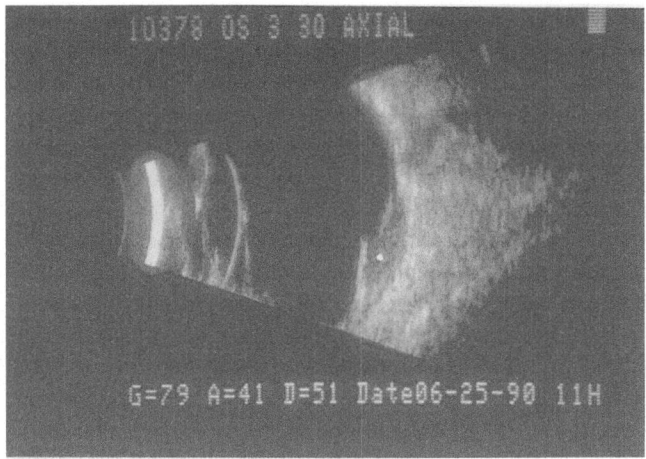

Fig. 6. B-Scan in one case of elevated metastatic choroidal lesion.

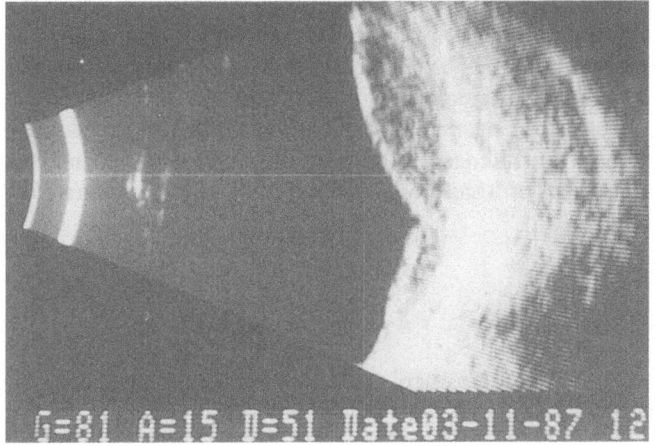

Fig. 7. B-Scan showing multiple choroidal lesions.

spontaneous movements of the spikes inside the lesion. This echographic pattern was found in 2 cases only, in which the echographic measurement showed a great increase in volume of the tumor in less than two weeks, and there was more than one lesion at the first examination or during the follow up. In B-Scan the metastatic tumor generally appears as a flat, concave, waxflow-like lesion (Fig. 5). In a lower percentage (35%), metastatic choroidal tumors are dome-shaped lesions, protruding from the scleral surface (Fig. 6). We have never found signs of Bruch membrane breaks. The presence of multiple focuses (Fig. 7) and fast growth without Bruch membrane rupture seems to be extremely important in ruling out a malignant melanoma in presence of a regular, low-to-medium reflective lesion, which also shows fast and spontaneous movements. In malignant melanomas we never detected such a fast growth in less than two weeks. In this type of neoplastic lesion an increase in volume needs at least one month to be significant, and a stage of fast growth is frequently associated with a rupture of the Bruch membrane, which gives the neoplasia the typical mushroom-shape. We have never detected a mushroom-shaped metastatic choroidal tumor, as described by Kerman et al. in 1987 in a metastatic carcinoma from parotid gland [7]. The low reflectivity of the three metastatic tumors (2 originated from a carcinoma, 1 from a cutaneous malignant melanoma), was probably related to a poor connective tissue amount and the prevalence of neoplastic cells [2, 13, 14]. We point out that all three of the mentioned patients died a few weeks after the choroidal metastatic tumor was diagnosed. When ocular metastatic tumors represent the first clinical sign of an unknown neoplasia, the echographic examination is of primary importance for the diagnosis and therapeutic approach, because the management is completely different for the cases of malignant melanoma, choroidal hemangioma or not neoplastic choroidal lesions.

Moreover the differential diagnosis of a disciform-like lesion is very important. Actually the disciform-like lesion should be more regular and layered than the metastatic one, but in some cases the echographic pattern could be very similar. A bilateral macular localization speaks more for a disciform lesion, but in case of peripheral localization, follow-up becomes necessary. In case of a disciform-like lesion the follow-up will show a change of reflectivity and a decrease of thickness. These data will allow us to rule out a metastatic tumor [5].

References

1. Cennamo, G., Foà, T. & De Palma, L. Studio clinico ed ecografico dei tumori metastatici della coroide. Clin. Oc. e. Pat. Oc. 9(4): 297–300 (1988).
2. Doro, D., Moschini, G.B. & Cardin, P. Low reflective choroidal metastatic tumor. In Hillman, J.S. & Le May, M.M. (eds.), Ophthalmic Ultrasonography. Doc. Ophthalmol. Proc. Ser. 38. The Hague: Dr. W. Junk (1983).
3. Ferry, A.P. Tumors metastatic to the eye and ocular adnexa. In Jakobiec, F.A. (ed.), Ocular and Adnexal Tumors, pp. 868–892. Birmingham: Ala, Aesculapius Press (1978).
4. Francois, J., Hanssens, H. & Verbraeken, H. Intraocular metastasis as first sign of generalized carcinomatosis. Ann. of Ophthal. April: 405–419 (1976).
5. Frazier Byrne, S. Differential diagnosis using Standardized Echography. In Hillman, J.S. (ed.), Ophthalmic Ultrasonography. The Hague/Boston/Lancaster: Dr. W. Junk (1983).
6. Freedman, M.I. and Folk, J.C. Metastatic tumors to the eye and orbit: Patient survival and clinical characteristics. Arch. Ophthalmol. 105: 1215–1219 (1987).
7. Kerman, B.M. & Fishman, M.L. Non melanomatous collar-button tumors. In Ossoinig, K.C. (ed.), Ophthalmic Echography. Doc. Ophthalmol. Proc. Ser. 48. The Hague: Dr. W. Junk (1987).
8. Nelson, C.C., Hertzberg, B.S. & Klintworth, G.K. A histopathologic study of 716 unselected eyes in patients with cancer at the time of death. Am. J. Ophthalmol. 788–793 (1983).

9. Ossoinig, K.C. & Blodi, F.C. Preoperative differential diagnosis of tumors with echography. In Blodi, F.C. (ed.), Part III. Diagnosis of intraocular tumors. Current Concepts in Ophthalmology, 4: 296. St. Louis: Mosby (1974).

10. Ossoinig, K.C. Standardized echography: basic principles, clinical application and results. In: Dallow, R.L. (ed.), Ophthalmic Ultrasonography: Comparative Techniques. Int. Ophthal. Clin. 19(4): 127–210. Boston: Little, Brown & Co. (1979).

11. Ossoinig, K.C. Advances in diagnosis ultrasound. In Henkind, P. (ed.), ACTA: XXIV International Congress of Ophthalmology, pp. 89–114. Philadelphia: J.B. Lippincott Co. (1982).

12. Ossoinig, K.C. Standardized Ophthalmic Echography of the Eye, Orbit and Periorbital Region. A comprehensive Slide Set (774 slides) and Study Guide, 3rd ed., pp. 29–36. Iowa City, Iowa: Goodfellow Company Inc. (1985).

13. Verbeek, A.M. A choroidal oat-cell metastasis mimicking a choroidal melanoma. In Thijssen, V.M. & Verbeek, A.M. (eds.), Ultrasonography in Ophthalmology, Doc. Ophthalmol. Proc. Ser. 29. The Hague: Dr. W. Junk (1981).

14. Verbeek, A.M. Differential diagnosis of intraocular neoplasms with ultrasonography. Ultrasound in Med. & Biol. 11(1): 163–170 (1985).

Address for correspondence: Eye Department, II School of Medicine, University of Naples, Via Panisi 5, I-80131 Naples, Italy.

28. Three cases of choroidal metastases with rapid growth and atypical echographic characteristics

L. RAVALLI, P. PERRI, P. MONARI, M. CHIARELLI,
M. ZIOSI and V. MAZZEO

(Ferrara, Italy)

Abstract. The Authors reproduce a series of echographs taken over a period of time in three cases of choroidal metastasis, clinically characterised by a turbulent growth rate, and echographically by anomalies when compared with typical metastases.

The first case, a thymoma metastasis, showed a very similar ultrasound pattern to that of a choroidal melanoma. The second, a flat-cell infiltrating carcinoma in the lung, at first sight this seemed an enormous angioma, owing to its domeshape and rather high reflectivity, but which showed a marked endotumorous vascularization. The third case, a bronchial adenocarcinoma, had a lenticolar mass with medium-high reflectivity, that in the follow-up showed a rapid growth with prevalent lateral extension.

Introduction

Uveal metastasis is certainly the commonest type of tumour in the eye. Bloch and Gartner (1971) and Nelson et al. (1983) came across histological instances of ocular metastases in 12 and 9.3%, respectively, of patients who had died from tumours, although only a small number of these tumours were clinically evident. Most metastasis are localised in the choroid, particularly at the posterior pole. Localisations in the ciliary body, in the iris, in the retina, or in the optic nerve are more rare. The site of origin of the metastasis is sex-linked: in males, 35–50% of all metastases are of pulmonary origin, roughly 25% of cases with unknown origin site, and 18% derive from skin tumours. In females, 75–85% originate in the breast, and 8–12% in the lung [12].

Clinical diagnosis is easier when this site is known, along with secondary localisations if possible, whereas it is more difficult when it is, as is often the case with pulmonary tumours, the first symptom. The most frequent early symptoms are worsening of sight and alterations in the visual field. However, the lesion often shows up in phosphenes or deep pain. Clinically, one can see at the back of the eye a not very thick, although extensive, mass, well delineated and separate from the choroid, and greyish-white or yellow. Even more than choroidal melanomas, a satellite serous retinal detachment is very common, as are multiple localisations, and the metastasis can be bilateral in roughly 20% of all cases [12].

The echograph can be different from case to case, given the variability of origins mentioned above. Traditionally, the most common forms are considered typical, i.e., the adenocarcinomas, and in particular that of the

P. Till (ed.), Ophthalmic Echography 13, pp. 285–290.

breast. The A-scan pathognomonic aspect is that of a very high reflective lesion (80–95%) with irregular distribution of echos [11–14]. When the lesion is thicker than 10 µs, the reflectivity may become lower, giving the typical 'V' shape [8].

Formerly it was thought that metastases had no echographically-visible internal vascularisation [7–13], but different cases of vascularised metastases have recently been described [2–15]. Metastases with low reflectivity have also been described by numerous authors in cases where the homogeneity of the internal structure, with no areas of acoustic impedance, stopped the production of highly reflective echoes, viz. seminoma [5], pulmonary microcytoma [15], uterine carcinoma [8], and follicular thyroid carcinoma [4].

The typical B-scan – in adenocarcinoma cases again – is that of a slightly elevated lesion, localised at the posterior pole, often multiple, and highly echogenic. It frequently associates with a satellite retinal detachment, which hides the lesion clinically [6]. Less frequent than the choroidal melanoma are dome-shape and choroidal excavations.

Clinical case histories

No. 1: C.E., a 60-year-old man complaining of a five-day-old floater, was found to have a greyish solid raised area at the back of his left eye, just above the disk, which had spread to the area around the macula. There was a serous satellite retinal detachment in the temporal regions. The patient had been suffering from lympho-epithelial thymoma for some time and bone, liver, and lung metastases had already been diagnosed. Echographic examination with A-scan showed the presence of a solid lesion, with low reflectivity and regular form, the thickness being 3.5 µs. The B-scan showed a slightly dome-shaped mass at the back of the eye, with very small internal echos, and with choroidal excavation. From the echograph it was therefore possible to diagnose either choroidal melanoma or ocular metastasis, with low reflectivity, but clinical anamnesis showed the second possibility to be more likely. Checks were carried out on the patient over a period of time, also to follow developments during a course of chemotherapy. In spite of this therapy, checks after 2, 4 and 6 months showed a net growth in the dimensions of the mass, an accentuated reflectivity and more echoes produced. (Fig. 1). After 6 months from diagnosis, the lesion occupied practically the whole eyeball. With A-scan, the sclera was seen to have lost almost all its reflectivity; vascularisation was present within the tumour, and the reflectivity, although medium to medium-low, was quite irregular. The high attenuation of ultrasound in the orbital tissue was very evident in B-scan. The patient complained of violent pain, and enucleation was planned. Histological examination revealed epithelial neoplasia, compatible with the neoplasia formerly ascertained. The patient died two months after enucleation.

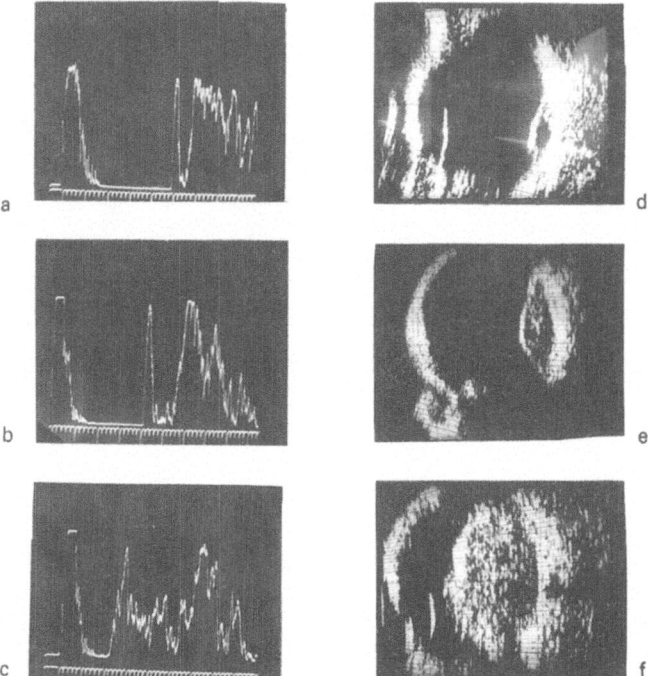

Fig. 1. Case No. 1: Lympho-epithelial thymoma choroidal metastasis. a, b, c: A-scan; d, e, f: immersion B-scan; a, d: at the time of diagnosis; b, e: two months later; c, f: six months later. Note the difficulty in distinguishing from malignant melanoma, especially with the first check-up; A-scan: lesion with low reflectivity and regular structure; B-scan: dome-shape lesion fairly echogenic, and with choroidal excavation.

No. 2: B.G., a 49-year-old man, had been having phosphenes in his left eye, and pain in the left trigeminal innervation. In the anamnesis, tobacco abuse (20–30 cigarettes per day) and the extirpation of fibrous mesothelioma from the lower lobe of the left lung four years previously were important. At the posterior pole of the left eye was a solid retinal raising, greyish-white in colour, spreading also to the macula and the upper part of the disk. There was also a serous satellite retinal detachment in the lower quadrants. Echography showed the presence of a solid mass at the posterior pole, very thick (about 11 μsec) with a wide base. In A-scan the reflectivity went from medium to high, showing a 'V' structure in some projections, and marked endotumoural vascularisation. B-scan showed a dome-shaped lesion, very thick and highly echogenic. Given that the echographic and clinical picture was suggestive of metastasis, although not actually pathognomonic, the site of origin was sought. On the right of the thorax a polycyclical mass was found in the upper lobe of the right lung, finding confirmed by thoracic CT. A bronchoscopy with biopsy was carried out, and a flat-cell infiltrating carcinoma was diagnosed. A brain CT also showed a metastatic-type nodular formation in the left occipital lobe. The patient was transferred to a medical ward for antiblastic, steroid,

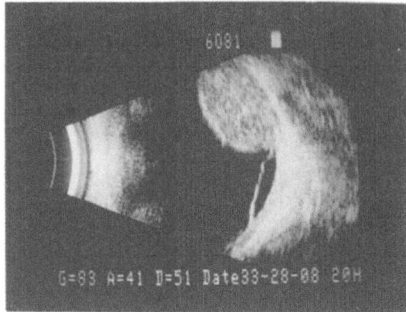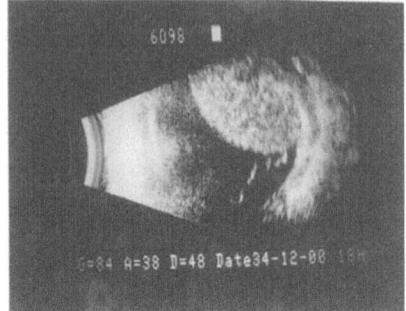

Fig. 2. Case No. 2: Choroidal metastasis from a pulmonary flat-cell – carcinoma. Contact B-scan: note the rapid increase in size in these two symmetrical images, one obtained 14 days after the other.

and antifungal therapies, with periodic checks on his eye problem. These latter checks showed an explosive rate of growth of the tumour, even with examinations only a few days apart (Fig. 2). After two months from diagnosis, the mass occupied almost all the eye. The patient died about two months after the last echographical examination.

No. 3: O.R., a 45-year-old man, had shown migraine-like headaches for some days, located at the back of his left eye. At the base, at the level of the posterior pole, in the upper parts, there was a solid, well-defined, greyish bump. The only anamnesis was tobacco abuse (20–25 cigarettes per day). Echography showed a lenticular lesion of about 4.5 μs thickness, medium to medium-high reflectivity according to the projection, with a fairly regular structure, and satellite retinal detachment. The strong suspicion of a metastatic lesion was confirmed by the presence of a polycyclical pulmonary formation in the lower part near the ileum, a finding confirmed by stratigraphy and thoracic CT. A bronchoscopy with bronchial washing permitted the diagnosis of a low-differentiation adenocarcinoma. Multiple bone metastases were also present, visible with scintigraphy. The patient was studied with a series of clinical and echographic examinations, which showed a rapid growth of the mass, in this case with prevalently lateral extension, and a worsening of the serous satellite retinal detachment (Fig. 3). At the last check-up, two months after diagnosis, the neoformation occupied all the upper parts, and most of the lower ones as well. The reflectivity of echoes was medium to medium-high, but the internal structure appeared more irregular. The patient is currently alive, a few weeks after the last examination.

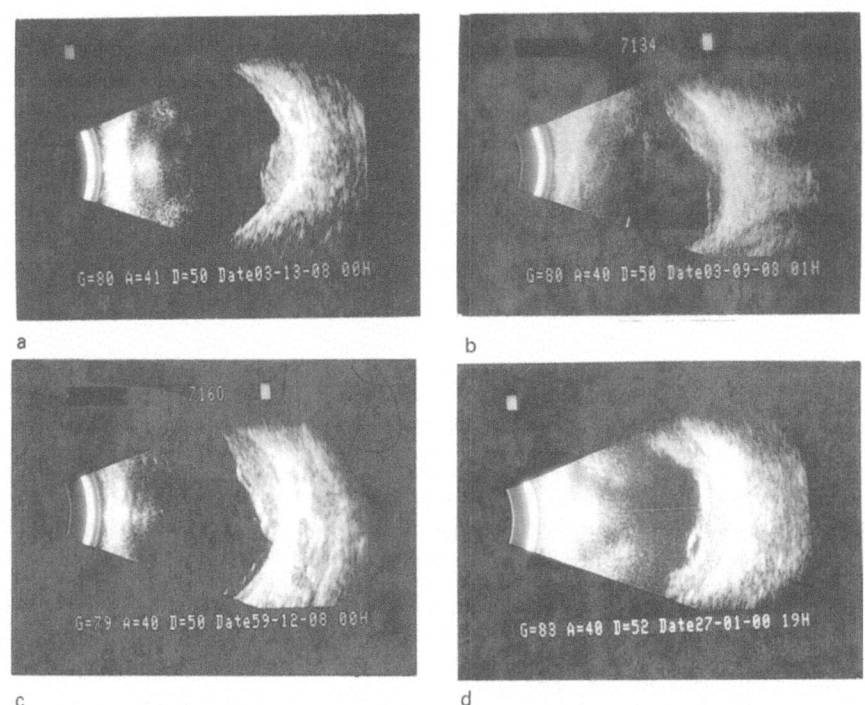

Fig. 3. Case No. 3: Choroidal metastasis from little-differentiated bronchial carcinoma. Contact B-scan: note the rapid growth of the lesion, with enlargement especially at the sides during follow-up. a: at diagnosis, b: two weeks later, c: 33 days later, d: 75 days later.

Conclusions

As has already been shown, clinico-echographic diagnosis of metastasis is usually fairly simple when a possible site of origin is known; it becomes more difficult when it is the first symptom of the disease, and/or when the echographic characteristics are especially atypical as in the first case, lympho-epithelial thymoma choroid metastasis where the echograph (at the beginning at least) did not distinguish it from a malignant melanoma. The low reflectivity of this lesion is, as always, bound up with its histological structure, with the epithelial and lymphatic cells evenly distributed within tightly packed units, one with another, without coarse structure or large lumps. A close follow-up of metastatic lesions, or suspect metastatic lesions, is fundamental in showing two types of variation in dimension, viz: A) moving towards a reduction in size up to the desappearance in these cases which respond well to antiblastic therapy [3–9], and B) towards an increase which can at times (as in the above cases) become explosive. The high growth rate of the lesion can be detected in examinations separated by only a few days or weeks, without moving across Bruch's membrane, and it is a pathognomonic characteristic of metastasis. The malignant melanoma, even in the rapid growth phase, is less rapid in evolution, and only checks on this growth several months apart show it to be accompanied by a movement across Bruch's membrane, assuming a mushroom-like shape [2].

One final datum that appears important is the endotumoural vascularisation visible with echography, present probably in the fastest-developing forms. This too might be considered an unfavourable prognostic indicator, especially when associated with rapid progression in the growth of the mass.

References

1. Bloch, R.S. & Gartner S. The incidence of ocular metastatic carcinoma. Arch. Ophthalmol. 85: 673–675 (1971).
2. Cennamo, G., Foà, T. & De Palma, L. Studio clinico ed ecografico dei tumori metastatici della coroide. Clin. Ocul. e Pat. Oc. 9(4): 297–300 (1988).
3. Dalia, T., Di Censo, B., Aiello, F. & Baquis, G. Ecographic and fluorangiographic controls in two cases of metastatic tumours of the choroid during chemotherapy. In Gallenga, P.E. et al. (eds.), Current Concepts on Ultrasounds, pp. 71–75. Roma: Novappia (1980).
4. Doro, D., Moschini, G.B. & Cardin, P. Metastasi coroideale da carcinoma tiroideo. In Masotti, L. et al. (eds.), VI Congr. Naz. SISUM, pp. 295–298. Roma: Novappia (1981).
5. Freyler, H. & Egerer, I. Echography and histological studies in various eye conditions. Arch. Ophthalmol. 95: 1387–1394 (1977).
6. Mazzeo, V., Galli, G., Perri, P. & Falco, L. Diagnostica bulbare. In Mazzeo, V. (ed.), Ecografia dell'apparato oculare. Testo Atlante, pp. 125–236. Milano: Fogliazza (1987).
7. Mazzeo, V., Ravalli, L. & Pistocchi, F. L'ecografia nei tumori del bulbo oculare. In Rossi, A. (ed.), Clinica dei tumori dell'occhio e dell'orirta, pp. 187–244. Ferrara: *SATE* (1981).
8. Mazzeo, V., Scorrano, R., Gallenga, P.E. & Rossi, A. Echographic pattern of choroidal metastatic tumours. In Gallenga, P.E. et al. (eds.), Current Concepts on Ultrasounds, pp. 67–70. Roma: Novappia (1980).
9. Mazzeo, V., Sebastiani, A., Bragliani, G. & Bertusi, M. Metastasi coroideale da carcinoma mammario regredita mediante chemio-ed ormonoterapia. II Riun. Scient. Reg. Ass. Ital. Oncol. Med. Abstract book 12 (1979).
10. Nelson, C.C., Hertzberg, B.S. & Klintworth, G.K. A histopathologic study of 716 unselected eyes in patients with cancer at the time of death. Am. J. Ophthalmol. 95: 788–793 (1983).
11. Ossoinig, K.C. Standardized echography: basic principles, clinical applications and results. In Dallow, R.L. (ed.), Ophthalmic Ultrasonography: Comparative Techniques, pp. 127–210. Boston: Little, Brown and Co (1979).
12. Schachat, A.P. Differential diagnosis of choroidal metastases. International Symposium on Intraocular tumors. Florence (1990).
13. Shammas, H.J. Atlas of ophthalmic ultrasonography and biometry. St. Louis: Mosby (1984).
14. Till, P. & Hauff, W. Differential diagnostic results of clinical echography in intraocular tumours. In Thijssen, J. & Verbeek, A.M. (eds.), Ultrasonography in Ophthalmology. Proceedings of the 8th SIDUO Congress, pp. 91–95. The Hague: Dr. W. Junk (1981).
15. Verbeek, A.M.A. Choroidal oat-cell carcinoma metastasis mimicking a choroidal melanoma. Case history. In Thijssen, J.M. and Verbeek, A.M. (eds.), Ultrasonography in Ophthalmology. Proceedings of the 8th SIDUO Congress, pp. 131–133. The Hague: Dr. W. Junk (1981).

Address for correspondence: Eye Clinic, Ferrara University, Corso Giovecca 203, I-4100 Ferrara, Italy.

29. Echographical examinations of patients with Coat's disease

J. DAMJANOVICH & L. KOLOZSVÁRI
(Debrecen, Hungary)

Abstract. Echographical examinations were performed on 6 patients with Coat's disease. The results were correlated with findings on routine clinical examinations and fluorescein angiography. In these cases the disease was well differentiated at least echographically, from the other retinal lesions causing leucocoria.

Introduction

Coat's disease is a rare lesion but it is one of the lesions causing leucocoria which – in early childhood – may increase the possibility of retinoblastoma [1].

Coat's disease occurs in children between the ages 5 and 12, generally in males and most frequently unilaterally and temporally.

The disease consists of vascular anomalies leading to a leakage – which means hemorrhagic and serous trans – and exudations – from the abnormal retinal vessels into the subretinal space and between the retinal layers [3].

Patients and methods

In the last 3 years, 6 patients with Coat's disease (5 males and one female) were examined echographically at our clinics.

The disease was localised unilaterally and temporally in each case.

The female patient was 33-years-old at the time of the examinations, the male patients were between 6 and 14 years.

In each case fluorescein angiography was made.

We used the 'A' as well as the 'B' method. The examinations were carried out with a Cooper Vision Digital B IV and previously on Sonometrics Ocuscan DBR 400 equipment.

P. Till (ed.), Ophthalmic Echography 13, pp. 291–295.

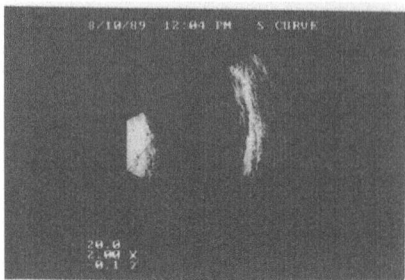

Fig. 1. Coat's disease: the first echographical sign is an increase in the thickness of retinal layers.

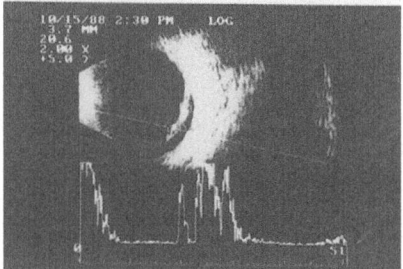

Fig. 2. Coat's disease: The retina is detached, the detached retina is thicker and the surface is uneven.

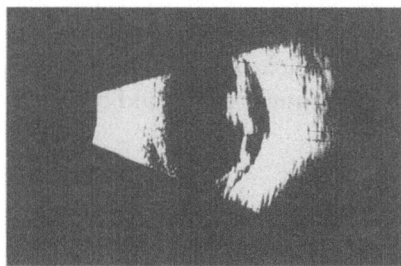

Fig. 3. Coat's disease: The thickness of the retina is uneven, and some places look like deposits.

Results

The earliest echographical sign was an increase in the thickness of retinal layers and this thickness of the retina was uneven in all of our cases (Fig. 1).

In five patients the retina was detached (Fig. 2). The cicatrix, the hemorrhages and exudates between the layers made a thicker retina and at some places it looked like deposits (Fig. 3).

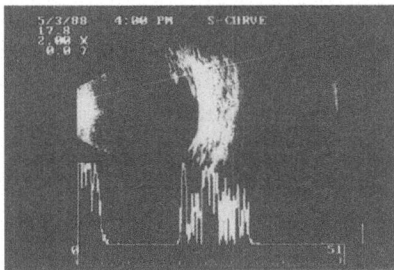

Fig. 4. Coat's disease: The subretinal space show an acoustical inhomogeneity.

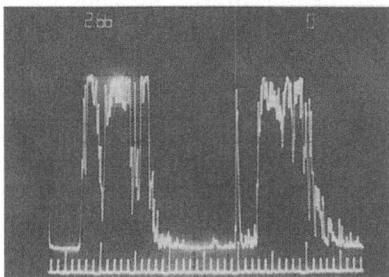

Fig. 5. Coat's disease: Low reflective echos (representing the cholesterol clefts and the erythrocytes) between the echospikes of the detached retina and the posterior ocular wall.

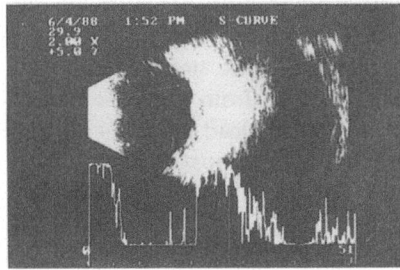

Fig. 6. Coat's disease: Echogenic opacities in the vitreous cavity, as the A-scan shows. The retina is uneven.

The subretinal space showed an acoustical inhomogeneity (Fig. 4). These small echogenic opacities, which were present in the subretinal space, represented the erythrocytes and the cholesterol deposits in the cases of four patients.

The echospikes caused by cholesterol clefts were clearly monitored by kinetic echography. Behind the echospike of the detached retina a number of fine lines were running into another during the eye movements.

The space between the detached retina and the posterior ocular wall, as observed with A-scan, characteristically contained low reflective echospikes, representing the cholesterol and the other components (Fig. 5).

The vitreous body may contain echogenic opacities with different intensities (Fig. 6), or may be relatively clear.

Comment

If the refractive mediums are optically clear, and exudations and teleangiectasies are present at the surface of the retina, the differential diagnosis is more difficult by common optical methods. These lesions may occur with retinoblastomas and hemangioblastomas as well.

If the refractive mediums are opaqued, ultrasonography is the only means for differentiation.

The echographical base of the differential diagnosis between the retinoblastoma and other lesions causing leucocoria (for example: persistent hyperplasia of primary vitreous; retinopathia of prematurity; von Hippel angiomatosis or Coat's disease) is, that these lesions display a membranous internal structure. These lesions do not cause shadowing but in phthisical eyes [2].

We list a few echographical signs which make an easier echographical differentiation between the lesions mentioned above:

In case of persistent hyperplasia of primary vitreous

A retrolental echogenic membranous structure is noted, which is regular in shape. Persistent hyaloid vasculature noted as an echogenic line, connecting the retrolental lesion and the optic nerve head. The abnormal vessels are tortuos and only a small part of them are monitored.

With A-scan the persistent hyaloid vessel is observed as a high spike. The axial length of the affected eye is shorter.

In case of retinopathia of prematurity

Fibrous bands are noted in the vitreous which are dense in the retrolenticular area. These bands cause a secondary traction retinal detachment, which can be localised or total. The axial length is generally shorter.

In a typical case of von Hippel angiomatosis

A temporally localised echogenic mass is observed with a honeycomblike structure, actually caused by the blood vessels. The blood flow in the vessels is well monitored by A-scan.

Finally it is interesting to mention that the disease generally occurs in an age group of boys between 5 and 12, but we diagnosed this disease in a 33-year-old female patient as well.

References

1. Koplin, R.S., Gersten, M. & Hodes, B. Real time ophthalmic ultrasonography and biometry, pp. 144–149. SLACK Incorporated USA (1985).
2. Ossoinig, K.C. Standardized echography: basic principles, clinical applications, and results. In: R.L. Dallow (ed.), Ophthalmic Ultrasonography Comparative Techniques, pp. 127–145. International Ophthalmology Clinics 19(4) (1979).
3. Shammas, H.J. Atlas of ophthalmic ultrasonography and biometry, pp. 94–108. CV Mosby Company (1984).

Address for correspondence: Department of Ophthalmology, University Medical School, Nagyerdei Krt. 98, H-4012 Decrecen, Hungary.

30. Different echographic aspects of retinoblastoma in two members of a family

L. PIERRO, C. CAPOFERRI, R. MAGNI & R. BRANCATO

(*Milano, Italy*)

Abstract. A 52-year-old woman presented in her right eye a whitish translucent mass, expanding from the retinal surface into the vitreous. Echography showed a hyperreflective lesion with a corresponding posterior shadowing. Fluorescein angiography confirmed the diagnosis of retinoma. Her grandson had been identified before birth as a carrier of the mutation of hereditary retinoblastoma. On his third day of life, the retinal surface was entirely covered with hemorrhages, echography showed a 1.2 mm thick, highly reflective membranous-like lesion in his left eye. A similar mass was detected three weeks later in his right eye. The lesions were successfully photo-coagulated. In the present study the authors report and discuss the echogaphic pictures obtained and the role of ultrasonographic examination in the diagnosis of different forms of retinoblastoma, considering clinical and genetic implications.

Introduction

Retinoblastorna (RTB) is the most frequent intraocular malignancy in childhood [1]. Recent advances in molecular biology have made it possible to identify the gene whose mutation predisposes to RTB, which is located within the q14 band of chromosome 13 [4]. Only 1% of cases of RTB regress spontaneously [3]. We report two cases of RTB in members of the same family, in which echography was determinant for diagnosis.

Case report

A married couple in their period of fertility were admitted for genetic counseling. The groom had been enucleated in his right eye at 13 months of age and then irradiated in the left eye for bilateral RTB. No complications had occurred in the ensuing years. At the time of consultation visual acuity in his left eye was light perception. One of his two sisters had died from bilateral RTB at the age of two months, whereas the other was alive in good health. His father was alive and in apparent good health, but five brothers of his father's had died during childhood of unknown causes. His mother had no family history of RTB and had always been in apparent good health. The bride had no anamnestic data of specific interest. One year later the couple, expecting a baby, asked for prenatal diagnosis. We examined the groom's parents. His father showed no evident alterations at fundus examination. His

P. Till (ed.), Ophthalmic Echography 13, pp. 297–299.

298

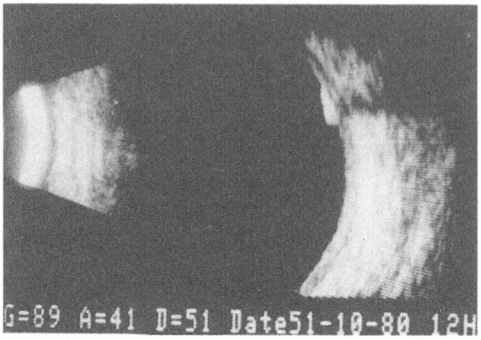

Fig. 1. B-scan ultrasonography with a small hyperreflective lesion 3 mm thick with shadowing because of calcification.

mother could see 10/10 in both eyes, but in her right eye a small area of chorioretinal atrophy in the nasal superior mid-periphery was evidenced, on which laid a globular whitish mass.

A-B scan ultrasonography showed a small hyperreflective lesion 3 mm thick: posterior acoustic shadowing confirmed the hypothesis of a calcified mass (Fig. 1). Retinal fluorescein angiography showed an area of chorioretinal atrophy, through which no dye leakage could be observed from the choroidal circulation; left eye fundus was normal. A diagnosis was made of spontaneously regressed RTB. DNA analysis from chorial villi at the eighth week of pregnancy was then performed. The risk of RTB was assessed to be 100%. The couple decided to continue the pregnancy. Subsequent trans-abdominal echographies of the fetus showed no alterations of the eyeballs. The baby was delivered at the 42nd week of pregnancy, healthy and lively. On the third day of life, fundus in both eyes was entirely covered by intra- and preretinal hemorrhages. Ultrasonography performed using Ophtascan S (Biophysic Medical) showed at B-scan examination (focused 10 Mhz probe) a small membranous lesion in the nasal parapapillary region in left eye (Fig. 2). At A-scan (non-focused 8 Mhz probe), a high reflectivity peak was evident 1.2 mm from the sclera. The lesion was too small to analyze tissue structure. Ultrasonography in right eye was normal. Diagnosis of suspected RTB was made and treatment was planned. One week later the tumor could be observed as a whitish mass, 1 disk diameter in size, and xenon photocoagulation was performed. Fundus in right eye was normal. Three weeks later, fundus examination showed a similar lesion at the posterior pole in right eye, which was also photocoagulated. Fundus examination performed at the last check (3 months of age) evidenced no signs of activity of the disease.

Discussion

Echographic pictures of RTB collected so far from patients aged from three months to 26 years, have been described as solid (highly echogenous, with

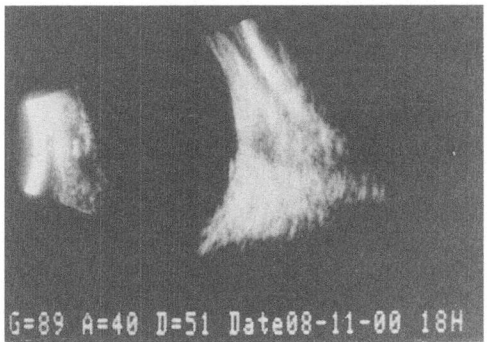

G=89 A=40 D=51 Date08-11-00 18H

Fig. 2. B-scan with a small membranous lesion in the nasal parapapillary region.

frequent calcifications), cystic (heterogeneous), mixed (both patterns), and diffuse (endophthalmitis-like appearance) [2, 5, 6]. The small membranous-like pattern observed in this case is probably due to the very early stage of progression of the tumor at the time of echography. We suggest that RTB be suspected when such a picture is obtained in the first days of life. Similar ultrasonographic images can result from other congenital diseases (such as persistence of Bergmeister papilla, drusen, oedema or tumors of the optic nerve nead, some forms of pseudoglioma): non papillary location and a normal axial length can be of help in differential diagnosis. Early diagnosis of RTB is important, since it can develop very rapidly. In our case the tumor, being smaller and shallower than usual at the time of diagnosis, could be treated with photocoagulation, thus avoiding intraocular complications of radio- or cobalt-therapy.

References

1. Devese, S.S. The incidence of retinoblastoma. Am. J. Ophthalmol. 80: 263–265 (1985).
2. Fernandez-Vigo Lopez, J. & Cuevas Alvarez, J. Formes échographiques typiques et atypiques de rétinoblastomes. J. Fr. Ophtalmol. 6: 43 (1983).
3. Gallie, B.L., Phillips, R.D., Ellsworth, R.M. & Abramson, D.M. Significance of retinoma and phtisis bulbi for retinoblastoma. Ophthalmology 89: 1393–1399 (1982).
4. Sparkes, R.S., Murphree, A.L. & Lingua, R.W. et al. Gene for hereditary retinoblastoma assigned to human chromosome 13 by linkage to esterase. D. Science 219: 971–973 (1983).
5. Sterns, G.K., Coleman, D.I. & Ellsworth, R.M. Ultrasonic characterization of retinoblastoma. Am. J. Ophthalmol. 78: 606 (1974).
6. Verma, N., Goshe, S. & Chadrasekhar, G. Ultrasonic evaluation of retinoblastoma. Japan. J. Ophthalmol. 28: 222 (1984).

Address for correspondence: Department of Ophthalmology, University of Milano, HS. Raffaele, Via Olgettina 60, I-20132 Milano, Italy.

31. Dysplastic retina and persistent primary vitreous simulating a retinoblastoma

R. SAMPAOLESI & J.O. ZARATE
(Buenos Aires, Argentina)

Introduction

At the SIDUO XI Congress we dealt with the errors in the diagnosis of retinoblastoma. In a period of 8 years, during which we studied 60 neoplasias, 40 of which were enucleated, we had 4 errors (2 false positives: choroidal hemangiomas and Coats' disease and 2 false negatives: panuveitis and vitrous hemorrhage). The differential diagnosis of retinoblastoma is closely associated with that of leucocoria.

The case presented corresponds to an association between persistent primary vitreous and dysplastic retina which was enucleated. The clinicoechographic diagnosis was retinoblastoma, due to its family antecedents, increased axial length and echographical features.

Case report

A boy of two months of age has leucocoria and enlargement of the right eye. He was born under normal labour after 40 weeks of gestation. The right eye presents a rigid and ectopic (towards low temporal) pupil. The anterior surface of the iris has radiated vessels which come together and form a peripupil circle. There is corneal oedema.

Intraocular pressure: *R.E.*: 23 mmHg; *L.E*: 8 mmHg.

Corneal diameter: *R.E.*: 14 mm; *L.E*: 11.5 mm.

Echometry length: *R.E.*: 22.75 mm.; *L.E.*: 19.27 mm.

C.T. scan: radiopaque mass at the posterior pole. In some sections the anterior surface is nodular.

The echography, in mode B, shows a mass that occupies two-thirds of the vitreous cavity. In mode A an echographic pattern of retinoblastoma is observed (Fig. 1, 2a and b, 3a and b).

In Fig. 1 we can observe the tracing obtained with mode A echography. This figure shows that there are several echoes of hich reflectivity (more than 90%) which lower the height of the scleral echo and produce a total orbital shadow evidenced by the absence of echoes.

Figs. 2a and b show echographies in mode B. In Fig. 2a, at 3 dB of system sensitivity, a solid lesion can be observed in the vitreous mass and in other

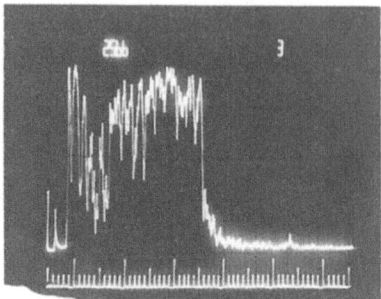

Fig. 1. Tracing obtained with mode A echography. There are several echoes of high reflectivity (more than 90%), which lower the height of the scleral echo and produce a total orbital shadow evidenced by the absence of echoes.

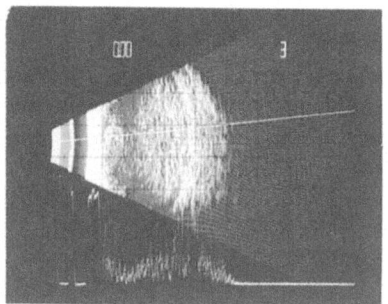

Fig. 2a. In mode A echography, at 3 dB of system sensitivity, a solid lesion can be observed in the vitreous mass and in other sectors.

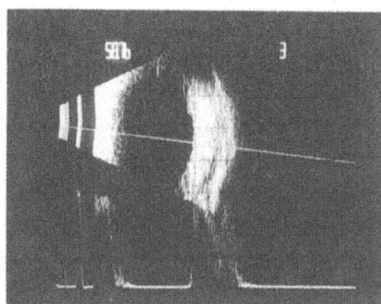

Fig. 2b. Mode B ecography also at 3 dB of system sensitivity. Posterior side of the eye with a mass of very reflective and dense tissue below it.

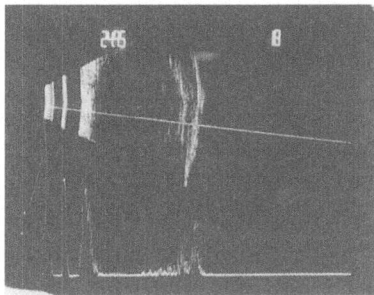

Fig. 3a. The intensity is further decreased (8 dB). Mode B echography which shows clearly the sclera with a very reflective coat in its front.

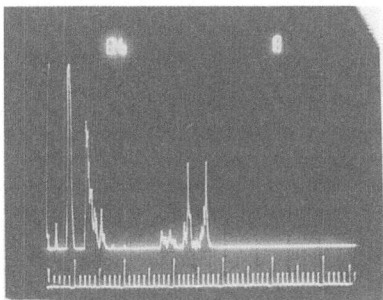

Fig. 3b. Mode A echography in which the 2 echoes corresponding to the above-mentioned coats, are observed.

sectors. In Fig. 2b, also at 3 dB of system sensitivity, the posterior side of the eye and a mass of very reflective and dense tissue below it, can be observed. In Fig. 3a the intensity is further decreased (8 dB). The sclera with a very reflective coat in its front, is clearly distinguished in mode B echography while in Fig. 3b, in mode A echography, the two echoes corresponding to the abovementioned coats, are observed.

The patient's cousin (in second grade) was enucleated, and the diagnosis was retino-blastoma. The same occured with the patient, the enucleation being performed at the same hospital.

Pathological findings

The external appearance of the eyeball from the temporal side shows an ectopic pupil and a big cornea. A horizontal cutting under the optic nerve shows absence of anterior chamber, white yellowish retrolental mass and cystic structure in the ciliary zone. Behind the retrolental mass there appear

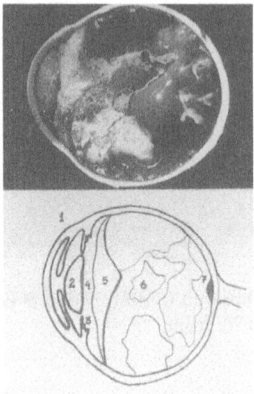

Fig. 4. Macroscopic cutting of the eyeball in which the following can be observed: (1) Anomalous development of anterior chamber (absence of trabecular meshwork and Schlemm's canal; Hypoplastic ciliary muscle; pupillary block and iridocorneal attachment; and anomalous vascularity of the iris. (2) Cataracts and dehiscence in the posterior lens capsule with liquefaction of the cortical fibers. (3) Elongated ciliary processes. (4) Persistent hyperplastic primary vitreous (retrolental connective tissue with remnants of the hyaloid vascular system). (5) Retinal gliosis and dysplastic retina. (6) Retroretinal hemorrhage; and hyperplasia of pigment epithelium. (7) Gliosis of optic disk.

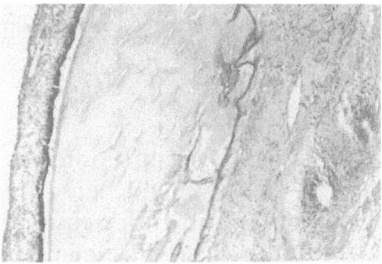

Fig. 5. Panoramic histologic cutting where there appears an abnormally vascularized iris; the lens with cataract behind it and the persistent primary vitreous and dysplastic retina.

partially organized blood clots. On the choroidal surface we find some formations of nodular appearance and coagulated blood origin (Fig. 4).

Fig. 4 shows a macroscopic cutting of the eyeball. An anterior cutting performed from a shorter distance shows a thin white area in the anterior part of the retrolental mass and a thick yellowish one in the posterior part.

The microscopic findings show: corneal oedema, hypoplastic iris, elongated ciliary processes, thin ciliary body and no sign of Schlemm's canal; anomalous vascularity of the iris: small and big vessels; cataracts in posterior

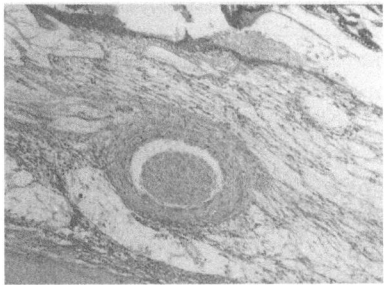

Fig. 6. Hyaloid remnants (magnified).

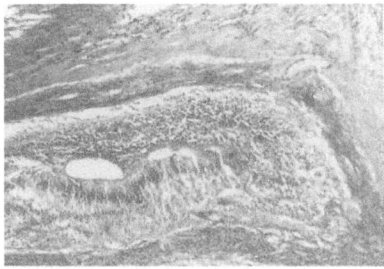

Fig. 7. Histologic cutting in which the retinal gliosis and the presence of dysplastic rosettes can be observed.

lens; persistent hyperplastic primary vitreous (retrolental connective tissue with remnants of the hyaloid vascular system; retinal gliosis and dysplastic retina; retroretinal hemorrhage, hyperplastic pigment epithelium and gliosis of optic disk.

Fig. 5 shows a panoramic histologic cutting where there appears an abnormally vascularized iris; the lens with cataract behind it and the persistent primary vitreous and dysplastic retina. Fig. 6 reproduces the hyaloid remnants (magnified). Fig. 7 shows a histologic cutting in which the retinal gliosis and the presence of dysplastic rosettes can be observed.

Conclusions

At the SIDUO XI Congress, held in Italy, we presented 4 errors in the diagnosis of retinoblastoma. We have now added a fifth case which was also erroneously diagnosed. The erroneous cases are explained below:

Echographic diagnosis	Histopathological diagnosis
Case 1: Retinoblastoma	Choroidal hemangioma
Case 2: Retinoblastoma	Coats' disease
Case 3: Panuveitis	Infiltrative diffuse retinoblastoma with pseudo-hypopyon in the vitreous body.
Case 4: Vitreous hemorrhage	Undifferentiated retinoblastoma.
Case 5: Retinoblastoma	Dysplastic retina and hyperplastic primary vitreous.

Cases 1, 2 and 5 are false positives. Cases 2 and 4 are false negatives.

References

1. Sampaolesi, R. Ultrasonidos en Oftalmología, pp. 307–342. Buenos Aires: Editorial Médica Panamericana (1983).
2. Sampaolesi, R. & Zarate, J.O. Errors in the diagnosis of retinoblastoma. In: Thyssen, J.M., Hillman, J.S., Gallenga, P.E. and Cennamo, G. (eds.), Ultrasonography in Opthalmology 11. Doc. Ophthalmol. Proc. Ser. 51: 189–196. Dordrecht: Kluwer (1988).

Address for correspondence: Parana 1239-1°A, 1018 Buenos Aires, Argentina.

32. Tumours of the choroid
Three unusual cases examined by ultrasound

H.C. FLEDELIUS, J.U. PRAUSE & E. SCHERFIG

(Hillerød and Copenhagen, Denmark)

Abstract. Ultrasound features are given for three choroidal tumours, two melanomas and one hemangioma. After enucleation, the latter case answered some of the questions raised in a previous paper (Fledelius & Scherfig 1988). The diagnosis could be confirmed histologically, but ultrasonically the tumour still appeared larger and thicker than estimated by the ophthalmoscope, and now also from the specimen. A melanoma in a 15-year-old female appeared like a cyst, also by ultrasound, but transvitreal biopsy gave the diagnosis. The last case study describes the spontaneous disintegration of a melanoma in an 83-year-old man, illustrated by current ultrasound examinations.

Introduction

For evaluation of tumours of the eye, the usefulness of diagnostic ultrasound is firmly established through many years experience. Ultrasonographers thus recognize the various acoustic patterns met in melanomas, for instance, thereby contributing to solving the differential-diagnostic problems. We want to present three cases, where ultrasound imaging was helpful, however not unambiguous.

Cases

Case No. 1. Eventually an 8-year-long clinical history found its solution when a young female, now in her mid-twenties, finally gave her consent to enucleation of a blind eye harbouring a solid tumour. Histologically it proved to be a choroidal hemangioma (Fig. 1) as suggested also from current ultrasound evaluations over several years (Fig. 2).

Initially the clinicians had considered a melanoma most probable, but at that time she refused the recommended removal of the eye. This part of the history was given at the SIDOU XI conference (Fledelius & Scherfig 1988). Trans-vitreal biopsy at that time showed only blood cells, no tumour tissue.

During a pregnancy two years later she developed a serous retinal detachment of the tumour eye. Surgery was unsuccessful, and one year later the eye was removed.

Over the years tumour thickness had been pretty constant. According to usual ophthalmoscopical rules of thumb, the 7–8 diopter prominence would

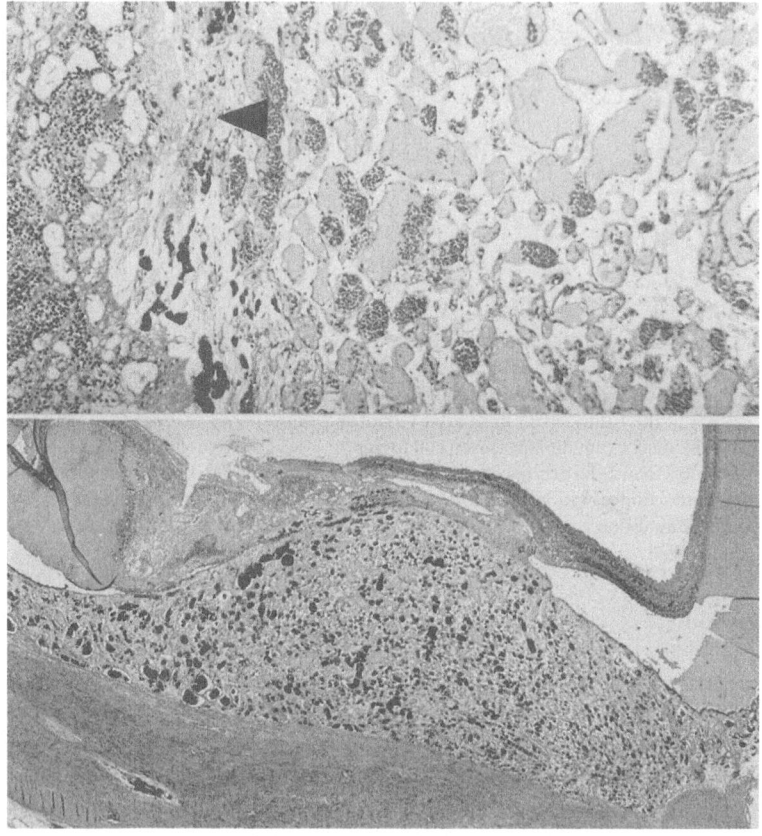

Fig. 1. Case No. 1, Choroidal hemangioma (Eye Path Lab No 1376/88), H-E stain, × 75 at top, × 50 at bottom. Rupture of Bruchs membrane (arrowhead, top).

correspond to 2–3 mm tumour thickness. In contrast, a 5–5.5 mm thickness was indicated by ultrasound (Fig. 2). The histopathologic specimen gave a measure of 3.8 mm. Even with allowance for tissue shrinkage due to preparation there is a discrepancy between methods, which is not yet fully understood.

Comment. Early in the course, ultrasound gave the correct diagnosis of the tumour, primarily based on the high inner reflectivity of the lesion. Choroidal hemangiomas are very rare in Denmark.

Case No. 2. A 15-year-old female attended the eye clinic of Rigshospitalet with a shadow in one eye. A cyst-like tumour was demonstrated by fundus examination. Ultrasound showed a prominence with a smooth rounded contour and only minimum reflectivity (Fig. 3). The presumed cyst, however, did not collapse when a trans-vitreal biopsy was taken. The removed tissue

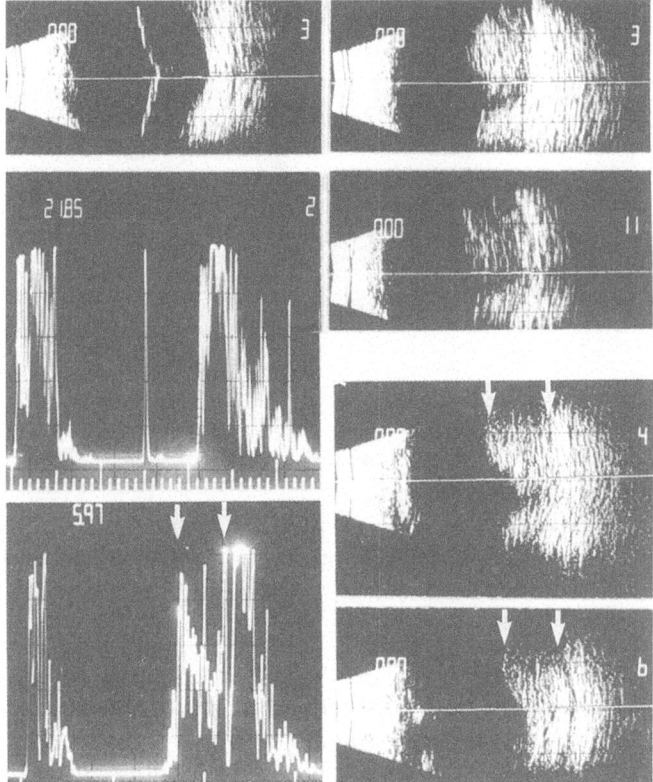

Fig. 2. At top, the highly reflecting hemangioma of Fig. 1, upwards in the eye (right), and the serous detachment downwards (left), shown by ultrasound. At bottom, status prior to enucleation. No change in outline and echodensity of the solid part of the tumour; thickness estimate near 6 mm. Interfaces vitreous/tumour and tumour/sclera indicated by white arrows.

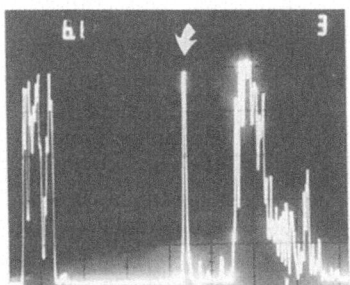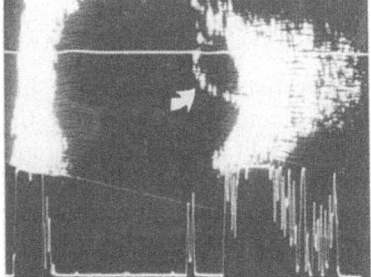

Fig. 3. Case No. 2. A cyst-like appearance due to low inner reflectivity of a rounded tumour in the fundus of a 15-year-old girl. Uveal melanoma was disclosed by transvitreal biopsy.

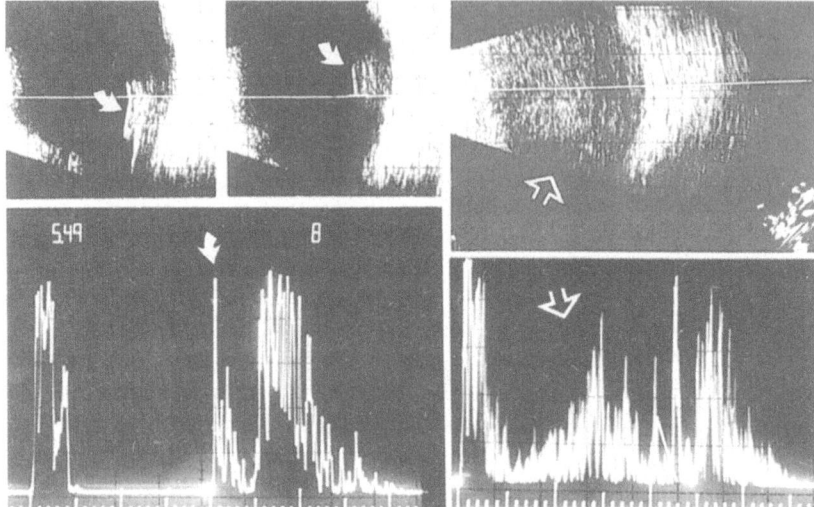

Fig. 4. Case No. 3. Choroidal melanoma with solid echopattern (solid arrows, left), to be followed by vitreous debris (open arrows, right) due to spontaneous tumour necrosis and disintegration, cf. text.

appeared solid; the texture was more homogeneous than typical for uveal melanoma, the diagnosis that was arrived at histopathologically. Subsequently she had local radiation treatment.

Comment. It is unusual to find a choroidal melanoma in a 15-year-old subject. Nor was the acoustic pattern typical. It however corresponded to the homogeneous appearance of the tumour tissue.

Case No. 3. In 1985 an 83-year-old man had uncomplicated intracapsular cataract extraction with insertion of an anterior chamber IOL. Initially he attained 6/12, but after a month there was visual loss due to vitreous clouding which made fundus evaluation impossible.

By ultrasound (Fig. 4) a solid tumour was demonstrated in the posterior eye segment, melanoma being the tentative diagnosis. This could be confirmed ophthalmoscopically, after Prednisone treatment and clearing of the vitreous.

A conservative approach was chosen and for two years there was no evidence of change in the size of the tumour. Painful glaucoma then developed. In the slit lamp a dense hemorrhage was observed before the pupil, and ophthalmoscopy could not be performed.

Ultrasound examination now showed vitreous opacities only. Apparently the tumour had disappeared. This was confirmed in the Eye Pathology laboratory; no tumour was visible after routine sections of the eye. All ocular tissue had to be sliced completely before a minimum rest-melanoma could be demonstrated (Fig. 5).

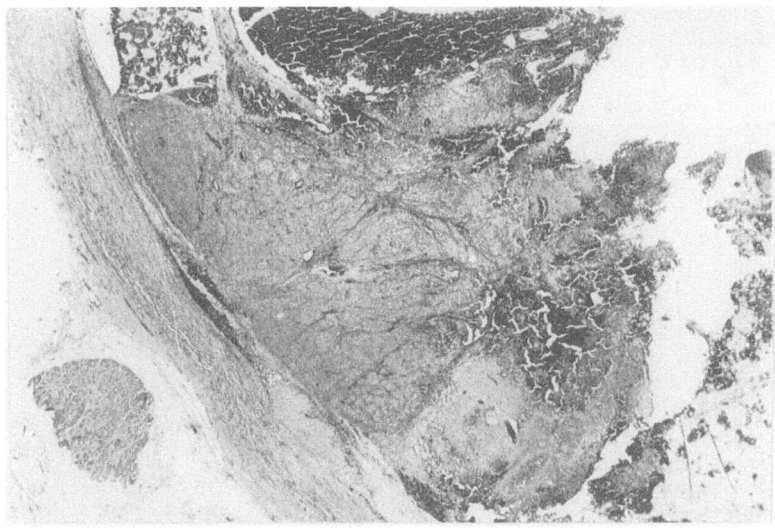

Fig. 5. Case No. 3, Survey × 25, H-E (Eye Path Lab No 412/187) of the tiny rest-melanoma that could be demonstrated after disintegration of the tumour, previously followed ophthalmoscopically and by ultrasound.

Comment: Internal vascular strangulation is the possible mechanism underlying the spontaneous tumour disintegration and transformation into vitreous debris. Partial or extensive necrosis in melanomas is well-known in literature (Duke Elder 1966) but tumour disappearance is unusual, and probably this is the first case to be demonstrated by ultrasound prior to enucleation.

References

1. Duke-Elder, S. & Perkins, E.S. System of ophthalmology, IX: Diseases of the uveal tract. pp. 888–892. London: Kimpton (1966).
2. Fledelius, H.C. & Scherfig, E. Choroidal haemagioma, king size or normal size by ultrasound. Doc. Ophthalmol. Proc. Ser. 51: 221–225 (1988).

Address for correspondence: Eye Department, Central Hospital, DK-3400 Hillerød, Denmark.

33. Echographic differential diagnosis of small choroidal solid lesions

G. MARCHINI & R. TOSI

(*Verona, Italy*)

Abstract. The differential diagnosis of small choroidal solid lesions is usually one of the most difficult problems for the echographist. In order to contribute to a rational solution of the problem the authors analyzed a series of 74 small (mean thickness ± S.D. = 2.7 ± 0.81 mm, min 1.8 mm, max 5 mm) choroidal 'tumors'. The echographic features of the solid lesions were evaluated in terms of sensibility, specificity, positive predictive value (PPV) and negative predictive value (NPV). This series was composed of 10 melanomas, 18 metastatic carcinomas, 12 nevi, 8 hemangiomas, 7 clotted hemorrhages and 19 disciform macular degenerations. In particular the attention was focused on the differentiation of melanoma with respect to other lesions. The most effective echographic characteristics for individualizing the small choroidal melanomas were the spongy internal texture (sensibility 90%, specificity 48%, PPV 21%, NPV 97%) and the choroidal excavation (sensibility 70%, specificity 97%, PPV 78%, NPV 95%) in B-scan; in A-scan they were: medium internal reflectivity (sensibility 100%, specificity 47%, PPV 23%, NPV 100%), regular internal structure (sensibility 70%, specificity 80%, PPV 35%, NPV 94%) and spontaneous vascular movements (sensibility 20%, specificity 100%, PPV 100%, NPV 89%). According to these results and those obtained from the analysis of the other choroidal 'tumors', the authors suggest an echographic algorithm for the correct diagnosis of each type of solid lesion.

Introduction

Exact and early diagnosis of a small choroidal melanoma is essential for two reasons: it allows conservative therapy and it gives a better chance of survival to the patient. It is well known that tumor size at diagnosis is an important prognostic factor (McLean et al. 1977; McLean et al. 1982). Nevertheless a small melanoma may be mimicked by several choroidal lesions such as metastatic carcinoma, nevus, hemangioma, clotted hemorrhage and disciform macular degeneration. These lesions have different prognosis and require different treatments. So the correct diagnosis may be missed. In fact the differential diagnosis of small choroidal solid lesions represents usually one of the most difficult problems for the echographist. The frequent finding of a poor thickness makes it an arduous task to verify all the effective signs for a correct diagnosis. In order to contribute to a rational solution of the problem we retrospectively analyzed the echographic features of our series of small choroidal 'tumors' in terms of sensibility, specificity, positive predictive value and negative predictive value. According to the results obtained

P. Till (ed.), Ophthalmic Echography 13, pp. 313–317.

from this study we suggest an echographic algorithm for differentiating each type of solid lesion.

Material and methods

We analyzed the ultrasonographic examinations of all choroidal solid lesions with an echographic thickness ≤5 mm performed at our institute.

This series was composed of 74 small 'tumors'. The final diagnosis was: 10 melanomas, 18 metastatic carcinomas, 12 nevi, 8 hemangiomas, 7 organized hemorrhages and 19 disciform macular degenerations. The thickness of the 74 solid lesions was ($\bar{x} \pm$ S.D.): 2.7 ± 0.81 mm (min.: 1.8 mm; max.: 5 mm).

Examinations were performed by Standardized Echography (T = 69 dB).

Contact technique (A-mode and B-mode) was employed following topographic, kinetic and quantitative diagnostic criteria. The measurement of max. thickness for each lesion was always determined using the same A-scan probe and US speed of 1550 m/sec. We looked for all the echographic features of the choroidal tumors reported in well-known studies of Ossoinig (Ossoinig et al.; 1974; Ossoinig et al. 1975; Ossoinig 1979) and in the major treatises of Ophthalmic Echography (Coleman et al. 1977; Shammas 1984; Mazzeo 1987). Then we calculated sensibility, specificity, positive predictive value and negative predictive value for each A-scan and B-scan characteristic of the single small choroidal solid lesions. In this type of analysis the gold standard is histology, but in our series it was impossible to obtain pathological specimens because the lesions were treated either by conservative therapy (not surgery) or by observation. Therefore the final diagnosis was clinically obtained and it was established on the basis of ophthalmoscopy and overall instrumental evidence. In uncertain cases the diagnosis was made only after a suitable follow-up. The characteristics of follow-up period were: mean.: 3.5 years; min.: 6 months (one case of metastasis); max.: 9 years (one case of nevus and one case of disciform macular degeneration). Attention was focused on those echographic features that resulted most effective to identify small melanomas with respect to other solid lesions. Furthermore, according to results gathered from this analysis we elaborated an echographic algorithm for the correct diagnosis of each type of small choroidal solid lesion.

Results

The most effective echographic features to identify small choroidal melanomas were: dome-shape, spongy internal texture and choroidal excavation in B-scan; in A-scan they were: 20–70% internal reflectivity, regular internal structure and spontaneous vascular movements. Sensibility, specificity, PPV

Table 1. Echographic characteristics resulted most effective to identify the small choroidal melanomas

Echographic characteristic		Sensibility %	Specificity %	PPV %	NPV %
B-Scan	Dome-shaped mass	80	63	25	95
	Spongy internal texture	90	48	21	97
	Choroidal excavation	70	97	78	95
A-scan	20–70% internal reflectivity	100	47	33	100
	Regular internal structure (°K)	70	80	35	94
	Spontaneous vascular movements	20	100	100	89

Table 2. Echographic characteristics resulted most effective to identify the following choroidal solid lesions: metastatic carcinoma, hemangioma, nevus, disciform macular degeneration and hemorrhage (solid)

Chor. solid lesion	Echogr. characteristic	(mode)	Sensibility %	Specificity %	PPV %	NPV %
Metastatic carc.	Irregular-multilobate shape	(B)	28	95	63	80
	Irregular internal structure	(A)	89	46	35	93
	Secondary retinal detachment	(A–B)	61	95	79	88
Hemangioma	High internal reflectivity	(A)	87	67	24	98
	Regular internal structure	(A)	87	80	35	98
Nevus	High internal reflectivity	(A)	83	18	16	85
	Regular internal structure	(A)	33	73	19	85
Disciform mac. deg.	High internal reflectivity	(A)	84	60	42	92
	Double internal stratification	(A)	84	100	100	95
Hemorrhage (solid)	Irregular internal structure	(A)	86	69	22	98

and NPV of these signs are reported in Table 1. Table 2 shows the results regarding the other solid lesions. Metastatic carcinomas were differentiated more efficiently by irregular-multilobate shape (B-scan – specificity of 95%), irregular internal structure (V-shaped or inverse angle K – A-scan – sensibility of 89%) and secondary retinal detachment (A- and B-scan – specificity of 95%). High internal reflectivity and regular internal structure (A-scan)

Table 3. Echographic diagnostic procedure suggested by the authors in case of a small choroidal solid lesion

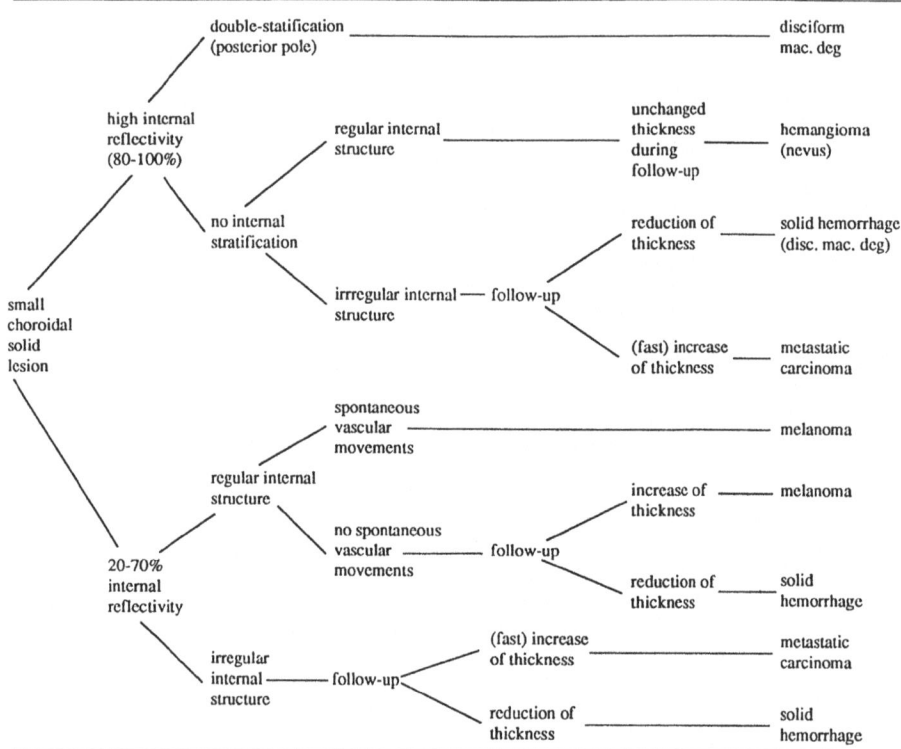

were the more effective signs in identifying hemangiomas and nevi, while to diagnose disciform macular degeneration two A-scan characteristics were important: high internal reflectivity and double internal stratification. Furthermore the more typical echographic feature of clotted hemorrhages (organized and solid) was the A-scan irregular internal structure. Finally in the scheme of Table 3 we report the echographic diagnostic procedure that we elaborated on the basis of our results.

Discussion

The mean thickness of the small choroidal solid lesion of our series is 2.7 ± 0.81 mm. This means that ultrasonographic pictures are often very difficult to interpret. To achieve the correct diagnosis of small 'tumors' there are several signs to be considered. On the basis of our results we found that three echographic features which are usually helpful are not useful in the cases that we studied: (1) the orbital shadowing is present both in large mass and in small calcified lesions as retinoblastoma and osteoma; (2) the high initial echo-spike and the absence of aftermovements are a pre-requisite of all solid lesions and obviously it is not useful in their differential diagnosis; (3) the internal acoustic vacuole depends on the type and the adjustment of the instrument employed. Other ultrasonographic signs are characterized by a valid diagnostic effectiveness. Medium (20–70%) internal reflectivity, regular internal structure (A-scan) and choroidal excavation (B-scan) are very important to individualize a small melanoma (Table 1). A-scan irregular internal structure (V-shaped or inverse angle K) and a secondary retinal detachment strongly suggest the diagnosis of metastatic carcinoma (Table 2). Finally two echographic features resulted pathognomonic (specificity of 100%): the double internal stratification for disciform macular degeneration (Table 2) and spontaneous vascular movements (SVM) for melanoma (Table 1). Nevertheless SVM have a low sensibility and in our series they have been noticed only in 2 cases out of 10.

Consequently only in a few cases is it possible to establish the correct diagnosis by a single echographic examination. Frequently in case of a small choroidal solid lesion the echographist may propose a probability diagnosis and the follow-up of thickness becomes necessary for sure diagnosis. From this point of view our diagnostic 'pathway' summarized in Table 3 and representing our experience and our effort is an attempt to resolve the problem of differential diagnosis.

References

1. Coleman. D.J., Lizzi, F.L. & Jack, R.L. Ultrasonography of the eye and orbit. Philadelphia: Lea & Febiger Ed. (1977).
2. Mazzeo, V. Ecografia dell'apparato oculare. Testo-Atlante. Milano: Fogliazza Ed. (1987).
3. McLean, I.W., Foster, W.D. & Zimmerman, L.E. Prognostic factors in small malignant melanoma of choroid and ciliary body. Arch. Ophthalmol. 95: 48 (1977).
4. McLean, I.W., Foster, W.D. & Zimmerman, L.E. Uveal melanoma: location, size, cell type and enucleation as risk factors in metastasis. Hum. Pathol. 13: 123 (1982).
5. Ossoinig, K.C. & Blodi, F.C. Preoperative differential diagnosis of tumors with echography. In: Blodi. F.C. (ed.) Current concepts in ophthalmology. St. Louis: The C.V. Mosby Co. (1974).
6. Ossoinig, K.C., Bigar, F. & Kaefring, S.L. Malignant melanoma of the choroid and ciliary body. A differential diagnosis in clinical echography. Bibl. Ophthalmol. 83: 141 (1975).
7. Ossoinig, K.C. Standardized echography: basic principles, clinical applications and results. Int. Ophthalmol. Clin. 19: 127 (1979).
8. Shammas, H.J. Atlas of ophthalmic ultrasonography and biometry. St. Louis: The C.V. Mosby Co. (1984).

Address for correspondence: Institute of Clinical Ophthalmology, University of Verona, Ospedale di Borgo Trento, I-37126 Verona, Italy.

34. Contribution of standardized echography to diagnostic work-up of intraocular lymphoma

D. DORO, E. MIDENA, E. MANTOVANI, M. SALA & F. MORO

(Padua, Italy)

Abstract. Standardized echographic examination of the right blind eye with neovascular glaucoma and cataract in a 52-year-old woman revealed solid retinal detachment with thickened retina and irregular mostly medium to high reflective subretinal echoes. After a few weeks the left eye developed ophthalmoscopically visible yellowish areas of solid retinal detachment at the posterior pole and multiple small peripheral choroidal infiltrates. Vitreous aspirate and retinochoroidal biopsy of the right eye failed to show evidence of intraocular tumor cells. Histological examination of the enucleated right eye showed massive subretinal lymphocyte infiltration with necrosis and hemorrhage. Immunohistochemistry confirmed the diagnosis of intraocular non-Hodgkin's large cell lymphoma. The results of standardized echography are discussed and correlated to the histological findings.

Introduction

Non-Hodgkin's intraocular lymphoma 'reticulum cell sarcoma' according to a dated classification [3, 5–7, 12, 13] can involve choroid, retina, vitreous, iris and the optic nerve. Due to the non-specific nature of the ophthalmic manifestations, a diagnosis of ocular non-Hodgkin's lymphoma is clinically difficult to make. According to Freeman et al. the mean delay from symptoms to the diagnosis by vitreous biopsy is 13 months [3]. In the ophthalmic echographic literature only one case of intraocular lymphoma without histological evaluation has been described [2]. We thought it interesting to report the diagnostic work up in the following case.

Case report

A 52-year-old woman, who had been suffering from therapy controlled arterial hypertension and type II diabetes mellitus for 15 years, was referred on January 1990 to our Clinic for 'bilateral exudative posterior uveitis'.

Since August 1989 she had been complaining for rapidly progressive visual acuity loss both in the right and a few weeks later, in the left eye.

She had been promptly evaluated elsewhere. Goldmann kinetic perimetry evidenced bilaterally inferior altitudinal defects involving the macula in the right eye. Fluorescein retinal angiography showed late hyperfluorescence of the right optic disc and patchy leakage from retinal capillaries more evident

P. Till (ed.), Ophthalmic Echography 13, pp. 319–326.
© 1993 *Kluwer Academic Publishers*.

in the right eye. Orbital CT scans were thought to be consistent with right choroidal hematoma or melanoma. Hemathological tests revealed elevated (40–60 mm/h) ESR, high (17,000/mm^3) white blood cells values, raised OKT-8 (37.4%). OKT-4, complement fractions, immunoglobulins were within the normal range. ELISA anti-viral hepatitis, anti-brucellosis, anti-toxoplasmosis IgM antibodies titers, VDRL, TPHA and tuberculin skin-test, reumathological evaluation were negative. HLA typing was positive for DRW-52. Systemic steroid therapy (50 to 25 mg prednisone/die) adminis-tered for about four months had not been effective.

On admission to our Clinic (January 1990), the right painful blind eye showed conjunctival and episcleral hyperemia, diffuse corneal edema, shal-low anterior chamber, Tyndall 2+, keratic precipitates, rubeosis iridis with angle neovascularization, fixed mydriasis, cataract and hazy vitreous that prevented fundus evaluation; IOP was 54 mm Hg. In the left eye corrected visual acuity was 20/100; there were 1+ flare and 1+ cells in the anterior chamber and 2+ haze and 2+ cells in the vitreous; IOP was 18 mm Hg. Goldmann perimetry confirmed left altitudinal inferior hemianopia.

Ophthalmoscopy revealed: elevated swollen optic disc with blurred edges and splinter hemorrhages; yellowish areas of elevated edematous retina at the posterior pole with several intraretinal hemorrhages along the superior temporal vessels; pigment epithelium mottling of the macula and the mid periphery.

Bilateral acute retinal necrosis or intraocular lymphoma was the suspected diagnosis on clinical grounds.

Hemathological tests revealed high (12,000/mm^3) white blood cell values with normal white cell formula, variable glucose plasma levels (3.0 to 15.8 mmol/L). ESR, OKT-4, OKT-8, protein fractions, immunoglobulins were within the normal range. CF anti-adenovirus, anti-ECHOvirus, anti-poliovirus, anti-coxsackievirus antibodies titers were not significant. Anti-cardiolipin antibodies and ELISA anti-HIV, anti-citomegalovirus, anti-her-pes zoster virus, anti-herpes simplex virus, anti-morbillivirus, anti-parotitis virus IgM antibodies titers were negative.

In the following weeks, the elevation and number of multiple apparently solid yellowish retinal detachments increased, and all quadrants from the posterior pole to the mid periphery of the left eye were involved. Peripheral multifocal confluent chorio-retinal infiltrates were observed; vitreous in-flammation and optic disc edema increased. Visual acuity of the left eye was gradually reduced to light perception.

Retinal fluorescein angiography of the left eye showed areas of early masked hypofluorescence at the posterior pole, late fluorescein leakage of optic disc and mid peripheral retinal vessels and staining of the subretinal lesions at the posterior pole (Fig. 1).

Contact B-scan of the right eye evidenced solid (no after movements) retinal detachments with different degrees of elevation at the posterior pole and mid periphery in all quadrants, irregular retinal surface, echogenic subre-tinal space but for some echofree temporal and nasal small areas (Fig. 2)

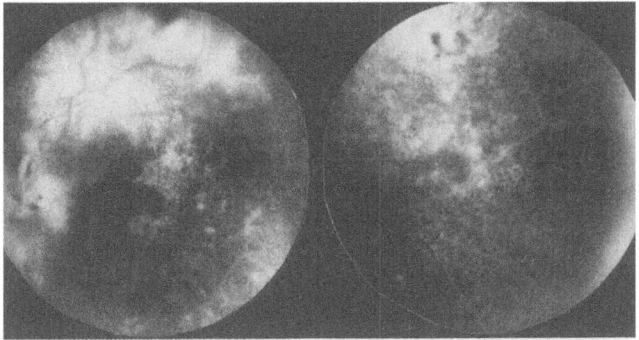

Fig. 1. Retinal fluorescein angiography of the left eye. Late fluorescein leakage from the optic disc (left) and mid peripheral retinal vessels (right); staining of an elevated subretinal lesion above the optic disc (left).

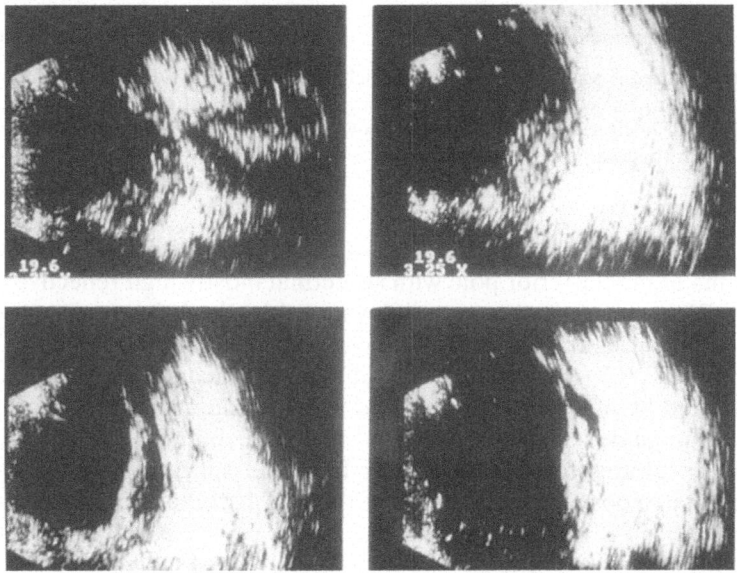

Fig. 2. Contact B-scan of the right eye. Solid retinal detachment with irregular retinal surface and various degrees of elevation at the posterior pole (top left) and peripheral echogenic subretinal mass inferiorly (top right). Some subretinal temporal (bottom left) and nasal (bottom right) areas are echo-free and disperse vitreous echoes are visible.

and disperse vitreous echoes at high system sensitivity setting. Standardized A-scan showed thickened retina with maximum elevation of 6 microseconds and medium to high subretinal echoes with irregular structure, but in some areas low and high reflective echoes co-existed (Fig. 3). No spontaneous vascular movements of the subretinal echo-spikes were present.

322

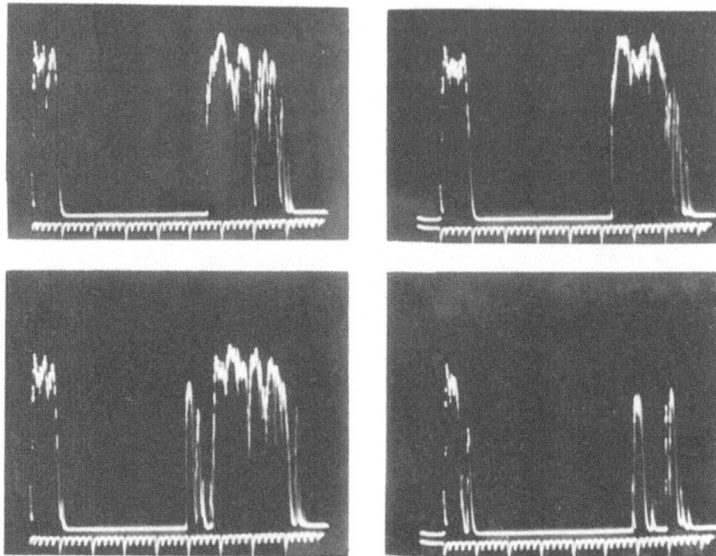

Fig. 3. Standardized A-scan echography of the right eye. Thickened retina and medium to high (top left and right) reflectivity with somewhat irregular structure of subretinal echoes at tissue sensitivity and T-20 dB setting (bottom right). Low and high reflective subretinal echoes in the same echogram (bottom left).

Similarly, standardized echography of the left eye displayed less elevated thick retina at the posterior pole with subretinal mostly high reflective echoes (Fig. 4). Right optic disc was more elevated than the left one.

Thickened perineural sheaths and increased retrobulbar optic nerve width (RE = 7.5; LE = 7 microseconds), but no subarachnoidal fluid could be demonstrated by means of standardized A-scan examination (Fig. 5).

Two echo-guided vitreous aspirates from the blind right eye failed to show cells; cultures for herpes viruses from the specimens were negative. Chorioretinal biopsy of the right eye showed lymphocyte infiltration and necrosis.

On NMR both hyperintense and hypointense T_2 weighted areas involving all the posterior segment of the right eye and slight thickening of the posterior pole of the left eye were detected. T_2 slightly hyperintense irregular area in the paramedian cerebellum and some similar areas bilaterally in the white substance were observed (Fig. 6). An inflammatory cause of the ocular lesions was suggested; cerebral abnormalities were considered aspecific, but intracranial lymphoma could not be ruled out.

For diagnostic purposes enucleation of the blind right eye was performed. Histology showed degenerated retina without necrosis and subretinal space grossly infiltrated by lymphocytes with necrotic debris and hemorrhagic areas (Fig. 7). Also the retrobulbar optic nerve was infiltrated by lymphocytes. The subretinal lymphocytes were large and had hypercromatic nuclei and

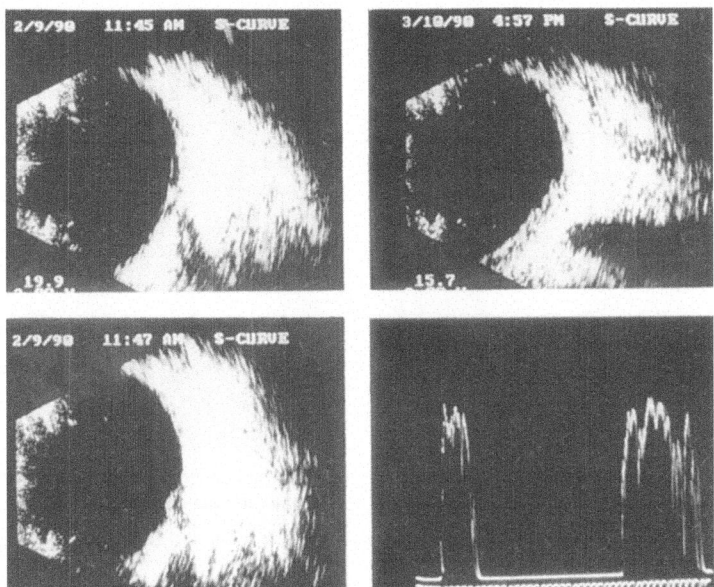

Fig. 4. Standardized echography of the left eye: B-scan shows progression of solid retinal elevation at the posterior pole within one month (top left and right) and protrusion of the optic disc (bottom left). Standardized A-scan shows high reflective subretinal echoes (bottom right).

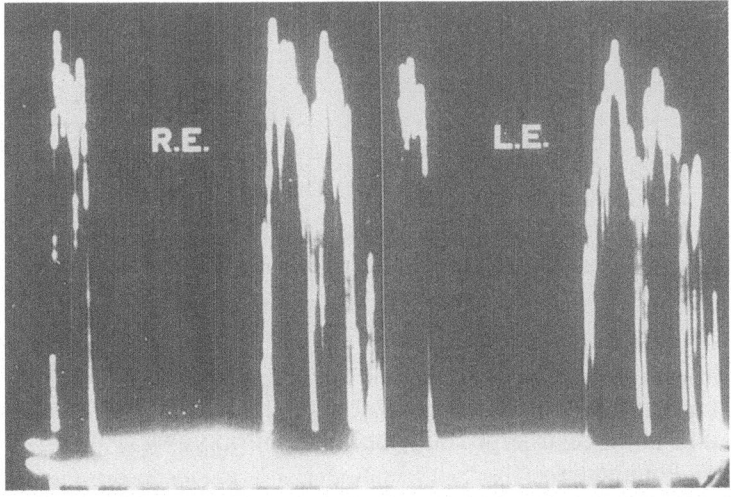

Fig. 5. Standardized A-scan. Solid optic nerve sheath thickening and increased transverse diameter of both retrobulbar optic nerves.

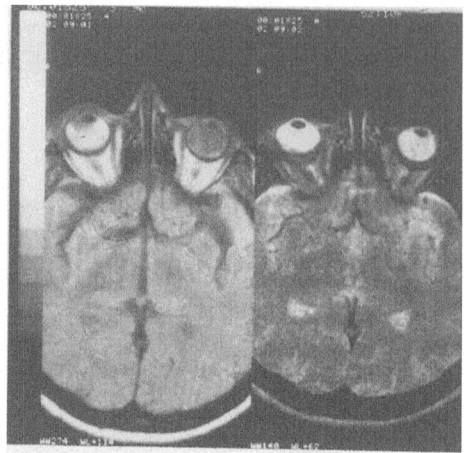

Fig. 6. NMR shows T₂ weighted hyperintense and hypointense areas at the posterior pole of the right eye and some T₂ hyperintense areas in the white substance mostly around cerebellum.

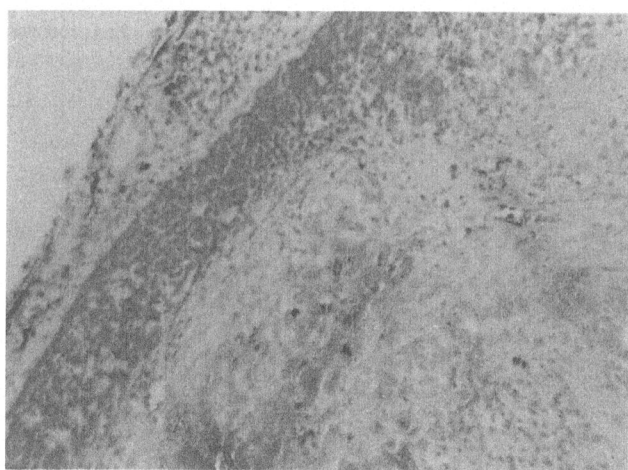

Fig. 7. Histological section of the right eye: degenerated retina and subretinal space with massive lymphocyte infiltration, necrotic debris and hemorrhagic areas (H.H. 200×).

scant cytoplasm. Monoclonal antibody staining evidenced B lymphocytes with cell membrane kappa immunoglobulin light chains, thus confirming the diagnosis of intraocular large cell lymphoma, also known as intraocular non-Hodgkin's lymphoma.

The patient was referred to oncologists to evaluate irradiation of central nervous system.

Discussion

Multifocal solid detachment of the retinal pigment epithelium and multiple small choroidal infiltrates are reported features of the rare introcular non-Hodgkin's lymphoma [3, 4, 7, 9, 13]. Unilateral or bilateral posterior uveitis unresponsive to steroids is a misleading sign that explains the delay of the diagnosis of intraocular non-Hodgkin's lymphoma [3, 5, 7–9]. Actually, our patient had been treated for several months for bilateral exudative posterior uveitis with progressive deterioration of the visual function. Neovascular glaucoma, as found in the right eye of our patient, has also been reported as a complication of intraocular large cell lymphoma [13].

The multifocal yellow-white confluent patches beginning in the periphery with spreading towards the posterior pole and the apparent exudative retinal detachment of the left eye of our patient suggested to us a possible diagnosis of bilateral retinal necrosis [11]. However, extensive serological investigations and vitreous aspirate failed to demonstrate viral infection.

The results of standardized echography of both eyes were difficult to interpret. Solid retinal detachment was evident in the right eye but some subretinal echo-free areas indicated possible exudative detachment. On standardized A-scan echography mostly high reflective subretinal echoes with irregular structure were found: these echo patterns were not akin to the low to medium reflective subretinal echoes reported in a case of reticulum cell sarcoma [2]. Also the echographic findings of the left eye with similarly thickened but less elevated retina did not suggest a clear diagnosis but a subretinal infiltration.

Magnetic resonance imaging could not rule out a cerebral involvement, typically associated with intraocular non-Hodgkin's lymphoma [3, 4, 7, 9, 13].

No useful diagnostic information was obtained by vitreous aspirate [1, 2, 5, 9] and chorio-retinal biopsy of the right eye of our patient. Lumbar puncture was not performed because of the reported low rate (25%) of positive findings in cases of intraocular non-Hodgkin's lymphoma [3]. Enucleation of the right blind eye and immunohistochemistry was needed to reach a conclusive diagnosis of intraocular large cell lymphoma.

Massive subretinal lymphocyte infiltration with necrosis and hemorrhage may account for the intriguing mostly high reflective subretinal echoes found on standardized A-scan. Also the retrobulbar optic nerve, which showed solid thickening on standardized A-scan echography [10], appeared infiltrated on histological evaluation.

Standardized echography failed to be conclusive in our patient, but showed solid subretinal lesions and signs of retrobulbar optic nerve infiltration. The peculiar echo patterns of this case should be taken into account by echographers who will encounter such a rare intraocular pathology, often presenting as a posterior uveitis unresponsive to steroids.

References

1. Bovey, E. Intérêt des biopsie oculaires dan la diagnostic etiologique des uveites. Klin. Mbl. Augenheilk. 194: 365–367 (1989).
2. Byrne, B. & Van Heuven, W.A.J. Echographic characteristics of a subpigment epithelial reticulum cell sarcoma. Ossoinig K.C. (ed.), Ophthalmic Echography, pp. 407–412. Dordrecht: Martinus Nijhoff/Dr. W. Junk (1987).
3. Freeman, L.N., Schachat, A.P., Knox, D.L., Michels, R.G. & Green, W.R. Clinical features, laboratory investigations, and survival in ocular reticulum cell sarcoma. Ophthalmology 94: 1631–1639 (1987).
4. Gass, J.D.M. Stereoscopic atlas of macular diseases: diagnosis and treatment, pp. 196–198. St. Louis: C.V. Mosby Co. (1987).
5. Kennerdell, J.S., Johnson, B.L. & Wisotzky, H.M. Vitreous cellular infiltration: association with reticulum cell sarcoma of the brain. Arch. Ophthalmol. 93: 1341–1345 (1975).
6. Klingele, T.G. & Hogan, M.J. Ocular reticulum cell sarcoma. Am. J. Ophthalmol. 79: 39–47 (1975).
7. Lewis, H. & Schachat, A.P. Non-Hodgkin's ('reticulum cell') lymphoma. In Ryan, S.J. (ed.), Retina, pp. 795–804. St. Louis: C.V. Mosby Co. (1989).
8. Minckler, D.S., Font, R.L. & Zimmerman, L.E. Uveitis and reticulum cell sarcoma. Am. J. Ophthalmol. 80: 433–439 (1975).
9. Nussenblatt, R.B. & Palestine, A.G. Uveitis. Fundamentals and clinical practice. Chicago: Year Book Med. Publ. 315–321 (1989).
10. Ossoinig, K.C., Cennamo, G. & Byrne, S.F. Echographic differential diagnosis of optic nerve lesions. Doc. Ophthalmol. Proc. Ser. 29: 327–331 (1981).
11. Pepose, J.S. Acute retinal necrosis syndrome. In Ryan, S.J. (ed.), Retina, pp. 617–623. St. Louis: C.V. Mosby Co. (1989).
12. Qualman, S.J., Mendelsohn, G., Mann, R.B. & Green, W.R. Intraocular lymphoma. Cancer 52: 878–886 (1975).
13. Sloas, H.A., Starling, J., Harper, D.G. & Cupples, H.P. Update of reticulum cell sarcoma. Arch. Ophthalmol. 99: 1048–1052 (1981).

Address for correspondence: Dr D. Doro, Ophthalmology Clinic, University of Padua, Via Giustiniani 2, I-35128 Padua, Italy.

PART FOUR

Intraocular disorders

35. Hemorrhagic and degenerative vitreal interfaces

V. MAZZEO, P. PERRI & L. RAVALLI
(Ferrara, Italy)

Abstract. The term 'pseudo-detachment of the posterior hyaloid in proliferating diabetic retino-pathy' was coined by Green and co-workers (SIDUO XII, Iguazu Argentina) to indicate that although echographic findings showed a detachment of the hemorrhagic vitreous, surgery revealed that the vitreous cortex was still attached. In light of these affirmations, and upon close examination of recent literature on the behaviour of the vitreous during hemorrhage, the authors have critically evaluated images of interfaces (one or more) met in vitreal hemorrhages.

Introduction

At the SIDUO XII Congress held in Iguazu (Argentina), Green and co-workers [3] introduced the term 'pseudo-detachment of the posterior hyaloid' in proliferative diabetic retinopathy. They described some cases where a splitting of the posterior vitreous was observed in diabetic patients with hemorrhagic vitreous. Echographic findings were those of a posterior detachment of a hemorrhagic vitreous, while at surgery the cortical vitreous was found to be in situ. Since then we have paid particular attention to a series of vitreal hemorrhages with different causes, showing some fairly exceptional echographic findings that so far have not been explained in the literature.

Descriptions of the echograms

We found a series of 'vitreous membranes' that co-exist with an image considered typical of a hemorrhagic vitreous detachment (Fig. 1). The differential diagnosis with a detached retina and/or a neovascular membrane was almost immediate in the screen using all the known acoustic criteria such as motility, topography, thickness and reflectivity. All the cases were then confirmed by follow-up. As far as motility is concerned, in several of these cases a motility typical of a posterior viteous detachment could be observed, while in others where the interfaces were quite near to the eyewall no after movements could be induced (Fig. 2).

P. Till (ed.), Ophthalmic Echography 13, pp. 329–332.

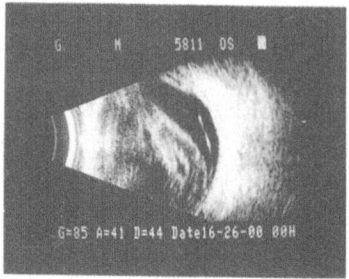 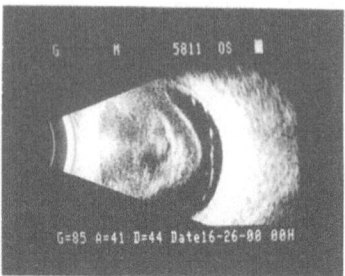

Fig. 1. Vitreous hemorrhage. Behind the hemorrhagic vitreous there is an acoustically empty space. A membrane-like structure shows all the characteristics of the detached hyaloid.

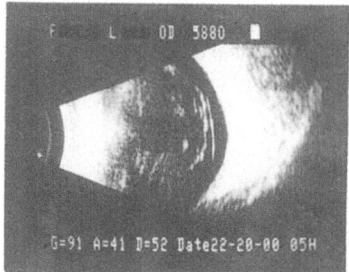

Fig. 2. 'Double vitreous detachment'. The end of the hemorrhagic vitreous simulates a hyaloid detached that is instead present after an acoustically empty space.

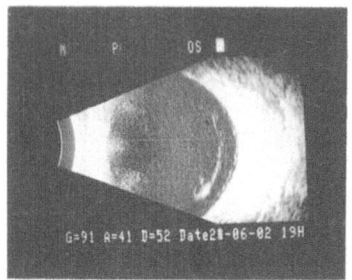 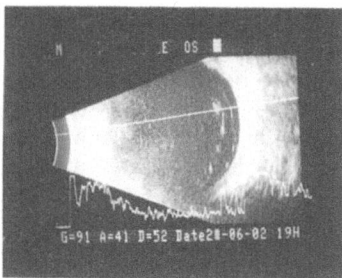

Fig. 3. Syneresis of a hemorrhagic vitreous. A very thin, membrane-like structure is clearly visible. Both these interfaces show after-movements typical of the vitreous body.

Discussion

The above echographs were obtained using contact B-scan of relatively recent manufacture (Ophthasonic, Tecknar and Ophthascan 5, Biophisic Medical). Both the apparatus has 10 MHz probes (nominal frequency) with linear amplification. Almost all the examinations were performed at maximum sensitivity setting, although this produces on-screen electronic noise.

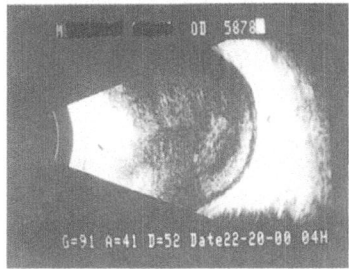 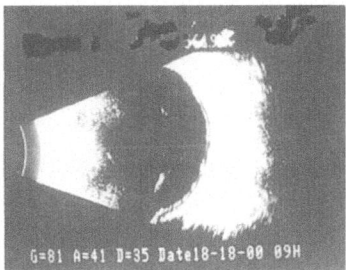

Fig. 4. Vitreous syneresis of hemorrhagic origin (left), and due to aging (right). The liquid/cortical vitreous interface is visible as a very thin line parallel to the ocular wall. No after-movements are present.

In the authors' opinion, this enables every piece of information to be gathered, as long as the user knows how to distinguish between noise and real interfaces. The attribution of these different 'membranes' to the vitreous appears justified in light of our knowledge of its ageing process [1, 2, 6, 8, 9] and of the pathological phenomena encountered in experimental hemorrhages to laboratory experiments on primates [4, 5, 7]. In cynomologus monkeys after injuries, two types of vitreous detachment take place. In the first, hemorrhagic syneresis occurs, leaving the cortical vitreous attached, and in the second it detaches from the retina along with the hemorrhagic vitreous.

In summary, in the presence of a significant post-hemorrhagic syneresis, the echographic image is that of a posterior hemorrhagic vitreous detachment while the cortex is *in situ* revealed by a very thin, immobile line. The latter probably originates from the liquid/cortex interface. In other subjects the cortical vitreous may then detach from the retina, in which case the echograms will show a kind of 'double posterior vitreous detachment'.

References

1. Denlinger, J.L., Eisner, G. & Balazs, E.A. Age-related changes in the vitreous and lens of Rhesus Monkeys. Ex. Eye Res. 31: 67–79 (1980).
2. Foos, R.J. & Wheeler, N.C. Vitreo-retinal juncture. Synchisis senilis and posterior vitreous detachment. Ophthalmology 89: 1502–1512 (1982).
3. Green, R.L., Cano, M.R., Lean, J.S., Thomas, E.L., Freeman, W.R. & Ligget, P.E. Pseudodetachment of the posterior hyaloid in proliferative diabetic retinopathy. XII SIDUO Cong. Program and Abstract 44 (1988).
4. Jakobieic, F.A. Ocular anatomy, embriology and teratology. Philadelphia: Harper and Row Pub. (1982).
5. Hsu, I.T. & Ryan, S.J. Natural history of penetrating ocular injury with retinal laceration in the monkey. Graefe's Arch Clinl Exp. Ophthalmol. 224: 1–6 (1986).
6. Larsson, L. & Osterlin, S. Posterior vitreus detachment. A combined clinical and physico-chemical study. Graefe's Arch Clin. Exp. Ophthalmol. 223: 92–95 (1985).

332

7. Miller, B., Miller, H. & Ryan, S.J. Experimental vitreous sineresis. Arch. ophthalmol. 103: 1385–1388 (1985).
8. Schepens, C.L. Il distacco di retina e malattie associate. Verducci Ed. (1985).
9. Spencer, W.H. Ophthalmic pathology an atlas and textbook, Vol. 2, Ch. 7, pp. 548–588. Philadelphia: W.B. Sauderders Company (1985).

Address for correspondence: Prof. V. Mazzeo, Eye Clinic, Ferrara University, Corso Giovecca 203, I-44100 Ferrara, Italy.

36. Is B-scan ultrasound useful in predicting the source of vitreous hemorrhage?

R.C. BOSANQUET & J.A. BELL

(*Newcastle Upon Tyne, United Kingdom*)

Abstract. Careful ultrasonography of the eye with vitreous hemorrhage can yield useful clues which indicate the source of bleeding in well over 50% of patients. We have described the most helpful signs and, in order to obtain the maximum information, we advise that ultrasonography is undertaken at an early stage of the vitreous hemorrhage and is regularly repeated until the clinical outcome is known.

Introduction

There have been a number of studies analysing the accuracy of ultrasound in eyes with vitreous hemorrhage (Fisher 1984; Müller-Breitenkamp 1984). These show that in experienced hands the ultrasound findings are a helpful indication of the true state of the posterior pole of the eye as judged by vitrectomy soon afterwards. At the SIDUO Congress in 1984, Green described the echographic features of spontaneous vitreous hemorrhage due to various causes other than diabetes (Green 1987). In this study we set out to see if the precise source of the hemorrhage could be deduced from an early echographic examination.

Method

We studied 20 patients who presented to the combined Ultrasound/Vitreo-Retinal Clinic at the Newcastle General Hospital with a vitreous hemorrhage sufficiently dense to obscure the fundus. The majority were fresh vitreous hemorrhages, but some were longstanding hemorrhages which had only recently been referred for fuller investigation. An ophthalmic and medical history was taken in the usual way and a full eye examination was carried out. B-Scan ultrasonogaphy was performed in a manner similar to that described by Green using a Sonometrics Ocuscan for the earlier examinations and a Biophysic Mini-B for the more recent examinations. Our technique was similar with the two instruments and the results obtained were comparable, but the attachment of a videoprinter to the Mini-B greatly simplified the process of obtaining representative prints for the patients' records.

Our technique was to look for echoes from the posterior vitreous surface.

P. Till (ed.). Ophthalmic Echography 13, pp. 333–336.

Table 1. Results (21 eyes)

Correct	11	(52.5%)
Non-contributory	4	(19.0%)
Unresolved	2	(9.5%)
Incorrect	4	(19.0%)

In all cases this was at least partly separated from the retina. It is only when the posterior vitreous is still attached to the disc that there may be difficulty in distinguishing a posterior vitreous detachment from a retinal detachment. Posterior vitreous detachments are mobile with extensive after-movements. They have low reflectivity, which decreases towards the periphery and they are often folded, particularly inferiorly.

Occasionally it can be extremely difficult to differentiate an incomplete posterior vitreous detachment, or a vitreous membrane inserting into the disc, from a retinal detachment and the more detailed techniques described by Ossoinig have to be employed (Ossoinig 1987). In a fresh vitreous hemorrhage the red cells are evenly dispersed throughout the vitreous so that vitreous gel appears acoustically empty. Usually, however, there will be weak echoes to indicate whether the hemorrhage is primarily intragel, retrogel, or both.

During the examination the eye is scanned through the closed lids, first vertically then horizontally while the patient looks to either side. In particular, the examiner is looking for areas of constant contact between the posterior vitreous face and the retina. Often the posterior vitreous face lies against the retina inferiorly due to the bulk of haemorrhage, but with eye movement it can be seen that the vitreous moves independently of the retina. Areas of constant contact between vitreous and retina are suggestive of new vessel formation or of a retinal hemorrhage breaking through to the vitreous. The signs can be very subtle. There may only be a few echoes in the vitreous but their positions relative to the retina during eye movements do not alter. When the hemorrhage originates from a mass lesion in the fundus this is obvious on B-scan, and Standardized A-Scan will differentiate between a disciform macula degeneration and a choroidal melanoma. New vessels inserting into the disc may appear quite extensive ophthalmoscopically without a correspondingly florid ultrasound picture and so echoes fixed to the disc need to be regarded as indicative of pathology. Membranes at the disc sometimes reattach themselves to more peripheral retina and so it is important to continue scanning the fundus carefully even though there are obvious vitreo-retinal attachments at the disc.

Results

We looked at 21 eyes of 20 patients (Table 1). We consider that in 11 we correctly localised the source of bleeding. In four patients the ultrasound

Table 2. Results (15 eyes), non-contributory and unresolved cases excluded

Correct	11	(73.3%)
Incorrect	4	(26.7%)

Table 3. Results grouped by underlying pathology

Ultrasound findings	Correct	Incorrect	Unresolved	Non-contributory
Disciform degeneration	2	0	0	0
Penetrating injury	2	0	0	0
Disc new vessels	4	1	1	0
Diabetic retinopathy without new disc vessels	2	3	0	0
Retinal tear	1	0	0	1
BRVO & BRAO	1	1	1	1
Retinal cyst	0	0	0	1
PVD alone (cause of hemorrhage unknown)	0	0	1	1

The total numbers exceed the number examined since some eyes showed multiple features and are included in more than one category.

was non-contributory in that there were insufficient features to indicate where the vitreous hemorrhage was coming from. In two eyes the vitreous hemorrhage is still present, so there is no clinical confirmation as to the source of hemorrhage. In four cases our predictions were incorrect.

When the 'non-contributory' and unresolved cases are excluded our success rate increases considerably. In other words, where we felt able to predict the source of vitreous hemorrhage and clinical confirmation was possible, we had a 73% chance of being correct (Table 2).

Discussion

Other authors (Butner 1982; Morse 1974; Green 1987) have looked at the causes of spontaneous vitreous hemorrhage. In an ultrasound clinic the population will be different since the patients usually have particularly dense and persistent hemorrhages and many are being seen repeatedly prior to vitrectomy. Our aim was to study not so much the cause of the hemorrhage, as to try and pinpoint its precise source. The difficulty that arose was that in some cases the source of the hemorrhage could never be determined even when a good view of the retina could be finally obtained. However, it is useful to look at the cases in groups according to their underlying pathology (Table 3). There is usually little difficulty in identifying vitreous hemorrhage due to a disciform macula degeneration. This is a particularly useful diagnosis to make at an early stage as vitrectomy is not indicated and frequent follow-up visits can be avoided.

In traumatic cases there is likely to be extensive membrane formation, which can be seen accoustically, and this will usually point to the region of retinal damage or bleeding.

In this series there was one case of a retinal detachment where we correctly localised the retinal tear. There was a second patient with a retinal detachment which was unusual in that the ocular pressure was extremely low and there appeared to be an associated choroidal effusion. In our view it would be unwise to rely on ultrasound alone to exclude a retinal tear in a fresh, recent dense vitreous hemorrhage. The cases in which our predictions were incorrect were mostly diabetics, either with background retinopathy only or with new vessels away from the optic disc. In such cases the retinal picture and the ultrasound findings can be complicated and the precise source of vitreous hemorrhage may never become clear. The findings can change substantially over time so that repeated detailed examinations are recommended in these patients.

References

1. Butner, R.W. & McPherson, A.R. Spontaneous vitreous hemorrhage. Ann. Ophthalm. 14: 268–270 (1982).
2. Fisher, Y.L. Contact ultrasonography in the evaluation of diabetic traction retinal detachment associated with vitreous hemorrhage. In Hillman, J.S. and Le May, M.M. (eds.), Ophthalmic Ultrasonography. Proceedings of 9th SIDUO Congress. Doc. Ophthalmol. Proc. Ser. 38: 93 (1984).
3. Green R.L. The echographic evaluation of spontaneous vitreous hemorrhage. In Ossoinig, K.C. (ed.), Ophthalmic Echography. Proceedings of 10th SIDUO Congress. Doc. Ophthalmol. Proc. Ser. 48: 233–238 (1987).
4. Morse, P.H., Aminlari, A. & Scheie, H.J. Spontaneous vitreous haemorrhage. Arch. Ophthalmol. 92: 297–298 (1974).
5. Müller-Breitenkamp, R., Trier, H.G., Völker, B. & Mester, U. Errors in diagnostic ultrasound. A critical review of 68 patients undergoing diagnostic ultrasound before vitrectomy. In Hillman, J.S. and Le May, M.M. (eds.), Proceedings of 9th SIDUO Congress. Doc. Ophthalmol. Proc. Ser. 38: 107–114 (1984).
6. Ossoinig, K.C., Islas, G., Tamayo, G.E. & Tamburelli, C. Detached retina versus dense fibrovascular membrane. Standardized A-Scan and B-Scan criteria. In Ossoinig, K.C. (ed.), Proceedings of 10th SIDUO Congress. Doc. Ophthalmol. Proc. Ser. 48: 275–284 (1987).

Address for correspondence: Department of Ophthalmology, Newcastle General Hospital, Westgate Road, Newcastle upon Tyne NE4 6BE, United Kingdom.

37. Echography in the study of vitreo–retinal interface pathology

T. AVITABILE, L. FRANCO, C. MARINO, A. PAPPALARDO,
A. LONGO, R. GHIRLANDA & A. REIBALDI
(*Catania, Italy*)

Abstract. In this study the authors point out the role of echography in vitreo–retinal junction diseases, considering the role that this pathology has in light of modern vitreous surgery. Physiologically, the vitreo–retinal interface is virtual and it cannot be studied by echography; it becomes echographically evident when it separates from the retina, or when it increases its thickness. The authors have focused attention on cases that have pathognomonic patterns: posterior vitreous detachment, macular epiretinal membranes, secondary epiretinal membranes, proliferative vitreo-retinopathy, retinopahy of prematurity. The authors emphasize the role of the latest generation B-scan in the study of this pathology; in fact new equipment allows the elaboration of frozen images in order to better study the vitreo–retinal interface.

Introduction

The vitreo–retinal interface can be defined as a surface that forms a frontier shared by two different territories (the vitreous body and the retina), but which is united by reciprocal exchange and interaction.

Under normal conditions, the vitreo–retinal interface is considerably beyond the resolution power of even the most sophisticated equipment, and it therefore cannot be appreciated through ultrasonography. Even less visible are the vitreo–retinal junctions which, in the opinion of several authors (Hogan et al. 1971; Foos 1972, 1974) are even below the resolution power of the electron microscope and occur only at the level of the chemical bond. The vitreo–retinal interface becomes visible only if the two neighboring structures are separated, as in the posterior detachment of the vitreous or, in the event of an increase in thickness, as seen in newly formed macular and extra-macular epiretinal membranes, in the course of proliferative vitreo-retinopathy (PVR) and in retinopathy of prematurity (ROP).

In the course of investigation of this interface, ultrasonography is indicated in the presence of opaque optical media of the eye or of transparent media. This test can complement other investigative techniques such as ophthalmoscopy and fluorangiography as an aid to the interpretations of reports.

Ultrasound examination of this particular border structure cannot be carried out easily using the traditional standardized A-scan method since a position perfectly perpendicular to the various structures forming the interface (vitreous – newly formed membranes – retina) will be exceedingly

P. Till (ed.), Ophthalmic Echography 13, pp. 337–343.
© 1993 *Kluwer Academic Publishers.*

difficult to achieve. Even the dynamic B-scan is seldom indicated (posterior detachment of the vitreous).

However, in this set of circumstances, the latest generation of equipment will certainly be of great assistance thanks to features that allow for more in-depth studies of the investigated structure. Indeed, this equipment has a higher resolution power than traditional equipment and it features a series of programs for the computerized processing of frozen images. Some of these programs, such as the 'saturate selected level' and the 'enhance contour' enable us to highlight all of those structures that present the same level of reflectivity. This is the first program, or the contour of the structure; the second one, which is particularly useful in this type of situation, involves the precise alteration of the contour. Naturally, since these lesions are often at the limit of the instrument's resolution power, a zoom can enable us to enlarge the image to twice the frozen size, thus allowing for an improved analysis of lesion features.

Considering the large number of diseases that can affect the vitreo–retinal interface, in this paper we focus on those diseases that present a pathogno-monic ultrasound picture and that can benefit from surgical treatment in particular, after first illustrating how a normal interface appears with this type of processing.

Normal interface

As noted above, the vitreo–retinal interface in physiological conditions is beyond the resolution power of any transducer. However, by using a program that highlights the contour and by selecting the reflectivity level that we know matches the posterior hyaloid (calculated in case of posterior detachment of the vitreous), we can obtain a perfectly regular curve.

Posterior vitreous detachment

The posterior detachment of the vitreous is the transformation of the vitreo–retinal interface from virtual into real, for which it will appear ultrasono-graphically as a surface splitting into two lines separated by an acoustically silent space, consisting of the posterior face of the vitreous and the profile of the anterior surface of the retina. Although the process of this detachment of the vitreous can be investigated using kinetic ultrasonography, the fine structure of its surface can be studied much more easily on a frozen image using the image processing programs that accompany these instruments. Clearly, since the two structures (vitreo–retinal) present different reflectivi-ties, it will be possible to highlight them at various levels of saturation and contour emphasis.

Macular epiretinal membranes

Macular pucker represents a contraction of the inner limit. During the initial phases, its ophthalmoscopic appearance is characterized by an irregularly shaped profile of the posterior pole; hence ultrasonography is a secondary test in these stages. In the more advanced forms there is a contraction of the newly formed epiretinal membranes with an increased alteration of the new posterior pole profile in the macular area. In these cases, thanks to the new generation of computerized equipment complete with programs for image processing and a zoom for enlarging, it will be easier to highlight these alterations.

The best program for this kind of study is 'enhance contour', which enables the user to select a given level to match the interface. The interface no longer appears as a thin and perfectly regular line, but presents thicker areas and a completely irregular and jagged profile. At times the double outline of the newly formed epiretinal membranes may be noticed at the posterior pole.

Secondary epiretinal membranes

Secondary epiretinal membranes (diabetic retinopathy, uveites, trauma, etc.) feature the appearance of complications altering the anatomic and functional integrity of the vitreo–retinal interface. Indeed, during the initial stage of the proliferative phase we may witness the appearance of thin epiretinal membranes that may gradually extend to the vitreous. In these cases, the ultrasound pattern is characterized by the presence of small, pre-retinal dense areas that can be properly highlighted by means of computerized image-processing programs. These programs enable the surface of the retina to be separated from that of the newly formed membranes, at the level of the lesion, since the reflectivity of the latter will be lower than that of the retina proper. During advanced stages, when the membranes are more widespread and organized, with multiple points of insertion on the retina, they may cause traction-induced detachment. In this case interpretation of the ultra-sound image is more complicated because of the continuity between the newly formed vitreous membranes and the retina (Hayashi et al. 1981). In these cases it is especially important to differentiate between the structure in light of a correct surgical approach.

The computerized examination gives us an opportunity, by means of the 'saturate selected level' program, to highlight only those structures that present the same level of reflectivity. Hence the newly formed membranes appear at the lower levels selected, whereas at higher levels the membranes disappear leaving only the more organized membranes along with retinal structures.

With the 'enhance contour' program it is possible to highlight either the membranes, the membrane–retina double interface, and finally only the contour of the retina, since these structures have progressively increasing reflectivity (Avitabile et al. 1988).

PVR

PVR is characterized, from the anatomopathological point of view, by the formation of vitreous membranes on the surface of the retina, or intra-retinally and sub-retinally. However, there are a number of stages that feature different ultrasound patterns.

During the initial stages we may be confronting a detachment of the retina with rigid folds at the level of the PVR. The retina, which appears as a uniform ultrasound structure once detached in these areas, is thicker and presents an irregular contour. Furthermore, it exhibits reduced motility in a B-scan kinetic test. Computerized processing is able to supply more infor-mation on the conditions of the interface. The areas with PVR can be identified more easily with the 'saturate selected level' program, where it is possible to appreciate an area of increased thickness that persist even at the highest levels. With the 'enhance contour' program it is possible to see two lines at certain levels, one of which will be the surface of the retina and the other the PVR (Avitabile et al. 1989; Reibaldi 1990).

During the more advanced stages characterized by the typical T-shaped ultrasound pattern, aside from an almost complete absence of motility at the dynamic test, resorting to the previously mentioned programs, it will be possible to differentiate the two structures forming the vitreo–retinal in-terface. First we highlight the membrane sealing the tunnel itself (vitreous), and later the surface of the retina, by increased reflectivity. During the terminal stages (echogenous triangle) the relationship between vitreous body and retina will be completely subverted.

ROP

Thanks to the greater diffusion of screenings, we have a lower rate of advanced cases (stages IV and V), where a differential diagnosis with the other leukokoriae becomes necessary.

During the initial stages, even though diagnosis is essentially ophthalmo-scopic, given the young age of the patients with whom such a procedure is implemented with difficulty, ultrasonography can be a valid aid to diagnosis. A typical ultrasound sign during the initial stages is the finding of mid-peripheral ridge, an expression of retinal thickening that appears echo-graphically as a thickening of the bulb profile. In this case the interface deformation appears only at the level of the ridge, as may be appreciated by means of the 'saturate selected level' and 'enhance contour' program.

During more advanced stages, B-scan reveal partial or complete detach-ment of the retina along with the presence of organization.

During the terminal phases (stages IV–V), there will be a subversion of the anatomical architecture of the bulb, with the presence of complete funnel-shaped detachment of the retina, sealed by a retro-lenticular membrane exhibiting a T-shaped ultrasound pattern. Obviously, during the initial stages and in those with traction-induced partial detachment of the retina, it is still possible to study the vitreo–retinal interface with the frozen image. It will indeed be possible to distinguish the surface of the retina from the newly formed membranes thanks to the different reflectivity levels. However, this will be far more complicated during the final stages given the considerable organization of the vitreous, which often prevents a distinct separation between the vitreous and the retina (in these cases a differential diagnosis with retinoblastoma for leukokoria may be more important).

Conclusions

Study of the vitreo–retinal interface is becoming increasingly important in that this virtual structure is now viewed as an active functional intermediate between the chorio-retina and the vitreous (Sahel et al. 1985; Schepens et al. 1987; Pallares et al. 1988; Bisantis 1990). Furthermore, the ophthalmological surgeon is confronted daily in clinical practice with a number of diseases originating from the vitreous and the retina involving the interface. We therefore believe it is appropriate to underline how, in view of the correct planning of a surgical procedure, ultrasonography, and especially the B-scan method, are essential means of diagnosis for these types of disease. This is especially true in cases of opaque optical media, but even under normal conditions to acquire a more detailed picture of the situation. This test indeed allows for the careful evaluation of the relationship between the retina and other endo-ocular structures and to highlight any condition that may be present along with all the relevant information for the benefit of the surgeon.

Furthermore, the new computerized B-scan instruments described above enable us to implement sophisticated image-processing programs, such as the 'enhance contour'. With this program we can now highlight the contour of a structure and in this case probe more deeply into the vitreo–retinal interface, or study parameters such as reflectivity, which, until a short time ago, were possible only with the A-scan method. All of the above supplies us with information that until now could only be obtained through the most attentive biomicroscopy, and could be performed only during surgery.

References

Avitabile, T., Guerriero, S., Scuderi, G.L., Veneziani, N. & Distante A. Recenti acquisizioni sulla diagnostica ecografica delle membrane vitreali. Roma: Atti LXIV Congr. Naz. S.O.I.: 307–311 (1984).

Avitabile, T., Cacciato, F. & Bonaccorsi, O. La diagnostica differenziale delle membrane vitreali up-date. Tavola rotonda su: 'Attualità in tema di strumentazione'. II Congr. Naz. S.I.E.O., Catania 1987. Cl. Ocul. e Pat. Ocul. 9(4): 249–252 (1988).

Avitabile, T., Cascone, G. & Reibaldi, A. Ecografia e P.V.R.: nostra esperienza. Comunicazione presentata al 4" Congresso S.I.E.O., Castrocaro Terme 25–26 novembre 1989. Atti su Clin. Ocul. in corso di stampa.

Avitabile, T. & Faro, S. Fisiopatologia e clinica dell'interfaccia vitreo-retinica. Diagnostica per immagini. Boll. Ocul. 69 (suppl) (1): 427–437 (1990)

Bisantis, C. Sistemazione nosografica della patologia e clinica dell'interfaccia vitreo-retinica. Boll. Ocul. 69 (suppl). (1): 403–417 (1990).

Cardia, L., Sborgia, C. & Miceli Ferrari, T. Pucker maculare. 'La chirurgia vitreo-retinica'. Simposio S.O.I. (1987).

Foos, R.Y. Vitreo-retinal juncture: topographical variation. Invest. Ophthalmol. 11: 801 (1972).

Foos, R.Y. Vitreo-retinal juncture: simple epiretinal membranes. Albrecht v. Graefes Arch. Ophthalmol. 189: 231 (1974).

Gallenga, R., Bellone, G., Gallenga, P.E. & Pasquarelli, A. Ultrasonografia clinica dell'occhio e dell'orbita. Malta: 53 Congr. S.O.I. (1971).

Gass, J.D. Stereoscopic atlas of macular diseases. St. Louis: Mosby (1970).

Hayashi, H., Oshima, K., Nakama, N. & Nishimura, Y. (1981) Ultrasonographic characteristics of operable massive periretinal proliferation. In Thijssen, J.M. and Verbeek, A.M. (eds.), Doc. Ophthalmol. Proc. Ser. 29: 5–12. The Hague: Dr. W. Junk (1981).

Hirokawa, H., Takahaswi, M. & Tremple, C. L. Vitreous changes in peripheral uveitis. Arch. Ophthalmol. 103: 1704–1707 (1985).

Hogan, M.J., Alverado, J.A. & Weddel, J.E. Histology of the human eye, 2nd ed., p. 687 Philadelphia: Saunders (1971).

Jaffe, N.S. Vitreous tractions at the posterior pole of the fundus due to alterations in the vitreous posterior. Trans. Am. Acad. Ophthalmol. Otolaryng. 71: 642 (1967).

Mazzeo, V., Ravalli, L., Falco, L. & Scorrano, R. Premature retinopathy on the B-scan. In Ossoinig, K.C. (ed.), Doc. Ophthalmol. Proc. Ser. 48: 431–435. The Hague: Dr. W. Junk (1987).

McLeod, D. & Restori, M. Rapid B-scanning in diabetic eye disease. In Thijssen, J.M. and Verbeek, A.M. (eds.), Doc. Ophthalmol. Proc. Ser. 29: 21–31. Dr. W. Junk (1981).

Ossoinig, K.C. Standardized echography: basic principles, clinical applications and results. Inter. Ophthalmol. Clin. 19: 127–285 (1979).

Pallares, M.R. Serrano de la Iglesia, J.M. Interfase vitreo-retiniana. Arch. Soc. Esp. Oftal. 54: 557–632 (1988).

Ponte, F. & Schifano, V. Fisiopatologia e clinica dell'interfaccia vitreo-retinica. Boll. Ocul. 69 (suppl). (1): 419–426 (1990).

Reibaldi, A., Avitabile, T., Guerriero, S., Distante, A. & Veneziani, N. Primi risultati sulla possibilità di differenziazione ecografica tissutale mediante falso colore. Clin. Ocul. e Pat. Ocul. 5(6): 9–12 (1984).

Reibaldi, A., Guerriero, S., Avitabile, T., Uva, M.G. Veneziani, N., Pasquariello, G. & Pasquali, F. Texture analisys di immagini ultrasonografiche in oculistica. Clin. Ocul. e Pat. Ocul. 8(1): 17–25 (1987).

Reibaldi, A., Avitabile, T., Guerriero, S. & Uva, M.G. Possibility of ocular tissue differentiation by means of false colour assisted echography. In Ossoinig, K.C. (ed.), Doc. Ophthalmol. Proc. Ser. 48: 201–206. The Hague: Dr. W. Junk (1987).

Reibaldi, A., Avitabile, T., Cascone, G. & Franco, L. Vitreous membranes up-date echographical diagnosis. In Sampaolesi, R. (ed.), Doc. Ophthalmol. Proc. Series 53: 225–231. Dordrecht: Kluwer Acad. Publ. (1990).

Reibaldi, A., Guerriero, S., Avitabile, T., Veneziani, N., Pasquariello, G. & Pasquali, F. Improvements on computer assisted echography. In Thijssen, J.M. (ed.), Doc. Ophthalmol. Proc. Ser. 51: 53–61. The Hague: Dr. W. Junk (1988).

Reibaldi, A. Patologia vitreo-retinica. Relazione al 'Seminario Internazionale di Ecografia B-scan del bulbo'. Ferrara 5 febbraio (1990).

Sahel, J. Pathologie de l'interface vitreo-retinienne. J. Fr. Ophthalmol. 8(4): 353–369. Paris: Masson (1985).

Schepens, C.L. & Neetens, A. The vitreous and vitreo-retinal interface. New York: Springer Verlag (1987).

Scullica, L. & Trombetta, C.J. Patologia dell'interfaccia retino-vitreale. Boll. Ocul. (69 (suppl) (1) (1990).

Spalton, D.J., Hitchings, R.A. & Hunter, P.A. Atlas of clinical ophthalmology (1984).

Steindler, P. Rilievi ecografici ed elettroretinografici nella fibroplasia retrolentale. In Orsoni, J.G. (ed.), Simposio Internazionale di Oftalmologia Pediatrica. A cura di M. Maione. pp. 96–101. Parma (1974).

Takeuchi, S. Ultrasonic diagnosis of massive periretinal proliferation. In Thijssen, J.M. and Verbeek, A.M. (eds.), Doc. Ophthalmol. Proc. Ser. 29: 13–20. The Hague: Dr. W. Junk (1981).

Tittarelli, R. & Mariotti, C. Il macular Pucker: recenti acquisizioni nella chirurgia vitreo-retinica. S. Margherita Ligure 26–28 Settembre (1988).

Address for correspondence: Institute of Ophthalmology, Catania University, Via Bambino 32, I-95124 Catania, Italy.

38. Tamponade substances in vitreo-retinal surgery
An echographical study

A. REIBALDI, T. AVITABILE, A. PAPPALARDO,
G. CASCONE, L. FRANCO & S. SILECI

(Catania, Italy)

Abstract. In this paper the authors describe the echographical aspects of internal tamponade substances (various kinds of gases and silicons). Because of its characteristics of innocuousness and repeatability, is possible to perform a correct echographic follow-up of surgical cases in which tamponade substances have been introduced, over all if we have cases with opaque media. The authors study various aspects of single tamponade substances that often are pathonomonic and their relations with the retina. They also point out how it is possible to perform computerized elaborations of images and correct measurements of dimensions and areas with new generation B-scan echography.

Introduction

In recent years, vitreo-retinal surgery witnessed a considerable expansion and an ever greater diffusion, in terms of both the availability of more sophisticated instruments, supplied by industries operating in the field of ophthalmic surgery and method perfecting. Among the latter, the use of internal tamponade substances has contributed enormously to the improvement of results, achieving a level of anatomic and functional success that at one time was not even dreamed of (Cibis et al. 1962, Cibis et al. 1963, Zivojnovic et al. 1982, Lincoff et al. 1983). Various internal tamponade substances are used in vitreo-retinal surgery, each with its own characteristics in terms of nature (liquid, gaseous, reabsorbable or not), and used according to the type of surgery planned. In this study the authors present their experience in monitoring eyes subjected to vitreo-retinal surgery using tamponade substances, and comment on the various echographic patterns for each type of substance used.

Echographic patterns

As stated above, the internal tamponade substances used in surgery are different in nature and in their echographic behavior once placed inside the bulb. This depends on their state (liquid or gaseous), density, specific gravity, and on the type of interface established between the vitreous and the substance itself, and thus supply typical echographic patterns that in most cases allow for an immediate identification of the substance.

P. Till (ed.), Ophthalmic Echography 13, pp. 345–350.
© 1993 *Kluwer Academic Publishers*.

Among internal tamponade substances we can distinguish those possessing physical and chemical features very similar to those of the vitreous body, such as saline solution and visco-elastic substances (healon and IAL) that are therefore more difficult to recognize echographically, while others, such as gaseous substances (air, SF6, C3F8) that are permeable to ultrasounds, give rise to typical artifacts that make them easy to recognize.

Even silicone oil presents a peculiar behavior from the point of view of ultrasound. This substance exists in two forms: the simple form (polydimethylsiloxane) and the fluorinated form (polymethyl 1-3,3,3,-trifluoropropylsiloxane). The fluorosilicone differs from normal silicone oil for the presence of a trifluoropropyl group in the place of a hydrogen radical. This group confers greater specific gravity to the molecule that goes from 0.972 g to 1.29 g, so that simple silicone oil is lighter than water by 3%, on which it will float in an aqueous environment (Petersen 1986). These physical characteristics enable us to differentiate their uses in vitreo-retinal surgery. The use of fluorosilicone oil is preferred when the retinal breaks are located in the lower sectors since they would not benefit from the use of normal silicone oil (Miyamoto et al. 1984, 1986).

Saline solution, hyaluronic acid

These agents are not very different from the vitreous body, for which they are excellent replacements. This is why their echographic patterns are quite similar to that of a normal bulb. Hyaluronic acid in the vitreous cavity creates a series of small interfaces presenting low reflectivity that can be detected echographically by means of an A-scan as very mobile echos with low reflectivity occupying the vitreous cavity; a B-scan shows minute vitreous corpuscles that are more visible through high reflectivity of the system.

Gaseous agents

The use of gaseous agents in vitreo-retinal surgery has been the subject of many previous papers, where we pointed out the importance of echographic monitoring in pneumatic retinopexy, as far as treatment of retinal detachments located in the upper sector are concerned, or in the treatment of retinal detachment with macular hole (Avitabile et al. 1988, 1990; Reibaldi et al. 1988).

Various gaseous agents can be used (air, SF6, C3F8), all of which, although presenting different types of behavior as far as expansion and persistence inside the bulb are concerned, present the same behavior from the echographic point of view.

It is well known that gaseous substances are impermeable to ultrasound, giving rise to the characteristic artifact that is easily recognizable with both A- and B-scans.

The gas bubble that the A-scan presents as a echo of extremely high reflectivity, at the vitreo–gas interface, causes shadowing of the posterior structures, and remains very high even lowering the sensitivity of the system. The B-scan is also typical; indeed, the upper portion of the tracing shows the presence of a large interface at the point of impact of ultrasound with the anterior surface of the bubble, while behind it, the profile of the posterior pole will be missing, once again because of acoustic shadowing; this way the profile of the sclera will present the characteristic lancing.

Our previous studies proved how, from echographically measurable parameters, thanks to the use of computerized equipment (surface of the largest bubble section, antero-posterior diameter of the bulb), it is possible to calculate the volume of the bubble, and hence to monitor its expansion over time.

Silicone oil

Silicone oil presents peculiar features from the point of view of ultrasound, due to the fact that it is very dense, slowing the spread of the ultrasound considerably, as shown by various authors (Poujol et al. 1978; Verbeek et al. 1981; Gallenga et al. 1985; Shugar et al. 1986). Indeed, the speed of ultrasound in silicone oil is approximately 980 m/sec, while in the vitreous it is 1532 m/sec. Hence the tracing of an eye full of silicone oil will be one-third longer than normal.

The echographic pattern of a bulb full of silicone oil may vary, depending on the amount of oil and the way in which it was placed inside the vitreous cavity. If there is just one huge bubble occupying the entire vitreous cavity, we will have a considerably longer echographic pattern both with A- and B-scans, with the loss of the signs concerning the orbit structures. With an A-scan, after an echo of maximum reflectivity there will be a return to the baseline at zero reflectivity, following by a scleral echo with reflectivity reduced to approx 30 dB (Clemens et al. 1984). With a B-scan, aside from the lengthening of the dimensions of the bulb, we will have flattening of the posterior profile.

On the other hand, when the bubble of silicone oil does not take up the entire vitreous cavity, there will be a part of vitreous body between its surface and the surface of the retina. Hence there will be a second interface that with either A- or B-scan could simulate retinal detachment. However there are criteria such as the absence of insertion to the optic nerve head or at other points on the eye surface, and especially the much larger size of the bulb with respect to normal, that would allow us to rule out retinal detachment.

Finally, under some conditions the interpretation of the echographic pattern of an eye treated with silicone oil is more difficult. This happens when the bubble breaks up during insertion into the bulb, giving rise to a number of interfaces that generate a series of artifacts occupying the entire vitreous cavity. Also when confronting eyes presenting considerable bulb profile changes for the apposition of plumb and/or scleral encirclement, aside from the presence of silicone oil. The echographic pattern of an eye containing fluorosilicone oil is completely different from one containing a series of echos with maximal reflectivity followed by a return to the baseline.

With a B-scan instead there was only one initial signal that decayed almost immediately behind the emission signal of the probe and no sign of bulbar structures could be seen. To rule out the possibility of this being a technical artifact we performed a biometric series using different types of equipment (Ophthascan's Biophysic Medical and Sonomed A-2000 B-3000) on a plexi-glass phantoma we filled with BSS, normal silicone oil (1000 cs) and then with fluorosilicone oil (1000 cs). In the case of BSS, we recorded a measurement with both instruments of 23.8 mm; using normal silicone oil we measured a typical lengthening of the pattern of 31.9 mm. Finally, we filled the phantoma with fluorosilicone oil and in this case we were not able to perform a biometric reading while we only measured a series of initial echos with high reflectivity, followed by a return to the baseline.

We then applied a similar procedure to a pig's eye, and obtained a normal pattern. Then we performed a vitrectomy with total removal of the vitreous body, replacing it with normal silicone oil. In this case, as expected, we noticed a considerable lengthening of the echographic pattern with a flattening of the profile of the posterior pole. Finally, when we replaced the normal silicone oil with the fluorosilicone oil we found a peculiar pattern, in every respect similar to that obtained in the case of operated eyes with fluorosilicone, with a total absence of echographic signs pertaining to the bulb.

Conclusions

In recent years, vitreo-retinal surgery has received a considerable impulse thanks to the setting up of new methods that also contemplate the use of tamponade substances. However, these agents, although contributing on one hand to the positive outcome of surgery, on the other, as can be seen in the case of gases for example, can sometimes make it difficult to examine the fundus with an ophthalmoscope, immediately after surgery or even later, due to the appearance of opaqueness in the optical media. This is verified by the appearance of cataracts in eyes with silicone oil. In all of these cases, and in others caused by complications such as vitreous hemorrhage, or in cases of insufficient dilation of the pupil, we could resort to ultrasonography. By supplying typical echographic patterns for the various types of agents used, ultrasonography allowed us to accurately monitor the situation even when, because of these special conditions, we could not adequately rely on more traditional methods. We wish to point out once again that ultrasonography performed using the most modern computerized devices allows us to implement test studies such as the study of bulbar areas and volumes after injection of special types of tamponade substances.

In conclusion, we feel it is important to highlight, as confirmed by our test studies, the considerable handicap of using fluorosilicone oil for echographic monitoring. The peculiar echographic behavior of this substance absolutely prevents one from acquiring information about the conditions of the bulb and the retina in particular. This happens in those cases when it is impossible to correctly explore the fundus using an ophthalmosope, because of peculiar situations that may occur (cataract).

References

Avitabile, T., Pappalardo, A. & Reibaldi, A. Il ruolo dell'ecografia nella retinopessia pneumatica. Atti II Cong. Naz. S.I.E.O., Catania 1987, In Clinica Oculistica e Patologia Oculare 4: 276–278 (1988).

Avitabile, T., Pappalardo, A. & Reibaldi, A. I mezzi tamponanti interni: Studio ecografico. Comunicaz. IV Congr. Naz. S.I.E.O. Castrocaro Terme 24–26 Novembre (1990).

Cibis, P., Becker, B., Okun, E. & Canaan, S. The use of liquid silicone in retinal detachment surgery. Arch. Ophthalmol. 68: 590–599 (1962).

Cibis, P. Vitreous transfer and silicone injections. In Symposium: Present status of retinal detachment surgery. Trans. Am. Acad. Ophth. and Otol. Oct. 20–25: 983–997 (1963).

Clemens, S., Kroll, P. & Rochels, R. Ultrasonic findings after treatment of retinal detachment by intravitreal silicone instillation. Am. J. Ophthalmol. 98: 369–373 (1984).

Gallenga, P.E. & Del Duca, M. Silicon oil and echography. In Advanced Course on Vitreo-Retinal Surgery. Rome (1985).

Lincoff, H., Coleman, J., Kreissig, I., Richard, G., Chang, S. & Wilcox, L.M. The perfluorocarbon gases in the treatment of retinal detachment. Ophthalmology 90(5): 548–551 (1983).

Miyamoto, K., Refojo, M.F., Tolentino, F.I., Fournier, G.A. & Albert, D.M. Perfluorather liquid as a long-term vitreous substitute. An experimental study. Retina 4: 264–268 (1984).

Miyamoto, K., Refojo, M.F., Tolentino, F.I., Fournier, G.A. & Albert, D.M. Fluorinated oils as experimental vitreous substitutes. Arch. Ophthalmol. 104: 1053–1056 (1986).

Petersen, J., Ritzau-Tondrow, U. & Vogel, M. Fluor-Silikonöl schwerer als Wasser: ein neues Hilfsmittel der vitreo-retinalen Chirurgie. Klin. Mbl. Augenheilk. 189: 228–232 (1986).

Poujol, J., Haut, J. & Fleury, P. Corrections a apporter dans l'examen échographique des yeux remplis de silicone liquide. Bull. Soc. Ophtalmol. Fr. 78: 367–369 (1978).

Reibaldi, A., Avitabile, T., Pappalardo, A., Franco, L. Gas retinal detachment treatment and echography. In Sampaolesi, R. (ed.), Ultrasonography in ophtalmology-12. Doc. Ophthalmol. Proc. Ser. 53: 249–255. Dordrecht: Kluwer Acad. Publ. (1988).

Shugar, J.K., De Juan, E., McCuen, B.W., Tiedeman, J., Landers, M.R. & Machemer, R. Ultrasonic examination of the silicone-filled eye: Theoretical and practical considrations. Graefe's Arch. Clin. Exp. Ophthalmol. 224: 361–367 (1986).

Tamburelli, C., Focosi, F., Oliva, G., Buratto, E. & Zagami, A. Tecniche ecografiche di posizionamento del tamponamento interno mediante gas, nel trattamento del distacco di retina con pneumoretinipessia. Atti III Congr. Naz. S.I.E.O. Napoli 13 Novembre 1988 in Clinica Oculistica e Patologia oculare. X (5) (1989).

Verbeek, A.M., Bayer, A.L. & Thijssen, J.M. Echographic diagnosis after intraocular silicone oil injection. In Thijssen, J.M. & Verbeek, A.M. (eds.), Doc. Ophthalmol. Proc. Ser. 29: 59–66. The Hague: Dr. W. Junk (1981).

Zivojnovic, R., Mertens, D.A.E. & Peperkamp, E. Das flüssige Silikon in der Amotiochirurgie (II) Bericht über 280 Fälle-weitere Entwicklung der Technick, Klin. Mbl. Augenheilk. 181: 444 (1982).

Address for correpondence: Institute of Ophthalmology, University of Catania, Via Bambino 32, I-95124 Catania, Italy.

39. Retinoschisis
Our Echographic Experience

L. KOLOZSVÁRI

(Debrecen, Hungary)

Retinoschisis gives a relatively little part of the membranous echo sources. It is often misdiagnosed echographically because echographic findings are similar to those in partial, circumscribed retinal or vitreous detachment.

Using A-method this alteration presents as a membrane echo of high reflectivity separated from the spikes of the posterior wall by a silent space representing intraretinal fluid.

Ossoinig [5] reported that the echo of schisis is thinner than that of detachment. Hillman & Ridgway [4] made quantitative measurements with the famous Kretz 7200 MA and showed a statistically significant difference between the acoustic reflectivities of the split retina in retinoschisis and a detached retina.

Applying the B-mode, many authors [1–3] emphasize that the elevation of the inner layer of the retina is cyst-like, dome-shaped in retinoschisis, and often bilateral. Its presence may be suspected especially when it is located infratemporally. The aftermovement of a separated retina is moderate in comparison with that of a detached one. All these are well known signs with which retinoschisis can be identified.

We have also seen such cases, but not all of them were so typical. Since 1986 we have examined echographically more than 2000 patients in our clinic using a Sonometrics Ocuscan DBR 400 and more recently a Cooper Vision Digital B IV. We found retinoschisis in 24 eyes of 22 patients (7 females, 15 males), comprising 20 unilateral and two bilateral cases. In each case diagnosis was confirmed by indirect ophthalmoscopy, by three-mirror contact lens examination, and by examination of visual fields. Even if a minimum progression of the schisis occured we applied laser coagulation.

The ages of our patients are shown in Table 1. Classifying the refraction of our patients (Table 2), six of them were emmetropic, other six were hypermetropic, and ten patients were myopic. In five of the 20 unilateral cases the fellow eyes were involved. These five patients were highly myopic and the fellow eyes had been operated on for retinal detachment with a successful outcome in four out of five eyes.

In one of our bilateral cases the splitting of the retina reached the macula causing 0.08 visual acuity. After scleral buckling with an encircling element and releasing the intraretinal fluid the retina reattached and the visual acuity was 0.9.

P. Till (ed.), Ophthalmic Echography 13, pp. 351–354.

Table 1. The age distribution of our patients

Age	No. of patients
3	1
11–20	4
21–30	7
31–50	4
51	6
Total	22

Table 2. Refraction

Diopters	No. of patients
0.0	6
−6.5−−14.0	10 (11 eyes)
+1.5−+4.0	6 (7 eyes)
Total	22 (24 eyes)

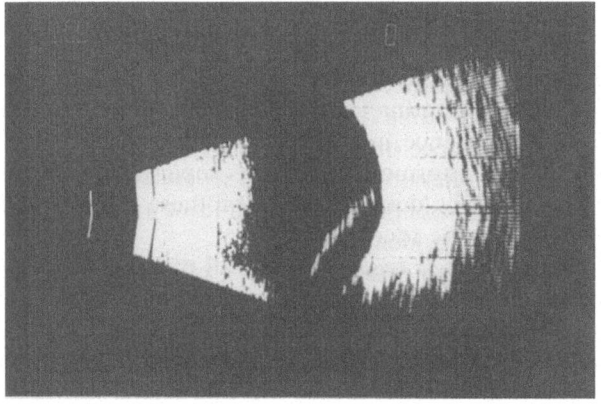

Fig. 1. Retinoschisis: dome-shaped.

The location of the elevated and separated retina was infratemporal in 22 eyes, but in seven of them the relatively large elevations extended even on the nasal part of the inferior retina. The alteration was supratemporal in one eye, and in another one it was nasal.

The cases with dome-shaped membranes (Fig. 1) were surprisingly few, that is in six eyes of five patients. In the other cases (13 eyes) the surface of the schisis looked chordlike (Fig. 2) on the screen, whereas in five eyes it appeared as a concave line (Fig. 3) toward the vitreous cavity.

The great number of our unilateral cases can be explained partly by the

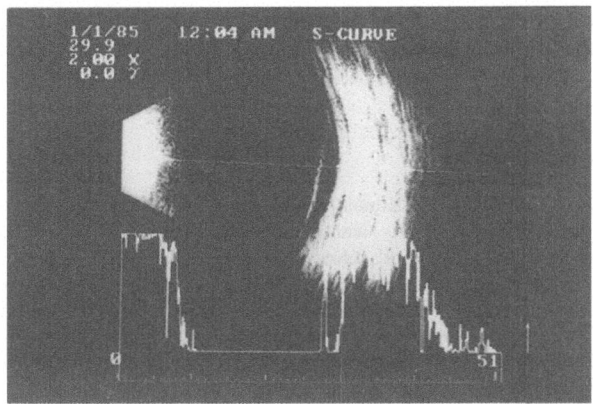

Fig. 2. Retinoschisis: chord-like.

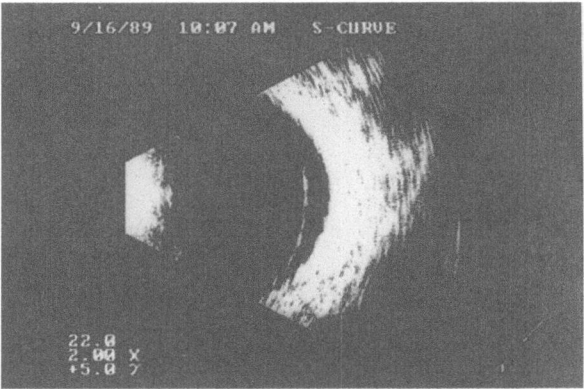

Fig. 3. Retinoschisis: concave.

few previous operations on the fellow eyes, as mentioned above, and partly by the relatively young age of our patients. In a recent case the alteration became bilateral, and that has led us to think that during regular follow-ups an involvement of the fellow eye is likely to be diagnosed.

It is significant that the number of highly myopic eyes is large. In our clinic we try to examine each highly myopic patient ultrasonically. We have found the myopic cases of this study among about 450 myopic patients we examined echographically. Summarizing our experience we can say that dome-shaped, more often chord-like, sometime, concave membranes with moderate aftermovement, located infratemporally, occasionally extending over the middle line, are very likely to be retinoschisis. These symptoms can often be found in relatively young, highly myopic patients.

The main task of echography is to follow such cases because the presence

354

and progression of schisis can be demonstrated very well ultrasonically, even compared with other optical methods.

References

1. Coleman, D.J. & Smith, M.E. Retinal and choroidal detachments. Handbook of clinical ultrasound. In de Vlieger, Holmes, Kazner, Kossoff, Kratochvil, Kraus and Poujol (eds.), Strandness, pp. 857–862. New York: John Wiley and Sons (1978).
2. Fisher, Y.L. Contact B-scan ultrasonography: A practical approach. In Dallow, R.L. (ed.), Ophthalmic Ultrasonography: Comparitive Techniques. International Ophthalmology Clinics, pp. 103–126. Boston: Little, Brown and Company (1979).
3. Guthoff, R. Ultraschall in der ophthalmologischen Ultraschalldiagnostik. Stuttgart: Ferdinand Enke Verlag (1988).
4. Hillman, S.H. & Ridgway, A.E. Retinoschisis and retinal detachment. An ultrasonic comparison. Ultrasonography in ophthalmology. Bibl. Ophthal. 83: 63–67 (1975).
5. Ossoinig, K. Ultrasonic diagnosis on the eye: an aid for the clinic. Symp. pp. 116–133. Münster: Ultrasonics in Ophthalmology (1967).

Address for correspondence: Department of Ophthalmology, University School of Medicine, Nagyerdei Krt. 98, H 4012 Debrecen, Hungary.

40. Further indications for the evaluation of the prescleral layer

N. ROSA & G. CENNAMO
(Naples, Italy)

Abstract. The evaluation of the so-called 'prescleral layer' has been introduced by K.C. Ossoinig to provide valuable information in making differential diagnoses between dense vitreous membranes and retinal detachment when the detached membranous surface gives borderline delta dB values. The authors have tried to establish whether this kind of examination can be helpful in making differential diagnoses in cases of retinoschisis.

Introduction

Quantitative A-scan echography II was introduced by K.C. Ossoinig in the early 1970s to help in making differential diagnoses between retinal detachments and dense vitreous membranes [3–4]. More recently, Ossoinig observed that if there is a retinal detachment, the first spike coming from the ocular wall is the surface of the pigmented epithelium, but if the retina is attached, the first spike will be the surface of the retina. He called these interfaces the 'prescleral layer' (PSL). He proposed to quantify not only the detached membranous surface but also the reflectivity of the PSL behind the detached membrane [5–6]. The obtained results indicated that the attached retina has a higher reflectivity than pigmented epithelium (Table 1).

On this basis we attempted to verify whether we could make differential diagnoses between retinal detachment and retinoschisis (Figs. 1 and 2) with this technique because it is not always possible to make a differential diagnosis with ophthalmoscopy or slit-lamp fundus examination or other echographic techniques [2].

Material and methods

By means of standardized A-scan echography we performed quantitative II technique in seven patients with retinoschisis, diagnosed with slit-lamp fundus examination, that showed no change in five years of follow-up. For this purpose we used a Kretz 7200 MA and measured the reflectivity of the retinoschisis, the attached retina, the PSL, and we compared these values with those of the sclera (delta dB) behind the retinoschisis (Fig. 3).

P. Till (ed.), Ophthalmic Echography 13, pp. 355–359.

356

Table 1.

PSL = retina	PSL = pigmented epithelium
9–12 delta dB	14–16 delta dB

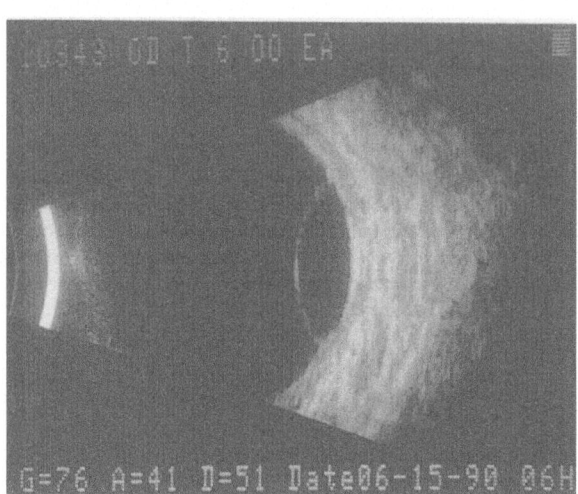

Fig. 1. B-scan showing a bullous retinoschisis.

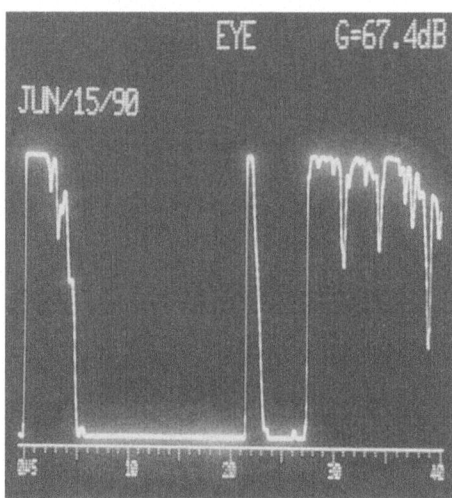

Fig. 2. A-scan of the same case of Fig. 1, showing a 100% sharply rising high spike from the inner layer of the retinoschisis.

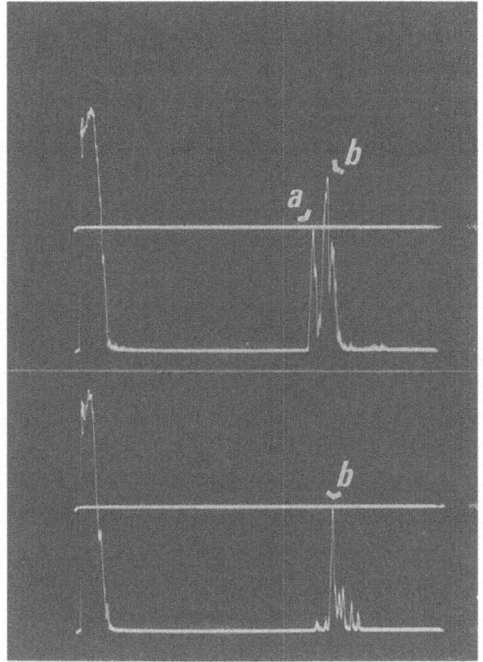

Fig. 3. The measures are taken by adjusting system sensitivity, in the way that the maximum spike from the PSL (a) and the maximum scleral spike (b) is shown by the height defined by the horizontal marker line.

Results

Our results (Table 2) show that the prescleral layer behind the retinoschisis has the same delta dB value as that of the normal retina. When we quantify the retinoschisis we find a wider range. In some cases we obtain the same values for retinal detachment, and borderline values in other cases. The attached retina presents values of delta dB ranging from 9 to 12.

Table 2.

Patients	1	2	3	4	5	6	7
Retinoschisis	16	20	14	14	13	15	16
Retina	11	9	10	9	10	11	12
PSL	12	12	10	12	11	9	12

Discussion

Several criteria can be used to make a differential diagnosis between retinal detachment and retinoschisis such as: ophthalmoscopic aspect, visual field

358

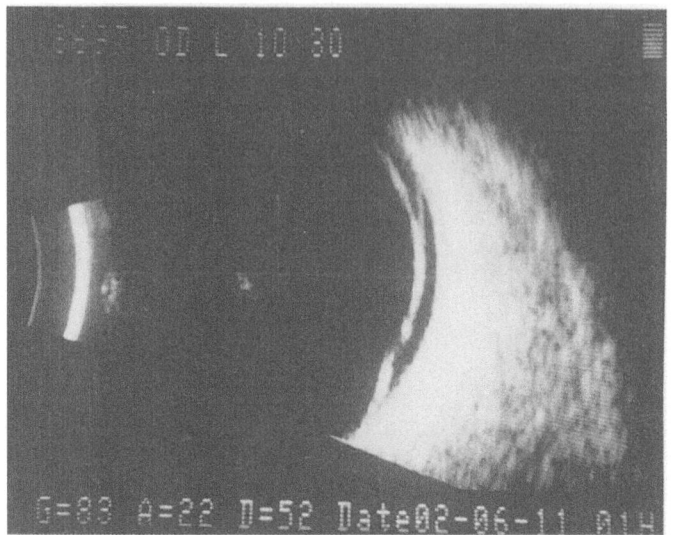

Fig. 4. B-scan showing a retinoschisis complicated by a retinal detachment.

with an absolute scotoma in case of retinoschisis, and a relative scotoma in the case of retinal detachment. Laser gives a white area in case of retinoschisis; moreover when we indent the schisis, it becomes whitish. Nevertheless, making differential diagnoses between retinal detachment and retinoschisis can sometimes be difficult. In the case of retinoschisis the rupture of the external layers forms a connection between the schisis cavity and subretinal space, and predisposes a retinal detachment (Fig. 4). In this case, a differential diagnosis is even more difficult. Sometimes the slit-lamp examination can show a yellow line that identifies the rim of the break at the external layer.

Senile retinoschisis has an incidence in the normal population of 7% after 40 years of age. In a study of 218 eyes with senile retinoschisis [1], Byer has described 25 eyes with retinoschisis and a break in the external layer, in which 14 cases (56%) underwent a retinal detachment. Byer also pointed out that non-treated patients with retinoschisis without retinal detachment have a lower probability of maculopathy with visual decrease in comparison with patients treated with surgical or parasurgical procedures. On the other hand, the percentage of retinal detachment in patients with retinoschisis is only 0.05; this means that among 2000 patients with retinoschisis, only one will have a retinal detachment. For this reason it is important to have an additional method that can add information in the differential diagnosis between retinoschisis and retinal detachment and that can distinguish a retinoschisis from a retinoschisis complicated by a retinal detachment.

Quantitative echography II of the prescleral layer gives different values in the case of retinal detachment or attached retina mainly because the inner retinal layer is smooth while the pigmented epithelium is rough. For this reason the retinal surface behaves as a mirror so that the maximum energy returns to the probe. In the case of pigmented epithelium, because the surface is rough, less energy returns to the probe and will be less reflective than the retina. With retinoschisis, our results indicate that in some cases it has the same reflectivity as the detached retina, but in other cases it has higher delta dB values. The latter results could be related to the convexity of the bollous retinoschisis surface. The evaluation of the reflectivity of the prescleral layer in cases of retinoschisis gives similar values to those obtained from the attached retina, may be because in retinoschisis the separation is at the level of external plexiform layer or fiber layer that is smoother than the layer of the pigmented epithelium.

References

1. Byer, N.E. Longterm natural history study of senile retinoschisis with implications for management. Ophthalmology 93: 1127–1137 (1986).
2. Gallenga, R., Bellone, B., Gallenga, P.E. & Pasquarelli, A. Ultrasonografia Clinica dell'Occhio e dell'Orbita. Malta: LIII Congresso SOI (1971).
3. Ossoinig, K.C. Standardized echography: basic principles, clinical applications and results. Int. Ophth. Clin. 19: 127 (1979).
4. Ossoinig, K.C. Standardized echography of the eye, orbit and periorbital region. Erd ed. Goodfellow Company Inc. (1985).
5. Ossoinig, K.C., Islas, G., Tamayo, G.E. & Tamburelli, C. Detached retina vs. dense fibrovascular membrane: standardized A scan and B scan criteria. In Ossoinig, K.C. (ed.), Ophthalmic Echography. Doc. Ophthalmol. Proc. Ser. 48. Dordrecht/Boston/Lancaster: Martinus Nijhoff/Dr. W. Junk (1987).
6. Rosa, N. & Cennamo, G. Studio Ecografico Della Membrana Pre Sclerale. Proc. IV SIEO Congress, in Clin. Ocul. e Pat. Ocul. XI(5) (1990).

Address for correspondence: Eye Department, II School of Medicine, University of Naples, Via S. Pansini 5, I-80131 Naples, Italy.

41. Recognition of retinal pigmentepithelium

S. CLEMENS & H. BUSSE

(*Münster, Germany*)

Abstract. The way of depicting the retinal pigmentepithelium by a commercial equipment is described with some characteristics. This further criterion of the situation of the retina turned out to be useful in the everyday diagnosis of retinal detachment. The possibility of measuring the thickness of retina and choroid separately makes it easier to recognize the choroidal effusion or the course of an endophthalmitis.

Introduction

In ultrasonographic diagnosis of retinal detachment the examiner orientates himself in the acoustic properties of the detached membrane. The main criteria for differentiation between retinal and vitreous detachment are the difference in reflectivity of the membrane related to the sclera; the shape of detached membrane; the relation to optical nerve and ora serrata; the sinusoidal aftermovements depicting of fine wrinkling of the retinal surface. In cases of proliferative diabetic retinopathy or after perforating injury, nevertheless about 20% of diagnoses are erroneous.

Jahlk (1983) pointed out the necessity for differentiated imaging of retina and choroid for routine purposes. We looked then for a constant reflecting structure at the borderline between retina and choroid.

Method

The examinations were done with a Tri-scan/Biophysic Medical with B- and AB-scan. We examined the axial resolution and found it to be 0.1 mm with the 6 dB criterion from Haigis and Buschmann (1980). In a fathom phantom especially for this purpose an axial resolution of 0.2 mm and better could be found. In this model several single fathoms are oriented parallel to each other with one double fathom. Depending on the angle of impact to the direction of the fathom the reflexes of surfaces has a different distance (Figs. 1 and 2). The axial resolution can be measured quite easily through the angle beta (β) between the plane of fathoms and the direction of the probe by the formula $b = a \times \cos \beta$, where b = the distance between surface echoes, a =

P. Till (*ed.*), *Ophthalmic Echography 13*, pp. 361–368.

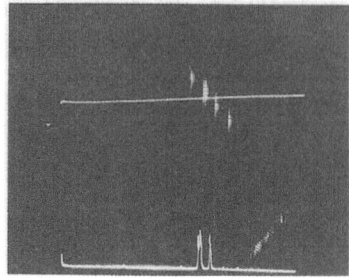

Fig. 1. Measurement of axial resolution with a wire model. AB-scan through a double wire with two separate echoes.

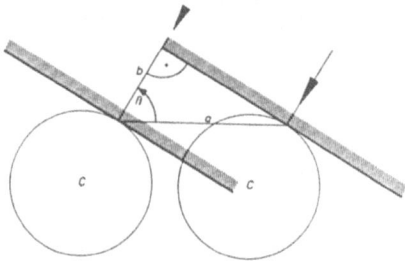

Fig. 2. Measurement of axial resolution. a = distance between impact of ultrasound; b = distance between echoes; c = wire. $\angle \beta$ = angle between wires and ultrasound.

the distance between points of impact, and β = the angle between the direction of fathoms and the direction of the probe.

The influence of the cornea, lens and pars plicata of the ciliary body turned out to hinder an exact measurement.

Results

We found a second curvilinear echo between the inner surface of the retina and the scleral echo. It could be depicted in all clinical examinations except cases of higher myopia and retinopathia pigmentosa. One prerequisite for depicting this second curvilinear echo is the right angle impact of the ultrasonic beam to the surfaces.

A maximum inclination of 10° is allowed; otherwise no second membrane-like echo could be obtained. When the ultrasound beam is directed through the cornea, lens or pars plicata the second membrane echo could not be found. Also in direction of examination directly through the sclera the shadowing is too strong for depicting the second echo. As a result, a zone between 20° and 90° distance from the posterior pole can be used for diag-

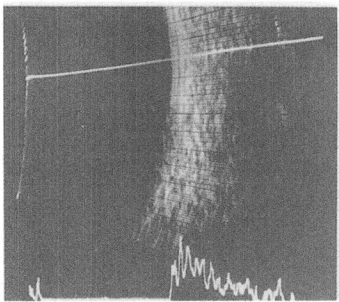

Fig. 3. Normal situation of the rear wall of the eye with three curvilinear echos, retina, pigmentepithelium and sclera.

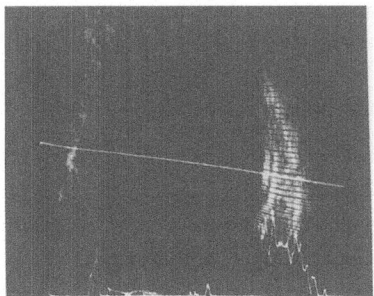

Fig. 4. Investigation of **vitreous bleeding, attached retina, pigmentepithelium** is visible as a second curvilinear echo with **lower reflectivity (diabetes).**

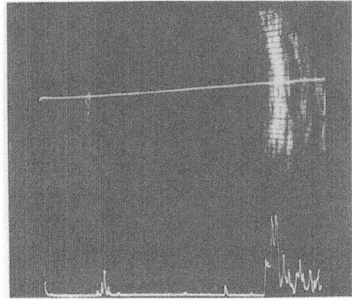

Fig. 5. **Four days after cataract surgery, thickening of choroid.**

nosis. In cases of concave surfaces like the normal posterior wall of the eye a wider field can be examined.

The second membrane-like echo between retina and sclera has about the same reflectivity in cases of attached retina as the retina itself, varying up to ±5 dB. Under normal circumstances the thickness of retina was 0.2 mm and

364

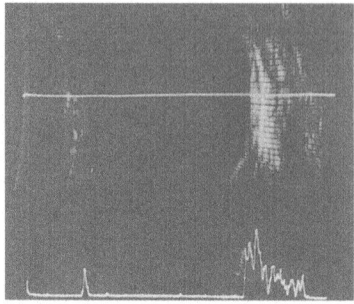

Fig. 6. Retinal and choroidal thickening after contusio bulbi.

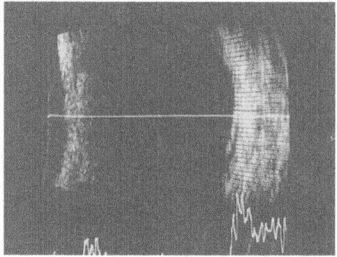

Fig. 7. Border of retinal detachment, no step in pigmentepithelium.

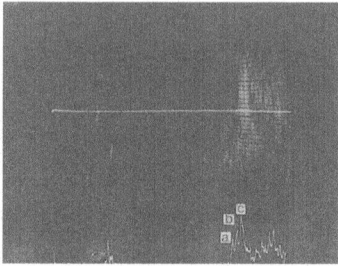

Fig. 8. Border of retinal detachment. a = retina; b = pigmentepithelium; c = sclera.

0.25 mm of the choroid. Measurements were taken 30° away from the posterior pole. To be sure not to depict choroidal vessels as a second membrane-like echo, a sideways movement of the probe for about 3° to 5° can be undertaken. The membrane-like second echo will be left, not so the choroidal vessels.

The differences in propagation of ultrasound in the different tissues at the posterior wall of the eye were not taken into account since they vary by not

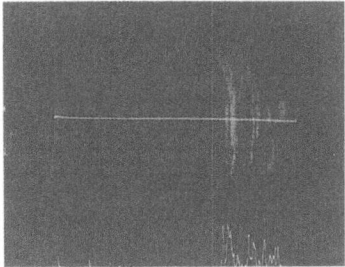

Fig. 9. Retinopathia pigmentosa without separation of retina and pigmentepithelium after scarring.

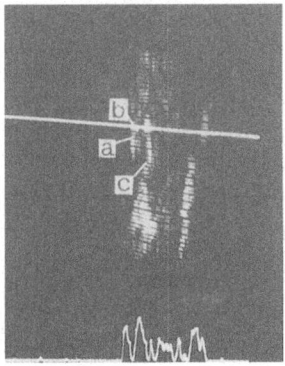

Fig. 10. Retinopathia diabetica proliferans after laser treatment. a = retina; b = pigmentepithelium; c = sclera. The AB-vector is in a gap of the pigmentepithelium where the laser scar is. The reflectivity of the pigmentepithelium is lower than that of the retina, and the choroid is swollen.

more than 5% (Coleman & Lizzi 1979). The second curvilinear echo represents the pigmentepithelium, because at the borders of retinal detachment, a stepless connection between attached and detached situation is visible.

In laser scars where only Bruch's membrane is left, the pigmentepithelium is scarred. In these cases we found a gap in the second curvilinear echo as a sign for the defect of pigment epithelium. The lateral resolution achieved with our equipment in reduced sensitivity was 1 mm. In higher reflectivity it is reduced to 3 or 4 mm. Since the examined structures are all in one plane the display is dependent only on the axial resolution.

Case reports

In Fig. 3 the rear wall of the normal eye is visible, with three curvilinear membranes: the retina (1) pigmentepithelium (2), sclera (3), and the tenon is also visible. The reflectivity of the pigmentepithelium is about 2 dB higher than that of the retinal surface.

In Fig. 4 an ultrasonic examination was performed because of vitreous bleeding. The retina is flat; the retina is depicted as a membrane-like echo, so the pigmentepithelium and the sclera with anterior and posterior surface. In this case the pigmentepithelium has a lower reflectivity in attached situations than the retina. We found a lower reflectivity of the pigment epithelium in all cases of proliferative diabetic retinopathy.

Fig. 5 presents the situation four days after cataract surgery with intraocular lens implantation. As a result of the wide opening of the eye, a choroidal thickening can still be observed which is more than twice as thick as the retina, which is not thickened. In all cases of opening of the eye, such as cataract or glaucoma surgery or vitrectomy or perforating injury, a choroidal thickening could be noticed which lasted for up to one week.

In Fig. 6 the situation five days after contusio bulbi is demonstrated with B- and AB-scans. The retina is swollen somewhat more than the choroid.

In Fig. 7 the border of a rhegmatogenous retinal detachment is depicted with an elevated retina in the lower part. The pigmentepithelium and the sclera are separately visible.

In Fig. 8 the border of a retinal detachment with retina (a), pigmentepithelium (b), and sclera (c). In the two cases of border of retinal detachment there is no step between detached and attached retina in the pigmentepithelium.

In Fig. 9 the scarred area of a retinopathia pigmentosa is depicted. It is not possible to distinguish between the retina and the pigmentepithelium separately.

In Fig. 10 the AB-vector is put through a laser scar of 1 mm (a = retina; b = defect in pigmentepithelium; c = sclera). A light thickening of the choroid compared to the normal thickness of the retina can be found. The reflectivity of the pigmentepithelium is in this case lower than that of the retina.

Discussion

In a B-scan a separated visualisation of the retina and choroid was only possible in routine echography in cases of retinal detachment (Rochels & Hackelbusch 1983; Cappaert et al. 1977). It was thought to be impossible to see the retina and choroid separately in cases of attached retina (Coleman & Lizzi 1979). The thickening of choroid and retina together was demonstrated by Ossoinig using a B-scan and was measured in an A-scan with reduced sensitivity (Ossoinig 1979). Separate imaging of retina and choroid is only possible with spectral analysis and negative filtering and RF-scanning. In spectral analysis a maximum axial resolution of 20 μm can be reached. A constant borderline echo which cannot be mismatched with choroidal vessels could not yet be found (Coleman & Lizzi 1979). Using this method the separate peaks have not yet been successfully analysed (Tane et al. 1988). Also, Sugata et al. have pointed out (1988) that an exact measurement of retina and choroid separately cannot be performed even in cases where the movements of the choroidal vessels are taken into account.

Up to now a thickened choroid was assumed if a thickened of retina and choroid was found together, since in histological examinations of cases with choroidal detachment the retina was not thickened (Wing et al. 1982).

The choroidal thickening was supposed when the distance between initial peak of retina and sclera in A-scan was 1 mm or more, or when in B-scan a double line was found (Jahlk et al. 1983) In cases of a beginning ophthalmitis the retina thickens first and then the choroid (Jahlk et al. 1983). The visualisation of the pigmentepithelium helps in the diagnosis of retinal detachment.

The negative influence of exact imaging by the lens was demonstrated by Baum (1965). A quite similar disturbance was found in the directic of ultrasound through pars plicata of the ciliary body and even through the cornea. In order not to depict a choroidal vessel as second curvilinear echo, a sidewards movement of the probe between 2° and 4° is necessary. The pigmentepithelium will be constant. No investigations were undertaken in experience to separate the several layers of the rear wall of the eye, because this would lead to other reflectivities.

Guthoff et al. (1988) have described a separated visualisation of the retina and choroid in one-third of their cases of measurement of the total volume of coates of the eye.

References

1. Baum, G. A discussion of acoustic artefacts in ophthalmic ultrasonography. Am. J. Ophthalmol. 60: 493–498 (1965).
2. Buschmann, W. & Haigis, W. Standards in ophthalmic ultrasonography. In Thijssen, J.M. et al. (eds.), Ultrasonography in Ophthalmology-11. Doc. Ophthalmol. Proc. Ser. 51. Dordrecht: Kluwer (1988).
3. Cappaert, M.D., Purnell, W.W. & Frank, K.E. Use of B-scan ultrasound in the diagnosis of benign choroidal folds. Am. J. Ophthalmol. 84: 375–379 (1977).
4. Coleman, J. D. & Lizzi, F.L. In vitro choroidal thickness measurement. Am. J. Ophthalmol. 88: 369–375.
5. Guthoff, R., Berger, R.W. & Draeger, J. Ultrasonographic measurement of the posterior coats of the eye and their relation to axial length. In Thijssen, J.M. et al. (ed.), Ultrasonography in Ophthalmology-11. Doc. Ophthalmol. Proc. Ser. 51: 327–329. Dordrecht: Kluwer (1988).
6. Haigis, W. & Buschmann, W. Die Bedeutung von Testreflektoren zur schnellen klinischen Überprüfung von Geräten für die ophthalmologische Ultraschalldiagnostik. In Biomed. Technik, Bd. 25. Berlin: Schiele Schön (1980).
7. Jahlk, A.E., Avila, M.P., Trempe, C.L. & Schepens, C.L. Diffuse choroidal thickening detected by ultrasonography in various ocular diseases. Retina 3(4): 277–283 (1983).
8. Ossoinig, K.C. Standardized echography: Basic Principles, Clinical applications and Results. In Dallow, R.D. (ed.), Ophthalmic Ultrasonography: Comparative Techniques, pp. 127–210. Boston: Little, Brown and Co. (1979).
9. Purnell, E.W. Ultrasonic biometry of the posterior ocular coats. Trans. Am. Ophthalmol. Soc. 78: 1027–1078 (1980).
10. Rochels, R. & Hackelbusch R. Echographische Befunde bei Aderhautabhebung. Klin. Mbl. Augenheilk. 182: 54–56 (1983).

11. Sugata, Y., Yamamoto, Y., Yano, M., Shibuya N. & Ito, K. Ultrasonic observations of ocular walls. In Thijssen, J.M. et al. (ed.), Ultrasonography in Ophthalmology-12. Doc. Ophthalmol. Proc. Ser. 51: 63–71. Dordrecht: Kluwer (1988).
12. Tane, S., Horikosho, J. Hargaya, A. & Mikaye, M. In vivo measurement of the thickness of the retino-choroidal layers by RF-signal analysis. In Thijssen, J.M. (ed.), Ultrasonography in Ophthalmology-12. Doc Ophthalmol. Proc. Ser. 51: 91–94. Dordrecht: Kluwer (1988).
13. Wing, G.L., Schepens, C.L., Trempe, C.L. & Weiter, J.J. Serious choroidal detachment and the thickened choroid sign detected by ultrasonography. Am. J. Ophthalmol. 94: 399–455 (1982).

Address for correspondence: University Eye Hospital, Domagkstrasse 15, W-4400 Münster, Germany

42. Effect of intraocular pressure on ocular wall volume

J. NÉMETH

(*Budapest, Hungary*)

Introduction

As concerns the diffuse-type alterations in the thickness and the volume of the ocular wall, the following facts are known from the literature: (1) There is a close inverse correlation between the ocular coat thickness and the axial length of the eye in healthy eyes with different refractive errors, and thus the volume of the ocular wall is constant [1, 2]; (2) In patients with glaucoma, the thickness of the ocular coats [9] and the volume of the coats [4, 6] are different from the normal data. The higher the intraocular pressure, the thinner is the ocular wall and the smaller its volume [4, 6, 8]; (3) In certain other eye diseases, diffuse alteration of the ocular wall can be detected. In cases involving ocular hypotony (uveitis, phthisis bulbi, after intraocular surgery or injury) and in patients with proptosis (with orbital congestion), the ocular wall thickness and volume were found to be significantly larger than in the normal control group [7].

In the first part of the present study, we investigated the dynamic aspects of the ocular wall changes in response to an artificially induced intraocular pressure elevation. In the second part, we examined the relationships between the intraocular pressure and the ocular wall dimensions in eyes with different diseases.

Patients and methods

In the first investigation, by using a Gmelin M-101 suction cup, we induced an intraocular pressure elevation in one eye of each of 5 subjects (see Table 1). Before pressure elevation, the intraocular pressure, the axial length of the eye and the ocular wall thickness were measured in both eyes of each subject. The intraocular pressure and the ocular wall thickness measurements were also performed in one eye of each subject during a short period (1–2 minutes) of suction and just after it. In each measuring set, 3–5 ocular wall measurements were carried out and the values were averaged.

In the second investigation, the intraocular pressure, the axial length of the eye and the thickness of the ocular wall were measured in 74 eyes of 50 subjects, comprising 10 healthy persons, 16 patients with ocular hypotony (6

P. Till (ed.), Ophthalmic Echography 13, pp. 369–374.

Table 1. Data on the subjects in the first investigation

Number	Sex	Age	Diagnosis
1	Female	37	Congenital glaucoma
2	Female	79	Chronic angle-closure glaucoma
3	Male	46	Open-angle glaucoma
4	Male	25	Contusio bulbi
5	Male	49	Healthy

Table 2. The intraocular pressure (IOP) and the thickness of the ocular wall in the five eyes in the first investigation before, during and after artificially induced IOP elevation

No.	Parameter	Before suction	During suction	After suction
1	IOP (mm Hg)	17	55	13
	Thickness (mm)	1.25	1.1	1.3
2	IOP (mm Hg)	18.5	51	16
	Thickness (mm)	1.45	1.1	1.4
3	IOP (mm Hg)	16	39	10
	Thickness (mm)	1.7	1.35	1.55
4	IOP (mm Hg)	7.5	43	6
	Thickness (mm)	1.75	1.4	1.8
5	IOP (mm Hg)	8.5	36	7.5
	Thickness (mm)	1.7	1.5	1.8

after intraocular surgery or injury, 4 with uveitis, 6 with phthisis bulbi), and 24 patients with glaucoma.

The axial length of the eye and the thickness of the ocular wall in the area of the posterior pole were measured by means of ultrasound at 10 MHz with Ultrascan Digital B System IV equipment. The precision of the echobiometric technique employed was found in earlier studies to be 0.1 mm as concerns the axial eye length and 0.07 mm as concerns the ocular wall thickness [5, 6]. The volume of the posterior half of the ocular wall was calculated in a manner similar to that used by Guthoff et al. [2].

Results

The intraocular pressures and ocular wall thicknesses of the 5 eyes examined in the first investigation before, during and after artificially induced intraocular pressure elevation are shown in Table 2. The volumes of the posterior half of the ocular wall before, during and after suction are displayed in Fig. 1.

In the second investigation, inverse exponential correlations were found between the intraocular pressure and the ocular wall thickness ($r = -0.68$; $p < 0.001$) and between the intraocular pressure and the ocular wall volume ($r = -0.71$; $p < 0.001$). The scatterplots of these relationships are presented

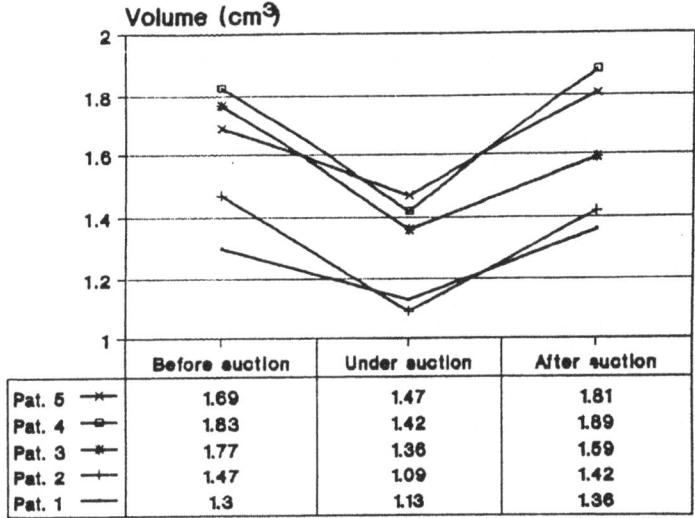

Fig. 1. Changes in the volume of the posterior half of the ocular wall in response to an artificial intraocular pressure elevation induced by suction.

in Figs. 2 and 3. In this material, the intraocular pressure ranged up to 69 mm Hg, the ocular wall thickness from 0.8 to 4.6 mm and the volume of the posterior half of the ocular wall from 0.68 to 3.74 cm³,

Discussion

Our results demonstrated that the ocular wall dimensions (thickness and volume) correlated strongly with intraocular pressure.

The first investigation revealed that the ocular wall was thinner during the artificially elevated intraocular pressure than before or after pressure elevation. The rapid change in intraocular pressure caused similarly rapid alterations in the eye wall thickness and volume. The changes in the ocular wall dimensions proved to be reversible.

The second investigation demonstrated the very wide ranges of the thickness and volume of the ocular coats in different diseases. In healthy eyes, even with high refractive errors, the volume of the posterior half of the ocular wall is fairly constant (about 1.6 cm³) [2], whereas in pathological conditions the volume of the eye wall may be changed considerably. In our mixed subject group (patients with ocular hypotony, inflammation or glaucoma and normal controls), the thickness and the volume of the ocular wall both exhibited a close inverse exponential correlation with the intraocular pressure.

The crucial point for the normal posterior wall volume (1.6 cm³) determined by Guthoff et al. [2] was at an intraocular pressure about 14 mm Hg,

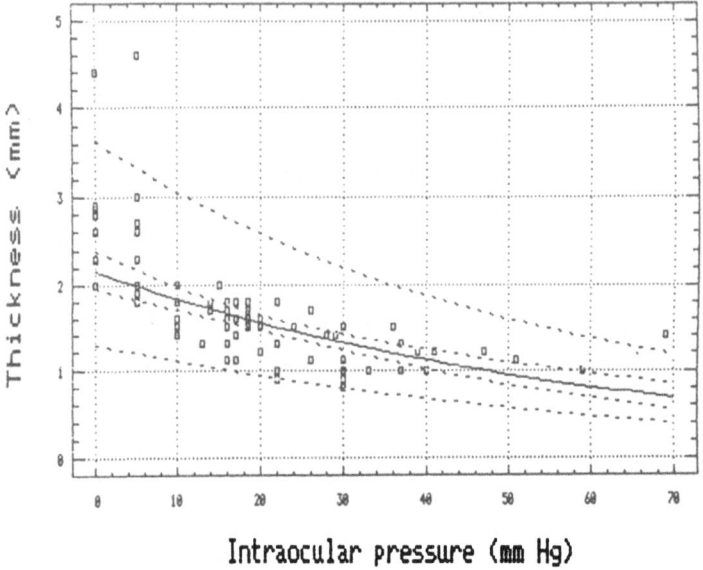

Fig. 2. Correlation between intraocular pressure and thickness of the ocular wall.

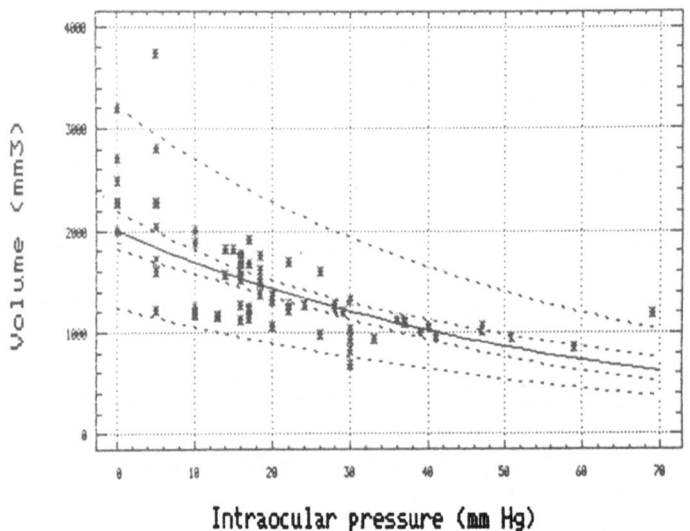

Fig. 3. Correlation between intraocular pressure and volume of the posterior half of the ocular wall.

with a 95% interval between 10 and 20 mm Hg (Fig. 3). Otherwise, in our control group the average volume of the posterior half of the ocular wall was found to be slightly lower (1.5 cm^3), corresponding to an intraocular pressure of 17 mm Hg. These intraocular pressure values are very close to the average intraocular pressure value found in a large normal population [3].

In our earlier studies of the ocular coats of glaucomatous patients, linear correlations were found between the ocular wall dimensions and intraocular pressure [5, 6, 8]. In contrast, the present investigation demonstrated that the best-fitting curve was an exponential one. The difference might be connected with the differences in the groups of patients involved in the two studies. The difference may also indicate that, in patients with ocular hypotony, the thickening of the ocular coats does not depend only on the low level of the intraocular pressure; other factors (such as inflammatory oedema and vascular congestion) may also play an important role.

Conclusion

The results of our study show that under pathological conditions (high or low intraocular pressure, inflammation or vascular congestion) the thickness and the volume of the ocular wall are altered. The changes in the ocular wall dimensions very closely and quickly follow changes in intraocular pressure. Thus, the intraocular pressure might be one of the most important factors which can cause diffuse-type alterations (thinning or thickening) in the ocular wall. Echobiometric detection of diffuse-type changes in ocular wall dimensions is of great clinical value, both in the diagnosis and in the follow-up of patients.

References

1. Guthoff, R. Ultraschall in der ophthalmologischen Diagnostik. Stuttgart: Ferdinand Enke Verlag (1988).
2. Guthoff, R., Berger, R.W. & Draeger, J. Ultrasonographic measurement of the posterior coats of the eye and their relation to axial length. Graefe's Arch. Clin. Exp. Ophthalmol. 225: 374-376 (1987).
3. Naumann, G.O.H. & Apple, D.J. Pathology of the eye, p. 771. New York, Berlin, Heidelberg, Tokyo: Springer-Verlag (1986).
4. Németh, J. A szemgolyó falvastagságának változása glaucomában. Szemészet 126: 107–111 (1989).
5. Németh, J., Szabó, Á. & Gyenes, Á. A digitális echobiometriáról. Szemészet 126: 153–158 (1989).
6. Németh, J. The posterior coats of the eye in glaucoma. An echobiometric study. Graefe's Arch. Clin. Exp. Opthalmol. 228: 33–35 (1990).
7. Németh, J. Thickness and volume of the ocular wall in different eye diseases. In Free paper, poster & video programme, p. 102. XXVI ICO Pte Ltd. Singapore: P. G. Publishing Pte Ltd (1990).
8. Németh, J. Augenhinterwandveränderungen bei Glaukom-Patienten. Fortschritte der Ophthalmologie 87: 138–139 (1990).

9. Tane, S. & Kohno, J. The microscopic biometry of the thickness of the human retina, choroid and sclera by ultrasound. In Acta XXV Concilium Opthalmologicum. Proceedings of the XXVth International Congress of Ophthalmology, pp. 275–277. Amsterdam, Berkeley, Milano: Kugler & Ghedini Publications (1987).

Address for correspondence: 1st Department of Ophthalmology, Semmelweis Medical University, Tömö u. 25–29, H-1083 Budapest, Hungary.

43. Ultrasonography in cryopexy of the retina

H. GERDING & S. CLEMENS

(*Münster, Germany*)

Introduction

Cryosurgical techniques have been established as the therapy of choice for a variety of retinal diseases. Today leading indications are prophylactic and therapeutical retinopexy as proposed by Lincoff et al. (1964) and antiproliferative or resorptive therapy of diabetic retinopathy (Osterhuis & Bijlmer-Gorter 1980; Paul 1982; Schimek & Spencer 1979; Mosier et al. 1985).

The duration of cryotherapy can be optimized applying the three grade criteria described by Lincoff & Kreissig (1971). In certain clinical situations (e.g. vitreal hemorrhages, cataracts) cryotherapy is desired without having the possibility of ophthalmoscopic control. In these situations the duration of cryotherapy has to be estimated on the basis of clinical experience. This may lead to an inadequate application since the necessary duration of cryotherapy is dependent on several parameters: intra- and interindividual variations of ocular wall thickness (Birch & Welch 1967), choroidal congestion, mechanical pressure of the application (Brihaye & Oosterhuis 1971), thermal conductivity of the environment, and inconstant performance of the technical equipment. Inadequate dosage of cryotherapy bears either the risk of insufficient effects or overdosage. As a consequence of overdosage severe complications (bleeding, retinal tears, pigment fallout, macular oedema, macular pucker, PVR) have been discussed (Böke 1965, Shea 1968, Tannenbaum et al. 1969, Chignell et al. 1971, Chignell & Shilling 1973, Kimball et al. 1978, Spitznas & Meyer-Schwickerath 1982, Robertson & Priluk 1979, Laqua & Machemer 1976). The aim of this survey has been first to investigate whether ultrasonography is a useful method for monitoring retinal cryotherapy, and second to establish criteria for the objective determination of the optimal cryotherapy duration for use without ophthalmoscopic control.

Material and methods

In vitro experiments were carried out on enucleated pig eyes which were obtained from a local slaughterhouse and used within two hours after death.

P. Till (ed.), Ophthalmic Echography 13, pp. 375–380.
© 1993 *Kluwer Academic Publishers*.

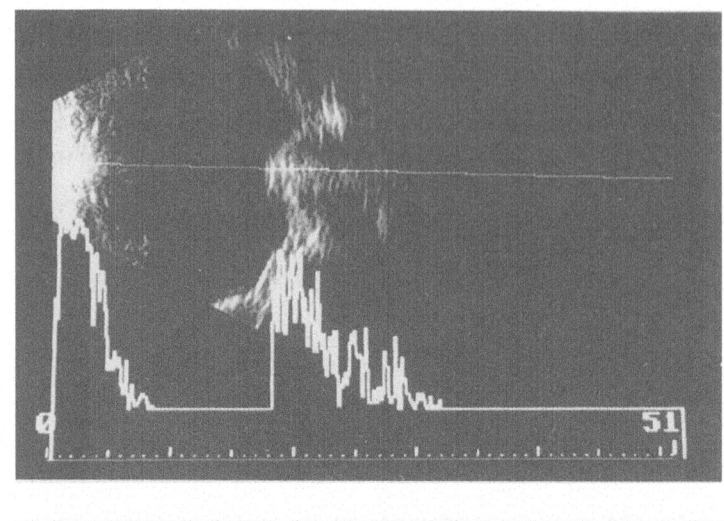

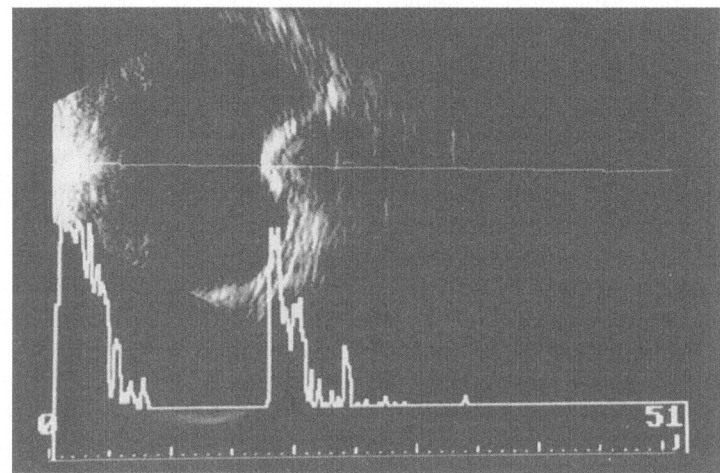

Fig. 1. In vitro cryopexy of a pig eye: (a) before and (b) after intensive freezing of the retina ('white' > 4 sec).

Eyes were mechanically stabilized in an U-shaped holder with the posterior pole on the basis. The transducer was fixed to the holder touching the sclera either in the equatorial region or up to 4 mm anterior to the equator. The indentating tip of the retinal cryoprobe was centered in the plane of the scan on the opposite scleral wall. A Keeler Amoils Cryo Unit ACU 14 MK.2 was used for cryosurgical application at a temperature between −50 ° and −80 °C. In vitro cryopexy was performed under indirect ophthalmoscopic control. Ultrasonographic monitoring was performed with a Cooper Vision Ultrascan Digital B 2000 unit. For the in vivo application of the method similar technical equipment was used.

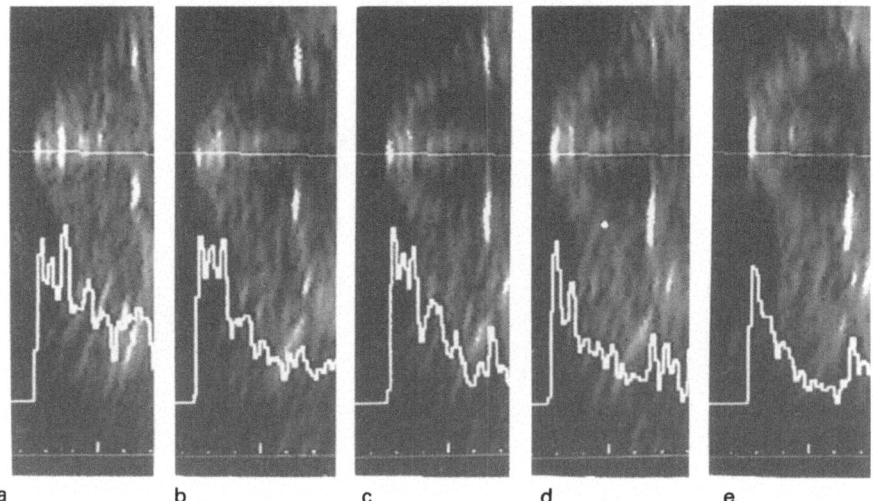

Fig. 2. Different stages of in vitro cryopexy of a pig eye. The sequence was performed at increased tip temperatures of −10 to −20 °C. (a) Situation before freezing, (b) ice ball within the sclera, (c) early, (d) intermediate and (e) intensive retinal freezing.

Results

The combination of A- and B-scan ultrasonography proved to be useful for the monitoring of retinal cryopexy. The B-scan allows a good orientation for the correct instrument localisation, while the A-scan enables the depth of the ice front to be determined. During the freezing process the progression of the ice ball to the inner retinal surface can be observed.

An example of in vitro testing (pig eye) is demonstrated in Fig. 1. Part (a) shows the situation before freezing. The tip of the cryoprobe can be localized by a relatively high reflex peak on the sclera. The convexity of the indented retina shows a posterior interference pattern. After intensive freezing (retinal 'white' on funduscopy for more than 4 sec; grade III according to Lincoff & Kreissig 1971) the retina delineates with a maximal reflection at the inner surface. The spatial progression of the ice ball extending from the tip of the cryoprobe to the inner retinal surface is demonstrated in Fig. 2.

The first sign after starting the application is an elevation of the scleral reflex (Fig. 2b). In Fig. 2(c–e) different stages of the futher freezing process are demonstrated. The progression of retinal freezing towards the inner limiting membrane is accompanied with a monophasic deformation of the reflex pattern and a deflection behind the ice peak. Clinically ultrasonographic control was applied for the cryotherapy of patients with diabetic retinopathy and vitreous hemorrhages. Fig. 3 demonstrates an example of a diabetic patient. The deformation of the retinal A-scan pattern served as

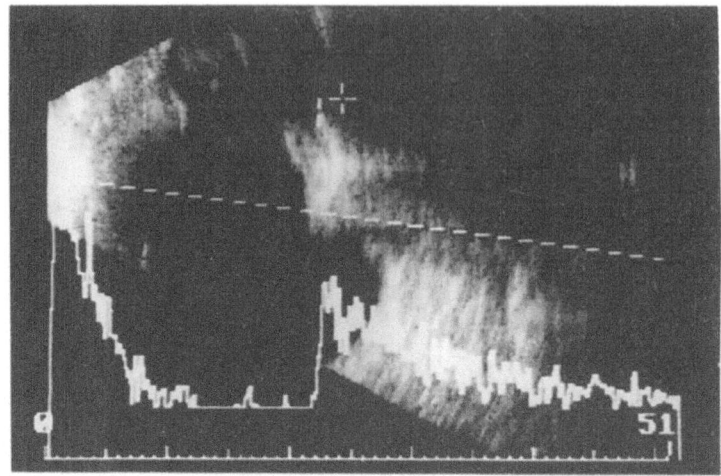

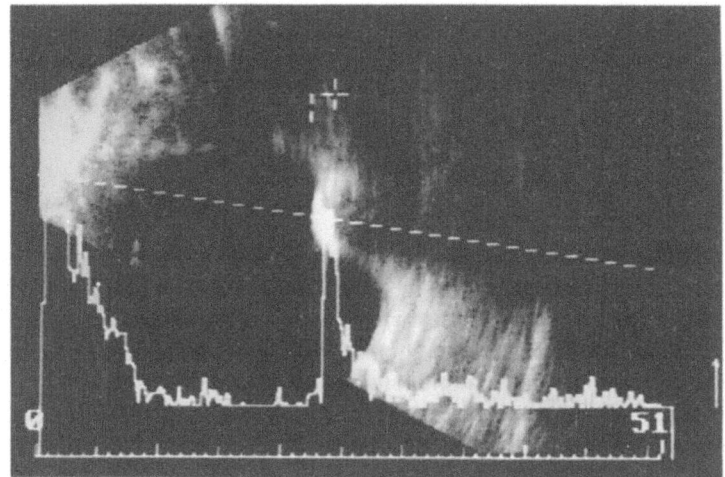

Fig. 3. Clinical example of cryotherapy monitoring: (a) before and (b) after complete retinal freezing.

a criterion for the temporal limitation of freezing and proved to be a useful parameter for objective cryotherapy control (Clemens et al. 1990).

Discussion

Cryotherapy has been established as an effective antiproliferative and resorptive treatment for diabetic retinopathy complicated by vitreous hemorrhages. The epidemiologic increase in diabetic retinopathy causes a quantitative expansion of the indication for this at least partially unmonitored cryotherapy. A clinically useful method for the objective dosage of ophththalmoscopically unmonitored retinal cryotherapy has so far been unavailable. Potential methods for the quantification of cryotherapeutic effects are thermometric or electrical conductivity measurements. As indirect methods, both have the disadvantage of relatively low precision. Generally unmonitored cryotherapy is timed either analogue to the necessary duration in visible portions of the fundus, or according to the experience of the surgeon. The potential overdosage of cryotherapy may contribute to an unfavourable outcome. Ultrasonographic A-scan montoring of ophthalmological cryotherapy was first applied by Koza & Matthäus (1986) for cyclocryothermy of glaucoma. Our results clearly show that A/B-ultrasonography is a useful and easy to handle method for ophthalmoscopically unmonitored retinal cryotherapy. The deformation of the echographic image of the retina during the progression of the ice ball can be used as a precise dosage criterion for the avoidance of overdosage.

References

Birch, P.G & Welch, R.B. Cryosurgery. Int. Ophthalmol. Clin. 7: 325–334 (1967).

Böke, W. Zur Cryopexie der Netzhaut. Klin. Mbl. Augenheilk. 147: 643–654 (1965).

Brihaye, M. & Oosterhuis, J.A. Experimentelle transsklerale Kryokoagulation der Netzhaut. Klin. Mbl. Augenheilk. 158: 171–174 (1971).

Chignell, A.H., Revie, I.H.S. & Clemett, R.S. Complications of retinal cryotherpy. Trans. Ophthal. Soc. (UK) 91: 635–651 (1971).

Chignell, A.H. & Shilling, J. Prophylaxis of retinal detachment. Br. J. Ophthalmol. 57: 291–298 (1973).

Clemens, S., Gerding, H. Emmerich, K.-H. Dosierung der retinalen Kryotherapie mit Hilfe der Echographie. Klin. Mbl. Augenheilk. 199: 12–15 (1991).

Kimball, R.E., Morse, P.H. & Benson, W.E. Cystoid macular edema after cryotherapy. Am. J. Ophthalmol. 86: 572–573 (1978).

Koza, K.-D. & Matthäus, W. Experimentelle und klinische Untersuchungen zur Optimierung der Kryotherpie des primären Glaukoms. Folia Ophthalmol. 11: 313–315 (1986).

Laqua, H. & Machemer, R. Repair and adhesion mechanisms of the cryotherapy lesion in experimental retinal detachment. Am. J. Ophthalmol. 81: 833–845 (1976).

Lincoff, H., McLean, J. & Nano, Cryosurgical treatment of retinal detachment. Trans. Am. Acad. Ophthal. Otol. 68: 412–432 (1964).

Lincoff, H.A. & Kreissig, I. The mechanism of the cryosurgical adhesion. Am. J. Ophthalmol. 61: 1227–1234 (1971).

Mosier, M.A., Del Piero, E. & Gheewala, S.M. Anterior retinal cryotherapy in diabetic vitreous hemorrhage. Am. J. Ophthalmol. 100: 440–444 (1985).

Oosterhuis, J.A., Bijlmer-Gorter. Cryotreatment in proliferative diabetic retinopathy. Ophthalmologica 181: 81–87 (1980).

Paul, H.-H Diathermie- und Kryokoagulation bei Glaskörperblutungen. Klin. Mbl. Augenheilk. 180: 282–285 (1982).

Robertson, D.M., Priluck, A. 360° prophylactic cryoretinopexy. Arch. Ophthalmol. 97: 2130–2134 (1979).

Schimek, R.A. & Spencer, R. Cryopexy treatment of proliferative diabetic retinopathy. Arch. Ophthalmol. 97: 1276–1280 (1979).

Shea, M. Complications of cryotherapy in retinal detachment. Can. J. Ophthalmol. 3: 109–112 (1968).

Spitznas, M., Meyer-Schwickerath, G. Indikationen zur Amotio-Prophylaxe. In: Meyer-

Schwickerath, G. & Ullerich, K. (eds.), Grenzen der konservativen Therapie. Stuttgart: Enke Verlag (1982).

Tannenbaum, H.L., Schepers, C.L. & Elzenarig, J. Macular pucker following retinal surgery. A biomicroscopic study. Can. J. Ophthalmol. 4: 20–23 (1969).

Address for correspondence: University Eye Hospital, Domagkstrasse 15, D-4400 Münster, Germany

44. Ultrasonography in cases of phthisis bulbi

Zs. LAMPÉ & L. KOLOZSVÁRI
(Debrecen, Hungary)

Since 1985, in the Department of Ophthalmology, Medical University of Debrecen, we have examined 52 patients with ultrasound with the diagnosis phthisis bulbi. We used both the A-scan and B-scan methods. Previously the examinations were carried out with a Sonometrics Ocuscan DBR 400 and CooperVisionDigital B IV equipment.

The classification of the shrinkage of the globe which is widely accepted today have been worked out by Yanoff & Fine [9]. This includes the definition of both of the most important conditions of the atrophy of the eye, i.e. atrophy and phthisis bulbi (Table 1). Group I, according to their classification, includes atrophies without shrinkage, and group II, consists of atrophy with shrinkage corresponding to atrophia bulbi. These hypotonic, cuboid eyes, which are smaller than normal, still maintain their histological structure. It is important to note that clinically this is called phthisis bulbi, although one of the main criteria of phthisis (i.e. histological disorganization) is not present. Group III includes cases with shrinkage and disorganization. Group IV, consists of cases with intraocular ossification. In the case of the 2 latter groups we can speak about phthisis bulbi also histologically [8, 9].

The classical clinical picture of phthisis bulbi can easily be recognized (Fig. 1). At the first survey enophthalmos and narrower interpalpebral fissure due to shrinkage of the globe are obvious. Hypotony is always present, and common findings are flattening and vascularization of the cornea [5].

Ultrasound diagnostics can be of the greatest help in cases without these characteristic symptoms, and where examination is difficult, for example because of the cloudiness of the optic media.

By means of the A-scan method the data which can be well characterized biometrically can be examined [2]. The first sign of the degenerative atrophy of the globe can be shortening of the axial length. Over the course of consecutive examinations such shortening enables not only an early diagnosis but also provides differentiation from stationary diseases such as microphthalmos, which has a similar clinical appearance [4].

The A-scan method is also adequate for the visualization of the thickening of the sclera and chorioretinal tissue, whereas the B-scan method is more suitable for the examination of these and other alterations.

By means of the B-method another early symptom in addition to the shortening of the axial length, i.e. hypotony and its consequences can be

P. Till (ed.), Ophthalmic Echography 13, pp. 381–384.

Table 1. Classification of the shrinkage of the globe (Yanoff & Fine)

I.	Atrophies without shrinkage
II.	Atrophies with shrinkage (atrophia bulbi)
III.	Atrophies with shrinkage and histological disorganization
IV.	Intraocular ossification

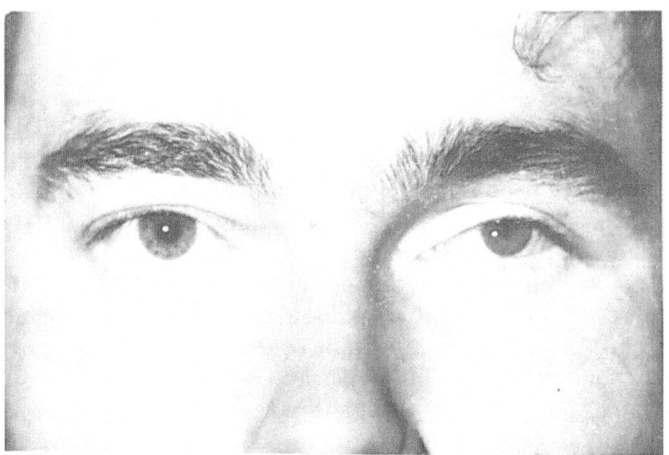

Fig. 1. Phtisis bulbi: classical picture of phtisis bulbi.

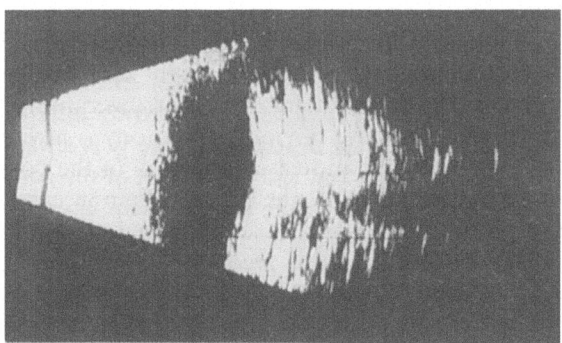

Fig. 2. Phtisis bulbi: shortened axial length with the B-scan method.

demonstrated (Fig. 2). As a result of the slight pressure on the globe in the course of the ultrasound examination the horizontal axis seems to be shortened and the vertical axis seems to be elongated [7].

Due to the thickening of the sclera and of the chorioretinal tissue which is a frequent consequence of hypotony, the two layers can be well differ-

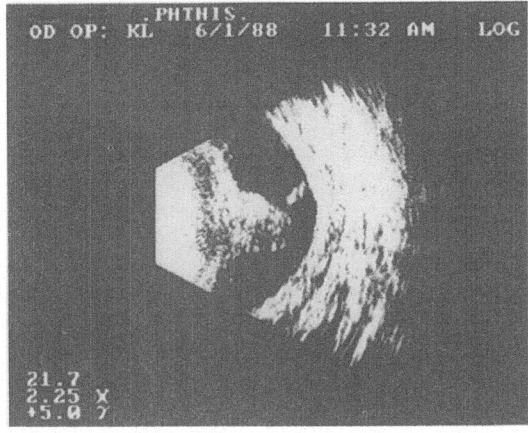

Fig. 3. Phtisis bulbi: thickened scleral, choro-retinal layer and proliferative vitreo-retinopathy.

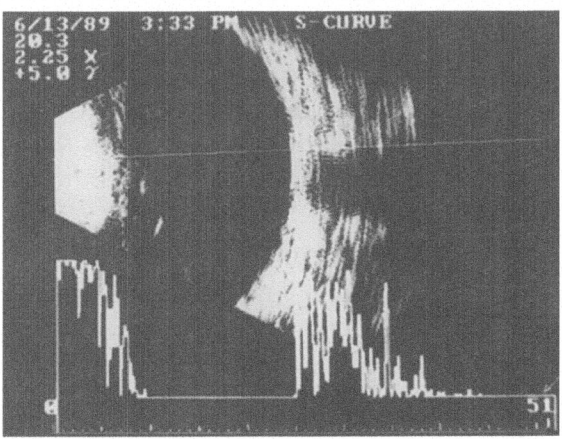

Fig. 4. Phtisis bulbi: papilloedema caused by hypotony.

entiated (Fig. 3.), and a papilloedema of small degree can be present (Fig. 4). Choroidal detachment frequently occurs (Fig. 5), and the often detached and folded retina runs from the papilla towards the center of the vitreous cavity [1, 6].

Beside the above symptoms vitreal hemorrhages and the presence of a cyclitic membrane are often seen.

Intraocular ossification is a special alteration. The bones in the vitreous cavity reflect characteristic echoes [1, 7].

With the A-method a high spike appears at the spot corresponding to the bone, but at the same time the characteristic spikes of the orbit behind the bone are missing. With the B-method the bone reflects an echo with high

384

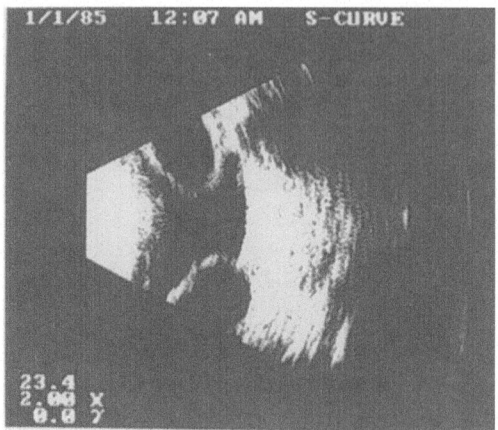

Fig. 5. Phtisis bulbi: choroidal detachment.

intensity and there is a characteristic repetition of echoes on the background. In the case of the echogram mentioned above we have to suspect the presence of an intraocular foreign body, especially if the atrophy of the globe started after a perforating injury.

Although we do not need ultrasound examination to diagnose phthisis bulbi, echography can be of a great help in the differential diagnosis in the follow-up of the alterations, in the choice of the cases to be operated, and in the choice of therapy.

References

1. Coleman, O.J., Lizzi, F.L. & Jack, R.C. Ultrasonography of the eye and orbit, p. 205 (1977).
2. Freyler, H. Beginnende Bulbusatrophie. Graefes Arch. Klin. Exp. Ophthal. 197: 203–208 (1975).
3. Guthoff, R. & Guthoff, K. Ultraschalldiagnostik in der Augenheilkunde. Z. für Prakt. Augenheilk. (1987).
4. Koplin, R.S., Gersten, M. & Hodes, B. Real time ophthalmic ultrasonography and biometry, pp. 69–71. USA: Slack Incorporates (1985).
5. Naumann, G.O.H. & Apple, D.J. Pathology of the eye, p. 317. Springer-Verlag (1985).
6. Ossoinig, K.C. Ophtalmic ultrasonography: comparative techniques. Intern. Ophtalmol. Clin. 19: 140 (1979).
7. Shammas, H.J. Atlas of opthalmic ultrasonography, pp. 180–274. CV Mosby Company (1984).
8. Stefani, F.H. Phtisis bulbi – an intraocular floride proliferative reaction. Dev. Ophthal. 10: 78–160 (1985).
9. Yanoff, M. & Fine, B.S. Ocular pathology, p. 74. Harper and Row (1975).

Address for correspondence: University Medical School, Department of Ophthalmology, Nagy-erdei Krt. 98, H-Debrecen 4012, Hungary.

45. Posterior pole configurations in progressive myopia

V. HIDASI, L. KOLOZSVÁRI & Z. NAGY

(Debrecen, Hungary)

Since 1979, in the Department of Ophthalmology, Medical University of Debrecen, scleral support operations on progressive myopic patients have been performed. Since then, 398 myopic patients have been examined with ultrasound, 149 males and 249 females. The number of eyes examined was 647: 525 high (>8.0 D), 112 moderate (4.0–8.0 D) and 10 low degree (<4.0 D) myopics. Most of them were young, between ten and twelve years (Fig. 1).

Myopic eyes were noted to have several shapes, so that in the last two years special attention has been focused on the examination of the posterior pole with B-scan method to classify the configurations, then axial length measurements were performed with A-scan method. Five successive readings were noted in the case of each eye. On the basis of the shape of 338 eyes the configurations were divided into two main groups and seven subgroups.

Group I contains the spherically enlarged type (Fig. 2). The first subgroup is the regular form, and the second subgroup consists of diffusely enlarged eyes with pointing of the papillar area. To the third subgroup belong eyes with a bulge somewhere on the posterior pole, except the papillar area. Finally, the fourth subgroup comprises globes with flattened posterior walls (Fig. 3).

Group II is the antero-posteriorly lengthened type (Fig. 4).subgroup is the regular oval form; the second is the same, but with the pointing of the papillar area; and the third subgroup consists of oval-shaped eyes with a bulge on the posterior pole adjacent to the papilla (Fig. 5) [5, 7].

Configuration distribution of the 338 eyes according to the degree of myopia indicates that the number of the spherically enlarged globes is much higher than that of the oval-shaped eyes, and within this group the regular form presents the most extensive subgroup [1]. There were no moderate-degree myopic eyes among the antero-posteriorly lengthened bulbs (Figs. 6a and 6b).

It is an interesting phenomenon that the same eyeball can show different shapes in the horizontal and sagittal planes (Fig. 7), respectively (except the regularly enlarged round bulbs).

In the course of our axial length measurements the values were noted to range between rather wide limits using the Cooper Vision Digital B IV

P. Till (ed.), Ophthalmic Echography 13, pp. 385–392.
© 1993 *Kluwer Academic Publishers.*

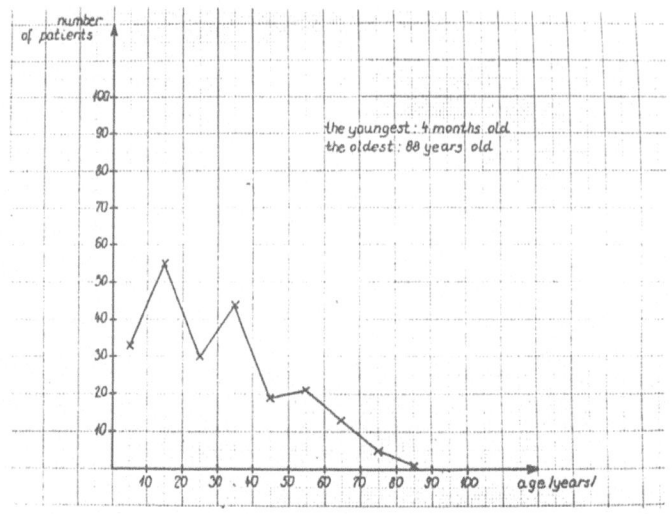

Fig. 1. The age distribution of our progressively myopic patients.

machine (Figs 8a and 8b). The mean value of the obtained differences within the different groups was calculated taking the highest and lowest of five successive measurements. The mean value of the differences proved to be much higher in the case of eyes with staphyloma and, thus, the standard deviation than in the case of the regular spherical or flattened moderately myopic eyes. This means that the authenticity of the axial length measure-

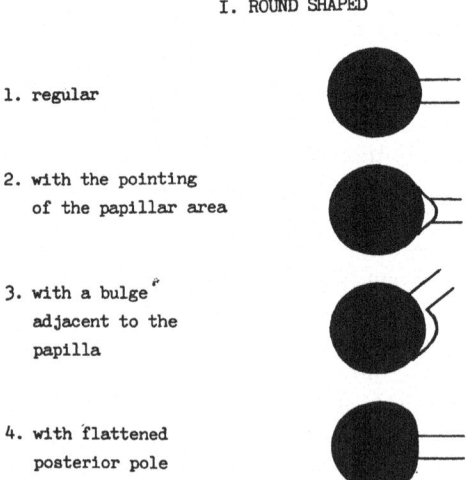

Fig. 2. Group I (round shaped) and the four subgroups of posterior pole configurations in progressive myopia.

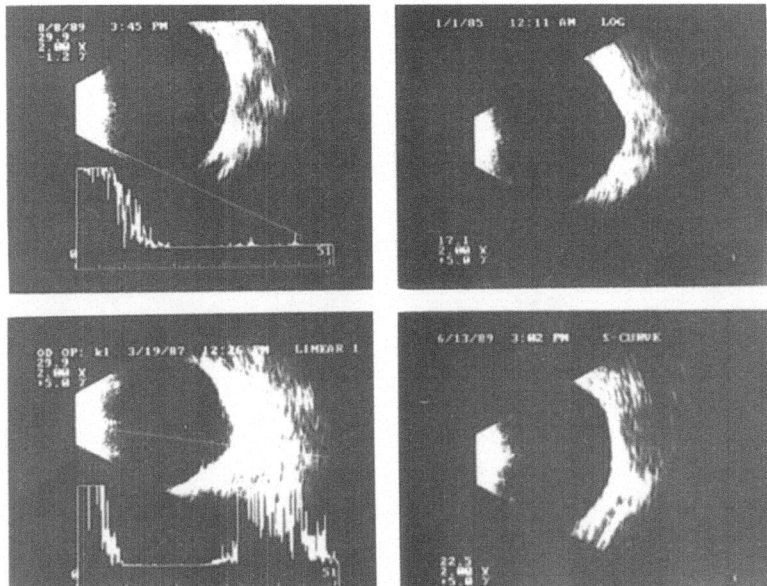

Fig. 3. The echographic pictures of the four subgroups of group I. The first subgroup is the regular, spherically enlarged bulb (*abovel left*). The second subgroup shows the pointed papillar area (*above right*). The third subgroup has a circumscribed bulge on the posterior pole except the papillar area (*below left*). The fourth subgroup is posteriorly flattened (*below right*).

ments with A-method is greatly influenced by the configuration of the globe in the case of progressively myopic eyes.

In examinations of anisometropic progressively myopic patients sometimes different forms of the two eyes were found [2, 3, 6]. In 31 patients the difference between the two sides was more than 3.0 diopters. The shapes of

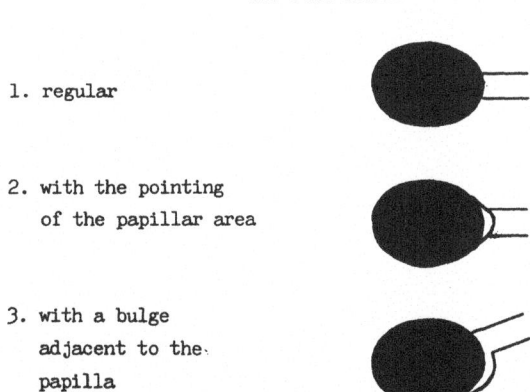

Fig. 4. Group II (oval shaped) and the three subgroups of posterior pole configurations in progressive myopia.

388

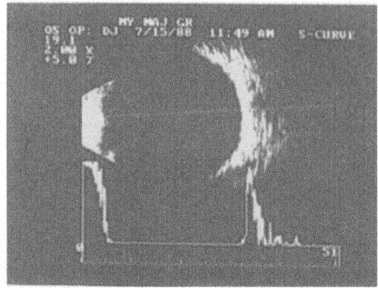

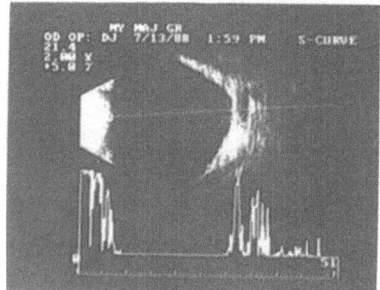

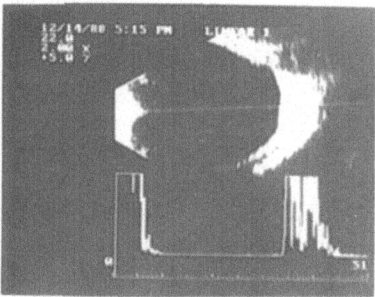

Fig. 5. The echographic pictures of the three subgroups of group II. The first subgroup is the regular oval form (*above*). The second subgroup shows the pointed papillar area (*below left*). The third subgroup has a bulge adjacent to the papilla (*below right*).

		I. Diffusely enlarged ROUND SHAPED				II. Antero-posteriorly enlarged OVAL SHAPED	
		high	moderate			high	moderate
1.	●	141	46	1.	●	43	0
2.	●	59	0	2.	●	13	0
3.	◐	32	3	3.	◐	10	0
4.	●	1	13				
sum total		233 +	62 =	295	sum total:	43 +	0 = 4:

(a)   (b)

Fig. 6. Configuration distribution of progressively myopic eyes according to the degree of myopia: (a) group I; (b) group II.

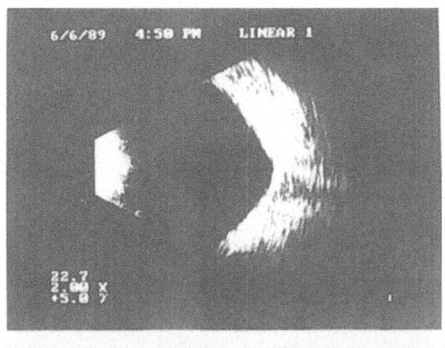

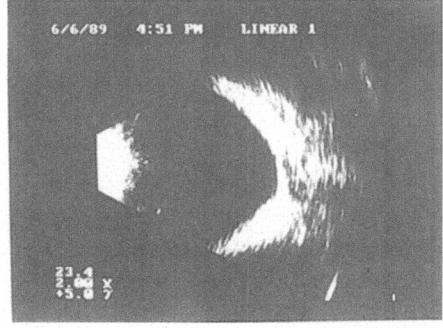

Fig. 7. Two echographic pictures of the same eye with the pointing of the papillar area in the horizontal (*above*) and vertical (*below*) planes.

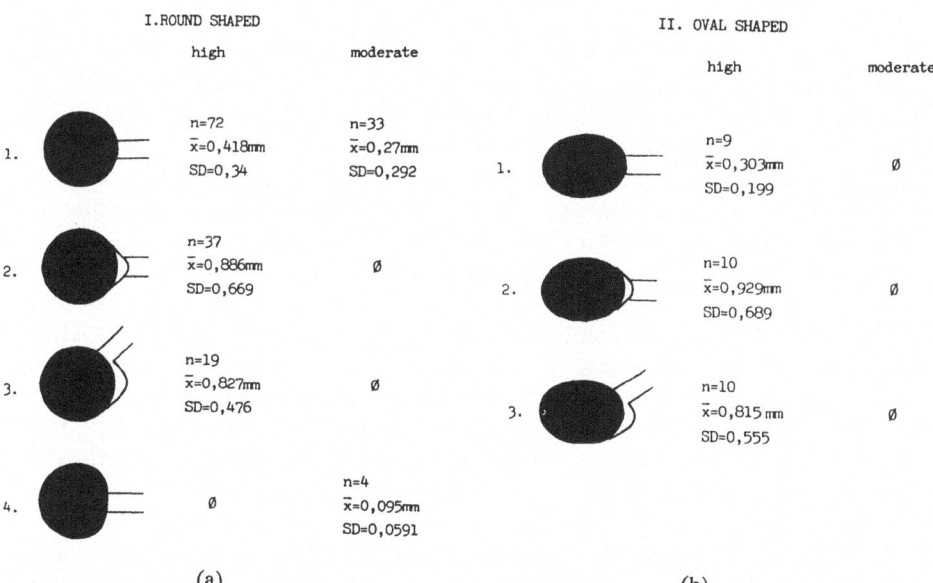

(a)   (b)

Fig. 8. The range of axial length values measured with A-method (Cooper Vision Digital B IV) in progressive myopia: (a) group I, (b) group II.

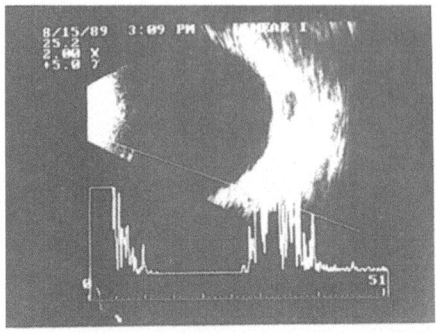

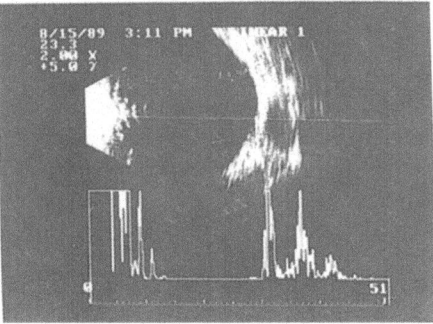

Fig. 9. Echographic pictures of two eyes of the same patient. The right eye (*above*) has a regular oval shape, the left eye (*below*) is regular spherical.

the two bulbs were different in nine cases. Fig. 9 shows the right and left eyes of the same patient. While the right eye has an almost regular oval shape with a myopia of − 16.0 diopters, the left is regular spheric with − 13.0 diopters of myopia. On the basis of these findings it can be supposed how certain configurations may develop. It is hardly possible to follow up the enlarging process on the same eye. In the case of high-degree myopic patients (independently of the patient's age) and recently in that of moderate-degree myopic patients, we perform the scleral support operation if the degree of myopia and the axial length were progressively increasing. The operation in turn changes the original configuration of the posterior pole (Fig. 10). After the operation in most cases the macular area was prominent because of swelling of the ocular wall, mainly the choroid. The same prominence can be seen one and two months later (on another patient) (Fig. 11). The improvement in visual acuity of both patients was 0.4 immediately after the operation, the initial values being 0.1 and 0.4, respectively. The presence of swelling could be supported by axial length measurements.

Still it cannot be stated whether the configuration of the posterior pole influences the result of the operation or not. On the basis of our few cases it is obvious that the greatest improvement in visual acuity immediately after the operation occurred in the subgroups where the bulb had a regular oval

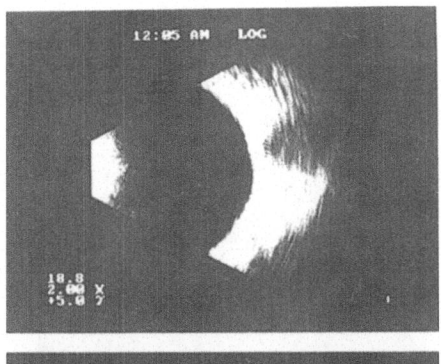

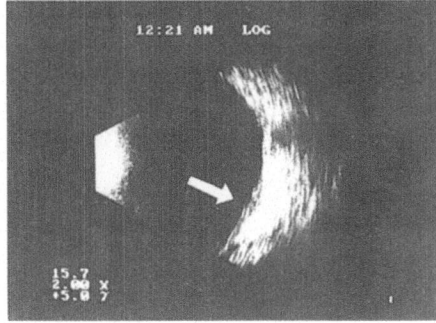

Fig. 10. Echographic pictures of the same eyeball before (*above*) and two days after (*below*) the operation (scleral support) in the horizontal plane. The macular area shows a swelling of choroid (arrow).

shape, with an average value of visual acuity 0.2, and where a temporal staphyloma was present (spherical or oval forms), where the average value of visual acuity had 0.1–0.15. The axial length reduction was greatest in the same subgroups, the average being about 0.3 mm immediately after the operation. The degree of myopia decreased by about 1.0 diopter in both main groups where bulges were adjacent to the papilla, and 2.0 diopters in the case of oval bulbs with pointed papillar areas [4].

These ultrasonographic findings are both interesting and useful in several aspects. Preoperative ultrasound examination eliminates the danger of the retrobulbar injections in the case of a large posterior staphyloma. Pre- and postoperative examinations allow the follow-up of the results of scleral support. Regarding the wide range of axial length values obtained with A-method, especially when the eye is cataractous, we have to be careful with the measurements. Finally, on the basis of the configuration type in connection with the postoperative results it might be possible to decide upon optimal cases for operation.

392

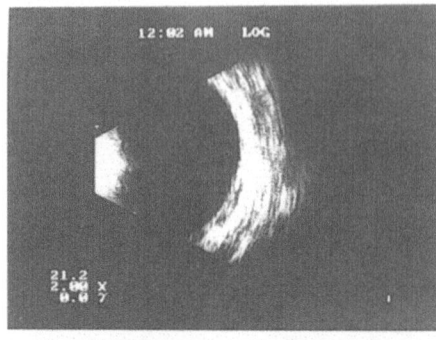

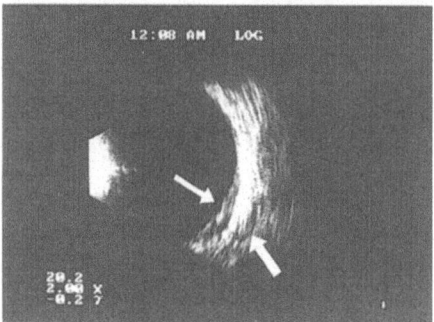

Fig. 11. Echographic pictures of the same eye one (*above*) and two (*below*) months after the operation (scleral support). Swelling in the macular area (thin arrow), the fascia lata band (thick arrow) and can be seen.

References

1. Fledelius, H.C. Ultrasound oculometry and exophthalmometry in high myopia with reference to the occurrence of retinal detachment. Acta Ophthalmol. 49: 707–714 (1971).
2. Fledelius, H.C. Refractive components in aniso- and isometropia. In: Fledelius, H.C. et al. (eds.), Doc. Ophthalmol. Proc. Ser. 28: 89–95 (1981).
3. Gernet, H. Oculometric findings in myopia. In: Fledelius, H.C. et al. (eds.), Doc. Ophthalmol. Proc. Ser. 28: 71–77 (1981).
4. Kolozsvári, L., Nagy, Z. & Alberth, B. The importance of echography in connection with sclera supporting surgical interventions. Szemészet 125: 59–62 (1988).
5. Nagy, Z. Some ideas on the surgical approach for reducing the refractive error in myopia. Szémeszet 118: 224–232 (1981).
6. Otsuka, J., Sugata, T. & Araki, M.: The ethyology of myopia as considered from differences in the refractive components of the right and left eyes. In: Fledelius, H.C. et al. (eds.), Doc. Ophthalmol. Proc. Ser. 28: 79–87 (1981).
7. Svirin, A.V., Serebriakova, T.V., Batmanov, U.E. & Nesterov, A.P. Dvuhmernaia echografia v issledovanii glaz s miopiei. Vestnik Oftalm. 5: 40–42 (1982).

Address for correspondence: Department of Ophthalmology, University School of Medicine, Nagyerdei Krt. 98, H-4012 Debrecen, Hungary.

46. Choroidal thickness in general anesthesia

P. RADEMACHER, S. CLEMENS & Ch. RADIG

(*Münster, Germany*)

Choroidal thickness is of clinical interest in connection with the anterior segment, especially cataract surgery. If the thickness of the choroid is known, its volume can be calculated approximately by the formula of the globe segment [1]. To prevent complications during operations such as hemorrhages or vitreous prolapse, a choroidal volume as small as possible should be planned.

By means of ophthalmic echography it is possible to perform separate measurements both of retinal and choroidal thickness by imaging the pigmentepithelium as a curvilinear echo between retina and choroid [2]. In contrast to other procedures (such as radioactive marked erythrocytes or inspection of choroidal vessels after resection of a scleral portion) ultrasound is a non-invasive, non-burdening method to measure the choroid and to calculate its volume, even during surgery.

During examinations of 15 patients, the choroidal thickness was measured before and during anesthesia while changing the narcotic parameters such as anesthetic concentrations and the position of the patient. Intraocular pressure and cardiovascular parameters (pulse and blood pressure) were also recorded. Just after the measurements in all patients a lacrimal passage surgery was performed. We used a 'Triscan' with an axial resolution of 0.1 mm in the B-picture, which we found experimentally. The ultrasonic probe was placed in four positions on the eyelids. In each quadrant the measurements were made and average values calculated. The first examination was done just after positioning the awoken patient on the operating table. Choroidal thickness, intraocular pressure and the cardiovascular parameter values were transcribed on a special protocol. Narcosis was induced with 0.3 mg/kg/KG Etomidate and 0.1 mg/kg/KG Fentanyl. After relaxation with 0.1 mg/kg/KG Vecuronium the patients were intubated. The next examination was made during the so-called 'steady-state' stage. This means constant inspiratory oxygen concentrations of 4.5 kPC. This phase was reached 10 min after intubation. Three further measurements were made adding to the volatile anesthetic Enflurane in increasing concentrations of 0.6, 1.2, and 1.8 vol.%. Final measurements were made after a 5-min chest and head elevation of 45 degrees.

Our results demonstrate a decrease in intraocular pressure with increasing concentrations of Enflurane. The continuously registered blood pressure

P. Till (ed.), Ophthalmic Echography 13, pp. 393–394.

values slowly fell during the 'steady-state' stage and with higher concentrations of Enflurane. The choroid swell in the 'steady-state' stage and Enflurane concentration of 1.2 vol.%. Then in the phase of chest and head elevation the choroidea was significantly less swollen.

Our results demonstrate a striking correlation between intraocular pressure, choroida thickness and blood pressure. We suppose that the increase in choroidal thickness is a consequence of a large ectasis of vessels and edematous dilatation of the entire choroidea due to an outfiltration of choroidal vessels into the interstitial tissue; we registered a simultaneous decrease in the systemic blood pressure and intraocular pressure, and therewith the tissue pressure fell still further [3]. The choroidal thinning after chest and head elevation could be the result of the decrease in central venous pressure.

As mentioned above, the choroidal volume can be calculated from its thickness. Due to the rigidity of the sclera the swelling choroid preferably extends into the vitreous body and moves it in the direction of the iris-lens diaphragm, especially after opening the anterior chamber. This could increase the risk of vitreous prolapse during intraocular operations. Also the literature refers to the greater danger of hemorrhages if the choroid swells.

As a result of our experiments, we believe that chest and head elevation could reduce the risk of vitreous prolapse and could produce more favourable conditions during intraocular, and especially cataract surgery.

References

1. Clemens, S., Rademacher, P. & Radig, Ch. Beeinflussung des Aderhautvolumens. Sitz.-Ber. 151. Vers. Verein Rhein. Westf. Augenärzte 151: 75 (1989).
2. Clemens, S., Kroll, P. & Meyer-Rüsenberg, H.-W. Interface Echos zwischen Netzhaut und Aderhaut. Klin. Mbl. Augenheilk. 192: 197–203 (1988).
3. Rademacher, P., Clemens, S. & Radig, Ch. Druckmessung und Bestimmung der Aderhautdicke bei Narkose. In: Anästhesie in der Augenheilkunde (Symp. Hannover), pp. 130ff. Stuttgart: Thieme (1988).

Address for correspondence: University Eye Hospital, Domagkstrasse 15, W-4400 Münster, Germany.

47. Echographic study of an episcleral reabsorbable explant

F.A. RODRIGUEZ, R.R. GOSALBEZ & R.B. MARTI

(Barcelona, Spain)

Abstract. We have studied through serial A and B mode echographic controls, series of 15 patients who underwent rhegmatogenous retinal detachment surgery with placement of episceral explants made of the reabsorbable material Dexon® (polyglycolic acid). In the last echographic controls (four months after surgery), we have found there is an absence of indentation of the ocular wall due to the complete reabsorption of the explant material, so that the eye recovers its normal contours and the retina remains attached.

Introduction

We studied a series of 15 patients who underwent retinal detachment surgery with episcleral explants of the reabsorbable suture Dexon®. In all cases, serial A and B echographic controls were performed preoperatively at four days after surgery, and thereafter at monthly intervals for the first four months after surgery (the longest follow-ups were nine months after surgery).

The amount of initial indentation produced with this type of explant ranged from 2 mm to 5 mm, with a mean value of 3.5 mm.

The three echographic parameters we determined to follow the evolution of the explant were: (1) the amount of indentation it produced; (2) the acoustic shadowing or sound attenuation that appeared behind the highly absorpive buckle; and (3) the sclera to explant distance.

Both the initial indentation and the sound attenuation gradually decreased as the explant was being reabsorbd, while the distance from the anterior sclera (under the tip of the ultrasound probe) to the vitreous-retina interface at the point of highest indentation slowly increased as indentation diminished. In the last echographic controls at four months after surgery, we have seen that there is an absence of indentation due to the complete reabsorption of the explant material, the eyeball has returned to its usual shape, and the retina remains reattached (Figs. 1 and 2).

Materials and methods

Our 15 patients (eight females and seven males) ranged in age between 30 to 69 years old (mean age 55 years). The surgical method we used was the

P. Till (ed.), Ophthalmic Echography 13, pp. 395–398.

396

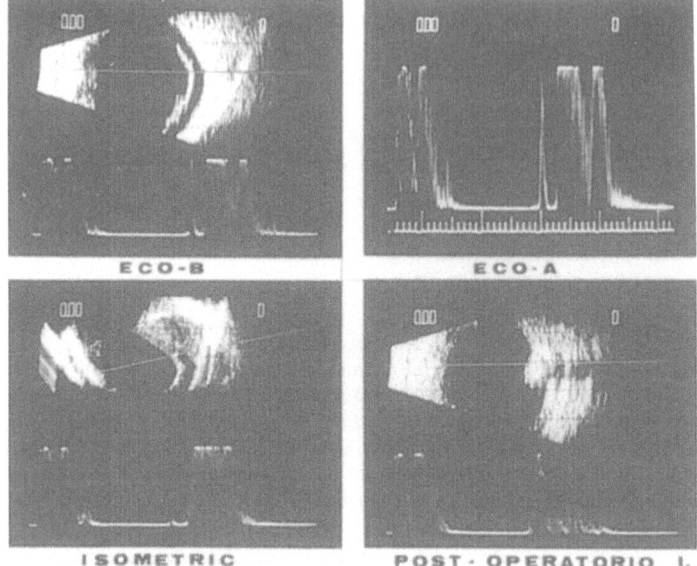

Fig. 1. B, A and isometric preoperative echograms of a retinal detachment (*above and below left*). Inmediate postoperative B echogram (*below right*) shows the amount of initial indentation, the sound attenuation behind the explant and the shortened anterior sclera-explant distance.

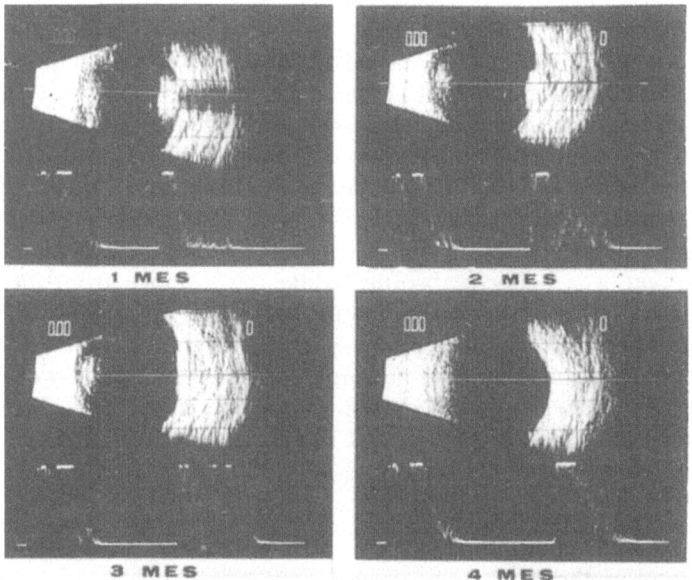

Fig. 2. Serial B echographic controls at monthly intervals after surgery show how both the indentation and sound attenuation gradually decrease, and the sclera-explant distance increases, as the explant reabsorbs four months after sugery, the globe regains its normal morphology.

Custodis–Lincoff technique placing an episcleral buckle made out of the reabsorbable suture Dexon® (a polymer of glycolic acid) over the site of the retinal breaks. In all 15 cases we performed transcleral cryoretinopexy prior to the buckling. Some cases required additional procedures such as drainage of subretinal fluid (10 eyes) or intravitreous injection of air (one eye).

The explant material we used was the reabsorbable suture Dexon®, a synthetic polymer of glycolic acid that is completely reabsorbed at a uniform rate, through simple hydrolysis, with minimal tissue reaction. It is well tolerated by ocular tissues, and complete reabsorption occurs within two to four months. Polyglycolic acid, because it is a synthetic product, is sterile, nontoxic and non-antigenic. It is available as braided multifilament sutures that are flexible and easy to handle. Our ultrasound unit is an Ocuscan DBR 400 ST model.

Results

The final visual acuity attained in our 15 cases ranged from 1/10 (previously amblyopic eye in a patient with anisometropia) to 10/10, with a mean value of 5/10. In follow-up controls (echographical and clinical up to nine months), we have had no redetachments, and have detected no significant complications that could be directly attributed to the explant.

Conclusions

We have studied a type of explant that can be used in the treatment of retinal detachment, which has the properties of being easily handled, well tolerated, nontoxic and completely and uniformly absorbable, so that in time the eye recovers its normal contours (this does not happen with conventional nonabsorbable explants such as silicone, teflon, or silicone sponge), with anatomical and functional recovery of the eye. Patients can also be spared the occasional trouble of the need to have extruded explants removed, discomfort on ocular movements, or long-term postoperative diplopia.

We consider that a permanence of indentation for about three months can be enough to achieve permanent retinal reattachment, in cases of uncomplicated rhegmatogenous retinal detachment, without signs of important vitreo-retinal traction and preferably cases with peripheral retinal breaks confined to one quadrant. Eyes with fixed retinal folds or other signs of significant traction should have permanent nonabsorbable buckles with a circling element, or vitrectomy techniques could be combined with the absorbable episcleral buckle.

398

References

1. Baum, G. Problems in ultrasonographic diagnosis of retinal disease. Am. J. Ophthalmol. 71: 723–739 (1971).
2. Blumenkranz, M.S. & Frazier Byrne, S. Standardized echography (ultrasonography) for the detection and characterization of retinal detachment. Ophthalmology 89: 7 (1982).
3. Coleman, J.D. & Jack, R.L. B scan ultrasonography in diagnosis and management of retinal detechment. Arch. Ophthalmol. 90: 000 (1973).
4. Coleman Jackson, D., Lizzi, F.L. & Jack, R.L. Ultrasonography of the eye and orbit. Philadelphia: Lea & Febiger (1977).
5. Espiritu, R.B. Absorbable suture in ophthalmic surgery. Philippine J. Ophthalmol. 6: 1.
6. Furgivele, F.P. Ophthalmic use of a new synthetic suture (Dexon): A preliminary report. Ann. Ophthalmol. 6(11): 6–11 (1974).
7. Jack, R.L. & Coleman, D.J. Diagnosis of retinal detachment with B scan ultrasound. Can. J. Ophthalmol. 8: 8–10 (1973).
8. Kerman, B.M. & Coleman, D.J. B scan ultrasonography of retinal detachment. Ann. Ophthalmol. 10: 903–911 (1978).
9. Offret, G. & Rousseelie, F. Diagnosis and surveillance of retinal detachment by means of time-amplitude ultrasonography. In Gitter, K. et al. (eds.), Ophthalmic Ultrasound, pp. 260–268. St. Louis: C.V. Mosby Co., (1969).
10. Oksala, A. & Lehtinen, A. Diagnostics of detachment of the retina by means of ultrasound. Acta Ophthalmol. 35: 461–467 (1957).
11. Postlewait, R.W. & Durhan, N.C. Arch. Surg. Vol. 101 (1970).
12. Poujol, J. Echographie en ophtalmologie. Paris: Centre National d'Ophtalmologie des Quinze-Vingts (1981).
13. Sampaolesi, R. Ultrasonidos en oftalmologia. Buenos Aires: Editorial Medica Panamericana (1984).
14. Sherman, S.E. Evaluacion de la sutura de Dexon en cirigia oftalmica. Ann. Ophthalmol. 7: 579 (1975).
15. White, R.H. & Parks, M.M. Polyglycolic acid sutures in ophthalmic surgery. Am. Acad. Ophthalmol. Otolaryngol. (1974).

Address for correspondence: C/Homero 40, 2° 1ª, 08023 Barcelona, Spain.

48. Ultrasound elaboration
Our position and results

L. FALCO, F. ANDREUCCETTI & S. ESENTE

(Florence, Italy)

Abstract. The authors present the results of ultrasound elaboration oriented towards vitreo-retina pathologies of the eye. The statistically processed data are presented and discussed to highlight the opportunities that this method can offer.

Introduction

We have further modified our previously described system for processing echographic signals [1–3]. The modification was required in order to facilitate comparison of results obtained. In fact, comparison of the data as presented previously was difficult: there was no clear typical pattern of the curves obtained in the single diseases, so it seemed that there were no typical patterns in the echographic tracings of the various diseases.

It was precisely this difficulty in comparing tracings that prompted us to make further changes in the system to obtain curve patterns, expressed with the 'best-fitting' method in two distinct lines correlated to numerical values that express their respective patterns. This representation, which is simply a different way of presenting the elaborated tracing, seems to distinguish similar tracings more effectively, leading to easier comparison and simplifying the diagnosis.

Materials and methods

We did not modify the acquisition system, the selection of the B-scan image vector or the FFT of the selected details as regards graphic representation, as described in previous papers [1–3]. Prior to this modification, the monitor showed four windows, which were utilized as follows: the first was the vector deduced from the frozen B-scan image; the second was the 'zoomed' detail of the selected marker on the vector; the third was the elaboration of the market selected with the FFT, and the fourth window was unused and empty. Our modification fills up the fourth window to show the mean of the spectral analysis. We divided the available space in the window into two parts, from 0 to 5.5 MHz and from 5.5 to 11 MHz.

P. Till (ed.), Ophthalmic Echography 13, pp. 399–401.

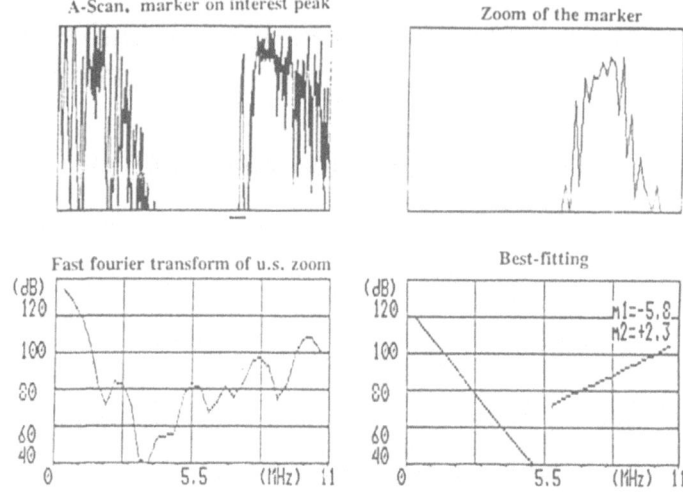

Fig. 1. Vitreal membrane structure.

We selected the 'best-fitting linear' method for the graphic representation of the spectral analysis pattern. This method's results are in the form of a straight line with a given angular coefficient. The value of the angular coefficient is shown on the right side of the window and is expressed as a numerical value with reference to each section of the line. The purpose of this representation is to obtain a simplified survey, based only on numbers as opposed to the dispersion of data as provided by spectral analysis.

Results

This new representation of the elaborated tracing has always been aimed at tracings of known diseases. In fact, interpreting a tracing represented by a new method is extremely easy when we know the pathological significance of the original image. For this reason we processed known pictures of vitreo-retinal diseases in spectral analysis is of the pathological vector derived from the B-scan image. In fact, we elaborated ophthalmoscopically known and unknown images of the vitreo-retinal membrane structure to define their characteristics in spectral analysis and according to the 'best-fitting' method.

At the beginning we were extremely enthusiastic. Subsequently the rough analysis of the data obtained did not reveal significant differences in the numerical values obtained from the patterns of the two lines as obtained with the 'best fitting' method. Therefore we processed the data in a different manner to see whether the system could yield adequate results. Later, after a different type of data analysis we noticed the difference between the numerical values for the two membranous structures. In fact the vitreal membranous structure's numerical value was greater for both the positive

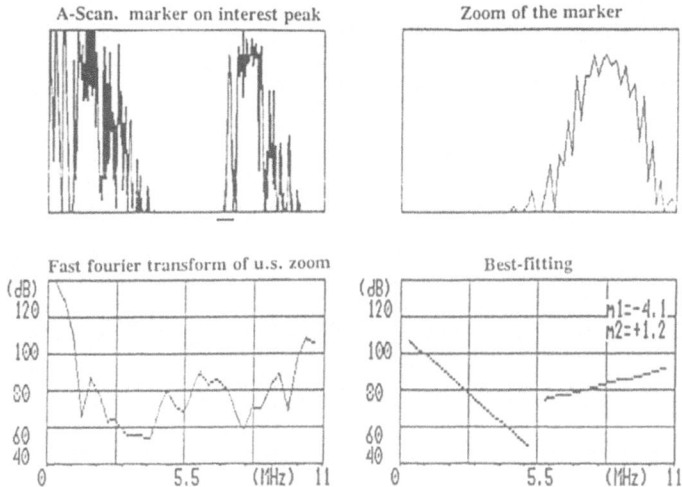

Fig. 2. Retinal membrane structure.

and negative components (Fig. 1) as compared to the best-fitting for the retinal membrane structure (Fig. 2). Although this casual objectivity does not prove the validity of the processing and presentation method, it does provide some positive outlooks for the future.

We are aware of the fact that, because of continued modifications to the system, we have not produced a statistically significant survey, and this is also partly the result of the difficulty in obtaining a relevant number of patients. We are hopeful that this latest modification will be able to provide statistically valid data. Currently, the research program calls for the acquisition of more data to analyse, comparison with other examiners and a statistical analysis of the data themselves.

References

1. Falco, L. & Andreuccetti, F. Analisi computerizzata del segnale ecografico: nostra esperienza. II Congresso Società Italiana di Ecoftalmologia, Catania, 1987. Proceedings: Clin. Ocul. 4: 257–259 (1988).
2. Falco, L., Andreuccetti, F., Esente, S., Passarelli, N., Mazzeo, V., Perri, P., Reibaldi, A. & Avitabile, T. Computerized analysis of echo signals: multicentric experience. In: Sampaolesi, R. (ed.), Ultrasonography in Ophthalmology 12. Doc. Ophthalmol. Proc. Ser. 53: 483–486. Dordrecht: Kluwer Acad. Publ. (1990).
3. Falco, L., Andreuccetti, F. & Esente, S. Nuovi sviluppi nell'elaborazione dell'immagine ecografica: note tecniche. III Contresso Società Italiana di Ecoftalmologia, Naples, 1988. Proceedings: Clin. Ocul. 5: 404–405 (1989).

Address for correspondence: Ophthalmology Centre, Corso Italia 2, I-50123 Florence, Italy.

PART FIVE

Anterior segment

49. Echographic evaluation of experimental cataractogenesis in rabbits by radio frequency signal

F. CENNAMO, G. CENNAMO, T. LIBONDI, G. IACCARINO,
N. ROSA & G. AURICCHIO

(Naples, Italy)

Abstract. X-ray irradiation and a galactose diet are two of the main approaches to experimental cataractogenesis that provide a useful model for examining the changes in the lens compared to human cataract. We measured the lens thickness in six sibling New Zealand rabbits with an RF signal, before and after irradiation and a galactose diet. In this paper we discuss our results and the importance of ultrasonic evaluation with an RF signal, to discover the early stages of cataract, before the appearance of lens opacities.

Introduction

In nuclear or cortical opacities of the lens the sound speeds are different. In human cataracts there is an increased sound speed in lenses with nuclear opacities, while there is a decreased sound speed in lenses with cortical opacities [2–8]. This difference is related to their different biochemical compositions: in nuclear cataracts there is an increased number of insoluble proteins, associated with a normal or reduced water content, while in cortical cataracts there is an increase in water content and a decrease in protein.

On the basis of these results we evaluated changes in sound speed along the optical axes of lenses in two types of experimental cataracts. This approach allowed us to verify a possible correlation between different pathogenetic mechanisms and the behavior of the sound speed in these lenses.

Material and methods

For this experimental study, we utilized six sibling four-week-old New Zealand rabbits. Three were X-ray irradiated with a single 2200 rad dose in the left eye. It has been demonstrated that in this way [4] the non-irradiated eye receives less than 50 rad, so that we could utilize the right eye of these three rabbits as a control group. The other three rabbits were fed with 20% galactose in water. The amount of the given galactose was 70 g pro die [5]. We examined the eyes of the six rabbits utilizing:
1. a Sonometric Ophthalmoscan 200 with a 15 MHz probe;
2. a data precision D 1000 pre-amplifer;
3. a data 6000 analog–digital converter; and
4. an IBM, AT personal computer 30 Mbyte hard disk.

P. Till (ed.), Ophthalmic Echography 13, pp. 405–410.

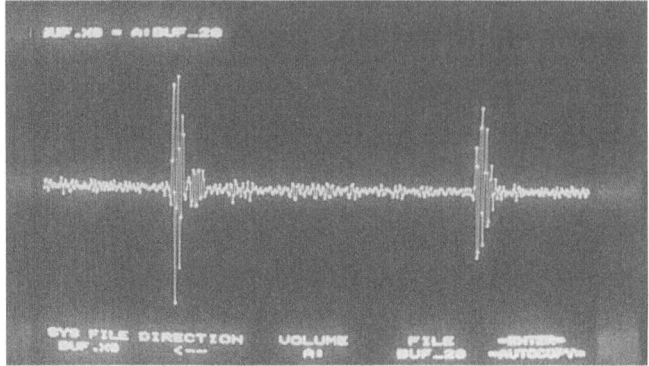

Fig. 1. RF signal obtained in a rabbit's lens with mild opacities.

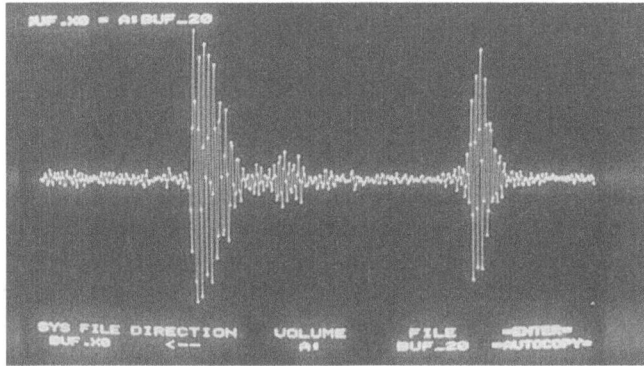

Fig. 2. RF signal obtained in a rabbit's lens with marked opacities.

Using a radio-frequency (RF) signal (Figs 1 and 2), we measured the lens thickness in microseconds with an immersion technique utilizing Ossoinig's immersion scleral shells [7]. Before the measurements, the rabbits were anesthetized with a mixture of ketamine-xylazine and their pupils were dilated with cyclopentolate and tropicamide. With more precision, we used two immersion shells (Fig. 3) in order to examine the lenses inside the focused zone of the beam.

We measured the lens thickness of the rabbits on galactose diets seven times: at the beginning of the experimental study, and 5, 12, 14, 20, 30 and 38 days after the diet started. The X-ray-treated lenses were measured at the same time as the previous ones, and again 45 days after irradiation. The final evaluation was performed in microseconds to indicate any difference in sound speed that could be related to the biochemical compositions of the lenses.

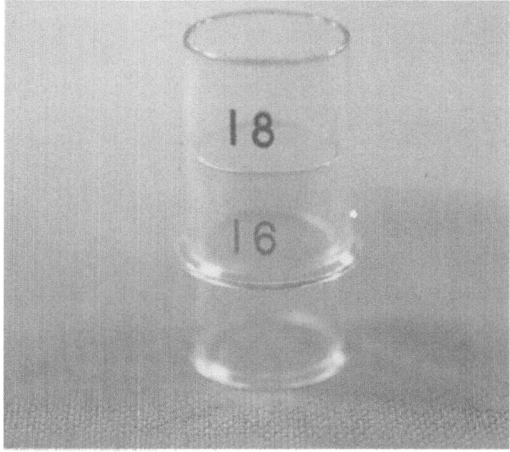

Fig. 3. Two immersion scleral shells. In this way the lens was inside the focused zone of the ultrasonic beam.

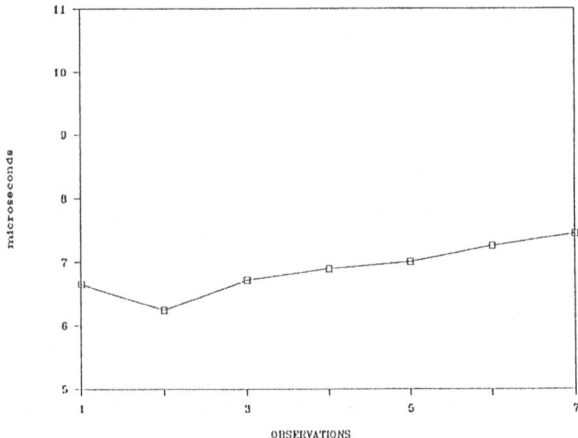

Fig. 4. Growth curve in case of normal rabbit's lens.

Results

The normal growth of the rabbit's lens (Fig. 4) points out that in the beginning there is a mild decrease in lens thickness followed by a moderate gradual–constant growth of the lens. This development seems to be the same as the human lens [3]. In the lens of the rabbits on galactose diets (Fig. 5) it is possible to point out a difference in lens growth because there is a mild increase in the growth curve a few days after the first administration of galactose. Later on, growth slows until the thirtieth day, at which point there is a sudden and marked increase in the growth curve of the lens. In an X-

408

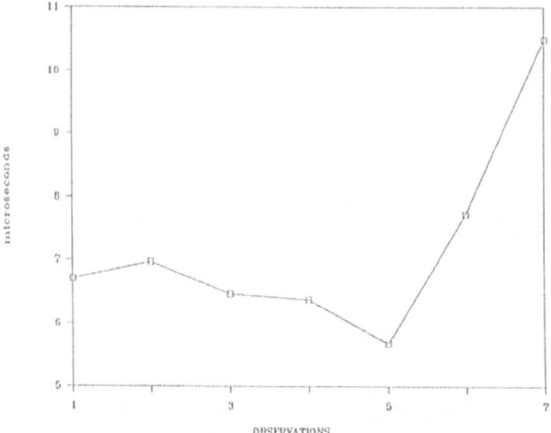

Fig. 5. Growth curve of the lens in rabbit on galactose diet.

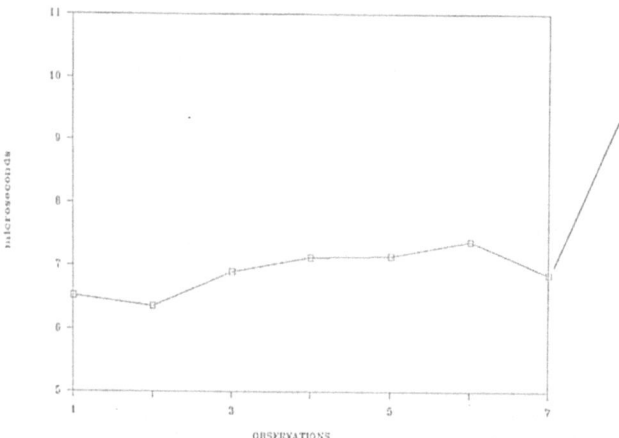

Fig. 6. Growth curve obtained in X-radiated rabbit's lens.

ray-induced cataract (Fig. 6) there is the same growth of normal lenses in the beginning, then a sudden and marked decrease in the growth curve around the fortieth day. The rabbits on galactose diets presented total cataracts six weeks after irradiation. In the irradiated rabbits mild lens opacities appeared three weeks after irradiation and total cataracts eight weeks after irradiation.

Discussion

Several studies have indicated that X-ray-induced cataracts in rabbits gives, among other phenomena an increase in membrane permeability with alteration of the Na/K ATPase with fiber hydration and destruction.

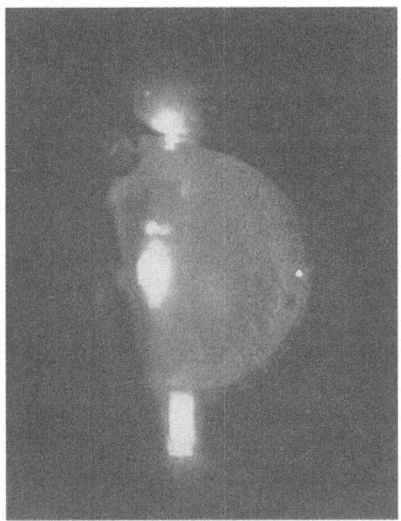

Fig. 7. Rabbit's cataractous lens at the slit lamp.

In galactose-induced cataracts there is an accumulation of dulcitol, the correspondent sugar-alcohol with an increase in lens water content, and finally osmotically induced cataracts. The exact mechanism of X-ray-induced cataracts is not well known. There is an impairment of membrane-permeability, together with disturbance of antioxidative mechanisms and the appearance of lens aggregates. This kind of mechanism may also be involved in human cataractogenesis. Senile nuclear cataract is characterized by macromolecular lens aggregates. In at least some types of human cataracts, membrane permeability and antioxidative mechanisms are also involved [1].

From our results it is possible to point out three different considerations. In the first one (within five days of the beginning of treatment) there is a difference in the behavior of lenses in the two groups. In particular, there is a decrease in the sound speed in the lenses of galactose-treated rabbits, while there is an increase in sound speed in the X-ray-irradiated lenses. Later on, although at different times, there is a coincidence of the phases between the X-ray-treated and galactose diet lenses. We saw increases of various degrees in the lens sound speeds, followed by a phase with a marked reduction in sound speed. In this phase a total intumescent cataract was present in both groups. We would like to point out that in a late stage we had the same kind of opacities (intumescent lens), even if different pathogenetic mechanism are involved.

By means of our method we were able to see the initial increase of the curve in galactose lenses at the beginning of the diet. At the end of the experiment when cataracts had developed (Fig. 7) different sound speeds in treated and control lenses were observed in both groups.

These preliminary data indicate that further studies to quantitate these differences would be worthwhile.

410

References

1. Auricchio, G. & Testa, M.: La patogenesi della cataratta. Redazione al 51 Congresso Nazionale della Società Oftalmologica Italiana 25–27/10/1986.
2. Bonavolontà, A., Cennamo, G., Rosa, N., Arienzo, G. & Corvino, C. Controlled clinical evaluation of bendazac lysine in senile cataract: comparison of different test proceedings. XXV International Congress of Ophthalmology. Roma 4–10/5/1986.
3. Cennamo, G., Rosa, N. & Daponte, P. Studio ecografico del cristallino catarattoso. Proceedings 2nd IACCR Int. Congress, Cefalù 17–19/10/1986.
4. Giblin, F.J., Chakrapani, B. & Reddy, V.N. High molecular weight protein aggregates in X-ray induced cataract. Exp. Eye Res. 26: 507–509 (1978).
5. Kinoshita, Jin H., Merola, L.O. & Dikmak, E. Osmotis changes in experimental galactose cataracts. Exp. Eye Res. 1: 405–410 (1962).
6. Loffredo, A., De Lellis, A. & Cennamo, G. Ultrasound velocity in different types of lens opacities. In J.S. Hillman and M.M. Le May (eds.), Ophthalmic Ultrasonography. Doc. Ophthalmol. Proc. Ser. 38. The Hague: Dr. W. Junk (1984).
7. Ossoinig, K.C. Standardized echography: basic principles, clinical applications and results. Intern. Ophthalmol. Clinics, 19: 127 (1979).
8. Pallikaris, I. & Gruber, H. Determination of sound velocity in different forms of cataracts. In J.M. Thijssen and A.M. Verbeek (eds.), Doc. Ophthalmol. Proc. Ser. 29: 165–169. The Hague: Dr. W. Junk (1981).

Address for Correspondence: Department of Computer Science, University of Naples, Via Claudia 21, I-80125 Naples, Italy.

50. Corneal thickness measured by ultrasound
A study of its variation with or without contact lens use

E. MORAGREGA, P. GARCIA-REZA & C. VELASCO

(Mexico City, Mexico)

Introduction

Day by day refractive surgery is being performed more frequently, and it is imperative to have a reliable measurements of the corneal thickness of our patients, in order to achieve a good post-surgical results. At the beginning we had only optical pachymetry, but since 1983 we have used ultrasonic devices to measure not only central corneal thickness but also paracentral and peripheral thicknesses. We believe that it is more reliable to use ultrasonic pachymetry to make the surgical plan for the depth of incisions in radial keratotomy, calibrating the diamond knife according to the thickness so measured, according to the papers presented at SIDUO X.

We believe that the thickness of the cornea could change according to the time of day, or between different days, and could lead to unpredictable errors in the radial keratotomy. We know from the Perk study that is the same to perform pachymetry in the operating room or days before, but this study was only made in central cornea.

With these data, we have studied changes in corneal thickness in central, paracentral and peripheral areas, in a normal population, and in contact lens users.

Material

We used a DGH 2000 ultrasonic pachymeter, an A-scan probe of 20 MHz with a sound velocity of 1640 m/sec, with a sample of 200 human eyes from the hospital of the Association to Prevent Blindness in Mexico. The three categories of patients are shown in Table 1.

Method

In Group I we measured each cornea upon first visit, and the second measurement 48 hours later. In Groups II and III, we measured each cornea during the first visit immediately after taking out the contact lens, and a second measurement 48 hours after discontinuing its use. Previous installation of

P. Till (ed.), Ophthalmic Echography 13, pp. 411–413.

Table 1. Sample details

Group	No. of eyes	Optic correction	Male	Female	Age min-max	Age mean
I	100	None	52	48	14–44	29.2
II	50	Hard contact lens	16	34	12–51	28.5
III	50	Soft contact lens	30	20	14–42	25.1

Table 2. Central corneal thickness, 200 eyes

Minimum	472 μ		
		Mean	547 μ
Maximum	609 μ		

topical anaesthetic drops (proparacaine), we use the optical center marker, to mark the 3 mm ring of paracentral measurement, always measuring in the same place. In the three groups, we also measured corneal thickness in the central portion, paracentral at 3 mm at three-hour intervals, and in periphery at 10 mm in the same meridians.

Results

The central corneal thickness in our population are reported in Table 2, and results obtained are given in Tables 3, 4 and 5.

We can see that in the non-contact lens users the corneal thickness in

Table 3. Results of Group I

		+001 μ		
	56 eyes		Mean	+007 μ
		+021 μ		
100 eyes			(central cornea)	
		−001 μ		
	44 eyes		Mean	−005 μ
		−013 μ		

Paracentral and periphery were the same

Table 4. Results of Group II

	−007 μ			
50 eyes		Mean	−034 μ	Central
	−055 μ			
			−019 μ	Paracentral
			−001 μ	Periphery

Table 5. Results of Group III

50 eyes	−007 μ			
	−048 μ	Mean	−028 μ	Central
			−022 μ	Paracentral
			−021 μ	Periphery

central, paracentral or periphery did not change in a statistically significant way, but in Group II, all corneas became thinner 48 hours after removal of the contact lens, but only in the central and paracentral portions; the periphery remained the same because this portion is not covered by a mobile small hard contact lens. In Group III all the corneas became thinner in the central, paracentral and peripheral portions because the whole cornea is covered by the soft contact lens.

With these results, we can consider that: (1) In patients who are not contact lens users, it is possible to perform ultrasonic pachymetry at any time before surgery; (2) In contact lens users, pachymetry needs to be performed at least 48 hrs after discontinuing contact lens use; and (3) Failure of radial keratotomy due to inaccurate corneal thickness measurement, could be the result of inadequate rest after contact lens use.

Address for correspondence: Hospital of the Association to Prevent Blindness in Mexico, Vicente Garcia Torres nr. 46, Mexico 04030 D.F., Mexico.

51. Corneal graft and echography

G. CENNAMO, A. LOFFREDO, N. ROSA, A. PEZONE & E. GUIDA
(Naples, Italy)

Abstract. The authors describe the role of a complete echographic examination with standardized echography before performing corneal graft surgery. During the examination it is important to establish vitreo-retinal conditions. When it is impossible to examine the anterior segment with a slit lamp, it is crucial to perform a careful examination of the anterior segment with echography, utilizing the immersion scleral shells according to K. Ossoinig.

Introduction

Before performing a penetrating keratoplasty (PK), it is crucial that the condition of the receiving eye is carefully studied. The results obtained from a complete echographic examination can influence the indications and prognosis of the implant. Echography can be performed in simple cases, but it is even more important when a triple procedure is planned and when it is impossible to evaluate the anterior segment with a slit-lamp examination (Fig. 1). In these cases echography allows the evaluation of vitreoretinal disease, but sometimes can be very useful for the study of the anterior segment.

It is difficult to calculate the IOL power in the case of a triple procedure. The three variables utilized for IOL calculations are axial eye length (AEL) post-operative anterior chamber depth and keratometry (K). The K value more influences the IOL calculation in this case, because there are only small changes in pre- and post-operative AEL and anterior chamber depth measurements.

To predict the post-operative corneal power, several methods have been proposed: recently Salam Eddin et al. [1] suggested that the corneal power of the donor globe is measured after an injection of ringer lactate solution into the vitreous chamber until the globe was felt to became firm. The post-operative K can then be calculated using the formula $K_2 = K_1 + 6\%\ K_1$, where K_1 is the pre-operative K value, and K_2 is the post-operative one. This formula can only be used when a 7.5 mm corneal button obtained from a donor globe is applied to a receiving bed 7 mm in diameter and the receiving bed is not heavily scarred, otherwise the authors advise that a penetrating keratoplasty and ECCE are performed, followed by a PC IOL when post-operative K values have been stabilized.

P. Till (ed.), Ophthalmic Echography 13, pp. 415–420.

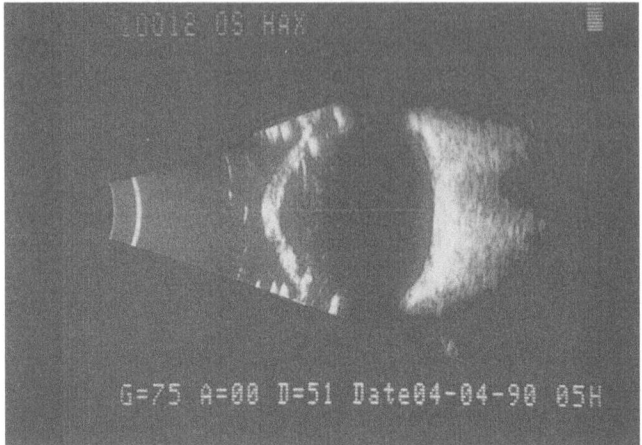

Fig. 1. Axial B-scan in one case of dense corneal leucoma showing a thick cornea, in which is evident the absence of the lens.

In our opinion this method does not allow the prediction of the post-operative K value for several reasons. First of all, to have a steady intraocular pressure (IOP) in an enucleated eye is very difficult; moreover, the difference in the diameters of the donor corneal button and the recipient bed will give unpredictable values for a different healing. Some surgeons use the pre-operative K of the operated or fellow eye in their formula. Others use average K values derived from their own series on the assumption that there is no correlation between pre- and post-operative K values [2–4].

Material and methods

In this retrospective study we evaluated the importance of echographic examinations in case of corneal graft and the K value that has to be used in case of triple procedure. For this reason we measured the post-operative K values in 40 eyes that had undergone penetrating keratoplasty in which the same diameters for the donor button and the receiving bed had been used. All these patients had undergone a complete echographic examination before the PK was performed.

Twenty-four males and 16 females were observed in our study; their ages ranged from 21 to 55. They underwent a PK in 24 cases for a keratoconus, in 8 cases for a herpes virus keratitis, in 4 cases for eye injuries, in 4 cases for bullous keratitis. The K values were evaluated after suture removal, and at least nine months after the surgery.

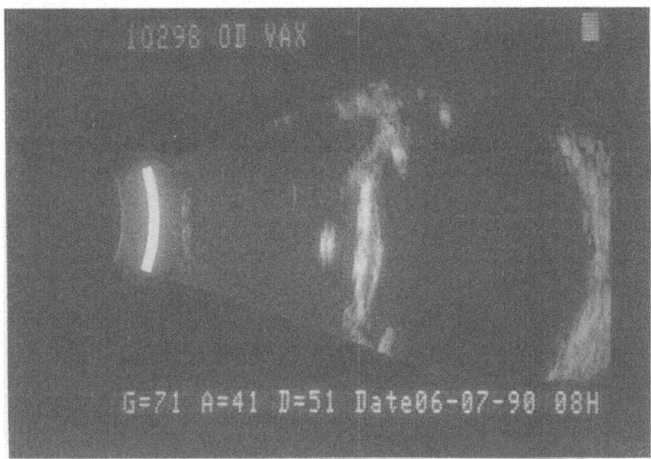

Fig. 2. B-scan showing a very thin lens.

Results

Our results indicate an average post-operative K value of 7.7 mm after suture removal; 76% of the values were in the range 7.4 and 8 mm, 16% less than 7.4 mm and 8% more than 8.0 mm.

Discussion

These results suggest, in the case of a triple procedure, the use of a K value of 8 mm in the calculation of IOL power. In this way if the *K* value is 7.4 mm for a standard AEL of 23.5 mm, a post-operative error of -3.5 D will be found. This is still a very good value for a comfortable near vision in 76% of cases. Only in 16% we will have a superior myopia, and in 8% we could have mild hyperopia.

In our experience, it is important to perform a complete examination of the globe with standardized echography before a PK in order to rule out the presence of vitreoretinal disease. Moreover, it may sometimes be very useful to evaluate the anterior segment with the immersion technique, utilizing Ossoinig immersion scleral shells. In this way it is possible to show the anterior segment with the A- and B-scan technique [5].

To achieve better healing in cases of dense corneal leucomas, it is very important to know the corneal thickness to trephine the cornea at a site where the thickness is normal. To be sure to trephine in normal thickness cornea, we can change the diameter of the receiving bed or we can perform an excentric trephination. The thickness of the cornea at the corneal apex can be measured with a standardized A-scan with immersion technique and at 3 and 4 mm from the apex with an ultrasonic pachymeter.

418

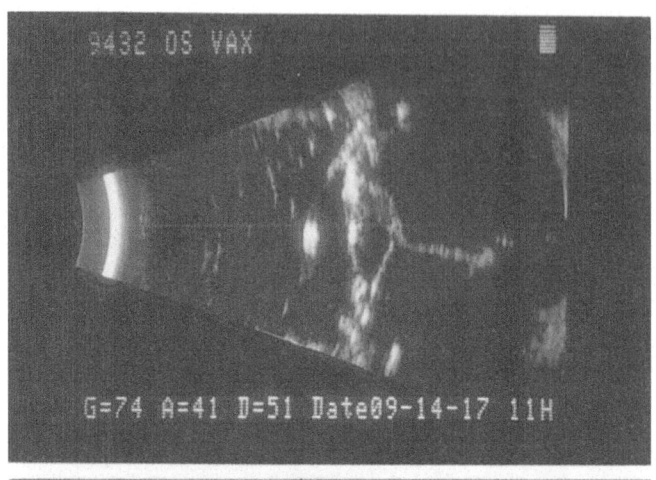

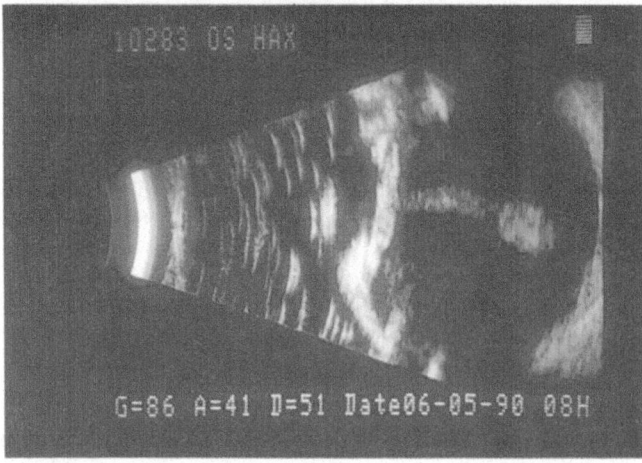

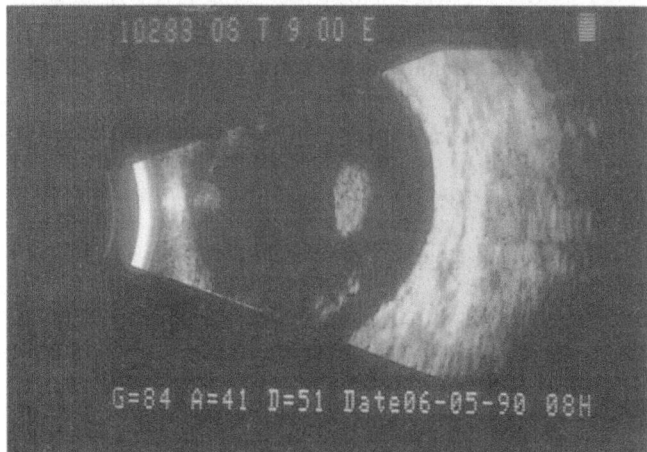

Fig. 3. Axial B-scan in two cases (A, B) with rupture of the lens posterior capsule showing lens material in the vitreous cavity. In (C) the nucleus of the lens in the vitreous cavity is displayed.

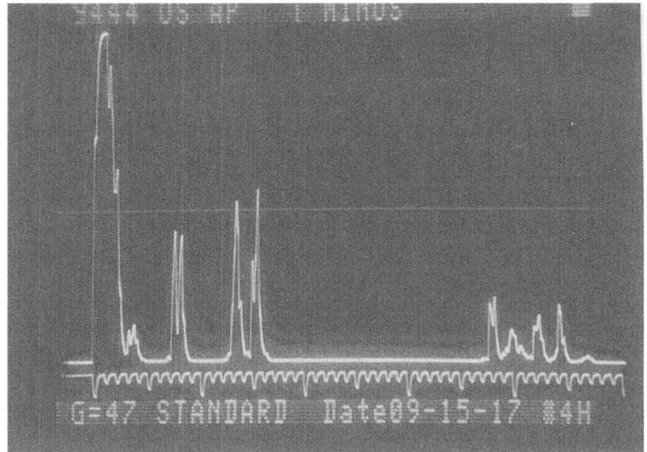

Fig. 4. Axial A-scan obtained with immersion technique. To obtain a better display of the peaks from the anterior and posterior surface of the cornea, anterior and posterior surface of the lens, and from the retina, T-20 sensitivity is used.

An irregular anterior chamber depth can suggest the presence of a plastic uveitis with anterior synechiae. These latter are better evaluated with the immersion B-scan technique. Immersion A-scan technique give us more information on lens conditions such as lens opacity or zonular lesions. In cases of phakodonesis, brief movements of the lens will be displayed on the screen as a trumbling of the spike from the anterior surface of the lens. Moreover in traumatized eyes, with standardized echography, it is also possible to identify dislocation of the lens, changes in volume, and lens shrinkage (Fig. 2).

In a lens with normal thickness and cataract opacities, an eventual rupture of the posterior capsula can be displayed (Fig. 3). This is a very important information in cases of a PC IOL when a triple procedure is planned. The A-scan immersion technique is effective in evaluating the axial eye length (AEL) (Fig. 4). Such data can be very important: a decrease in AEL, together with other echo findings such as choroidal thickening with or without calcification or vitreo-retinal membranes, can suggest the presence of a bulbar phthisis.

On the other hand an increase in AEL can be compatible with the presence of a glaucomatous lesion. Several authors have showed that an increase in intraocular pressure (IOP) during the first years of life (until 16 years) will give an increase in AEL. The presence of anterior chamber irregularities, together with a history of ocular trauma during youth, and an increase in volume in comparison with the fellow eye can suggest a glaucomatous damage even if the IOP is normal. In these cases of normal IOP the AEL measurement has a prognostic meaning for an optic nerve damage, more than B-

420

scan echography, because we can see the disappearance of the glaucomatous excavation with a normalization of the IOP.

References

1. Salah-Eddin, Amr, Abdel-Hakin & Khalil, Ahmad. Intraocular lens power calculations in the triple procedure. Br. J. of Ophthalmol. 73: 709–713 (1987).
2. Casey, T.T. Corneal grafting and intraocular lenses. In Rosen, E.S., Haining, W.M. and Arnott, E.J. (eds.), Intraocular lens implantation, p. 609. St. Louis: Mosby (1984).
3. Katz, H.R. & Forster, R.K. Intraocular lens calculations in combined penetrating keratoplasty, cataract extraction and intraocular lens implantation. Ophthalmology 92: 1203–7 (1985).
4. Musch, D.C. & Meyer, R.F. Prospective evaluation of determined formula for use in triple procedure surgery. Ophthalmology 95: 79–85 (1988).
5. Ossoinig, K.C. Standardized echography: basic principles, clinical applications and results. Intern. Ophthal. Clinics 19: 127 (1979).

Address for correspondence: Eye Department, II School of Medicine, University of Naples, Via Pansini 5, I-80131 Naples, Italy.

52. Diagnostic ultrasonography of the anterior segment of the eye

A.M. VERBEEK

(*Nijmegen, The Netherlands*)

Abstract. Because the part of the globe in direct contact with the transducer cannot be visualised (blind zone) and focused transducers have poor imaging qualities in the near sound field, diagnostic ultrasound of the anterior eye segment has been treated in a stepmotherly fashion. With a simple immersion technique we can visualize quite accurately a variety of pathologic conditions of the cornea, the anterior chamber, the iris, the lens, the ciliary body and the total eye. The B-mode information is superior to the A-mode in this method and in this part of the eye.

Introduction

The ultrasound transducer intermittently transmits sound pulses and receives the reflected energy (echo) after interaction with the tissue. The equipment cannot register echoes during the transmission of a pulse. The system is 'blind' in that short period of time and consequently the tissue in direct contact with the transducer cannot be 'seen' (a).

For optimal echographic imaging, structures must be hit perpendicular by the sound beam and must be of a certain minimal size. The structures of the anterior segment are curved and have small dimensions (b).

The mostly used B-scan transducers are focused in such a way that they give maximal axial and lateral resolution in the posterior part of the eye (c).

Because of the above-mentioned limitations (a, b, c), which result in poor imaging qualities in the near sound-field, diagnostic ultrasound is hardly used for anterior in the eye located lesions [4, 11, 13]. However, examination of the globe with an immersion technique instead of the contact method by-passes these problems. The quality of the image of the anterior segment is improved so much that it gives us detailed information on the cornea, the anterior chamber, the iris, the lens and the ciliary body with normal available A- and B-mode equipment.

Materials and methods

Instead of the time-consuming and patient inconvenient waterbath immersion method, we adapted an old and simple technique involving a contact eye cup held in position by the lids, which was used by Coleman and Ossoinig

P. Till (ed.), Ophthalmic Echography 13, pp. 421–430.

for their biometric measurements. The patient is placed in a horizontal position and after topical anaesthesia of the cornea/conjunctiva with oxybuprocaine (Novesine R 0.4%) the sclera-supported eye cup is well tolerated. The cup (perspex cylinder, well polished conical bottom circle, diameter 20–22–24 mm, height 20 mm) is filled with air-bubble-free methylcellulose 2%. The B-scan transducer is placed in a positive meniscus of the coupling agent and the globe is scanned clockwise. The instruments used are the Bronson-Turner (Storz Inc.) contact B-scan and the Ophthascan 'S' (Biophysic Medical) A/B-scan system with the normal 8 MHz A-mode and the 10 MHz B-mode transducers. The results are photographed (Polaroid film type 667) with (Ophthascan) and without magnification of the echographic picture. The examination can be performed within a few minutes without the help of extra hands.

Patients

Approximately 1200 patients per year are seen for a diagnostic ultrasound examination. Because most of the pathology is located in the vitreous cavity or the posterior segment contact A/B-scan ultrasonography alone gives satisfactory results. When the cornea is opaque, the anterior chamber is filled with blood or debris, pupillary dilatation is poor or absent, the iris/ciliary body shows a prominent lesion or the posteriorly located pathology can be related to the anterior segment, immersion ultrasonography is indicated in addition. This latter procedure was used on 10% of our patients. The indications for anterior segment ultrasonography are compiled in Table 1.

The cornea

The anterior and posterior surfaces of the normal cornea can be seen as two just separated spikes using the conventional 8 MHz A-probe. For more accurate corneal thickness measurements (such as radial keratotomy) ultrasonic pachymeters have been developed with a special designed 20 MHz transducer [5, 8]. Only the central part of a normal cornea is depicted by the 10 MHz B-scan transducer as two convex curved signals (Figs. 2AB, 3B, 4ABC). When the cornea is opaque and/or thickened (hematocornea, cornea decompensation, edema, leucoma, burned) the peripheral part and also the anterior chamber angle are visible on the B-mode image (Fig. 1A). Corneal size (micro-megalo-) and shape (keratoconus, (Fig. 2A), globus, ectasie (Fig. 1C)) can be determined, while calcium deposits, iris adherence (Figs. 1C, 3A) or retrocorneal membranes (Fig. 1D) can be seen well.

Table 1. Indications for anterior segment ultrasonography

Structure	Assessment	Path. condition
Cornea	Thickness	Corneal disease pachymetry
	Shape	Keratoconus/globus/ectasia
	Reflectivity	Calcification, foreign body
Ant. Chamber	Depth/Shape	Congenital deformities
		trauma, glaucoma lens-swelling
	Reflectivity	Blood, debris, cortex, foreign body
Iris	Shape	Trauma, bombans synechia, pup.
		reactions, ciliary body related p.a
	Reflectivity	Cyst, mass
Lens	Thickness	Accomodation
	Size, shape	Microspherophakia, 'bag' size,
		capsular integrity
	Presence	Aphakia
	Position	(sub)luxation, artif. lenstype
	Reflectivity	Cataract type, artif. lens,
		foreign body, calcification

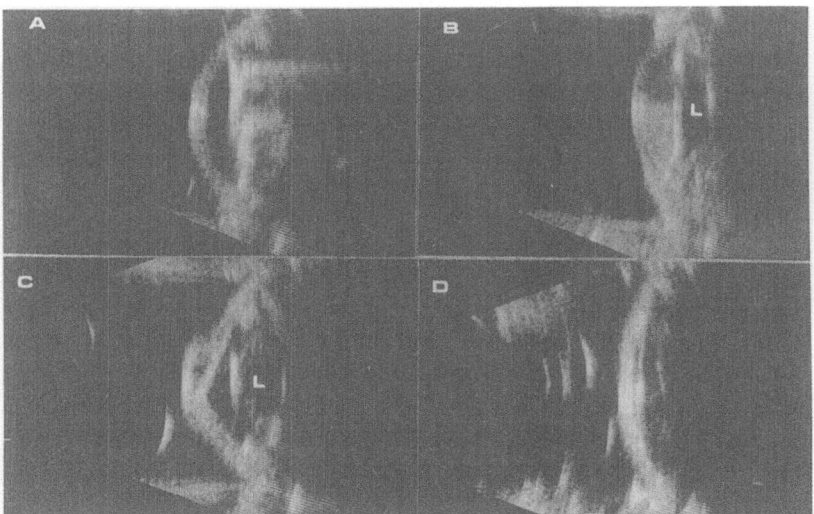

Fig. 1. Cornea All corneas thickened. *A.* Decompensated cornea after AC-IOL surgery. *B.* Hematocornea, hyphema, clear lens. *C.* Ectasia, anterior synechia, clear lens. *D.* Decompensated cornea, retrocorneal membrane, aphakia.

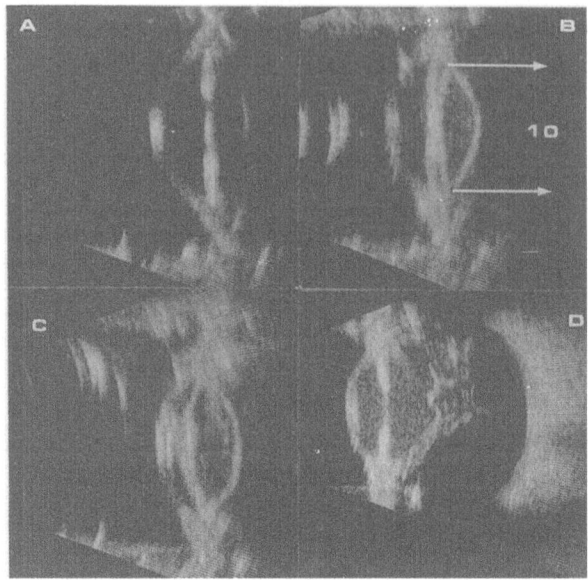

Fig. 2. *Anterior chamber* (AC), *A*. Deep AC, keratoconus. *B*. Normal AC, posterior chamber visible, capsular cataract. *C*. Shallow AC, traumatic cataractous lens, anterior lens capsule rupture, cortex in AC. *D*. Hematocornea, hyphema, aphakia, vitreous hemorrhage.

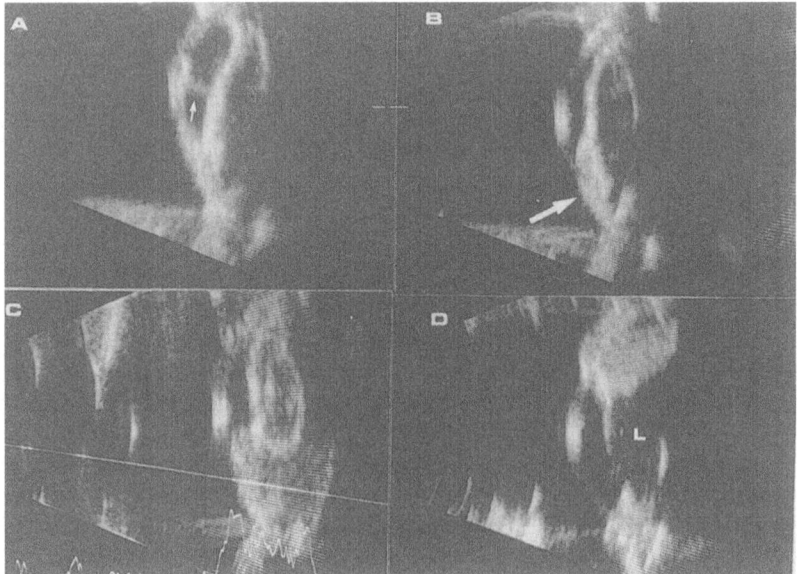

Fig. 3. *A*. Iris cyst (white arrow). *B*. Iris mass (white arrow). *C*. Iris-ciliary body mass lesion, cataract. *D*. Iris-ciliary body mass lesion with epibulbar extension (L = lens).

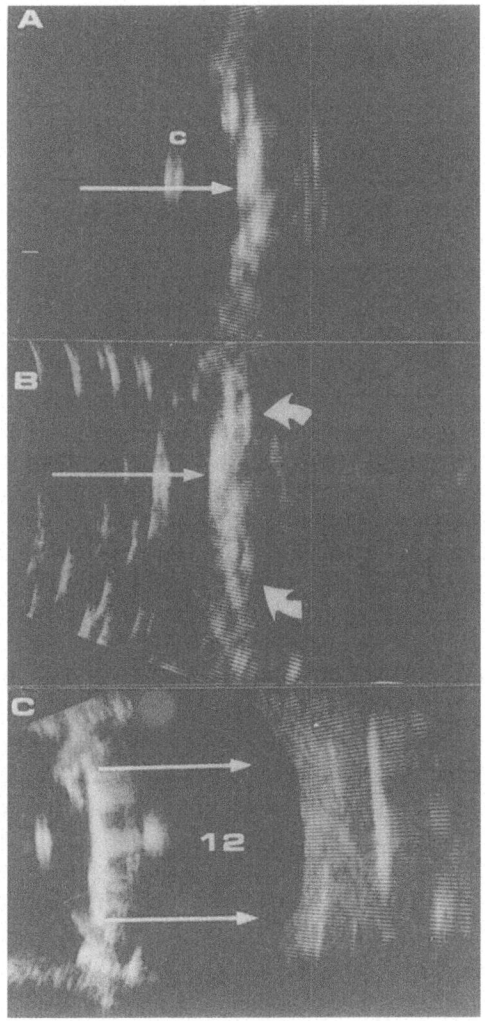

Fig. 4. Intra ocular lens types. A. Posterior chamber lens (J-loop). *B.* Irido-capsular lens (Binkhorst). Arrows point to haptics. *C.* Rota-disc lens ±12 mm diameter.

The anterior chamber (A.C.)

The anterior chamber depth (3–3.5 mm) varies with age [3], and can be measured accurately by A-mode echography. An shallow anterior chamber is easily recognizable. Between the posterior corneal and the anterior lens spike normally no echoes are visible even with very high frequencies and sensitivity settings. Blood, debris or lens cortex in the anterior chamber are clearly depicted (Figs. 1B, 2C, 2D). An impression of the angle and the likelihood of the occurrence of angle recession can be obtained while in the condition of capsular cataract even the posterior chamber can be seen (Fig. 2B).

The iris

In the normal eye, using 10 MHz transducers, the axial resolution of the system is usually insufficient to 'see' the iris separate from the lens. The pupil can be determined by finding the location where only the anterior lens capsule is visible (Fig. 2A). In aphakia this gives no problems (Fig. 2D). Then consensual pupillary reactions can be controlled when optically impossible [4]. Anterior synechiae and iris bombans can be easily demonstrated (Fig. 1C). Posterior synechiae and iridodialysis are more difficult to assess. In case of a lesion suspected for iris melanoma, the probability of dealing with pseudomelanoma is 76% [14]. With anterior segment ultrasonography we can differentiate adequately massive versus cystic and iris versus combined iris ciliary body pathology (Fig. 3).

The lens

The axial A-mode of a normal lens shows only spikes from the anterior and posterior lens surfaces (capsule) because the lens contents are homogeneous [9]. In the normal emmetropic eye the thickness varies from 3.7 to 5.0 mm [3]. In the B-scan image we see a small central convex and a larger central concave curved segment (Fig. 2A). With high-resolution echography it is possible to study accommodative changes [7]. As the cataract develops, more details of the lens are revealed on the echogram caused by acoustic heterogeneity of the lens capsule, the cortex or the nucleus (Figs. 2B, 3C). Different types of cataract can be distinguished (Fig. 5BC), and the integrity of the lens capsule can be controlled (Figs. 2C, 5D) [16].

In trauma cases in particular, the presence, dislocation or absence of the lens can be diagnosed (Fig. 2D). An estimation of the meridional size of the capsular bag can be made (Fig. 2B). Intralental foreign bodies or calcifications give rise to very strong signals followed by a reverberation 'tail' or and/or an acoustic shadow, respectively. When the patient's history is incomplete and the cornea opaque the position and type of artificial lenses can be shown [12]. A differentiation in anterior chamber, iridocapsular and posterior chamber IOL type can be made (Figs. 4ABC).

Total eye

In many pathological conditions it is largely artificial and quite incomplete to perform a contact-scan examination of the posterior segment without imaging the eventual anterior segment connections. Cyclitic membranes,

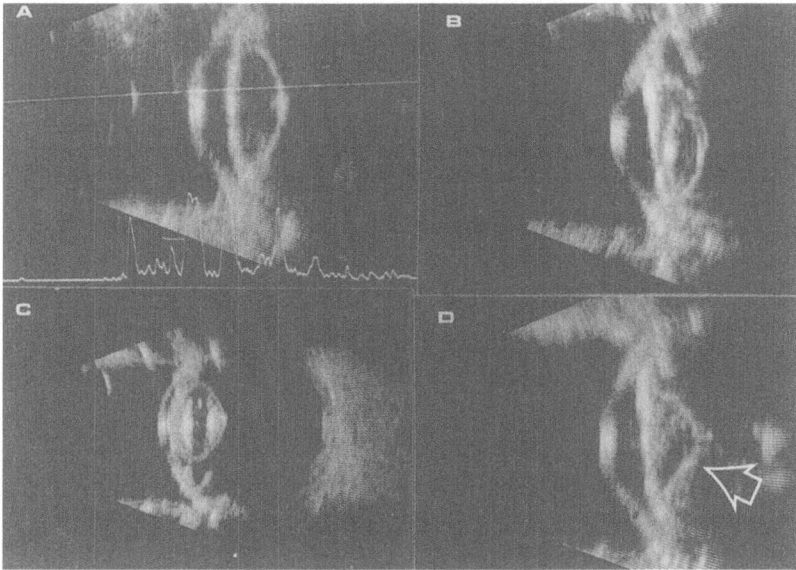

Fig. 5. Lens. A. Capsular cataract. *B.* Cataracta Morgagni. *C.* Swollen lens. *D.* Traumatic cataract with posterior capsular rupture (arrow) and foreign body.

retinal desinsertion (Fig. 6) or ciliary body detachment can be visualised much better employing an immersion technique.

Total eye imaging can help the surgeon in planning keratoprothesis operations or to find the dislocated lens in the anterior part of the vitreous. Hemorrhages or inflammations can be limited to the anterior segment or affect the whole eye. Very often just one photograph can show the referring colleague an overall picture and good idea of the most important anatomic details of his patient's eye (Fig. 6).

Discussion

Immersion echography of the eye is a well-known technique that is used mostly for biometric measurements but for diagnostic purposes its use is quite limited [2, 6]. The contact-scanners do not visualise the anterior segment and for this reason the ultrasonographic diagnostic interest for this part of the eye faded away. Calling to mind the simple technique of Coleman and Ossoinig with small modification (methylcellulose 2% filled cup instead of laborious waterbath), the author tries to promote this way of examination not for biometric but for diagnostic purposes.

The B-scan image gives easy recognisable topographic information. The acquisition of quantitative data, aiming the one-dimensional A-scan (without the guidance of the B-scan) to the area of interest, is relatively difficult.

428

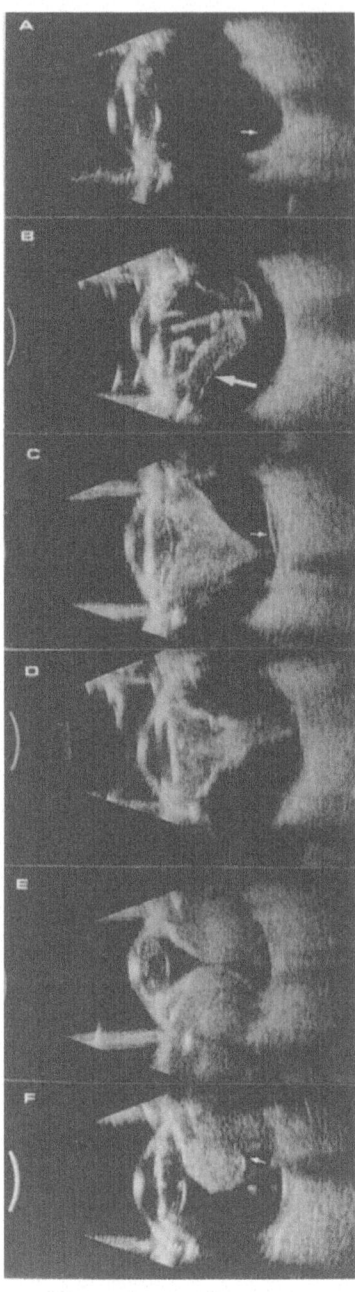

Fig. 6. Total eye. A. Staphyloma posticum. *B.* Total posterior vitreous detachment, intragel hemorrhage. *C.* Triangular posterior vitreous detachment, localised tractional retinal detachment (arrow). *D.* Funnel-shaped retinal detachment, vitreous hemorrhage. *E.* Kissing hemorrhagic choroidals. *F.* Mushroom-shaped choroidal melanoma (arrow points to break through Bruchs membrane).

The A-mode orientation in the anterior segment with strong physiological reflectors close to the pathologic conditions is limited. A combined A–B-scan with standardized vector A-scan analysis does not exist, but would give further improvement [10]; at present most quantitative data are derived from B-scan gray-scale information. For the same reasons the A-scan kinetic aspects of the echogram cannot be obtained as well as in posterior segment lesions. The lack of quantitative and kinetic information makes a further differentiation of mass-lesions hazardous also because the gross histologic architectures of the ciliary body melanoma, adenoma and leiomyoma resemble each other [15]. Until now we have been unable to differentiate these three tumours, so special care should be taken to avoid unnecessary enucleations.

The use of higher frequencies can improve the resolution of the system and will be subject to further investigation. With the immersion method we get easy interpretable (photographic) results that can help to popularize diagnostic ultrasound, which is still experienced as a difficult examination technique by many people.

References

1. Coleman, D.J. Ultrasonography of the eye and orbit, p. 101. Philadelphia: Lea-Febiger (1977).
2. Coleman, D.J. Ultrasonography of the eye and orbit, pp. 173–182. Philadelphia: Lea-Febiger (1977).
3. François, I. & Goes, F. Ultrasonographic study of 100 emmetropic eyes. Ophthalmologica 175: 321–327 (1977).
4. Guthoff, R. Ultraschall in der ophthalmologischen Diagnostik, pp. 36–37. Stuttgart: Enke Verlag (1988).
5. Kremer, B. et al. Determination of the corneal thickness using ultrasonic pachometry. Ann. Ophthalmol. 17: 506–507 (1985).
6. LeMay, M. B-scan ultrasonography of the anterior segment of the eye. Br. J. Ophthalmol. 62: 651–656 (1978).
7. Lepper, D. & Trier, H.G. Measurements of accomodative changes in human eyes by means of a high-resolution ultrasonic system. In Ossoinig, K. (ed.), Opththalmic Echography, pp. 157–162. Dordrecht: Dr. W. Junk (1987).
8. Lepper, R.D. & Trier, H.G. Optical and acoustical measurement of the corneal thickness. A study on phantoms and living human eyes. In Ossoinig, K. (ed.), Ophthalmic Echography, pp. 101–106. Dordrecht: Dr. W. Junk (1987).
9. Oksala, A. & Varonen, E.R. The echogram of the normal and opaque lens. Acta Ophthalmol. 43: 272–280 (1965).
10. Ossoinig, K.C. Standardised echography: basic principles, clinical applications and results from ophthalmic ultrasonography comparative techniques. Int. Ophthalmol. Clin. 19(4): 127–210 (1979).
11. Poujol, J. Echography in ophthalmology, p. 34. Paris: Masson (1985).
12. Scherer, U. & Rochels, R. Artefakte im A- und B-Bild-Echogramm nach Implantationen von Kunstlinsen. Ophthalmologica 187: 192–195 (1983).
13. Shields, J.A. Diagnosis and management of intraocular tumors, p. 14. St. Louis: Mosby Company (1983).
14. Shields, J.A. et al. The differential diagnosis of malignant melanoma of the iris. Ophthalmology 90: 716–720 (1983).

15. Shields, J.A. et al. Mesectodermal leiomyoma of the ciliary body managed by partial lamellar iridocyclochoroidectomy. Ophthalmology 96: 1369–1382 (1989).
16. Skalka, H.W. Ultrasonic diagnosis of posterior lens rupture. Ophthalmic Surgery 8: 72–76 (1977).

Address for correspondence: A.M. Verbeek, Department of Ophthalmology, University of Nijmegen, Philips van Leydenlaan 15, 6500 HB Nijmegen, The Netherlands.

53. Ultrasonography of the posterior lens capsule in trauma

S. CLEMENS & K.-H. EMMERICH
(*Münster, Germany*)

Abstract. The characteristics of different possible defects of the posterior lens capsule are demonstrated and discussed. Planning the implantation of an intraocular lens is facilitated by examining the posterior capsule with ultrasonography. The necessity of a vitrectomy can be foreseen.

Introduction

In 30% of perforating injuries involving the interior segment a trauma of the lens can be found (Mugar 1978). Implanting an intraocular lens during wound repair is contradicted (Oppong 1978). The implantation of an intraocular lens 6–10 days later avoids complications that may result from synechia that develop later (Fjodorov 1981). In the following cases an ultrasonographic diagnosis of the lens could be made: cataract (Okasala 1961; Metz & Bronson 1969), subluxation or luxation, wide opening of posterior lens capsule with prolapsing lens material (Coleman 1977), topography, amount of opacities, age-related changes, closed-angle glaucoma, malignant glaucoma, phacolytic glaucoma, measurement of accommodation under pharmacological influence of the ciliary muscle (Poujol 1985).

Others mention the necessity of an intact posterior lens capsule for implantation (Trinkmann & Runde 1985; Ohrloff 1982; Binkhorst 1969).

Method

In 31 cases of perforating injuries of the anterior segment after one week of primary surgery a transpalpebral examination by B- and AB-scan was performed to analyze the situation of the posterior lens capsule. Compared to the intact eye, criteria for traumatism of the posterior lens capsule have been worked out. The anterior capsule could not be examined exactly due to a flat anterior segment or contact with the iris. By shifting the probe a systematic examination of the posterior lens capsule was performed, since a rectangular impact of ultrasonic beam is a prerequisite for the analysis.

In normal cases a posterior lens capsule is a high reflecting curvilinear line. Concerning the situation of the posterior lens capsule, after cataract

P. Till (ed.), Ophthalmic Echography 13, pp. 431–435.
© 1993 *Kluwer Academic Publishers.*

432

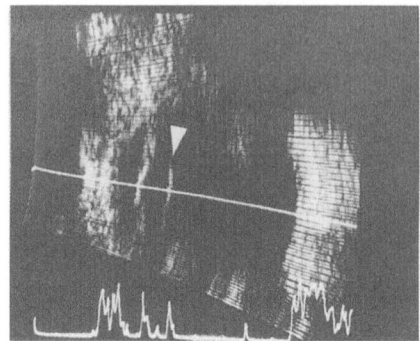

Fig. 1. Intact posterior lens capsule (arrow) after windshield injury of anterior segment.

surgery of the injured eyes, the surgeon was asked about the situation or it was predictable through the mechanism of trauma.

Results

The following criteria could be used to detect defects in the posterior lens capsule:
1. totally or partially missing curvilinear echo, especially in cases of echogenic posterior lens material;
2. steps in the curvilinear echo;
3. bending;
4. protrusion of the posterior lens capsule, eventually localized, and
5. track of lens material in vitreous.
   The following criteria could not reveal defects:
1. reflectivity within the lens;
2. thickness of the echogenic posterior lens material; and
3. flattening of the anterior chamber through forward dislocation of the iris – lens diaphragm and swelling of the lens material.
   In all situations exact analyses of the posterior lens capsule could be performed. The predicted situation was verified by the surgeon or, in cases where surgery was not necessary, by the mechanism of trauma-like intravitreal foreign body.

Cases

The first case (Fig. 1) represents the situation one week after primary surgery for windshield injury involving the cornea, iris and lens. The posterior lens capsule is intact. In a second step a posterior chamber lens was implanted.

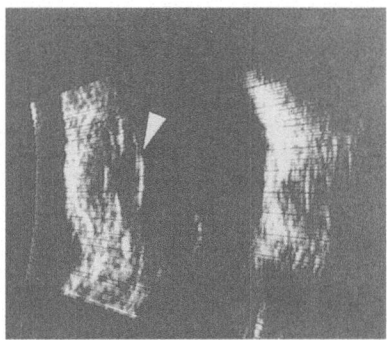

Fig. 2. Step and defect in posterior lens capsule localized after injury with wire (arrow, Tri-scan).

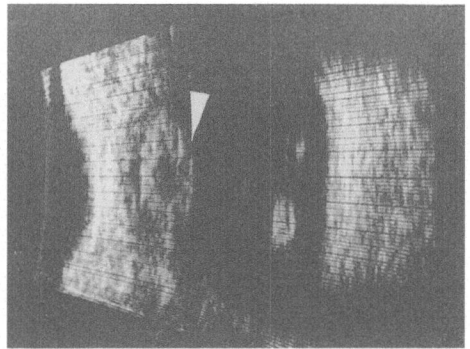

Fig. 3. Protrusion of lens material, lens capsule with large opening, intravitreal foreign body.

The second case (Fig. 2) shows a step in the posterior lens capsule after perforation by a wire that was pulled out directly after trauma. The curvilinear echo is interrupted (arrow) and a step is visible. Since the cataract did not progress, no further surgery was necessary.

The third case (Fig. 3) was a perforating injury with intravitreal foreign body of 3 mm in X-ray. Instead of a curvilinear echo a protrusion of lens material was found (arrow).

In the fourth case (Fig. 4) another intraocular foreign body was found. In the primary wound repair also to prevent retinal detachment a cerclage was laid around the equator. The posterior lens capsule is visible only in parts with steps and gaps. The implantation of a posterior chamber lens was not possible and after a lensectomy an anterior chamber lens was implanted.

The fifth case (Fig. 5) was a perforation injury with foreign body perforation of lens and track of lens material into the vitreous cavity. The linear echo is visible only in parts. In this case a lensectomy had to be performed with anterior lens implantation.

434

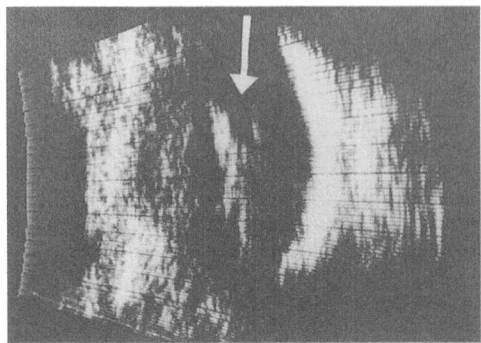

Fig. 4. Interrupted curvilinear echo, steps (arrow) after trauma with intravitreal foreign body. To prevent amotio a cerclage was laid.

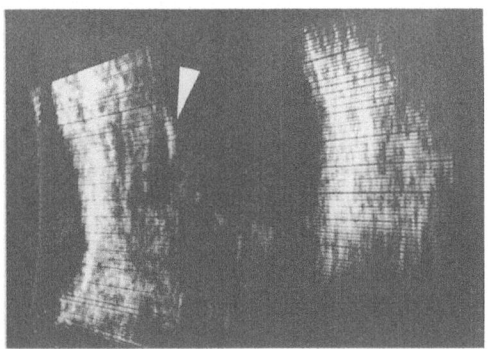

Fig. 5. Curvilinear echo of posterior lens capsule in the upper part (arrow), below track of lens material into the vitreous cavity.

Discussion

The examination has led to several criteria for predicting and analyzing the situation of the posterior lens capsule after trauma, especially in smaller defects. In all cases the predicted situation was correct, as has shown the second step surgery or the mechanism of trauma.

In cases where despite smaller defects in the posterior lens capsule a posterior chamber lens was implanted, the situation was predicted correctly. The examination by ultrasound is helpful in planning a second surgery for implantation because by slit-lamp examination the posterior lens capsule is usually not visible due to cataract. In cases of later defects of the posterior lens capsule a lensectomy with anterior vitrectomy has to be performed and, depending on the situation of the retina, an anterior chamber lens can be implanted.

When there is found to be a defect in the sclera or the retinal situation is unclear an intraocular lens should not be implanted in this situation until the retina is stable after a cryotherapy, cerclage or posterior vitrectomy.

References

1. Binkhorst, C.D., Gobin, M.H. & Leonard, P.A.M. Posttraumatic artificial lens implants (pseudophakoid) in children. Br. J. Ophthalmol. 53: 518–529 (1969).
2. Coleman, C.J., Lizzi, F.L. & Jack, R.L. Ultrasonography of the eye and orbit. Philadelphia: Lea & Febiger (1977).
3. Fjodorov, S.N., Egorova, E.V. & Zubareva, L.N. 1004 cases of traumatic cataract surgery with implantation of an intraocular lens. Am. Intraocular Implant. Soc. J. 7: 147–153 (1981).
4. Metz, G. & Bronson, N. Ultrasound appearance of senile lens changes. In Gitter, K. et al. (eds.), Ophthalmic Ultrasound. pp. 218–223. St. Louis: Mosby (1969).
5. Muga, R. & Maul, E. The management of lens damage in perforating corneal lacerations. Br. J. Ophthalmol. 62: 784–787 (1978).
6. Ohrloff, C., Dardenne, M.U., Konen, C. & Sherif, A. Erfahrungen mit den ersten 1400 Hinterkamerlinsenimplantationen nach Phakoemulsifikationen. Klin. Mbl. Augenheilk. 181: 253–256 (1982).
7. Oksala, A. Acoustic structure of the opaque and of the transparent lens. Klin. Mbl. Augenheilk. 138: 374–380 (1961).
8. Oppong, M.C., Kern, R., Schipper, J. & Käppeli, F. Zur Korrektur der traumatisch bedingten einseitigen Aphakie bei Kindern und im Erwerbsleben stehender Erwachsener mit intraokularen Linsen. Klin. Mbl. Augenheilk. 172: 431–434 (1978).
9. Poujol, J. Echography in Ophthalmology. New York – Paris: Masson (1985).
10. Trinkmann, R. & Runde, H. Zur Problematik der Doppelperforation der Linse durch intraokulare Fremdkörper. Klin. Mbl. Augenheilk. 186: 307–309 (1985).

Address for correspondence: University Eye Hospital, Domagkstrasse 15, W-4400 Münster, Germany.

PART SIX

Instrumentation

54. A newly developed A- and B-scan device for ophthalmic ultrasonography

A. SAWADA, J. FUKIYAMA, F. MARUIWA & Y. BABA

(Miyazaki, Japan)

Abstract. An A- and B-scan ultrasonic diagnostic device (US 3000, Nidek Co., Japan) has been developed, with the following important facilities: (1) alignment of vector A shown on the B-scan; (2) variability of the dynamic range in the stored B-scan, which is very useful in traumatized eyes, particularly in perforating injury; and (3) direct reading of ultrasonic reflectivity in stored vector A. The last two functions have been unavailable so far.

Introduction

For successful ophthalmic ultrasonography, specially designed ultrasonic equipment, as well as experience and skill, are essential. A- and B-scan echography have their own advantages. A-scan echography is superior to B-scan echography from the viewpoint of reflectivity evaluation, whereas B-scan echography is excellent to obtain morphological understanding. To make the best use of them in ocular diagnosis, we have recently developed a new apparatus in which A- and B-scans are combined in one unit. The new equipment has many important facilities; their clinical benefits will be discussed.

Materials and results

The equipment, US 3000, is manufactured by the Nidek Co. in Japan. Of three kinds of facilities described in the following, the last one is equipped only in very limited one.

1. Alignment of vector A is shown on the B-scan. It has been recognized that an A-scan indicates the ultrasonic reflectivity of the tissue most precisely, but the problem is that recognition of the alignment of the ultrasonic beam is not always distinct. To solve the problem, combined A- and B-scan equipment has been developed.

In the new equipment, vector A is displayed with the B-scan image at the same time, and its alignment is shown on the B-scan image. Vector A can be swung in any direction within the scanning angle. As the alignment is swept, the shape of vector A varies in concert with the quality of the B-scan

P. Till (ed.), Ophthalmic Echography 13, pp. 439–444.

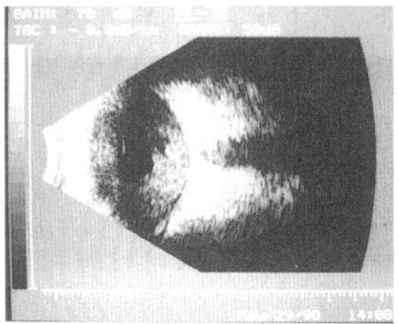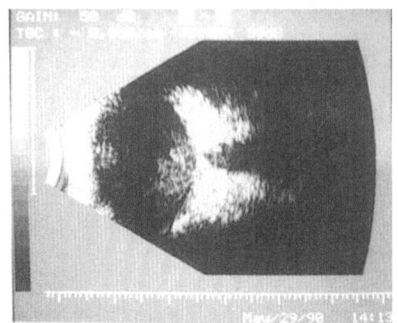

Fig. 1. (A) In a case of vitreous hemorrhage, all the signals are displayed with the gain of 70 dB and with the dynamic range of 50 dB, which is the standard setting; (B) With the dynamic range of 30 dB and with the gain of 50 dB, only stronger signals are left.

images of the tissue, through which the vector A is passing. Such variability of vector A can be maintained even after the image is stored. A function of this kind is already available in several ophthalmic diagnostic ultrasonic devices.

2. Variability of the dynamic range in the stored B-scan. Up to now it has not been possible to change the sensitivity setting after the image is stored. When a different sensitivity setting is required, other images with the desired setting need to be displayed again. Thus the examiner needs to hold the probe on the lesion as long as the scanning and recording is repeated. Sometimes this takes a long time and is not safe in ocular trauma, particularly in perforating injury. It is also difficult to reproduce exactly the same image the next time.

In the new equipment, the dynamic range and gain can be changed in the stored B-scan. After a B-mode image is stored, quantitative analysis can be done by the adequate arrangement of the dynamic range and the gain. Until now it has not been possible to change the dynamic and gain after storage in any kind of equipment. The dynamic range can be changed from 50 dB (the standard setting) down to 10 dB in steps of 10 dB. While the dynamic range is fixed, the gain can also be changed at intervals of 2 dB. The extent of gain change is dependent upon the fixed dynamic range; the gain corresponds to the window level of X-CT and the dynamic range to the window width. Both are useful in quantitative analysis of ultrasonic reflectivity.

In a case of vitreous hemorrahge, when the dynamic range is set at 50 dB, as shown in Fig. 1A, all the signals, higher and lower reflectivity, are displayed. With a dynamic range of 30 dB, all the signals are confined within the narrower dynamic range. As the gain is reduced, only stronger signals are left and the others disappear, as shown in Fig. 1B. The procedure with reduced sensitivity has been used so far by many to evaluate the ultrasonic reflectivity so precisely.

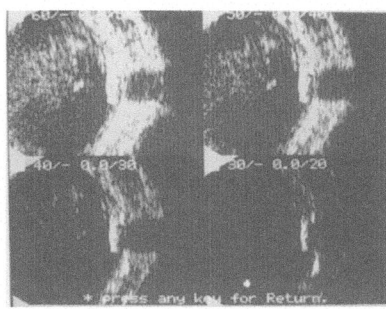

Fig. 2. A large foreign body just in front of the fundus is displayed with the standard setting. At more reduced dynamic range of 20 dB and the gain of 30 dB the foreign body signal still remains.

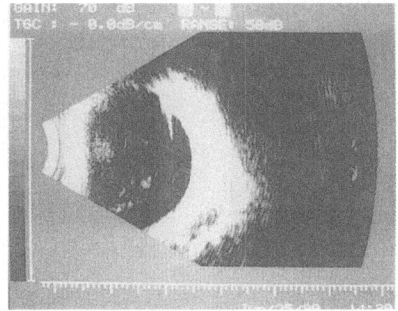

Fig. 3A. A case of vitreous hemorrhage with the standard gain and dynamic range.

The case of a foreign body is one of the best examples. After an image is stored, the dynamic range was reduced successively and the gain was reduced. By the adequate arrangement dynamic range and gain, quantitative analysis of the reflectivity is available. As shown in Fig. 2, a large foreign body is displayed just in front of the fundus structure with marked acoustic shadow at the standard dynamic range and gain. At a more reduced dynamic range of 20 dB and gain of 30 dB, the foreign body signal remains. With this facility the frequency and the time required to hold the probe on the lesion can be minimized and the ultrasonic reflectivity from the lesion can be quantitatively evaluated.

Fig. 3A shows a case of vitreous hemorrhage with the standard gain and dynamic range. Fig. 3B shows the change with reduced sensitivity. In these pictures the focus is adjusted to the stronger signals. Almost all signals in the vitreous disappeared with a gain of 30 dB and a dynamic range of 10 dB. On the other hand, when the focus is adjusted to the weaker signals, signals of a different character are produced. When the dynamic range is reduced and gain is increased, weaker signals are more strongly displayed and the

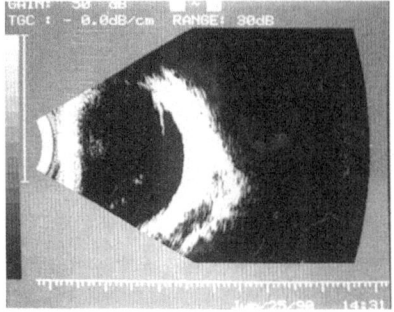 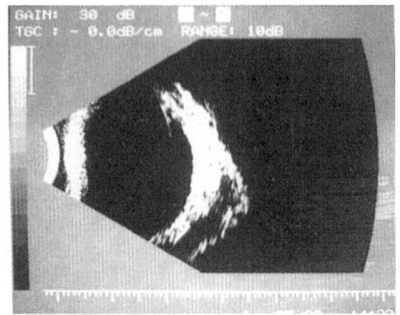

Fig. 3B. At the reduced gain and dynamic range, signals in the vitreous disappeared.

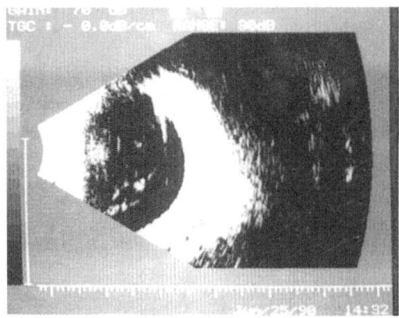 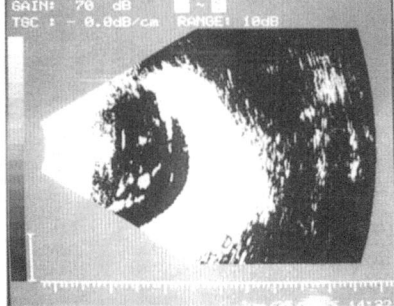

Fig. 3C. At the reduced dynamic range of 30 dB or 10 dB and at the highest gain of 70 dB weaker signals are strongly displayed.

others are overloaded, as shown in Fig. 3C. In this process weaker signals are weighted and those weaker signals which are not displayed with standard gain, are manifested. In a certain sense this is the so-called supersensitivity setting.

On the same original stored image, we can adjust the focus on either the stronger or weaker signals by shifting the gain level upwards or downwards.

3. Direct reading of ultrasonic reflectivity in stored vector A. It is not necessary here to describe the concept and significance of quantitative echography in ultrasonic tissue differentiation of the lesion. The method of performing quantitative analysis of ultrasonic reflectivity of a lesion using the newly developed equipment is as follows. The stored vector A can be enlarged and displayed with a dynamic range of 25 dB. Because the amplification is logarithmic, the reflectivity value of the ultrasonic wave to the target tissue can be read directly, as well as the value of reflectivity to the standard tissue, the sclera, using a gain variation of 2 dB difference.

The difference between them can be used in diagnosing retinal detachment and other membrane-like lesions. The results of Ossoinig (1984) and Sawada

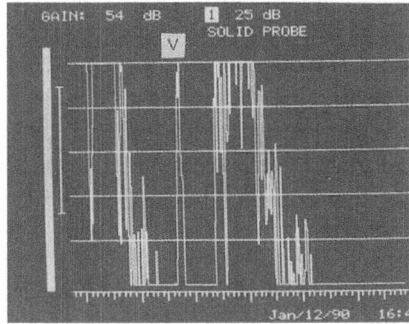

Fig. 4A. The peak (V) from vitreous hemorrhage reaches to the top line, which corresponds to the gain of 54 dB.

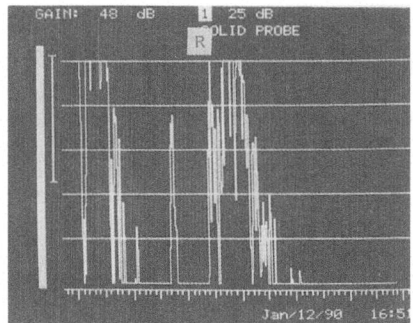

Fig. 4B. The peak (R) from the detached retina reaches to the top line, which corresponds to the gain of 48 dB.

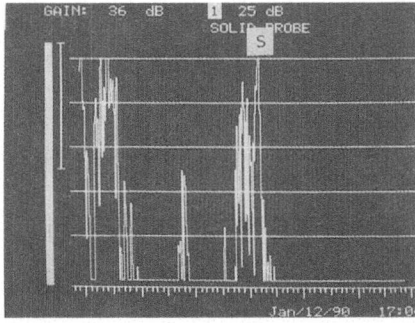

Fig. 4C. The peak (S) from the sclera reaches to the top line, which corresponds to the gain of 36 dB.

444

(1986) using the Kretztechnik 7200 MA have been used as criteria to differentiate retinal detachment from vitreous membrane formation and proliferative diabetic retinopathy. However, new criteria for using this equipment still need to be established.

Fig. 4 shows the enlarged vector A in a case of vitreous hemorrhage and retinal detachment. The highest reflectivity of a membrane-like lesion in the center of the vitreous is 54 dB in the enlarged A-mode. On the other hand, the highest reflectivity of the membranous lesion just in front of the fundus structure is 48 dB. The highest reflectivity of the sclera is 36 dB, as shown in Fig. 4C. Then the ΔdB between the sclera and the membrane in the center of the vitreous is 18, and that between the sclera and the membrane just in front of the fundus structure is 12. At the vitrectomy vitreous hemorrhage and retinal detachment with subretinal hemorrhage was found. By direct reading of ultrasonic reflectivity, the ultrasonic quantitative differentiation between vitreous membrane formation and retinal detachment, or between foreign bodies and other point-like lesions, can be done easily and exactly.

In conclusion, among three components essential to standardized ultrasonography, the two, topographic and quantitative, can be put into practice with the new equipment. The remaining kinetic evaluation can be done partly by comparing images before and after postural changes using a four-image display system, which are discussed in the separate paper in these proceedings.

Acknowledgements

The study was supported in part by Grants-In-Aid for Scientific Research C-01570978 from the Ministry of Education, Science and Culture of the Japanese Government.

References

Sawada, A. Study on ultrasonic tissue characterization of intraocular membranous structures. Acta Soc. Ophthalmol. Jpn. 90: 43–66 (1986).
Sawada, A. et al. Usefulness of simultaneous display of four different B-scan images in ocular diagnosis. This volume, Chapter 60, pp. 489–494.

Address for correspondence: Department of Ophthalmology, Miyazaki Medical College, 5200 Kihara, Kiyotake, Miyazaki, 889-16 Japan.

55. Power spectrum analysis of ultrasonic radio-frequency signals on cataracts

S. TANE, M. HASHIMOTO & Y. KIMURA

(Kawasaki, Japan)

Abstract. The ultrasonic RF signal power spectra of various types of cataract were analysed to detect differences between the types of cataract. Individual specific decreased absorption patterns were obtained in the high-frequency domains. These were considered to be helpful in the differential diagnosis of cataracts.

We have carried out Fourier's transformation of ultrasonic radio-frequency (RF) signals for the power spectrum analysis of frequency components, which could not be adequately collected by conventional methods such as A-mode and B-mode. Our subsequent experiments were done in order to gain more information and improve the diagnostic accuracy of ultrasonography in ophthalmological examination.

In the present study we applied this method to the diagnosis of lenticular diseases. Various types of cataract were subjected to power spectrum analysis, and correlations were made between the types of cataracts classified according to the difference in the pattern of lens opacities, which has conventionally been performed by slit-lamp microscopy, and the results obtained by this method. Figure 1 shows the method used.

Echo signals are transmitted vertically onto the cornea either by the immersion method or the contact method using focused PZT transducers 5 mm in diameter at 10 MHz from a St. Marianna's high-resolution ophthalmic ultrasonic diagnostic equipment. The A-mode of the lens thus obtained was converted to a radio-frequency (RF) signal using a Hitachi 650-type ocilloscope. The signal was then subjected to Fourier's transformation using a DATA 6000 type computer waveform analyzer (Universal Waveform Analyzer). Frequency power spectrum analysis was also done. These power spectrum curves were summed to obtain the average for each individual cataract type.

The number of patients examined is shown in the Table 1. In addition to 18 eyes of 18 normal persons ranging in age from 22 to 45 years, 74 eys of 74 patients with only senile cataract ranging in age from 36 to 78 years were examined in the present study. The morphology of the cataracts showed that they could be divided into three types, as shown in Table 1: subcapsular cataracts, nuclear cataracts and total cataracts.

Cases representative of each type are now described. Slit-lamp exami-

P. Till (ed.), Ophthalmic Echography 13, pp. 445–450.

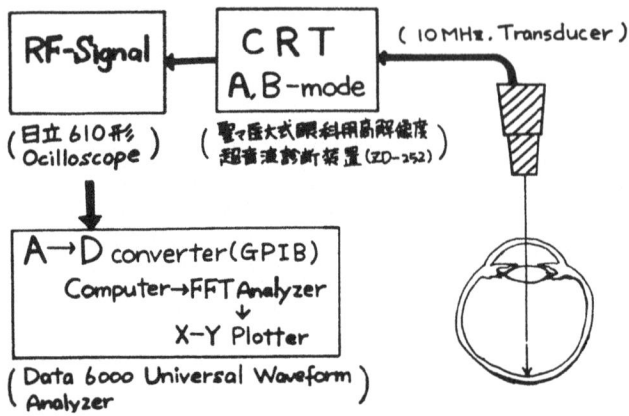

Fig. 1. Block diagram of the data acquisition system.

Table 1. The case of power spectrum analysis of ultrasonograms in cataract lesions

	Cases	Eyes
Normal eyes	18	18
Cataracta subcapsularis (Cat. capsularis)	34	34
Cataracta partialis (Cat. nuclearis)	22	22
Cataracta totalis	18	18
Total	74	74

nation findings of a normal lens observed with a Schimpfug camera in a healthy 25-year-old male subject are shown in Fig. 2A. A large transparent nucleus can be observed behind the thin bright cortical layer. In Fig. 2B are shown the B-mode, the A-mode scans, the RF signal wave pattern and the power spectrum wave pattern of the normal lens.

The A- and B-mode scans show that the lenticular parenchyma is echographically transparent and echo-free. However, ultrasonic power spectrum analysis showed a small-wave type of frequency spectrum pattern without gradient within the range −18.0 dB to −42.0 dB over the domain 11–50 MHz, as shown on the right lower part of Fig. 2B. The difference between the maximum and minimum decibel levels was about 24 dB.

The slit-lamp examination findings of the cortex and capsular cataract observed in a 62-year-old male patient are shown in Fig. 3A, and the relevant ultrasonic imaging findings are shown in Fig. 3B. The A- and B-mode scans revealed thickening of the cortex, and the RF power spectrum analysis provided a pattern showing a descending gradient within the range of

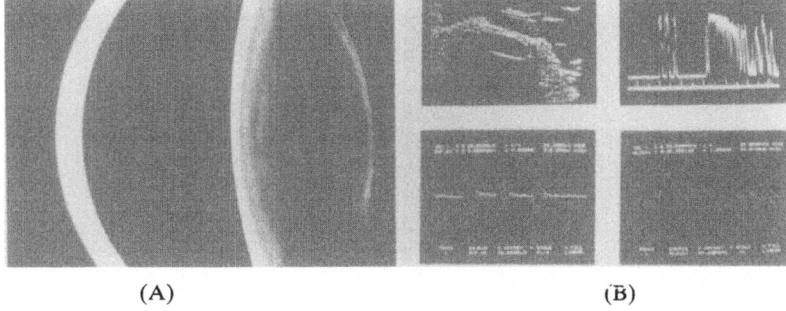

(A)   (B̄)

Fig. 2A,B. The slit-lamp examination finding of normal lens observed with a Schimpfug camera (A), and the A- and B-mode, the RF signal wave pattern and power spectrum wave pattern of the normal lens (B).

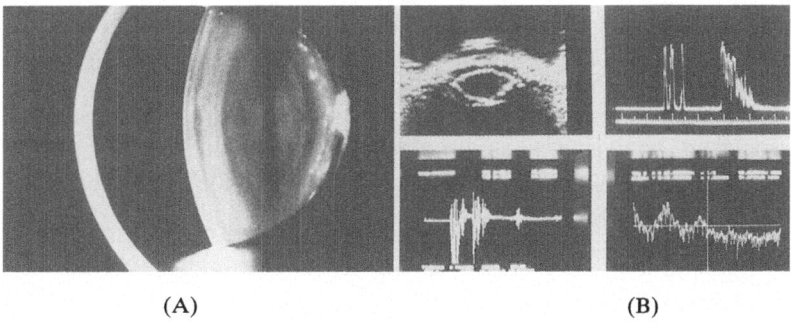

(A)   (B)

Fig. 3A,B. The slit-lamp examination finding of the cortex and capsular cataract (A), and the A- and B-mode revealed thickening of the cortex and the RF spectrum analysis (B).

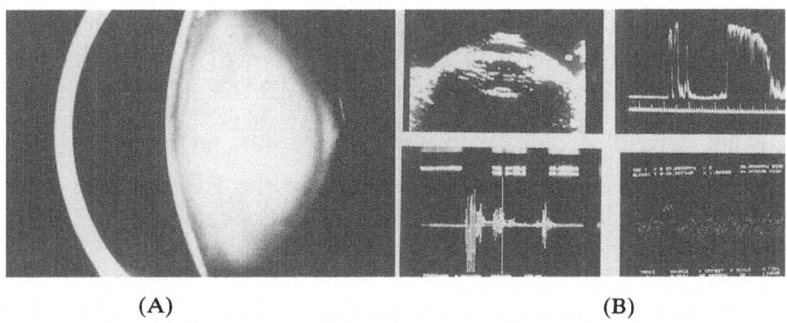

(A)   (B)

Fig. 4A,B. The slit-lamp examination finding of the nuclear cataract (A), and the A- and B-mode, the RF signal wave pattern and power spectrum wave pattern of the ultrasonogram of opacity inside the lens (B).

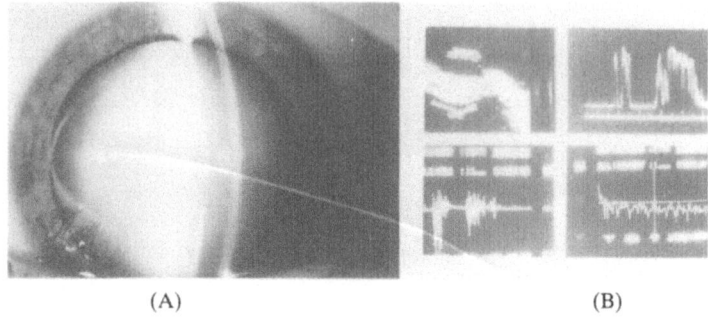

(A)   (B)

Fig. 5A,B. The slit-lamp examination finding of the total cataract (A), and the A- and B-mode, the RF signal wave pattern and power spectrum wave pattern of the ultrasonogram of total opacity of the lens (B).

−22.0 dB to −65.0 dB over the whole domain 11–50 MHz. The difference between the maximum and minimum decibel levels was about 43 dB.

Next the slit-lamp examination findings, a 55-year-old female patient with nuclear cataract are shown in Fig. 4A, and ultrasonic imaging in Fig. 4B. The A- and B-mode scans show an echo of opacity inside the lens. The RF power spectrum analysis revealed a gradient-free, small-wave RF spectrum pattern within the range of −16 dB to −62 dB throughout the domain 11–50 MHz. The difference between the maximum and minimum decibel levels was about 46 dB.

In all patients with total cataracts, the A- and B-mode scans showed an echo of opacity of the entire lens. RF power spectrum analysis revealed a gradient-free, small-wave frequency spectrum pattern within the range of −37 dB to −62 dB throughout the domain 11–50 MHz. The difference between the maximum and minimum decibel levels was about 25 dB (Fig. 5).

RF signals and RF spectrum patterns of normal eyes and eyes with each type of cataract are shown in Fig. 6. The ultrasonic RF signal spectrum patterns obtained by each summed average in the spectrum frequency domains 11–50 MHz varied for each type except for a peak at 10 MHz which occurred with the transducer used. A flat pattern of −30 dB was obtained in normal lenses, a descending pattern of −40 dB to −45 dB in cortex cataracts, a flat pattern of −40 dB in nuclear cataracts, and a flat pattern of −50 dB in total cataracts.

In particular, the intensity of reflex (dB) of the RF spectrum curves for each time point at 20, 30, 40 and 50 MHz, in every cataract was significantly less than that of a normal lens.

The histopathological findings of a senile nuclear cataract are shown in Fig. 7, and those of a subcapsular cataract in the Fig. 8. The cortex is deeply stained, and dense nuclear sclerosis, which is less deeply stained than the cortex, is seen. At these sites each frequency component of an echo seems

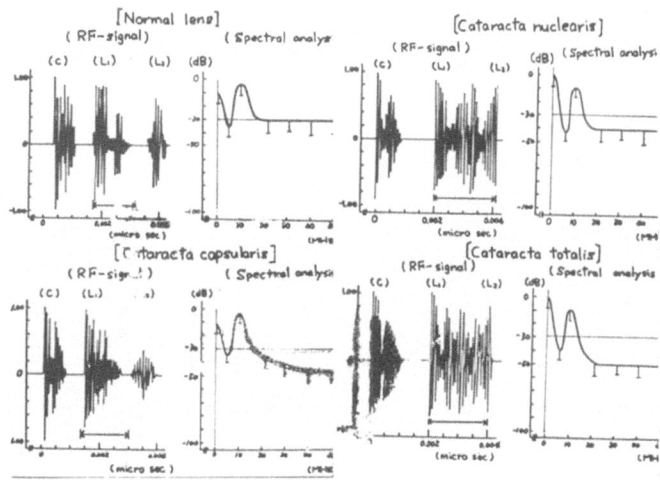

Fig. 6. RF signals and RF spectrum patterns of normal eyes and with each type of cataract.

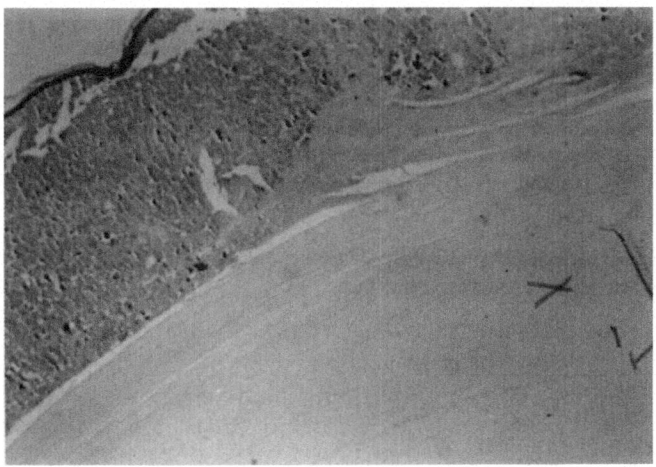

Fig. 7. The histopathological finding of a senile nuclear cataract.

to be absorbed, but the absorption was considered acoustically to reflect the quantitative difference rather than the qualitative difference, as described previously. The correlations between the histology of cataracts and the power spectrum patterns are under investigation.

450

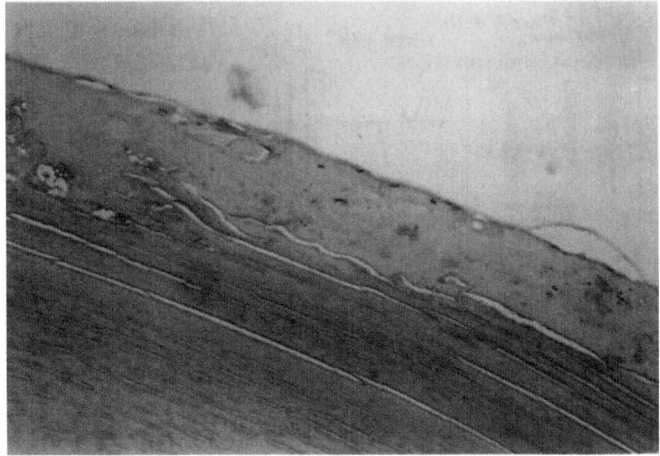

Fig. 8. The histopathological finding of a subcapsular cataract.

References

1. Thijssen, J.M., Cloostermans, M.J.T.M. & Verhoef, W.M. In Thijssen, J.M. and Nicholas, D. (eds.), Ultrasonic Tissure Differentiation in Ophthalmology, Ultrasonic Tissue Characterization, pp. 146–158. The Hague: Martinus Nijhoff Publishers (1982).
2. Tane, S. & Kimura, Y. Power spectrum analysis of ultrasonic radio-frequency signals in vitreous diseases. In Ferray di Oliveira, L.N. (ed.), Ophthalmology Today, Proceedings of the VIII Congress of the European Society of Ophthalmology (held in Lisbon, Portugal), pp. 357–359. Amsterdam: Excerpta Medica (1988).
3. Thijssen, J.M. & Oosterveld, B.J. Texture in Tissue Echograms, J. Ultrasound Med. 9: 215–229 (1990).

Address for correspondence: Department of Ophthalmology, St. Marianna University, 2-16-1 Sugao, Miyamae-ku, J-213 Kawasaki-shi, Japan.

56. Three-dimensional display and its application to stereoscopic representation

Y. SUGATA, K. MURAKAMI, M. ITO, T. SHIINA
& Y. YAMAMOTO
(*Tokyo, Japan*)

Abstract. We have developed a three-dimensional display system by spiral scanning ultrasonography and parallel scanning using an array transducer. Processing the resultant three-dimensional (3D) echo signals, it becomes possible to observe the shape of the ocular region from any desired direction, as well as to obtain a section profile with color gradation on CRT. 3D analysis of the structure and volume measurement are also made in this system. The rotation display of a 3D image makes it possible to visualize the relationship of the structure from any viewing direction and angle with the aid of joystick. The direct application of the rotation process presents a stereoscopic view of the structure of interest. A parallel set of 3D images observed from approximately 10 degrees outward each other gives a stereoscopic view by looking them simultaneously. A set of angled 3D images on the same CRT or an overlaid reconstruction of angled images with different colors give similar effects. The stereoscopic representation has an advantage in that it can store 3D information on prints and restore them in most simple way.

Introduction

Three-dimensional (3D) display involves some aspects on useful clinical information, so that 3D display systems have been reported many times together with clinical applications and results. In this report a stereoscopic representation is presented as another application of the developed system.

Method

3D ultrasound data are collected by an immersion method in supine position with the aid of the spiral scanner interfaced with the conventional ultrasound diagnostic equipment documented elsewhere (Yamamoto 1987, 1988, 1990).

To visualize naturally occurring pathological states, we have developed a 3D display system in ultrasonography. As an extension of the B-mode display, 3D-mode is especially meaningful in describing the pathology of a sonically empty ocular region with or without transparent light pass, such as the spatial extension of the structure and their spatial relationships. It may be helpful to describe or follow the clinical course quantitatively, such as the fate of retinal detachment or a tumor.

In addition to the spiral scanning of a single transducer, the parallel

P. Till (ed.), Ophthalmic Echography 13, pp. 451–457.

452

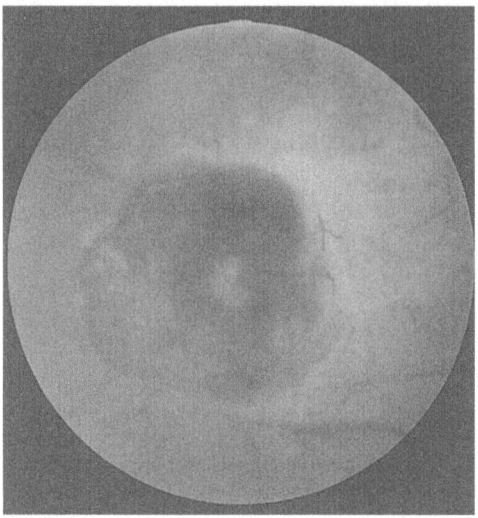

Fig. 1. Fundus photograph of suspected choroidal melanoma.

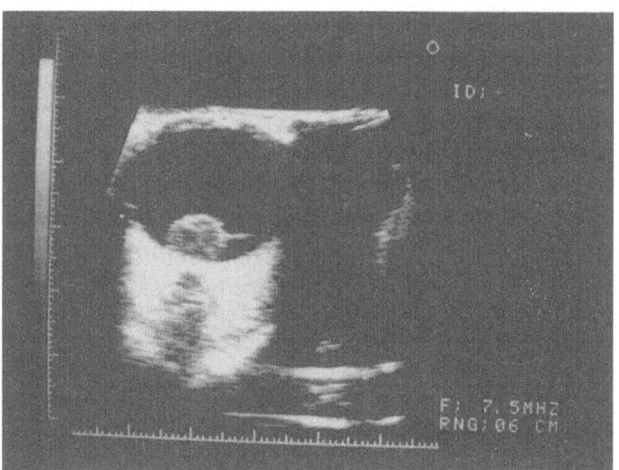

Fig. 2. B-mode image of the tumor.

scanning of an array transducer is also employed to collect 3D echo information. The former has the advantage that it can give a precise description of a region, and the latter is better for faster scanning and a smooth image.

In addition to realistic 3D imaging, 3D information provides other possibilities over B-mode. They are measurements of distance, area and volume, and reconstruction of a section profile with gradation code. It also gives relative locational information, such as A- and B-mode qualitative images,

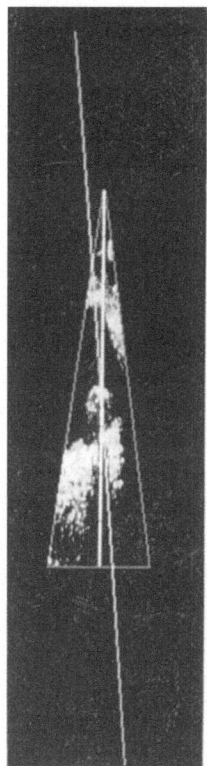

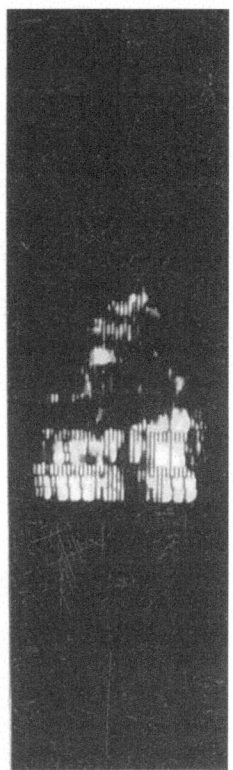

Fig. 3. An antero-posterior guide line on the
sectional reconstruction of the ocular region.

Fig. 4. The sagittal section of the tumor.

the total shape, etc. The rotation program generates the 3D image as seen from any desired direction.

As a direct implementation of the rotation program, a pair of two images obtained as seen slightly outward, give a stereoscopic representation on a paper as well as on a monitor. It is one of the most concise ways to store or recover 3D information such as is frequently used in stereoscopic fundus photographs, compared with other image processing systems, which naturally require the assistance of a computer.

Results

A suspected choroidal melanoma (Fig. 1) protruded inside the vitreous cavity with secondary retinal detachment around the optic disc is shown in a conventional B-mode section (Fig. 2). From 3D data the section profile with color gradation was reconstructed on CRT and an antero-posterior guide line was superimposed (Fig. 3) for extracting the section profile of the tumor (Fig.

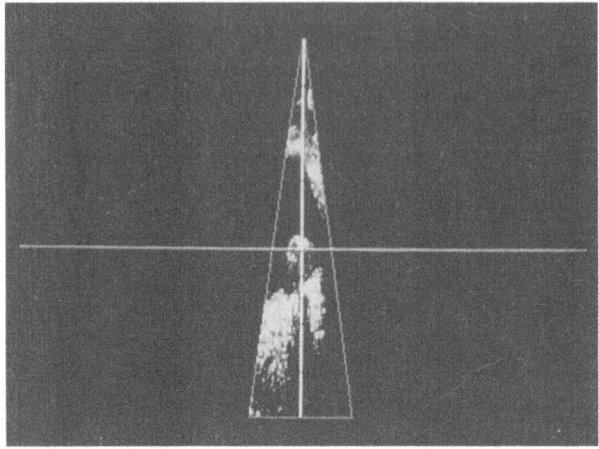

Fig. 5. A. transverse guideline on the sectional reconstruction of the ocular region.

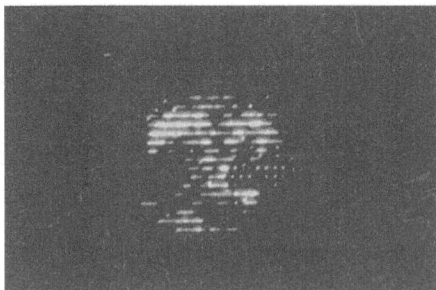

Fig. 6. The transversal section of the tumor.

4). The transversal dissection across the stalk of the tumor (Fig. 5) gives the idea of hypothetical section profile (Fig. 6) as scanned in this direction.

The pseudo-3D reconstruction of the posterior fundus as seen by an ophthalmoscope (Fig. 7) helps direct perception of the pathological structure.

According to the rotation program of a 3D image on CRT (Sugata 1989, 1990), a pair of angled 3D images after the reconstruction process on a CRT presents a stereoscopic view of the structure on a plane (Fig. 8). Two differently colored reconstructions overlaid on a CRT give also the stereoscopic view when seen through red and green filters (Fig. 9).

Since a vitreous membrane usually reflects weak echo signals, they sometimes form a discontinuous, speckled image rather than a clear B-mode image. However, scattered weak echoes from the vitreous may find a useful application in the stereoscopic representation. A funnel-shaped vitreous detachment (Fig. 10) presents weak echoes around the optic disc even in the maximal gain (Fig. 11). A parallel set of two photographs of sectional images,

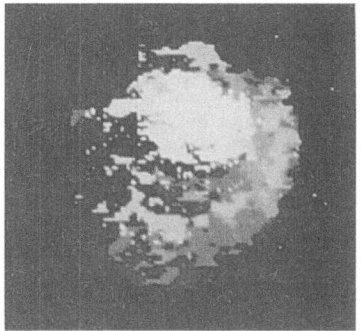

Fig. 7. 3D-reconstruction of the tumor.

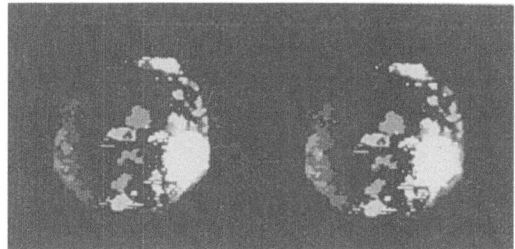

Fig. 8. An angled pair of 3D-images for stereography.

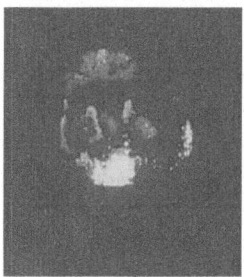

Fig. 9. An overlaid reconstruction of 3D-images for a green–red stereoscope.

which are reconstructed from scattered vitreous echoes, display a cluster of dots showing the shape of the vitreous cavity (Fig. 12).

Discussion

Although the precision of 3D display system is weak, it exceeds that of the B-mode in many respects except that it allows dynamic diagnosis. In the

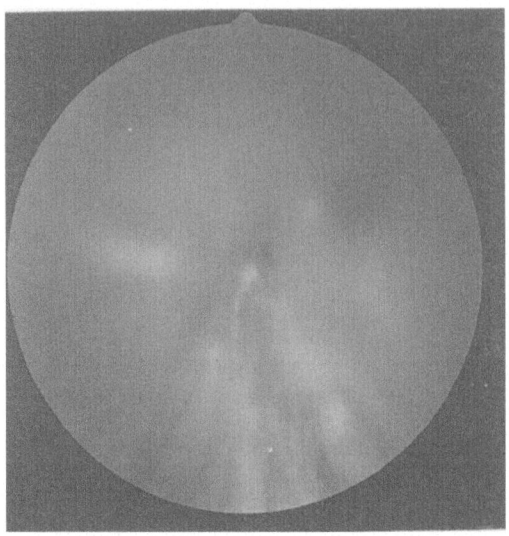

Fig. 10. The fundus photograph of funnel-shaped vitreous detachment.

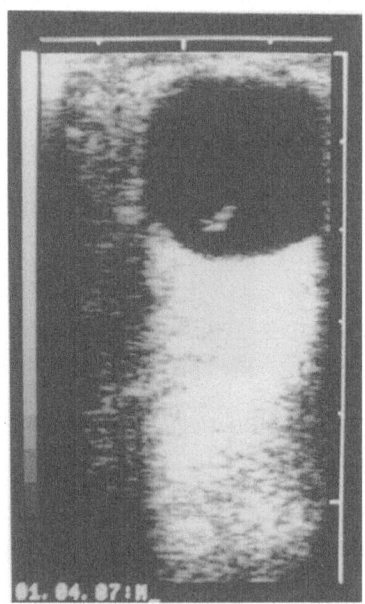

Fig. 11. B-mode image of the vitreous detachment.

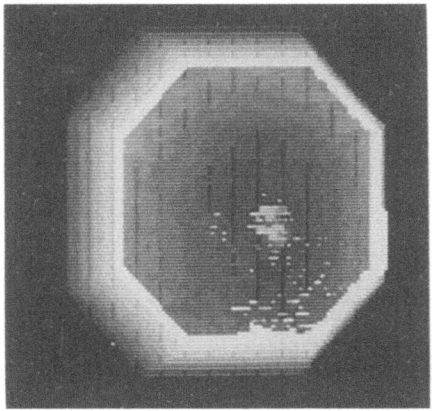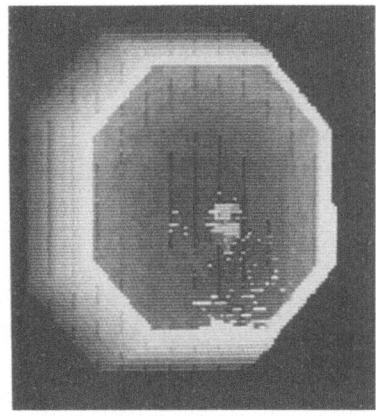

Fig. 12. A parallel set of the 3D-reconstruction of the vitreous detachment for stereography.

direct application of 3D-mode, the stereoscopic representation is a useful and concise way of preserving and restoring 3D information on paper. When this method is applied to weak echoes from the vitreous, scattered dots will be displayed in the image. But they can be positively used and evaluated for the structural components in the space, even though in the past they were regarded as noise and neglected.

References

Yamamoto, Y., Sugata, Y., Tomita, M. & Ito, M. Three dimensional display of the ocular region: Improvement of scanning method. In Ossoinig, K.C. (ed.), Ophthalmic Echography. Doc. Ophthalmol. Proc. Ser. 48: 207–214. Dordrecht: Martinus Nijhoff/Dr. W. Junk (1987).

Yamamoto, Y., Kubota, M., Sugata, Y., Matsui, S. & Ito, M. Three dimensional ultrasonography of ocular region. In Thijssen, J.M., Hillman, J.S., Gallenga, P.E. and Cennamo, G. (eds.), Ultrasonography in Ophthalmology. Doc. Ophthalmol. Proc. Ser. 51: 11–18. Dordrecht: Kluwer Acad. Publ. (1988).

Yamamoto, Y., Sugata, Y., Tomita, M. & Ito, M. Three dimensional scan using a single transducer and image construction. In Sampaolesi, R. (ed.), Ultrasonography in Ophthalmology. Doc. Ophthalmol. Proc. Ser. 53: 455–460. Dordrecht: Kluwer Acad. Publ. (1990).

Sugata, Y., Yamamoto, Y. & Ito, M. Three dimensional display of ocular region using an array transducer. In Sampaolesi, R. (ed.) Ultrasonography in Ophthalmology. Doc. Ophthalmol. Proc. Ser. 53: 461–466. Dordrecht: Kluwer Acad. Publ. (1990).

Sugata, Y., Murakami, M., Fukuyo, T. Fukuyo, T. & Yamamoto, Y. Image processing and clinical significance in ocular ultrasonography (22nd report). Image reconstruction of posterior fundus. Jpn. J. Clin. Ophthalmol. 43: 1126–1127 (1989).

Address for correspondence: Department of Ophthalmology, Komagome Hospital, Bunkyo-ku, Honkomagome, Tokyo, J-113 Tokyo, Japan.

57. From computer-assisted echography to a multielement linear curtain ultrasonic system
Our experiences

S. GUERRIERO, G. MINERVA, L. CARDIA, F. NIRCHIO,
G. PASQUARIELLO & N. VENEZIANI
(Bari, Italy)

Abstract. This paper describes research within the CNR's Progetto Finalizzato 'Tecnologie Biomediche e Sanitarie', subproject 'ultrasounds'. The aims of this study were as follows: (1) in the field of digital processing of B-scan images, aimed at tissue characterization by means of texture analysis; and (2) in the design and implementation of an echographic unit for ophthalmology, with advanced technical features. The prototype of the electronic interface between a 64-element linear curtain transducer, at 10 MHz, and the videofrequency section of the last unit is working actually, included in a commercial echograph produced by ESAOTE-Biomedica. In this paper, experimental results obtained with the developed hardware are shown. The integration of hardware and software modules within a single advanced unit is currently in progress. It will be based on a personal computer, supported by a video interface and by the hardware modules now under test.

Introduction

In the last ten years the ultrasound imaging technique has become one of the most common diagnostic tools in medicine. The success of this technique is due not only to its simplicity and non-invasive nature, but also to the significant improvements in the echographic units and their diagnostic capabilities. Better performance has been achieved by advances in different fields, such as ultrasonic transducer technology, microelectronic and computer applications, and in software technology resulting a wider flexibility from hardware structures.

At present, small and powerful microcomputers make it possible the design of echographs allowing to perform not only biometric operations on the echographic tracks and optimizations of their display, but also the computation of physical parameters. With digitally processed video and radiofrequency signals, it is now possible to develop software methods that can characterize biological tissues traversed by an ultrasonic field.

Ophthalmology has taken advantage of global improvements in the fields related to the echographic technology. Several different units are now available, generally provided with a single-element probe, mechanically scanned, allowing real-time B-mode imaging. Only one echograph, made by Storz (USA) in 1983, has been provided with a 7.5 MHz linear array transducer, using 35 unfocused elements and an acoustic beam electronically scanned in the direction transverse to the ultrasound propagation.

P. Till (ed.), Ophthalmic Echography 13, pp. 459–473.

In this paper the implementation and testing of an advanced echograph for ophthalmology are described. This has been the result of a research project to design the best performing prototype that would allow exploitation of the advantages introduced by new technologies. The focus of this work was to improve geometrical resolution (mainly in the transverse direction) and to develop software techniques to obtain more objective diagnoses of pathology. In fact, the correct evaluation of echographic images still depends too much on the operator's experience and ability to identify and correlate information such as contours, shapes, dimensions and the texture of patho- logical structures.

From the first point of view, the design and implementation of electronic modules have been appointed, with the aim to use a multielement ultrasonic probe, expressly developed for this prototype by the Istituto di Acustica of the Italian CNR, in Rome.

From the second point of view, some software techniques have been developed, at different levels of complexity in the following fields:
- spectral and statistical analysis of radiofrequency ultrasonic signals, to provide a numerical characterization of these, connected with selected areas of an echogram;
- texture analysis of selected areas in a B-mode image, to further improve the discrimination of different ocular pathologies;
- interactive use of color scales, to enhance the intensity variations with respect to their appearance in a grey level image.

Before prototype implementation, all the software techniques based on the processing of videofrequency signals were tested using images from other available units. The specifications of software and hardware implementations are described in the following, such as the preliminary results of experiments to validate the potential performance of the final unit. This will be based on a personal computer, supported by a video interface and by the electronic modules now under test. The integration of the developed techniques within a single echograph is now in progress.

False color coding of B-mode images

In B-mode echographs providing grey scale images, the monitor image is formed of dots whose intensity is proportional to the amplitude of reflected echoes. From these images, it is very difficult to distinguish different tonalities when they represent echoes with similar amplitudes. In fact, according to the Weber and Fechner law, the human eye is able to distinguish differences in brightness ranging up to 1% only in ideal conditions so that the two densities to be distinguished are spatially close and of medium value. In the range of high and low light levels, the resolution power of the human eye decreases significantly, especially if the two densities are far apart or hazy. These are the conditions in which B-mode echographic images are usually evaluated.

In order to extract the greatest amount of information from an echogram false color coding was adopted to make it more readily interpretable. The steps in the false color processing were as follows:
- B-mode sequence recording on videotape;
- real-time sampling of the entire B-mode sequences with data storage on a memory buffer (frame grabber);
- computation of the grey level frequency histogram of the single image inside the frame buffer;
- automatic attribution of pre-established color codes to known grey level bands;
- modification of the attributed colors by means of interactive tools, allowing the operator to define new false color scales as segments in a 3D color space; these segments were coded on the basis of red, green and blue coordinates of their extremity, with values ranging from 0 to 255 (one byte for each coordinate);
- B-mode sequence re-examination assigning in real-time the color coding previously defined.

Texture analysis for tissue characterization

Tone and texture are two components of vision; they are correlated and are present with different weights within an image. More specifically, we can say that texture is related to the spatial distribution of grey levels, i.e. to the roughness or smoothness created by the variation in tone or by the repetition of visual schemes. In the analysis of digital images, the tone and texture measurement procedures require a quantitative characterization of these two quantities. Image tone variations constitute a kind of information that can be directly obtained through digital electro-optical devices. Conversely, the qualitative texture information can not be directly perceived through the acquisition system and has to be drawn from the digital image data. Most of the procedures to quantify image texture reported in the literature are based on the measurement of spatial correlations among the image grey levels. The most frequently used methods are:
- PSM: (Fourier) power spectrum method, based on the subdivision of the spectrum in anular and sectoral regions for examining the roughness of the area and direction of structures;
- SGLDM: spatial grey level dependence method, or second-order grey level statistic, based on a $M(d, \theta)$ matrix calculation of the grey level spatial dependences, also mentioned as grey level co-occurrence method (GLCM);
- GLDM: grey level difference method, in which the analysis is made with first-order statistics on local frequency vector defined by $f_d(x, y) = |f(x, y) - f(x + \Delta x, y + \Delta y)|$, with $\vec{d} = (\Delta x, \Delta y)$;
- GLRM: grey level run-length method, based on 'run-length' statistics, i.e. on values $P(i, j) =$ length-i runs number (in a prefixed direction) related to pairs of grey levels belonging to range j.

In the case of synthetically produced textures, Conner and Harlow showed, both theoretically and experimentally, that the best results are given by GLCM compared with other methods. For this procedure, which we used, we now present a more detailed description.

SGLDM

Consider a rectangular image with N_x elements along each line and N_y elements in each column, and take N_L as the highest brightness value to be given to a pixel. If we indicate with $L_x = 1, 2, \ldots, N_x$ the horizontal spatial field, with $L_y = 1, 2, \ldots, N_y$, the vertical spatial field and with $G = 0, 1, 2, \ldots, N$, the grey levels as a whole, we can represent our image as a function I, defined in the $L_x * L_y$ field with values in G, which assigns to every pair (i, j) with elements in the field $L_x * L_y$, a tone value G_K, so that $I(i, j) = G_K$. Now suppose that all information about the image texture is in the co-occurrence matrix M, which is also defined as a second-order calculated probability matrix, built according to the spatial distribution of the grey levels on the image.

Each element (d) of the matrix represents the frequency $P(i, j)$ wherewith transition occurs between the grey levels i and j comparing two pixels at distance d in the direction θ. Such matrices, which contain level coupling frequencies, depend on the chosen direction and on the distance between the pixels being compared.

In our investigation we considered only the direction $\theta = 0$, shiftings along the lines, whereas for distances between pixels we took values from 1 to 10. In 'low-frequency' images, pixels presenting slight spatial separations show similar grey levels; this implies that the most meaningful values in the co-occurrence matrix M will be concentrated along the main diagonal and next to it. Conversely for the 'high-frequency' fine texture, corresponding to more meaningful differences in the pixel's grey levels, then in the M matrix the values spaced outside the main diagonal become important.

In our investigation we used four different parameters, calculated on the co-occurrence matrix and defined as follows:

Contrast

$$\text{Con} = \sum_{i=0}^{NL} \sum_{j=0}^{NL} (i - j)^2 P(i, j),$$

which represents a measurement on matrix M dispersion value with the main diagonal; it is null if it results in $P(i, j) = 0$ for $i \neq j$; or its value is low if concentration occurs next to the principal diagonal.

Entropy

$$\text{Ent} = -\sum_{i=0}^{NL}\sum_{j=0}^{NL} P(i,j)\log[P(i,j)],$$

which has very low levels when $P(i,j)$ have very different values.

Second angular moment

$$\text{ASM} = \sum_{i=0}^{NL}\sum_{j=0}^{NL} P(i,j)^2,$$

whose values are inversely proportional to the number of $P(i,j) \neq 0$ in the matrix.

Inverse difference moment

$$\text{IDM} = \sum_{i=0}^{NL}\sum_{j=0}^{NL} \frac{P(i,j)}{(i-j)^2 + 1},$$

which shows the presence of $P(i,j) \neq 0$, in which $i \simeq j$. None of these parameters considered individually can show the whole content of co-occurrence matrix information; it is clear that for a good estimate of image texture they have to be used together. In our investigation texture parameters have been calculated for various values of distance d among pixel pairs in the $\theta = 0$ direction (along the lines). Before calculating the $M(d,\theta)$ matrix, we normalized the contrast of the image through the histogram equalization in order to stress the structures contained within it.

Prototype of an electronic scanning echograph

Mechanical features

The prototype is supplied with a 64-element linear array transducer, which is 55 mm long, 35 mm wide, and 10 mm high. Each element is 6 mm high and 0.48 mm wide, and the gap between each element is 0.03 mm (Fig. 1). The central frequency of the transducer is 10 MHz and its bandwidth 5 MHz (Fig. 2).

The cord connecting the transducer with the receiving electronics (made by Gore) has 66 coaxial wires with total diameter of 7.9 mm. The diameter of each central wire, as well as that of the shielding wire is 0.15 mm (Fig. 3a, b). Such a cord has good flexibility and permits easy use of the device.

The transmitting and receiving electronics comprise both modules of ESAOTE commercial units and some custom-made units (Figs. 4 and 5). These latter were built using a wire-wrap technique; although this allows easy integration of the modules, is not the best solution as far as noise immunity is concerned. The commercial ESAOTE unit hosting the prototype is an AU-1000; it is no longer produced because it has been replaced by new

464

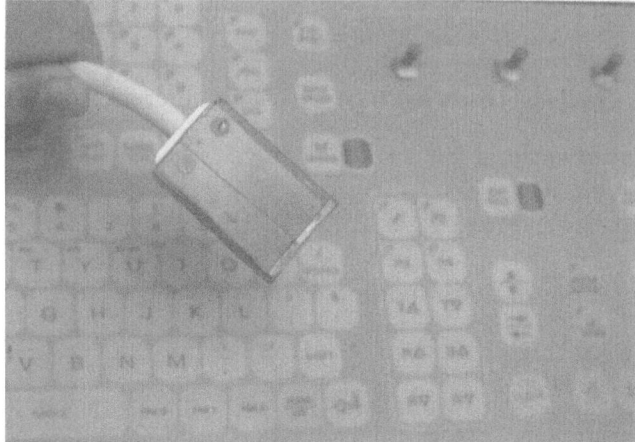

Fig. 1. The probe: note the useful and the manageable size.

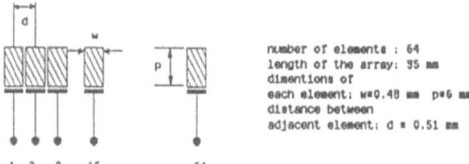

number of elements : 64
length of the array: 35 mm
dimentions of
each element: w=0.48 mm p=6 mm
distance between
adjacent element: d = 0.51 mm

Fig. 2. Characteristics of the probe.

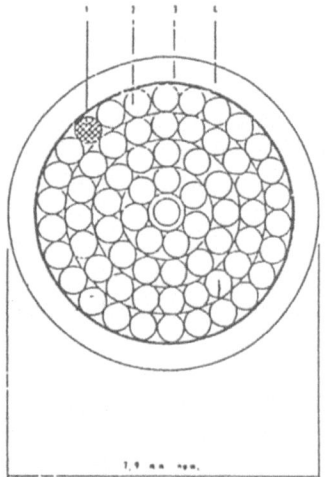

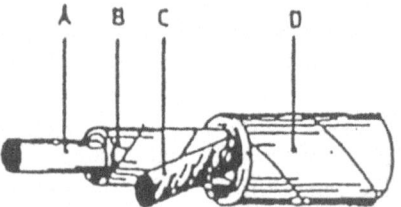

Fig. 3a,b. Section of the cord connecting the transducer with the receiving electronics.

models with more sophisticated circuit solutions that allow better echographic images.

Functional characteristics

The linear array has 64 active elements electronically focused either in transmission or reception. The number of elements, their transverse dimensions and the driving technique used permit echographic images with a large number of nontrivial lines and a transverse resolution of 1 mm. Fig. 6 shows some simulations of the acoustic beam generated by a group of eight elements of the array. The -3 dB contour of the transmitted beam shows how the resolution changes along the beam depth.

Driving technique of the transducer

Every image line is obtained by the excitation of eight adjacent elements in the array which are not excited simultaneously, but according to their relative positions within the active group. In order to produce an ultrasonic focalized beam at the depth of 25 mm, close to the bottom of the eye, first the outer elements are excited, and then the inner ones, with a maximum delay of 32 ns (Fig. 7). Using eight elements at a time, 57 groups are possible. The line repetition frequency (the reciprocal of two successive line acquisitions) is 2.94 kHz, while the image repetition frequency (the number of images per second) is 24 Hz.

The signals received by the inner elements of the active group are in an opportune way delayed in reference to those received by the outer ones, in order to focalize the image and keep the resolution within its optimal values (Fig. 8a). The first seven elements of each active group are used to obtain the odd lines of the images, while the elements from the second to the eighth are used for the even ones (Fig. 8b). In this way, even lines are neither replicas of odd ones nor obtained by interpolation between two adjacent odd lines. The displayed images are much more detailed because they are composed of 114 effective different lines of view. Signal reception is performed by exploiting the dynamic aperture technique: at first, only the central element is used, and then the adjacent ones are activated in sequence. This permits image saturation to be reduced in the front part and to have a comparable resolution along all of the image. The prototype bandwidth of 5 MHz and central frequency of 10 MHz allow an axial resolution of 0.4 mm. Fig. 9 shows a comprehensive view of the technique characteristics.

Preliminary tests and conclusions

Figs. 10, 11, and 12 show a normal human eye, an orbit with a right muscle, and an orbit with the optic nerve. In these three figures the ocular fundus outline is well evident; in Fig. 11 the right muscle is well outlined in the

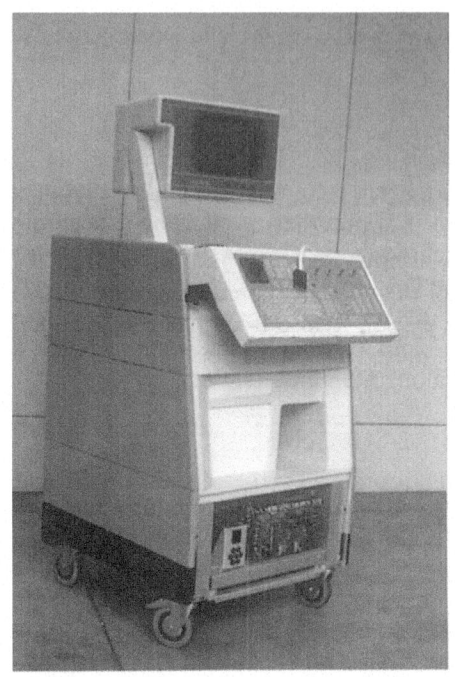

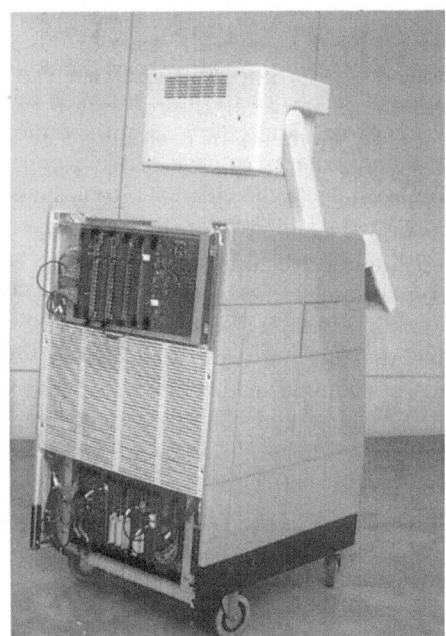

Figs. 4–5. The prototype.

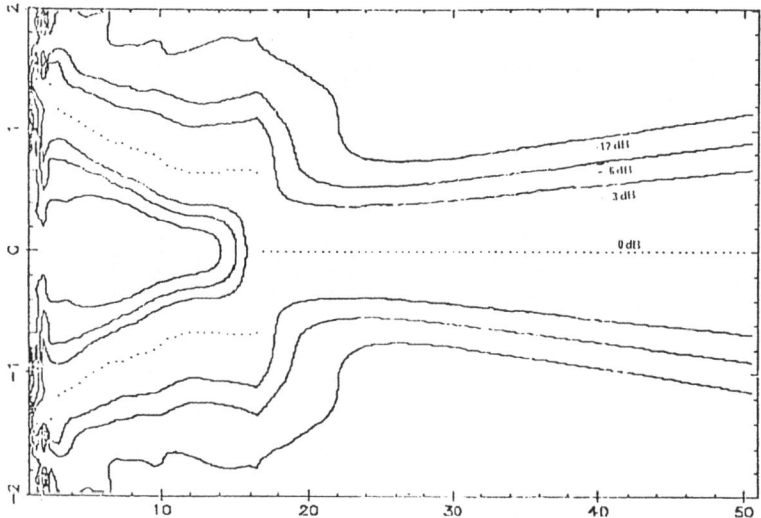

Fig. 6a. Computer simulation of the contour pressure field generated by 8-element array, focalized at 25 mm depth (off-axis distance and distance from the transducer are in mm).

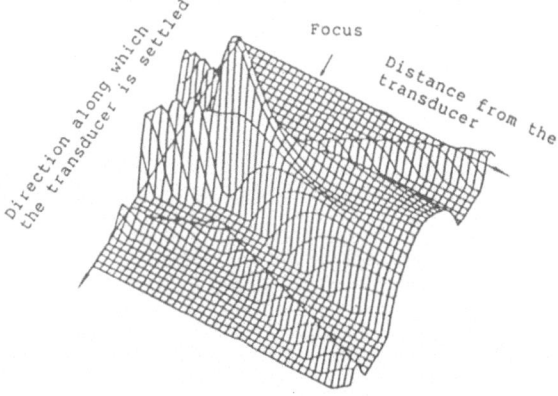

Fig. 6b. Computer simulation of the pressure field generated by eight elements of the array.

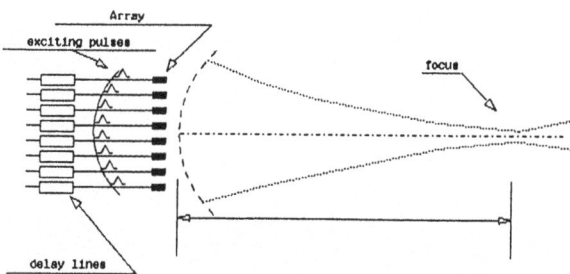

Fig. 7. Electronic focusing.

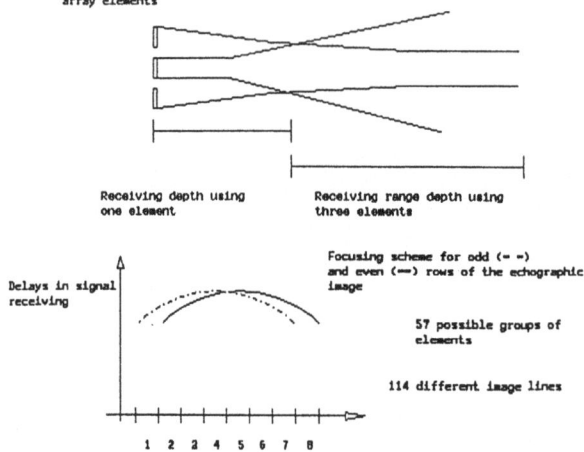

Fig. 8a,b. Receiving using a dynamic aperture technique.

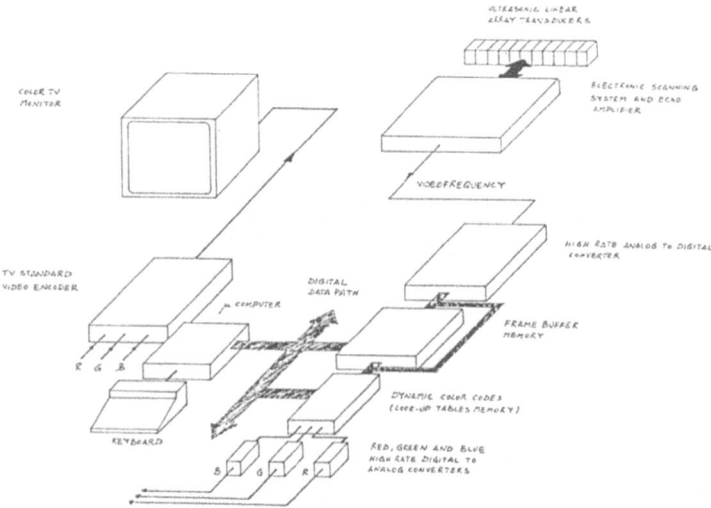

Fig. 9. Comprehensive view of technique characteristics.

orbit and its edges are precise. In Fig. 12, where the immage is smaller than in Fig. 11, we can see the optic nerve and its sheaths. In Figs. 13 and 14 the retinal detachement is evident. In Fig. 15 there is proliferative retinopathy. In Fig. 16 we can see a vitreous hemorrhage.

In Figs. 17, 18, and 19 we show a horse eye. In Fig. 17 we can see an anterior segment: the two corneal surfaces, the iris surface and the lens posterior faces are clearly represented. In Fig. 18 the horse eye vitreous body was injected with blood, and in Fig. 19 blood and a foreign body are present in the vitreous chamber.

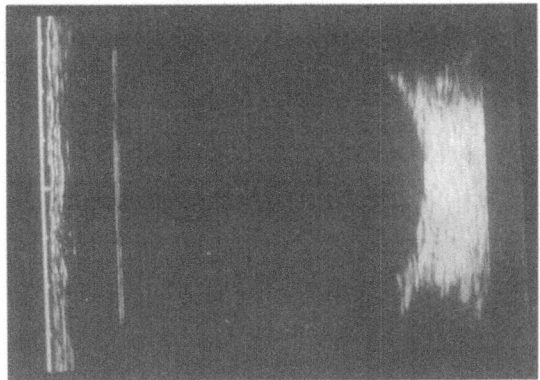

Fig. 10. The normal human eye.

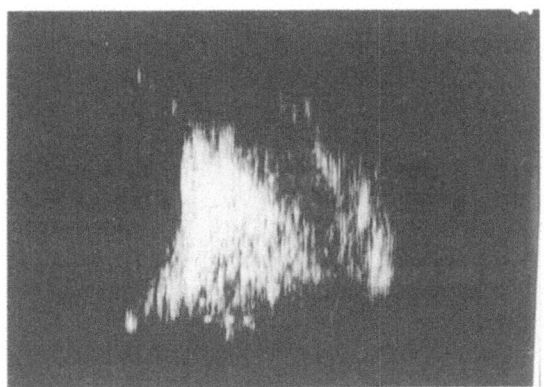

Fig. 11. Eye orbit with a right muscle.

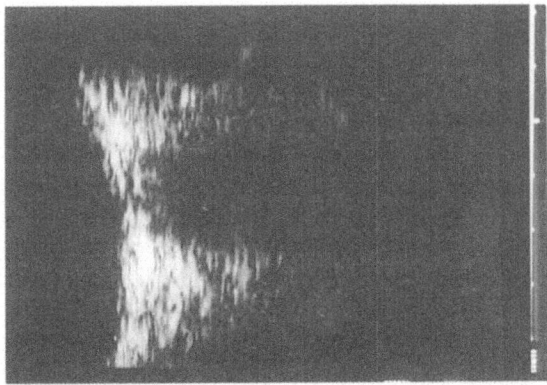

Fig. 12. Eye orbit with the optic nerve.

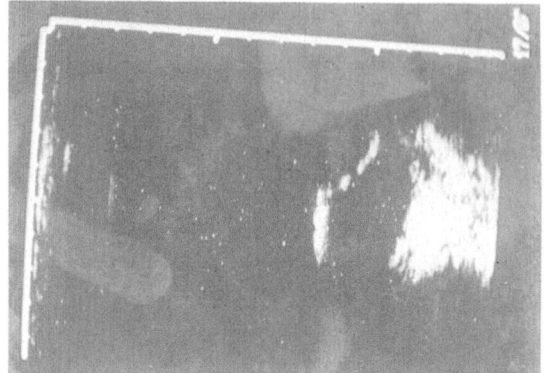

Fig. 13. Retinal detachment.

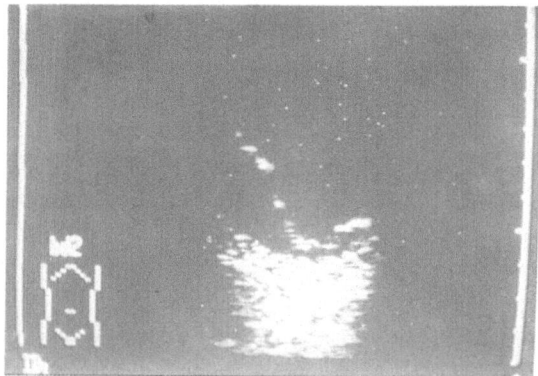

Fig. 14. Retinal detachment.

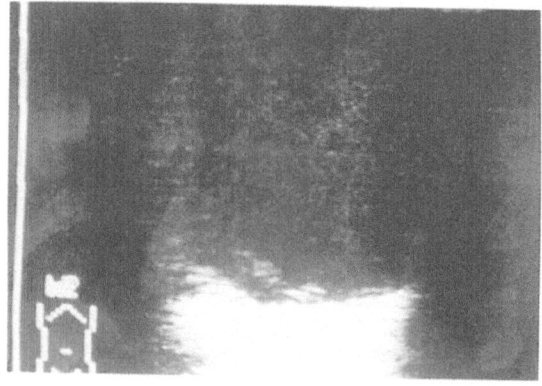

Fig. 15. Proliferative retinopathy.

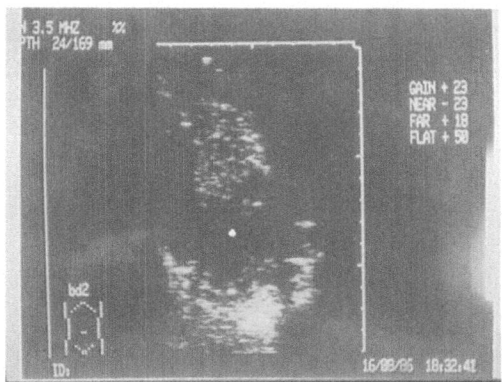

Fig. 16. Vitreous hemorrhage.

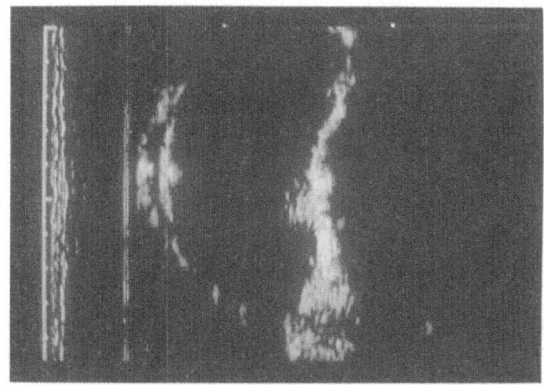

Fig. 17. Horse eye: anterior segment.

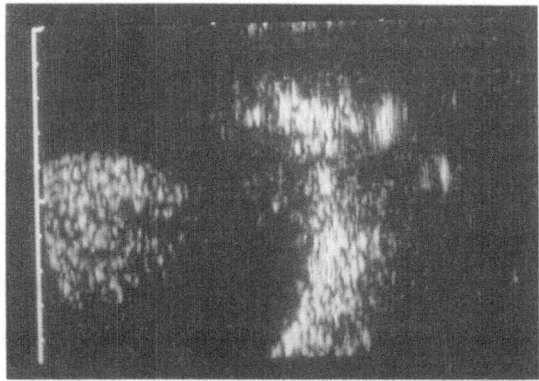

Fig. 18. Horse eye: vitreous body injected with blood.

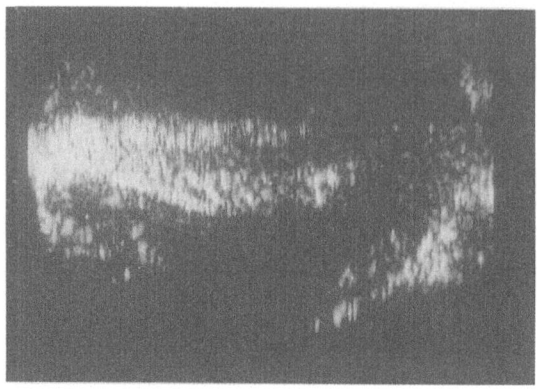

Fig. 19. Horse eye: vitreous cavity with blood and a foreign body.

All the images are of good quality, especially if we consider that they were obtained from a prototype working for one week. When the prototype is improved, the images quality will no doubt be better because of the acoustic characteristics and the electronic pilotage of the probe. It is important to outline the reduced dimensions of the probe so that it is useful and manageable for ophthalmic use.

References

1. Wyszecki & Judd. Color in business, science and industry. John Wiley and Sons Inc. (1975).
2. Liebesny, J.P. & Lele, P.P., Enhancement of ultrasonic B-scans by chromatic encoding. Proceedings of IEEE Ultrasonic Symposium, pp. 37–38 (1973).
3. Coleman, D.J. & Katz, L., Color coding of B-scan ultrasonograms. Arch. Ophthalmol. 91 (1974).
4. Reibaldi, A., Avitabile, T., Guerriero, S., Distante, A. & Veneziani, N. Primi risultati sulle possibilità di differenziazione ecografica tissutale oculare mediante falso colore. Clinica Oculistica e Patologia Oculare. 5(6): 9–13 (1984).
5. Cardia, L., Reibaldi, A., Avitabile, T., Guerriero, S., Veneziani, N. & Distante, A. First result about echographical ocular tissue characterization by false colours. Poster Session, 7th Congress of the European Society of Ophthalmology, Helsinki (1984).
6. Reibaldi, A., Guerriero, S., Avitabile, T. & Veneziani, N. Validazione dell'ecografo A e B-scan Renaissance della STORZ. Technical Note of the Istituto di Clinica Oculistica. University of Bari (1984).
7. Reibaldi, A., Guerriero, S., Avitabile, T., Veneziani, N. & Distante A. Primi risultati di ecografia assistita. Bollettino di Oculistica, 64(5–6) (1985).
8. Haralick, R.M., Shanmugam, K. & Dinstein, I. Textural features for image classification. IEEE Trans. Syst. Man. Cybern. SMC-3: 610 (1973).
9. Haralick, R.M. Statistical and Structural Approaches to Texture. Proceedings of the IEEE. 67: 768 (1979).
10. Conners, R.W. & Harlow, C.A. A Theoretical comparison of texture algorithms. IEEE Trans. on Pattern Analysis and Mach. Intell. PAMI-2: 204 (1980).
11. Pasquali, F., Pasquariello, G. & Veneziani, N. Package per il calcolo di parametri di tessitura su porzioni di immagini digitali. Bari: Technical Note of IESI/CNR (1985).

12. Pasquali, F., Pasquariello, G., Veneziani, N., Selvaggi, F.P., Martino, P., Reibaldi, A. & Guerriero, S. Texture analysis di immagini ultrasoniche in medicina. Lipari: Proceedings of the 7th Congress of GNCB (1985).

13. Reibaldi, A., Guerriero, S., Avitabile, T., Uva, M., Veneziani, N., Pasquariello, G. & Pasquali, F. Texture analysis di immagini ultrasonografiche in oculistica. Ferrara: Proceedings of the National Congress of Ophthalmology (1985).

14. Reibaldi, A., Guerriero, S., Avitabile, T., Veneziani, N., Pasquariello, G. & Pasquali, F. Improvements to computer assisted echography. In Thijssen, J.M., Hillman, J.S., Gallenga, P.E. & Cennamo, G. (eds.), Ultrasonography in Ophthalmology 11: 53–61. Dordrecht: Kluwer Acad. Pub. (1988).

15. Guerriero, S., Montrone, F., Durante, G., Pasquali, F. & Pasquariello, G. Diagnostica ecografica orbitaria assistita dal computer. Clinica Oculistica e Patologia Oculare. IX(4): 305–311 (1988).

16. Thijssen, J.M., Bayer, A.L. & Verbeek, A.M. Computer support for ultrasonic diagnosis. Documenta Ophthalmologica 48(2): 315–318 (1979).

17. Brigham, E.O. The Fast Fourier Transform. Englewood Cliffs, N.J.: Prentice-Hall Inc. (1983).

18. Oppenheim, A.V., Willsky, A.S. & Young, I.T. Signals and systems. London: Prentice-Hall International Inc. (1983).

19. Coleman, D.J. & Lizzi, F.L. Computerized ultrasonic tissue characterization of ocular tumors. Am. J. of Ophthalmol. 96: 165–175 (1983).

20. Gardner, W.A. Statistical spectral analysis: a nonprobabilistic theory. Englewood Cliffs N.J.: Prentice-Hall Inc. (1988).

21. Macovski, A. Medical imaging systems. Englewood Cliffs, N.J.: Prentice-Hall Inc. (1983).

22. Panella, E., Spalierno, G. & Veneziani, N. Studio di fattibilita di un ecografo B-mode a scansione elettronica per applicazioni oftalmiche. Bari: Technical Note of IESI/CNR (1986).

23. Nirchio, F., Panella, E., Spalierno, G. & Veneziani, N. Ecografo per oftalmologia: progress report. Bari: Technical Note of IESI/CNR (1986).

24. Guerriero, S., Montrone, F., De Carolis, G., Nirchio, F. & Veneziani, N. Ecografo a cortina lineare multielemento per applicazioni oftalmiche: caratteristiche e prestazioni preliminari. Clinica Oculistica e Patologie Oculare X(5): 397–403 (1989).

25. Duerinickx, A.J. Modeling wavefronts from acoustic phased arrays by computer. IEEE Transactions on Biomedical Engineering. BME-28(2) (1981).

26. Hunt, J.W., Arditi, M. & Foster, F.S. Ultrasound transducers for pulse-echo medical imaging. IEEE Transactions on Biomedical Engineering. BME-30(8) (1983).

27. De Carolis, G., Nirchio, F., Posa, F. & Veneziani, N. Image computer simulations of echographic linear array imaging systems: a synthetic aperture approach. Submitted to Acustica, Int. Journal on Acoustics (1989).

Address for correspondence: Department of Ophthalmology, University of Bari, Policlinico, Piazza G. Cesare, I-70100 Bari, Italy.

58. Telediagnosis by faxed ophthalmic ultrasonogram

S. TANE & M. HASHIMOTO
(*Kawasaki, Japan*)

Introduction

It would be clinically very useful if we could send ultrasonograms, which are taken by technicians or are diagnostically difficult, to remote central hospitals within moments, and request accurate diagnosis by specialists. In this study, we attempted to telephotograph ophthalmologic A-mode and B-mode film imaging pictures using an ordinary facsimile apparatus, as clearly as possible without impairing gray scales, and to read the telephotographed pictures.

Methods

The type of facsimile transmitter and receiver used in this study was NEFAX-3EX (NEC, made in Japan), which divides shading between black and white into 16 grades of gray scale, and makes medium-grade telephotographing possible (Fig. 1). The telephotographed ultrasonogram pictures were monochrome, A-mode and B-mode polaroid pictures of the eyes, photographed with ZD-252, ZD 255, and Topscan (ES-100 type) ultrasonic diagnostic equipment. In addition, color pictures obtained by a color scan converter were telephotographed. The pictures were sent to both nearby places within the city limits and remote places outside the city limits, in order to compare the results in relation to distance. Telephotographing took only 15 seconds. Pictures telephotographed under the following conditions were compared.

1. With letter keys fixed at the normal position: (a) pictures alone, (b) pictures placed between carrier sheets, and (c) xerox copies of pictures, were telephotographed.

2. With letter keys fixed at the photograph position: (a) pictures alone, and (b) pictures placed between carrier sheets, were telephotographed.

P. Till (ed.), Ophthalmic Echography 13, pp. 475–482.
© 1993 *Kluwer Academic Publishers*.

476

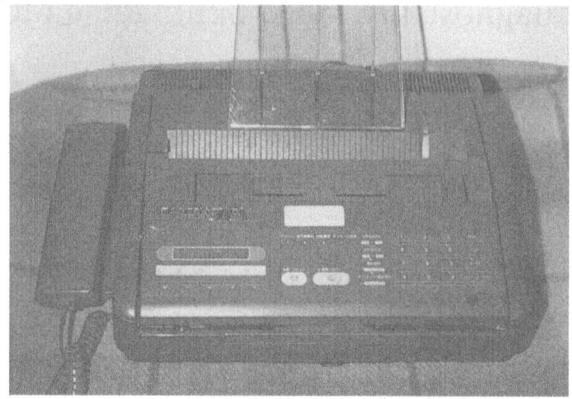

Fig. 1. Facsimile transmitter and receiver (NEFAX-3EX, NEC, made in Japan).

Results

Thirty photographs were chosen at random from approximately 12,000 photographs obtained during ultrasonic examinations over the last five years, and fax telephoto-transmission was conducted under the above conditions. Telephoto-ultrasonograms of some cases are described in the following.

Patient 1 was a 58-year-old man with diabetic retinopathy with vitreous hemorrhage (Fig. 2). The left column (top) shows the original picture from immersion B-mode using St. Marianna's ophthalmic high-resolution ultrasonic diagnostic equipment. The right column (top) shows the original picture from contact B-mode using ophthasonic A- and B-scan III type equipment. The two pictures in the middle row are facsimile display pictures with letter keys in the normal position, of which black and white contrast is excessive and shading is lacking. In contrast, the two bottom pictures show telephotographed facsimile pictures with letter keys at the photographic position. This technique provided neutral shading, corresponding well to that in the original photographs, and was considered not to be problematic for diagnostic purposes.

Patient 2 was a 38-year-old man with old retinal detachment (Fig. 3). Shown at top left is the original D-mode display in this case. The detached retina is shown in an easily understandable way in the form of a false stereographic display. At top right is the telephotographed facsimile picture with letter keys at the photographic positions, showing shading corresponding more to that in the original photograph and is more diagnostically advantageous than the facsimile display picture (bottom left), with letter keys at the normal position.

Patient 3 was a 63-year-old woman with retinal detachment (Fig. 4). The top row (left and right) show B-mode and A-mode display, respectively. In A-mode both the facsimile picture with letter keys at the normal position

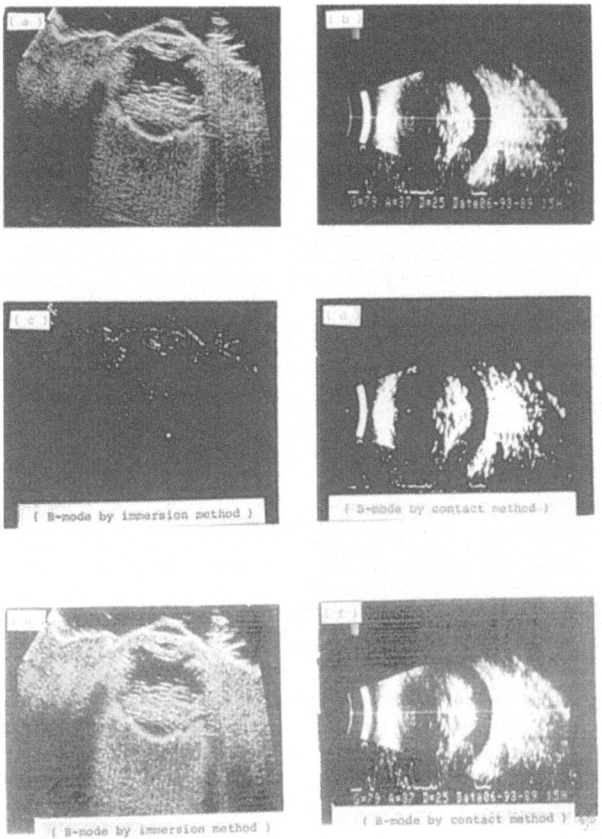

Fig. 2. B-scan ultrasonogram and fax pictures of a 58-year-old man with Diabetic Retinopathy with vitreous hemorrhage. TOP: *Left*, original picture taken by B-mode tomographic immersion ultrasonography; *right*, original picture taken by B-mode tomographic contact ultrasonography. MIDDLE: Fax pictures transmitted with letter keys at the normal position. *Left*, B- mode by immersion method; *right*, B-mode by contact method; BOTTOM: Fax picture transmitted with letter keys at the photographic position. *Left*, B-mode by immersion method; *right*, B-mode by contact method.

(bottom row, left and right), and the facsimile picture with letter keys at the photographic position (middle row, left and right), are clearly displayed. Thus, there are no problems in using A-mode, in which no shading is required, for diagnosis.

Patient 4 was a 65-year-old man with trauma complicated by massive vitreous hemorrhage and retinal detachment (Fig. 5). The color display enables easy diagnosis of retinal detachment, due to the differences in shading. In this case also, it can be seen that the facsimile picture with letter keys at the photographic position (middle row, left and right) provides more

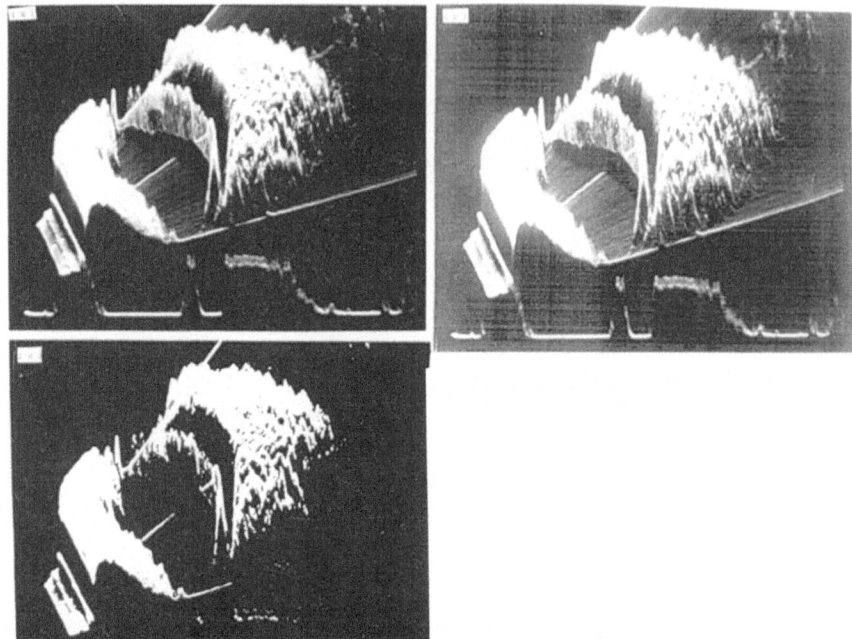

Fig. 3. D-scan ultrasonogram and fax pictures of a 38-year-old man with old retinal detachment. TOP: *Left*, Original picture taken by D-mode tomographic immersion ultrasonography using St. Marianna's ophthalmic high-resolution ultrasonic diagnostic equipment. TOP: *Right*, Fax picture transmitted with letter keys at the photographic position; BOTTOM: *Left*, Fax picture transmitted with letter keys at the normal position.

satisfactory shading and is more useful for diagnosis than the facsimile picture with letter keys at the normal position (bottom row, left and right).

Fig. 6 shows two cases with orbital diseases. The top row (left and right) shows immersion B-mode displays of orbital lymphoma and cavernous hemangioma, respectively. The bottom row (right and left) shows telephotographed facsimile pictures with letter keys at the normal position, which display no shading and are unsuitable for diagnostic purposes, while the telephotographed facsimile pictures with letter keys at the photographic position (middle row, right and left), have satisfactory shading, making diagnosis easy. This technique is very useful for reaching a diagnosis.

Discussion

The authors have pointed out that it is useful for mass screening to entrust picture-taking procedures to technicians in ultrasonography as in X-ray pho-

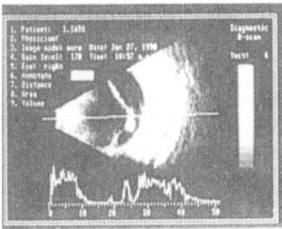 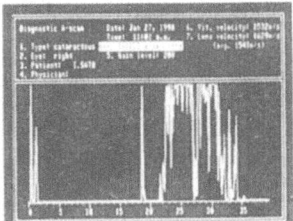

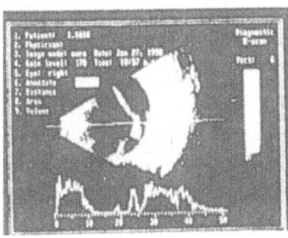 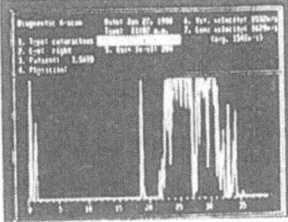

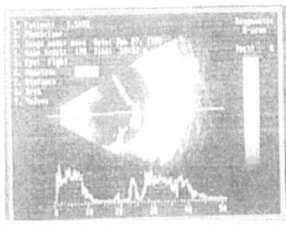 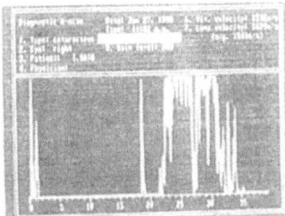

Fig. 4. B-mode ultrasonogram and fax pictures of the retinal detachment in a 63-year-old woman. TOP: *Left*, original picture taken by B-mode tomographic contact ultrasonography; *right*, original picture taken by A-mode contact ultrasonography. MIDDLE: Fax pictures transmitted with letter keys at the photographic position. *left*, B-mode by immersion method; *right*, A-mode by contact method. BOTTOM: Fax pictures transmitted with letter keys at the normal position. *Left*, B-mode by contact method; *right*, A-mode by contact method.

tography, and to have specialists undertake the reading and diagnosis of the picture. Shibuya and Ito have been aware of this for a long time, and reported a method of quick diagnosis by connecting signals and power sources from depopulated remote places with a single line. In this study, we attempted transmission of ophthalmologic pictures, using a type of moderately priced fax apparatus (NEFAX-3EX, NEC) which is commonly used at home or in offices, and proved its usefulness. With this method, it is presumed possible that photographs can be telephotographed from remote clinics to central hospitals, and for accurate diagnoses by specialists to be obtained promptly.

480

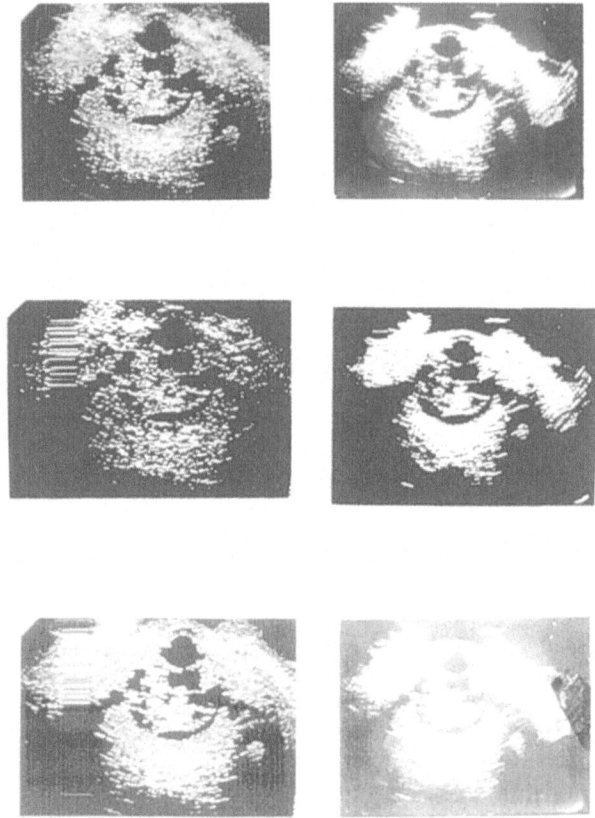

Fig. 5. B-scan ultrasonogram and fax pictures of the massive vitreous hemorrhage with retinal detachment in a 65-year-old man. TOP: *Left,* Original picture taken by B-mode tomographic immersion color display ultrasonography; *right,* original picture taken by B-mode tomographic monochromatic display ultrasonography. MIDDLE: Fax pictures transmitted with letter keys at the photographic position. BOTTOM: Fax pictures transmitted with letter keys at the normal position.

Conclusion

1. A-mode film imaging pictures could be telephotographed with preservation of the original image.

2. In B-mode pictures, the gray scale was rather poor, because fax provides 8 dots/1-mm picture. Moreover, images of thin original pictures received were unclear. The original pictures were xeroxed and transmitted, and images with sufficient clearness for diagnosis could be received.

3. Telephotographed fax images sent with letter keys at 'photograph' yielded

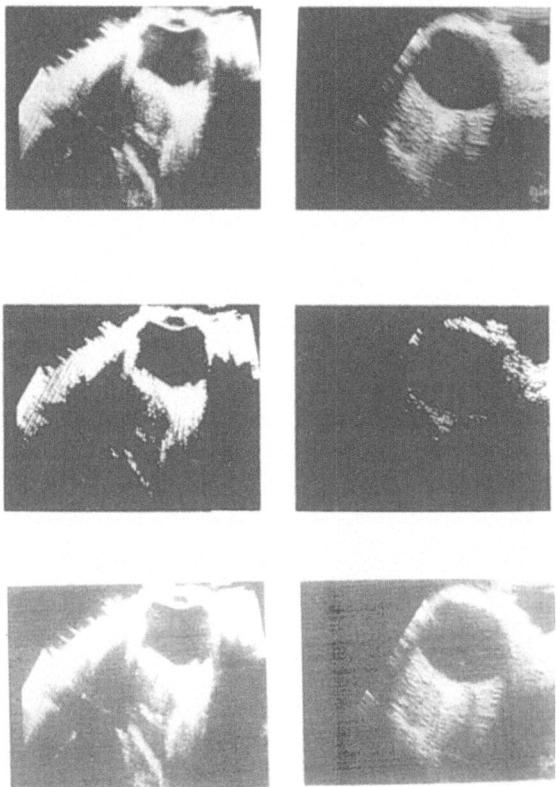

Fig. 6. B-scan ultrasonograms and fax pictures of orbital tumors. TOP: *Left,* Original picture of lymphoma taken by B-mode tomographic immersion ultrasonography; *right,* original picture of cavernous meningioma taken by B-mode tomographic immersion ultrasonography. MIDDLE: Fax pictures transmitted with letter keys at the photographic position. BOTTOM: Fax pictures transmitted with letter keys at the normal position.

a gray scale of medium grade which corresponded well with the original pictures, and were useful for diagnosis.

4. By using method described above, images similar to the original pictures could be obtained, in spite of the rather light color.

Thus, remote telephotographing of ultrasonic images by fax proved useful for diagnosis, without any specific problems in practical use.

References

1. Shibuya, N. & Ito, K. New systems of ultrasonic diagnostic equipments, Medical Ultrasound 38: 139–140 (1981).

2. Tane, S., Hashimoto, M., Hashimoto, T., Hirata, M. & Kimura, Y. Studies on ultrasonic diagnosis in ophthalmology (Report 23): Telediagnosis by faxed ultrasonogram. Clinical Ophthalmology 43: 1128–1129 (1989).

Address for correspondence: Department of Ophthalmology, St. Marianna University, 2-16-1, Sugao, Miyamae-ku, Kawasaki-shi, 213 Japan.

59. The differential diagnosis of endobulbar tumors by means of false colors

T. AVITABILE, G. CASCONE, C. MARINO, C. GAGLIANO,
O. BONACCORSI, F. MARANO & C. BUCCHERI
(*Catania, Italy*)

Abstract. The differential diagnosis of endobulbar tumors has been performed up to now, prevalently by means of A-scan standardized echography. Thanks to our school, which recognized the use of technological development in regards to false colours, in 1984, today we have computerized B-scan equipment in false colours, with programs that give us the opportunity to perform frozen image elaborations. By means of such programs is possible to study the characteristics of reflectivity, the texture and the contours of the structures that we are examining. Furthermore such equipment is able to perform accurate measurements of dimensions and areas. The authors in this work report their experience on the possibility to perform the differential diagnosis of the principles of endobulbar tumors by means of B-scan in false colours and analyze their various echographical aspects.

Introduction

Until now, the diagnosis of the nature of endobulbar tumors has been considered a hard testing bench for the opthalmologist. The most frequent bulbar neoformations are retinoblastoma in pediatric age and melanoma, choroidal angioma and metastasis in adult age.

Considering that, in case of transparent media, ophthalmoscopy and the fluorangiography are still fundamental to the study and diagnosis of these pathologies, echography, unique in case of opaque media, is also important in such circumstances either for differential diagnosis or follow-up.

Until some time ago, the echographic technique chosen to make diagnoses of endobulbar tumors was the standardized A-scan, according to Ossoinig. In fact, this method gives us information about reflectivity, which is a very useful parameter in such ocular pathologies. But, in spite of these undoubted advantages, this method presents some difficulties, because it requires an execution which is characterized by the examination of a series of meridians. Consequently, it is also difficult to carry out this examination, which needs moreover an active collaboration from the patient that, in case of retinoblastoma in a child, is obtainable with difficulty. To obtain a correct diagnosis from this method, the examiner must have a good training and a good deal of experience; if a test is mismanaged it can cause artifacts with the possibility of false negatives and false positives.

To obviate the inconveniences caused by A-scan, for several years our school has pointed out the value of last generation B-scan (Reibaldi et al.

P. Till (ed.), Ophthalmic Echography 13, pp. 483–488.

1984, 1987; Avitabile et al. 1987) as foretold by Coleman. The impossibility of studying the reflectivity, a key parameter in the diagnosis of tumors, is a great gap which has already been attributed to B-scan.

In another delicate field of the bulbar echographic diagnostics concerning the differentiation of vitreous membranes, we proved that it is also possible to obtain information about reflectivity and then the correct diagnosis with only the B-scan. We used, at first, experimental techniques and subsequently last generation computerized B-scan which are provided with different programs to elaborate the frozen image in false colors.

With this study, we want to start to consider the utility of B-scan in false colours in the field of tumors, because our school has gained many years of experience in the use of false colour techniques (Reibaldi et al. 1984) and in the characterization of endobulbar tumors texture by texture analysis (Reibaldi et al. 1984).

Elaboration programs

The peculiar characteristics of this last generation equipment is the substitution of the traditional gray scale with another one in false colours. Moreover, with these instruments, it is possible to obtain a computerized elaboration of a frozen image which, by using a series of programs in the menu, allows us to easily carry out a texture characterization to obtain a more accurate diagnosis.

The apparatus now on the market is the practical realization of an intuition of our school, which several years ago conducted some experimental studies in collaboration with CNR's IESI Institute. With this technique we see the representation of different ocular structures, pathological or not, with different colours to which correspond different reflectivities and therefore different pathologies. With the 'saturate selected level' program, we can only show those areas with the same pre-selected reflectivity. With the 'saturate above level' program, we can point out all those structures with a higher reflectivity at the selected level.

Another particularly useful program is 'enhance contour', which shows the contours, allowing us to determine the limits of a bulbar neoformation. A further program, 'enhance texture', is particularly useful in case of tumors, and can point out the inner texture of the lesion. Moreover, in this peculiar kind of pathology, programs that allow us to perform the follow-up appear important. In fact, by placing the markers it is possible to obtain accurate measurements or even to calculate surfaces drawing polygonals. This is particularly useful to follow-up, the development of a neoformation or to consider the effects of a possible conservative therapy (radiation and chemotherapy, laser, etc.).

Furthermore, just in case of very small neoformations, we can use a zoom which allows us to enlarge the image to study their characteristics better.

Retinoblastoma

Retinoblastoma's peculiar echographic picture, which allows us an easy identification in case of classical form, is obviously connected with its histological nature. In fact, retinoblastoma is characterized by a neoformation which occupies the vitreous body with the presence of calcificated and necrotic areas. This anatomo-pathologic structure justifies the traditional echographic A-scan pattern where there are numerous peaks with a low irregular reflectivity in relation with a shadowing of posterior structures in the presence of calcifications.

The echographic B-scan picture is characterized by the presence of one or more than one mamillary mass with regular acoustic structure which however, in the presence of necrotic and calcificated areas, can become irregular with a pathognomic shadowing.

Programs of computerized elaboration in false colour allow us to point out, in addition to the typical characteristics of B-scan mentioned above, a series of information about reflectivity and texture, which permits us to make diagnosis of nature like A-scan. In particular, using the saturate selected level program, we shall easily be able to show the calcificate areas which will persist even at the highest levels of saturation, while the echos of the remaining mass will disappear. By also using the saturate above level program, we shall be able to show all those structures which will have received the highest reflectivity at the selected level. Of course, using the other programs at our disposal we can study better still the neoformation either in its texture (enhance texture) or in its contours (enhance contours).

Choroidal neoformations

In our study, we have also examined the choroidal neoformations (melanoma, angioma, metastasis). To make a diagnosis we used echography, CT, NMR and above all, in case of transparent media, fluorangiography and, of course, opthalmoscopy. Nevertheless, echography is generally considered the best means to make a correct diagnosis of the nature of the choroidal mass, reminding us that, in some cases, lesions which present similar clinical characteristics need a quite different therapy. Therefore it is plain that a correct diagnosis is very important (Coleman et al. 1977). As we have discussed above, reflectivity is the fundamental echographic parameter which is able to make the differential diagnosis in such pathologies. Until some years ago, only A-scan could show this data, but now, in our opinion, it can also be displayed by B-scan, in which we find the substitution of the traditional gray scale with colours, where a different colour corresponds to a different gray level. Moreover, these B-scans allow us to study the inner texture of the lesion, and a series of other parameters, whose analysis leads us to its probable nature (Avitabile et al. 1989). The echographic parameters that we can study by B-scan in case of a probable choroidal neoformation are:

reflectivity, shape, location, measurement (dimensions), acoustic vacuole, choroidal excavation, inner texture and follow-up. Accurate analysis of all the echographic parameters given through B-scan, will enable us to make a correct diagnosis of its nature when we are in the presence of a choroidal mass. Nowadays, some of these parameters can be still better studied with the latest generation of B-scan.

Of course, we can distinguish reflectivity better with a scale in false colours than with one in black and white; we can also distinguish it thanks to some programs of elaboration (saturate selected, saturate above, reject level) with some numbers that, each of them, correspond to a different colour. In fact, we can point out the inner reflectivity of the neoformation excluding other bulbar structures that are not important for use at that moment.

On the other hand, we can select a reflectivity level and display, on the monitor, only those structures which present a particular level, in order to compare the neotransformation's reflectivity with another bulbar structure's one. Therefore, we would find out a very high reflectivity (95–100%) in case of hemangioma; a slightly lower reflectivity in the case of metastasis and a remarkably lower reflectivity in the case of melanoma (5–60%).

Shape: it can be considered an echographic parameter which precisely pertains to B-scan. Angioma will appear to be a roundish formation with definite limits. Melanoma may be a variable shape according to whether Bruch's membrane is intact or not. In the first case, it will be dome-shaped, while in the second case it will be typically mushroom-shaped (Shammas 1984). On the contrary, metastasis present a confused shape with indistinct limits, like a waxflow (Cennamo et al. 1988).

Location: it can also offer a further tool to make a differential diagnosis. Angioma is often located in the posterior pole near optic nerve's head as well as metastasis, which often affects the left eye more than the right one. This event is probably due to left carotid's direct origin from the aorta, while right carotid originates from the brachycephalic trunk. On the contrary, melanoma may appear in any zone of choroid.

Dimensions: among the various elaborations offered by this equipment, we have the possibility to execute, thanks to the motion of two markers, an accurate measurement of the mass. These devices also allow us to draw some polygonals around the formation, giving us the volume of the mass. Angioma's dimensions are not usually over 5–6 mm. On the contrary, melanomas and metastasis are various dimensions, reaching such growth that sometimes it occupies the whole eye ball (Poujol & Chaintron 1988).

Acoustic vacuole is another parameter which pertains to B-scan and is characteristic of choroidal melanoma. It presents a prevalently cellular structure and scarcity of interfaces which will cause the acoustic vacuole on the display.

Choroidal excavation appears when a certain area of normal choroidal is replaced by a pathologic tissue with a low reflectivity (Mazzeo 1987). Therefore it is the echographic representation of tumor's invasion in the choroid, which we have found in 80% of the cases with the same incidence either in the case of a melanoma or in the case of metastasis but never in the case of an angioma (Poujol & Le Roy 1983).

Inner texture is characterized by the echos of the considered structure; it will be the result of a lower or a higher homogeneity of the studied texture. The presence of a less or most remarkable cellular component, the presence or the absence of vessels full of blood will naturally give rise to a different inner texture. Among the considered formations angioma generally appears with a fine and regular texture. On the contrary, metastasis have a very coarse inner texture while melanoma present a fairly spongy one.

Follow-up is an important parameter which has to be considered in these kinds of pathologies. In fact, the field of the tumor's, unlike others, diagnosis of nature, is very often pointed out by tumor's temporal evolution. Thanks to last generation of B-scan, we have the possibility to screen the examined image, as expounded above, and to consider the answer to an eventual conservative therapy.

After reiterated measurements, either of thickness or of surface, we deduce that angioma and metastasis tend to grow very slowly. On the contrary, melanoma is characterized by a growth which becomes evident in the case of a breakage of Bruch's membrane and we then notice that the tumor is typically shaped like a mushroom (Cennamo et al. 1988).

Conclusions

Up to the present, the diagnosis of a tumoral endobulbar pathology is anything but simple. The clinical evaluation must be supported by other semeiotic research such as fluoroangiography, retinal angiography with green indocyanine and in the second place echography, CT and NMR (Falco et al. 1988).

Evidently this sequence of semeiotic research, reported in order of importance, is modified in case of opaque dioptric media in favour of echography, which becomes fundamental, or if we must treat very young patients, for whom other examinations are difficult to carry out.

In this study, we want to point out the importance of B-scan in the diagnosis of the nature of the main tumoral endobulbar lesions (retinoblastoma, angioma, metastasis, melanoma) considering that, until some time ago, this kind of diagnosis was entrusted only to standardized A-scan.

We are now continuing a study that our school (Reibaldi et al. 1984–87) had begun several years ago, in which we assert that the information contained in an A-scan picture is also present, even if in a different way, in a B-scan pattern. If this statement has already been well coded in the differential diagnostics of vitreous membranes, we are at the first attempts at the field of tumor pathology (Reibaldi et al. 1987).

Moreover, we want to stress the utility of the latest generation of B-scan equipment which shows the representation of a B-scan image either by gray levels or by false colours. With these devices it is possible to make a computerized elaboration of the frozen image which, by using a series of programs, allows one to easily carry out a characterization of the textures in order to obtain a more accurate diagnosis, resulting in a briefer training period from the examiner.

References

Avitabile, T., Cacciato, F. & Bonaccorsi, O. La diagnosi differenziale delle membrane vitreali up-date. Atti II Congr. Naz. S.I.E.O. Catania 7 Nov. (1987).

Avitabile, T., Pappalardo, A. & Spina, A. Il B-scan a contatto nel retinoblastoma. Boll. Ocul. 68, (suppl 6) (1989).

Avitabile, T., Cascone, G., Marino, C. and Gagliano, C. Primi risultati con il B-scan in falsi colori nel retinoblastoma. Poster at International Symposium on Intraocular Tumors, Firenze 2–4 February (1990).

Cennamo, G., Fao, T. & De Palma, L. Studio clinico ed ecografico dei tumori metatatici della coroide. Clin. Ocul. 4: 297–300 (1988).

Coleman, D.J., Lizzi, F.L. & Jack, R.L. Ultrasonography of the eye and orbit. Philadelphia: Lea & Fabiger (1977).

Falco, L., Esente, S., Fanfani, S., Passarelli, N. & Pierro, L. Risonanza nucleare magnetica e diagnostica differenziable tra melanoma maligno ed emangioma della coroide. Atti III Congr. Naz. S.I.E.O. Napoli 13 Nov. (1988).

Mazzeo, V. Ecografia dell'apparato oculare. Testo atlante. Fogliazza editore (1987).

Poujol, J. & Le, Roy M. Echographic modifications of the choroid in its tumors and pseudo-tumors. In Hillman, J.S. and Le May, M.M. (eds.), Opthalmic Ultrasonography, pp. 57–62. The Hague: Dr. W. Junk Publishers (1983).

Poujol, J. & Chaintron, M.C. Analysis of a recent series (254 cases) of choroidal tumours. In Thijssen, J.M. (eds.), Ultrasonography in Ophthalmology, pp. 157–164 (1988).

Reibaldi, A., Lo Russo, V.V. & Delle Noci, N. 8 years of A- and B-scan ultrasonography in tumoral diagnostics of the globe and orbit. Atti VIII Symposium S.I.D.U.O. Nijmegen (Netherlands) 16–19 Settembre (1980).

Reibaldi, A., Avitabile, T., Guerriero, S., Distante, A. & Veneziani N. Primi risultati sulle possibilità di differenziazione ecografica tissutale oculare mediante falso colore. Clin. Ocul. e Pat. Ocul. V(6) (1984).

Reibaldi, A., Guerriero, S., Avitabile, T., Uva, M.G., Veneziani, N., Pasquariello, G. & Pasquali, F. Texture analysis di immagini ultrasonografiche in oculistica. Clin. Ocul. e Pat. Ocul. VIII(1) (1987).

Reibaldi, A., Avitabile, T. & Cascone, G. Emangioma coroideale: ecografia B-scan. International Symposium on Intraocular Tumors, Firenze 2–4 February (1990).

Shammas, J.H. Ultrasonografia e biometria oftalmologica. Medical Books (1984).

Address for correspondence: Institute of Ophthalmology, Catania University, Via Bambino 32, I-95124 Catania, Italy.

60. Usefulness of simultaneous display of four different B-scan images in ocular diagnosis

A. SAWADA, J. FUKIYAMA, F. MARUIWA & Y. BABA

(Miyazaki, Japan)

Abstract. The simultaneous display of four different B-scan images is one of the most distinguished functions of the new ultrasonic diagnostic equipment. The equipment can be used for many purposes: four images of different directions; four images of different sensitivity settings; or four images in comparison between two eyes and others.

Introduction

Ultrasonography is one of the important modalities for the diagnosis of various kinds of ophthalmic disorders. Usually ultrasonic A- and B-scan images are evaluated on monitor, films, prints, or other materials, and occasionally videotapes are used. All of these images are separately taken and shown, so that when the same pictures with decreased or increased gain are needed, it is necessary to hold the probe in the same position while pictures with different gain are taken. This is rather dangerous in some cases, particularly in traumatised eyes, and it is not so easy to repeat. In the new diagnostic equipment we have recently developed, gain and dynamic range can be changed after the images have been stored, as described elsewhere in this volume. It would be valuable if two or more images could be displayed on one monitor at the same time, and in our new ultrasonic diagnostic equipment four different B-scan images can be displayed at the same time. In this paper we discuss the method of using this facility and the advantage of the new function of the equipment in clinical use.

Methods

The new equipment (US 3000, Nidek Co., Japan) is the A- and B-scan ultrasonic diagnostic equipment. The probe frequency is 10 MHz.

The method for the simultaneous display of four different B-scan images is as follows. In a first step, one B-scan image is displayed on the monitor, with the most important part of the target tissue in the center. Then the

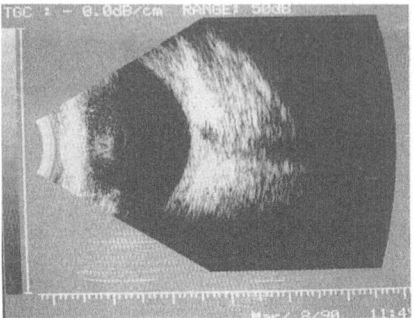

Fig. 1A. The original image is stored.

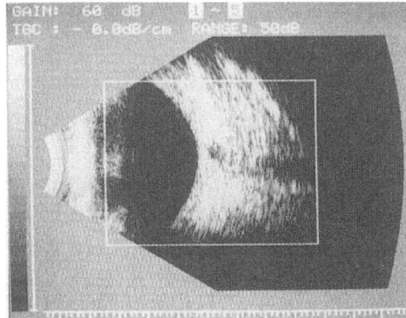

Fig. 1B. The area to be transferred is enclosed within a box.

image is stored (Fig. 1A). The initially stored image should be the original, after which the area to be transferred is enclosed by a box (Fig. 1B). The position of the box on the original image can be shifted to any direction (Fig. 1C). The enclosed boxed image is transferred to the monitor and displayed in the one-fourth portion of the monitor. The position of the transferred image on the monitor can be freely selected and changed with the function buttons.

Materials and results

Simultaneous displays of four different B-scans can be used, for many purposes.

1. Four images of four directions or quadrants of the eye and the orbit. Four images of four directions (superior, inferior, nasal and temporal) are simultaneously displayed. Four images in four quadrants are also available.

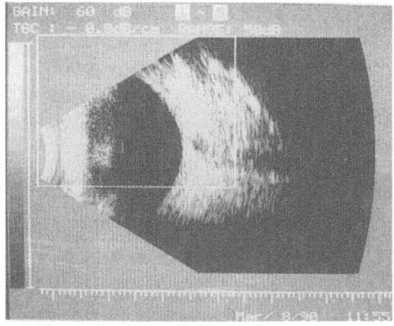

Fig. 1C. The position of the box on the original can be shifted in any direction.

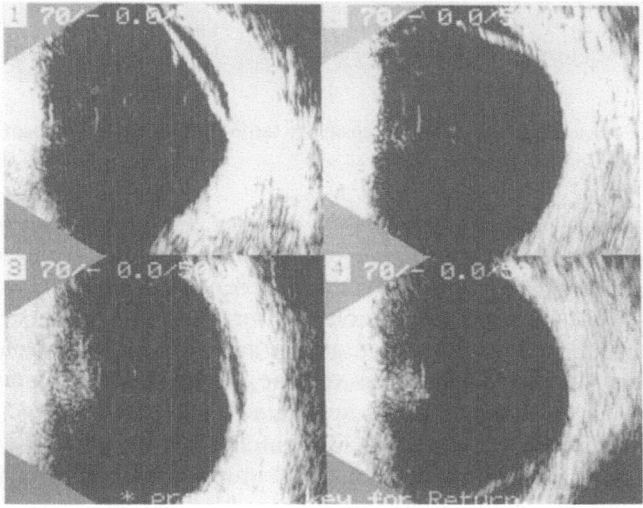

Fig. 2. Four images of four directions in a case of retinal detachment.

Some of these four images can be composed of the different original images successively, so that images of different areas can be composed and displayed simultaneously. Four images in the different parts are useful for showing localization and extent of intraocular lesions as well as orbital lesions. In the same manner, oblique scanning is also available. A topographic description of the lesion can be easily done. This kind of image arrangement is very useful in showing localization and extent of the lesion. Fig. 2 shows a case with vitreous hemorrhage and retinal detachment. The topographic relation between both lesions and the fundus structure is well documented.

This kind of image arrangement is very suggestive in those cases, in which the shape in two sections crossing at right angle is quite specific for diagnosis. Arterio-venous fistula is one of the best examples.

492

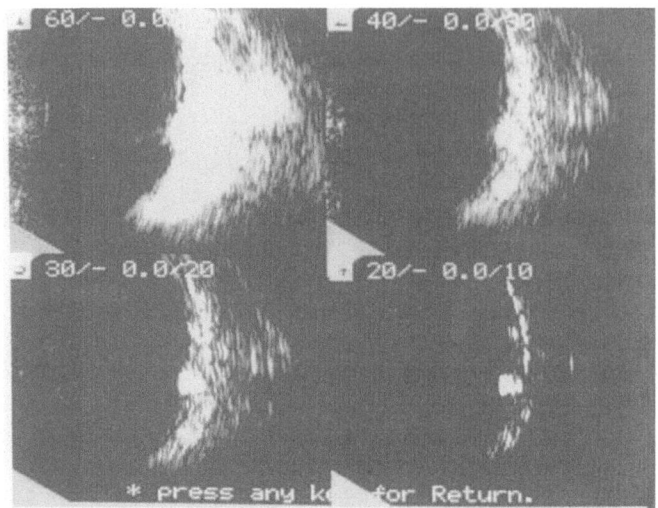

Fig. 3. Four images with different sensitivity settings in a case of a foreign body.

2. Four images with different sensitivity settings. It is unnecessary to emphasize the importance of quantitative evaluation of the ultrasonic reflectivity with different sensitivity settings in the differential diagnosis. It is useful in membrane-like lesions such as vitreous hemorrhage and retinal detachment, and is also applicable to tumor diagnosis and foreign body detection. As described in a separate paper in this volume, in the new equipment, imaging parameters such as dynamic range and gain can be changed and the corresponding images can be displayed. The images to be transferred and displayed can be selected at will from those images with different settings of dynamic range and gain. These multiple-graded images can be produced from the same stored image as well as from different stored images.

A case of foreign body is one of the best examples, in which the quantitative evaluation of ultrasonic reflectivity is needed. As shown in Fig. 3, a foreign body just in front the posterior eye coat is clear. The reflectivity is extremely strong. In traumatized eyes as these, mutiple-graded images can be produced from only a single image. In cases of asteroid hyalosis or vitreous hemorrhage, with reduced gain, signals from the vitreous almost disappear. However, in the former granule-like signals are left.

In cases of choroidal detachment (Fig. 4) or posterior scleritis, the inner reflectivity of the thickened membrane-like lesion is very high, which is one of characteristics of these lesions as well as the shape.

In cases of orbital tumors, findings with reduced sensitivity are very useful in defining the boundary and revealing the details of the content.

3. Four images for comparison between two eyes. Ultrasonographic findings

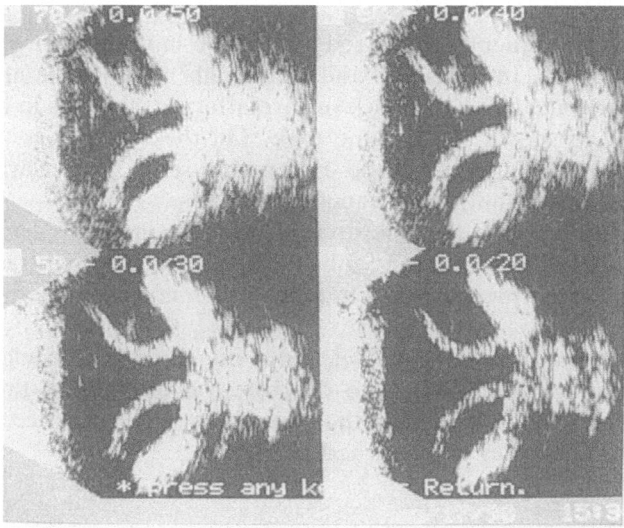

Fig. 4. Four images with different sensitivity settings in a case of choroidal detachment.

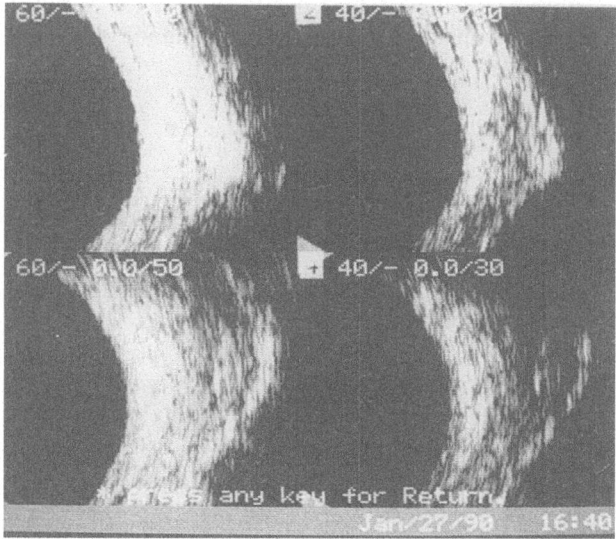

Fig. 5. Four images of the medial rectus muscles with high and low amplification in comparison between two eyes. The upper two are from the right eye. The lower two are from the left eye. The right two are at a gain of 60 dB, the left at 40 dB.

494

in one eye are frequently compared with those in the other eye, particularly in orbital lesions. In a case of unilateral high myopia, the affected eye is long and protruded. When both eyes are affected, findings in both eyes are required to be shown at the same time. On these occasions, simultaneous displays of four images would be extremely useful, particularly in cases of hypertrophy or swellings of extraocular muscles.

Fig. 5 shows a case of hyperthyroidism. The upper two are the medial rectus muscle of the right eye with high and low amplification. The lower two are of the left medial rectus muscle, which is more hypertrophic.

4. Four images for other purposes. Four-image displays could be used for many other purposes, such as to describe the mobility of the lesion with postural change, lens luxation in the vitreous, or to record successive images, such as a tumor under the detached retina.

Conclusion

In conclusion, the four-image display system that is provided by the newly developed equipment, is very useful in the ultrasonic diagnosis of various ocular lesions. Further extention of application is much expected.

Acknowledgement

The study was supported in part by Grants-In-Aid for Scientific Research C-01570978 from the Ministry of Education, Science and Culture of the Japanese Government.

Reference

Sawada, A. Study on ultrasonic tissue characterization of intraocular membranous structures. Acta Soc. Ophthalmol. Jpn. 90: 43–66 (1986).

Address for correspondence: Department of Ophthalmology, Miyazaki Medical College, 5200 Kihara, Kiyotake, Miyazaki, 889-16 Japan.

61. Area and volume calculation by three-dimensional echography of the eye

E. MOTOLESE, M. BURRONI, G. ADDABBO, G. DELL'EVA,
B. D'ANIELLO & N. PATERRA
(*Siena, Italy*)

Abstract. The authors discuss their experience regarding the three-dimensional reconstruction of the echographic image, firstly of an orbital angioma and secondly, of a malignant choroidal melanoma. Of the latter, they calculate the volume and the total external surface. Reference is also made to data regarding reproducibility, the errors of reconstruction methodology and volume calculation. However, it is more reliable than the commonly used echographic procedures.

Introduction

The new diagnostic needs in ophthalmology have created a constant stimulus for research in echography. We have recently become interested in the possibilities of using three-dimensional images originating from two-dimensional echograms obtained from B-scan echograph Mod. 200 Sonometric System with a probe of 10 MHz. These images enable the volume of the reconstructed lesions to be calculated in a precise manner. This is very important in the area of ocular tumors, such as malignant choroidal melanoma where, if the volume is correctly calculated, it permits observation of the tumor's evolution and its eventual sensitivity to control therapy.

Materials and methods

A case of orbital cavernous angioma and one of choroidal melanoma have been studied, and both the total surface and the volume of the latter have been calculated.

The examination was calculated by having the patient fix his eye on a small torchlight. Both vertical and horizontal seriated scans distanced at 1 mm apart for the angioma, and 0.5 mm for the melanoma, were made. Each scan was recorded as a digitized reading. The images of the lesion's surroundings were manually reconstructed in a connected manner, in order to improve visual quality. The surroundings of the previous lesion were vectorized and superimposed onto the intial echogram.

Subsequently, it was progressed to a three-dimensional elaboration. In the image of the orbital angioma the reconstruction of the eyeball and that

P. Till (*ed.*), *Ophthalmic Echography 13*, pp. 495–498.

of the muscular cone appears stylized, since they were not those of the examined patient, although the lesion is actual, both in its dimensions and its morphological reconstruction. In the case of the choroidal melanoma, only the specific pathological zone was considered.

Discussion

The manual extraction of the surroundings of a lesion is one of the most delicate phases of this procedure, which could be subject to variability both intraobserver and interobserver. To reduce the extent of accidental error in both cases, multiple readings of the surroundings of each single section was taken. In this way all the surroundings could be processed to the end with the 'AND' binary operator.

It should be noted that the possibility of error is negligible with a medium value of 'O' of Gaussian distribution. The correct interpretation of what has been discussed is solely related to the quality of the image, i.e.,

(a) *Intrinsic quality* depends on the relationship between the signal/sound of the echograph, due to which the echograph with the 'reject' function gives better intrinsic quality.

(b) *Comparative quality* is inversely proportional to the error of the quantization data of:

$$Eq = \sum_{i=1}^{n} \sum_{i=1}^{m} (li_{(x,y)} - lr_{(x,y)})^2,$$

where $li_{(x,y)}$ is the ideal image, and $lr_{(x,y)}$ is the real reference image. For small values of Eq, the quality is noticeably better.

(c) *Diagnostic quality*. On the basis of the results, the better the probability of correctly recognizing a lesion, the better is the diagnostic quality. It also depends on the sensitivity of the echograph used to recognize the lesion, in this case about 87%.

The limits of the lesion sections between numbers 20 and 45 were taken into consideration for the choroidal melanoma.

The pathological area of each single section was reconstructed. The measurements were noted taking into account that in an area of $2500\,mm^2$ ($50\,mm \times 50\,mm$) in the entire echographic video, there are 311^2 pixels of digital frequency and that the pixel frequency is balanced with dimensions of $1:1$. Thus it has been possible to calculate the scale factor of each individual pixel according to the ratio

$$F_{scale} = \frac{50^2}{311^2} = 2.58 \times 10^2.$$

Once the scale factor is known, it is possible to calculate the total area of the sections according to the formula

$$A_{\text{tot}} = \sum_{i=1}^{25} A_i \times F_{\text{scale}}.$$

$A_{\text{tot}} P\ 132.27 \times 2.58 \times 10^{-2} = 3412.75 \text{ mm}^2 = 34.13 \text{ cm}^2.$

The total area of the calculation is found with:

$$\text{Vol}_{\text{tot}} = A_{\text{tot}} \times 0.5 \text{ mm (section interval)}.$$

In this case, $\text{Vol}_{\text{tot}} = 34.13 \times 0.05 \text{ cm} = 1.70 \text{ cm}^3.$

It is possible to calculate the total external surface of the lesion according to the formula

$$S_{\text{tot}} = 2 \sum_{i=1}^{25} p_i \times \text{linear scale factor} \times 0.5,$$

where the linear scale factor is equal to 1.6×10^{-1}, of which

$$S_{\text{tot}} = 2 \sum_{i=1}^{25} p_i \times 1.6 \times 10^{-1} \times 0.5.$$

$$S_{\text{tot}} = 688.02 \text{ mm}^2.$$

Each single perimeter section can be calculated by counting the surrounding pixels and reproducing them with the linear conversion factor.

It is important to remember that in the calculation of the areas of each section it is possible to make an error that can reach a maximum value equal to the semiperimeter in pixel of the section generically considered. In synthesis:

$$0 \leqslant \text{error} \leqslant p_i.$$

where p_i = semiperimeter of the generic section. The result is that the maximum total relative error made in the calculation of the section areas is given by the formula

$$E_{\text{rel.tot.}} = \sum_{i=1}^{25} \frac{P_i \cdot F_s}{A_i \cdot F_s}.$$

$$E_{\text{rel.tot.}} = \sum_{i=1}^{25} \frac{P_i}{A_i}.$$

It seems that the errors in the volume calculation has a relation to the total relative errors of the area calculation if the number of sections tends towards infinity. If it has in fact:

$$\lim_{n \to} E_{\text{vol.tot.}} = \sum_{i=1}^{25} \frac{P_i}{A_i},$$

498

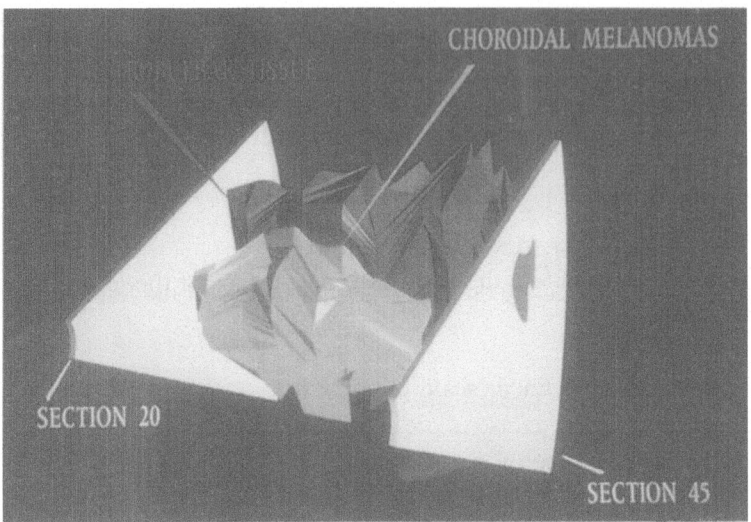

Fig. 1. An example of a 3-D reconstruction of a choroidal malignant melanoma.

where $E_{vol.tot.}$ is the maximum possible error in the calculation of the lesion volume (Fig. 1).

We have valued experimentally the calculation process inserting 1 cc of gel and H_2Mg_3 $(SIO_3)_4$ under the chorio-retina, after scleral incision, in a pig eye and estimating the volume by three-dimensional echography.

Results: known volume = 1 cc; estimated volume = 0.951 cc.

We believe that the calculated error of volume (<0.05) would encourage further studies.

References

1. Pratt, W.K. Digital images processing. Wiley and Sons (1978).
2. Nagao, M. & Matsutama, T. Edge preserve smoothing. Computer Graphics and Image Processing 9: 334–407 (1979).
3. Azriel, R. & Avinash C.K. Digital picture processing. London: Academic Press (1982).
4. Harrington, S. Computer graphics. McGraw-Hill (1983).
5. Yamamoto, Y., Kubota, M., Sugata, Y., Matsui, S. & Ito, M. Three-dimensional ultrasonography of ocular region. In Documenta Ophthalmologica Proceedings Series 51, Ultrasonography in Ophthalmology 11. Dordrecht: Kluwer Acad. Publ. (1986).

Address for correspondence: Department of Ophthalmology, University of Siena, Via A. Nannizzi 4, I-53100 Siena, Italy.

PART SEVEN

Biometry

62. Extracapsular cataract extraction with posterior chamber lens implantation

Comparison between preoperative lens power calculation and postsurgical refraction

F. SAYEGH, Z. SHAMAYLEH, G. JAYYOUSI & A. SHAHEEN

(Amman, Jordan)

Abstract. In this paper we determine the difference between the lens power calculated to produce emmetropia and a standard +20 diopter lens, and, if such a difference exists, what will be the magnitude and the practical significance. The average value of calculated lens power was found to be +18.2 ± 4.26 D. A negative correlation was found between the calculated lens power and corneal refraction ($r = -0.25$) and between the calculated lens power and axial length ($r = -0.84$). 35% of examined cases had a lens power of less than +18.0 D or more than +22.0 D. 30.5% of operated cases did not show astigmatism after one year of observation. 20.3% were found to be emmetropic, 50.9% had minor errors of refraction. The use of spectacles for distance in this group could be discounted. 28.8% of operated cases needed eyeglasses for distances of $> + 1.0$ sph. comb. > -1.5 cyl. The expected error of refraction was -0.45 ± 0.88 D. The postoperative spherocylindrical equivalent was found to be -0.23 ± 1.42 D.

Introduction

The practical value of posterior chamber lens implantation after extracapsular cataract extraction aims to achieve the best physiological optical results, minimizing the aniseikony and avoiding the need for spectacles for distance. Eyeglasses are unlikely to be used in most developing countries. Estimation of the lens power can be done if the patient's error of refraction is known before the cataract has developed, or it can be calculated from keratometry and ultrasound biometric measurements. It has been suggested that if standard +20 D lenses are used in patients with a preoperative refractive error of less than 5 D at myopia or hypermetropia, the results are equivalent to those seen if preoperative biometry is used [1, 2, 3]. In contrast, others have found that a routine lens calculation before surgery is indicated and useful [4, 5]. In this paper we compare the calculated lens power for emmetropia and postsurgical refraction, to determine whether a significant difference exsists between the calculated lens power for emmetropia and a standard +20.0 D, and, if such a difference exsists, what is the magnitude and practical significance?

Material and methods

Extracapsular cataract extraction (ECC) with posterior chamber lens implantation was performed on 400 consecutive cases. Keratometry was done by

P. Till (ed.), Ophthalmic Echography 13, pp. 501–506.
© 1993 *Kluwer Academic Publishers*.

502

Table 1. Age and sex distribution of operated cases (male : female = 1.7 : 1)

Age in years	Male 54.3 ± 14.8	Female 57.7 ± 12.8	Total 55.7 ± 14.2
10–19	4	4	10
20–29	10	2	12
30–39	20	4	24
40–49	56	20	76
50–59	59	40	99
60–69	64	57	121
70–79	28	16	44
80–89	11	5	16
Total	252	148	400

two different examiners using two different keratometers. The ultrasound biometric measurements were made using a Sonometrics system BR400. The average of three readings was considered and the Binkhorst formula was used to calculate the posterior chamber lens for emmetropia. In cases with unilateral cataract, the IOL was selected to avoid aniseikony.

The ECC was done by using the expression of the nucleus and automatic irrigation aspiration technique. The corneoscleral incision was adapted with seven interrupted stitches. Dexamethasone and gentamycine were injected subconjunctivally at the end of surgery. The refraction was examined 1, 2, 3, 6 and 12 months after surgery. Patients with calculated lens power of equal or less than +10.0 D were excluded from IOL implantation. In cases with high astigmatism, the corneoscleral stitches were removed 2 months after surgery.

Results

The age and sex distribution of operated cases are shown in Table 1. The mean age of operated cases was 56 years with a male : female ratio of 1.7 : 1. This confirms the results of a previous study on the incidence of cataracts among 5000 consecutive cases examined at an outpatient clinic [6]. Before surgery 31% of the patients used eyeglasses for distance. The error of refraction for this group was found to be −1.28 ± 2.44 sph. and −1.53 ± 0.3 cyl. A comparison between the normal distribution of spherical error of refraction (Fig. 1) submitted in the ophthalmic outpatient clinic (−0.37 ± 3.24 D) and the preoperative errors of refraction for this group (−1.28 ± 2.44 sph.; 1.53 ± 0.3 cyl.) shows that the distribution curve is shifted to the myopic side. It indicates that either a large number of cataract patients are myopic, or that myopia has been induced by the cataract.

The biometric results and the linear correlation between the examined parameters are shown in Table 2. As expected, a negative correlation was found between the calculated lens power and corneal refraction, between

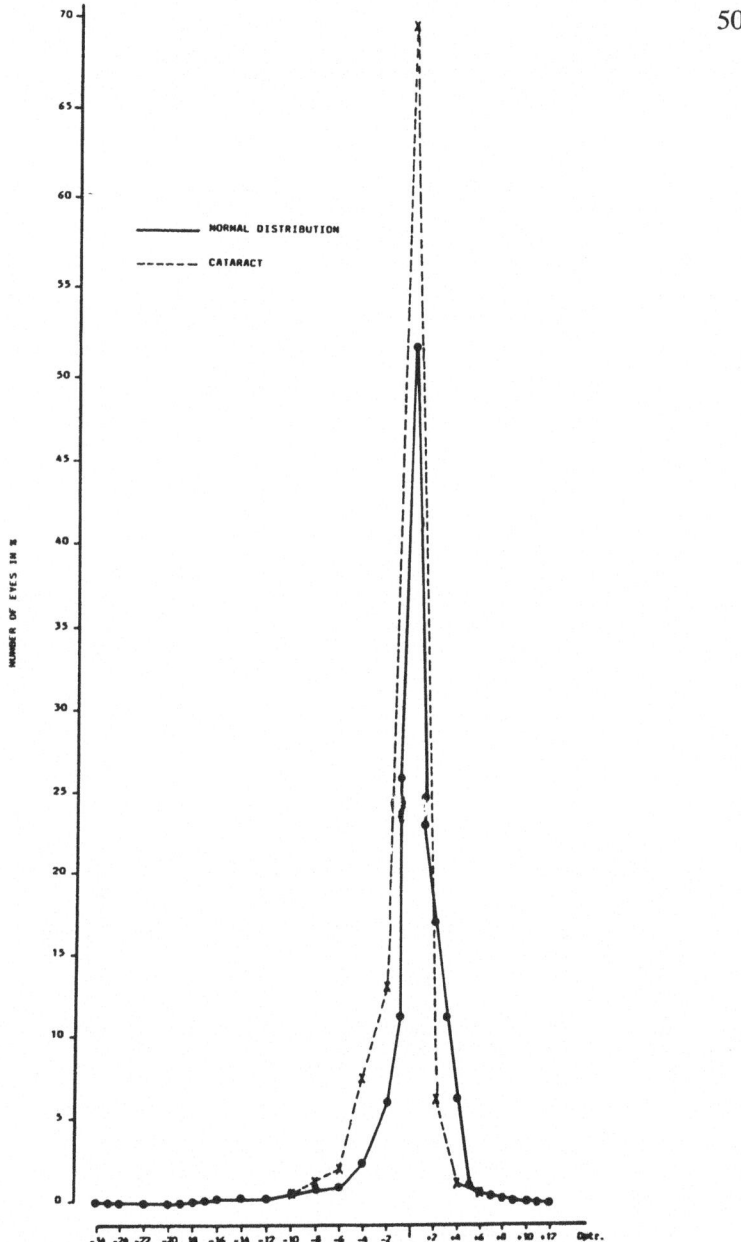

Fig. 1. Comparison of the normal distribution of spherical refractive errors and preoperative spherical errors of refraction.

the lens power and axial length, and between the corneal refraction and axial length. The higher the calculated lens power, the lower was the corneal refraction and axial length, and vice versa.

The preoperative calculated lens power was found to be 18.2 ± 4.26 D, ranging between −8.5 D and +33.5 D (Fig. 2). In 35% of cases we found

Table 2. Mean values, and correlation between examined parameters

Parameter	m + SD	Correlation coefficient (r)				
		k_1	k_2	$k_1 + k_2/2$	AL	LP
k_1	43.32 ± 1.89	1.0	0.82	0.95	−0.21	−0.19
k_2	44.24 ± 1.99	0.82	1.0	0.96	−0.16	−0.27
$k_1 + k_2/2$	43.78 ± 1.86	0.95	0.96	1.0	−0.17	−0.25
Axial length	23.57 ± 1.57	−0.21	−0.16	−0.17	1.0	−0.84
Lens power	18.22 ± 4.26	−0.19	−0.27	−0.25	−0.84	1.0

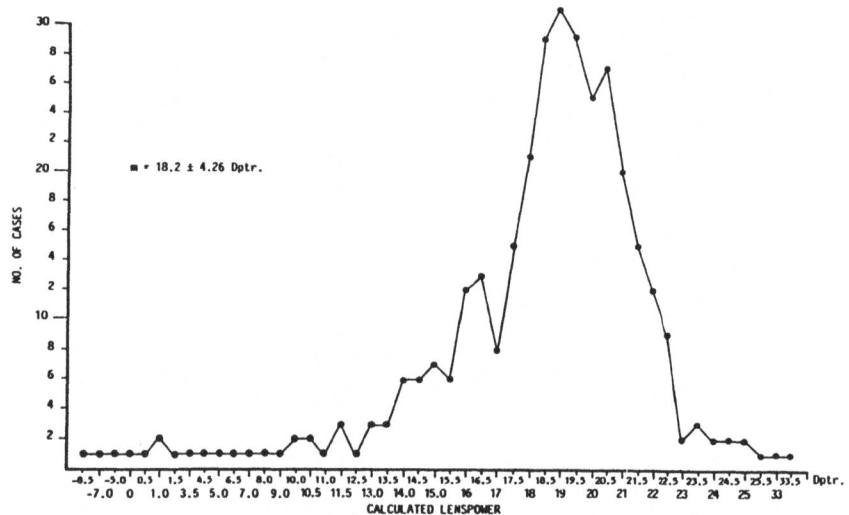

Fig. 2. Calculated lens power in cases with senile cataract.

less than +18.0 D or more than +22.0 D, confirming the importance of biometry for intraocular lens implantation.

Table 3 shows a comparison between the expected and postoperative errors of refraction. One can notice a relatively high astigmatism during the first week after surgery, although this decreases with time. The difference between expected and postoperative errors of refraction was found to be only 0.22 D.

Table 4 compares the angle of astigmatism before and after surgery. In comparison to preoperative findings (36.8%) a high incidence of astigmatic angles between 165° and 15° (62.1%) was found one month after surgery. A relatively tight suture at 12° and a swelling of the corneoscleral margin were found to be responsible for this astigmatism. Removal of this stich after 8 weeks causes normalization of the condition and a shifting of the angle from 180° to 90° in 13.4% of cases.

The refraction one year after posterior chamber lens implation is shown in Table 5. 20.3% were emmetropic, 50.9% had a visual acuity without

Table 3. Expected and postoperative errors of refraction

Postoperative errors of refraction	Spherical	Astigmatism
After		
1 week	$+2.66 \pm 1.48$	-5.21 ± 1.65
1 month	$+1.82 \pm 1.61$	-4.34 ± 1.91
2 months	$+1.10 \pm 1.44$	-2.72 ± 2.13
3 months	$+0.45 \pm 1.30$	-1.60 ± 1.46
6 months	$+0.34 \pm 0.45$	-1.07 ± 0.71
1 year	$+0.32 \pm 1.53$	-1.11 ± 1.33
Spherocylindrical equivalent	-0.23 ± 1.43	
Expected error of refraction	-0.45 ± 0.88	$t = 2.20, p = 0.05$
Theoretical error of refraction with a $+20.0$ D lens	-1.78 ± 0.24	$t = 7.48, p < 0.0010$

Table 4. Angle of astigmatism (in minus cyl.) before and after extracapsular cataract extraction

< Astigmatism (%)	Before surgery	1 month after surgery	1 year after surgery
0–10	33.8	41.2	31.9
15–20	1.5	11.9	12.8
25–30	3.1	9.3	8.5
35–40	–	2.3	–
45–50	6.2	1.1	2.1
55–60	6.2	1.5	4.2
65–70	1.5	1.8	–
75–80	1.5	–	–
85–90	23.1	3.7	17.1
95–100	–	0.4	2.1
105–110	1.5	1.9	2.1
115–120	9.3	1.1	4.4
125–130	–	1.4	2.1
135–140	7.7	1.1	–
145–150	1.5	7.4	2.1
155–160	–	4.9	–
165–170	3.0	9.5	8.5

Table 5. Postoperative errors of refraction

Error of refraction	%	
Absence of astigmatism	30.5	
Emmetropia	20.3	
+1.0 sph. only	10.2	
+1.5 cyl. only	13.6	50.9
+1.0 sph. comb. < −1.5 cyl.	27.1	
> +1.0 sph. comb. > 1.5 cyl.	28.8	

correction between 0.5 and 0.8, these eyes did not require spectacle correction. Only 28.8% needed eyeglasses for distance.

Discussion

Extracapsular cataract extraction and posterior chamber lens implantation were performed on 400 consecutive cataract cases, and we compared the calculated lens power to produce emmetropia, the expected postoperative refraction, and the theoretical refraction if +20 D lens were used. Our results here were as follows:

1. A large number of cataract patients are either myopic, or myopia has been induced by the cataract.
2. The mean value of calculated lens power is +18.2 ± 4.26 D.
3. There is a significant difference between the lens power calculated for emmetropia and the expected refraction if a + 20 D lens had been used.

In some developing countries, the use of spectacles is not accepted by the community and patients will visit the ophthalmologist only when a mature cataract has developed. It is therefore not possible to select cases with refractive errors of less than 5 D. In our study, 35% of cases were found to have a calculated IOL-power of less than +18 D or more than +22 D. One can conclude that keratometry and ultrasound biometry are important and mandatory.

Acknowledgements

I would like to thank Dr. Talib Sarie, Director of the Computer Center, University of Jordan, and Samira Jaradat and Butheina Awwad for their assistance.

References

1. Singh, K.A., Sommer, A.D. & Jensen, J.W. Payne: Intraocular lens power calculations. Arch. Ophthalmol. 105: 1046–1050 (1987).
2. Thompson, S.M. & Mohan-Roberts, V.A. A comparison of postoperative refractive results with and without intraocular lens power calculation. Br. J. Ophthamol. 70: 22–25 (1986).
3. Prior, C., Day, J.O., Ramsay, R.J. & Stephens, R. IOL prediction: an evaluation of preoperatively determined intraocular lens power accuracy. austr. and New Zealand J. of Ophthalmol. 16: 111–117 (1988).
4. Hope-Ross, M. & Mooney, D. Intraocular lens power calculation. Eye 2: 367–369 (1988).
5. Boerrigter, R.M.M., Thijssen, & Verbeek, A.M. Intraocular lens power calculations: the optimal approach. Ophthalmologica (Basel): 191: 89–94 (1985).
6. Sayegh, F., Arafat, N. & Ashoury, I. Cataract, a major cause of curable blindness in Jordan. Lens Research 3: 182, 271 (1986).

Address for correspondence: Head Department of Ophthalmology, Director of the Jordan Eye Bank, University of Jordan, P.O. Box 13371, Amman-Jordan.

63. Clinical results of preoperative intraocular lens power calculation by the Binkhorst formula

P. LEWANDOWSKI & M. SKURCZYŃSKI

(*Warsaw, Poland*)

Introduction

We have used Binkhorst formula for IOL power calculation in our clinic since 1987. In our work we aim to make clinical opinion on Binkhorst's formula for planning preoperative IOL power. IOL power was calculated for emetropia and a small amount of myopia – 0.5 D. The postoperative analysis was based on visual acuity and spherical refraction. We did not investigate postsurgical astigmatism.

Material

Two hundred twenty-nine patients were in our postoperative observation. Surgery was performed between February 1987 and October 1989. We observed 122 women – 73.6 years old, 107 men – 71.9 years old. In 199 cases ECCE was made and in 30 cases ICCE was made. In these groups 145 IOLs were implanted into the posterior chamber and 84 IOLs were implanted into the anterior chamber. Intraocular lenses for operations were used from various firms.

Equipment

We used Ultrascan Sonometric DBR-300 and Sonomed A-2000 for ultrasound examination. OPTON and Carl Zeiss Jena CL-100 for keratometry. Texas Instrument – 58C and Sonomed for IOL power calculation.

Results

The first group concerns patients with AC IOLs – 84 patients. ICCE was discovered in 30 cases. ECCE was discovered in 54 cases. Axial lengths ranged from 21.5 mm to 26.5 mm. Corneal radius range from 6.86 to 8.54. The range of power AC IOLs was from 13 D to 23 D. The biggest number

P. Till (ed.), *Ophthalmic Echography 13*, pp. 507–510.

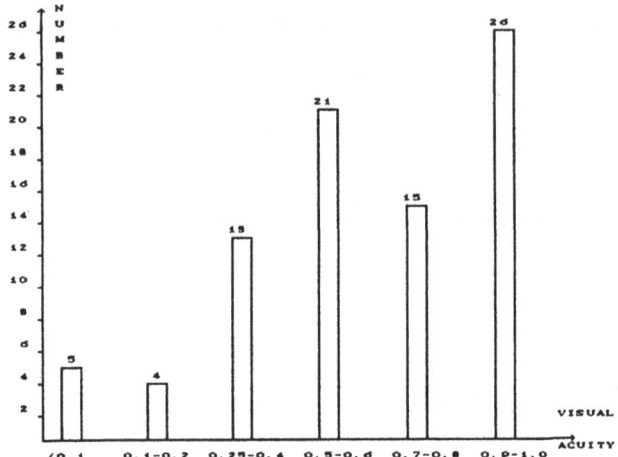

Fig. 1. Postoperative visual acuity after 6 months for AC IOL group.

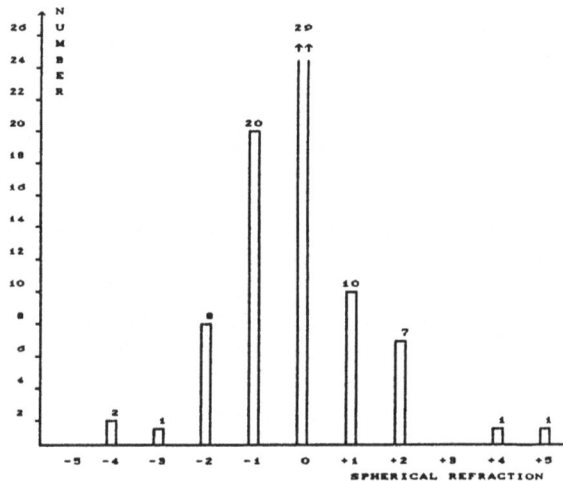

Fig. 2. Postoperative spherical refraction after 6 months for AC IOL group.

of IOLs inserted into the anterior chamber was in the group of power between 20 D and 19 D.

After six months, 62 patients (74%) had corrected or uncorrected visual acuity of more than 0.5; 22 patients (26%) had corrected or uncorrected visual acuity of less than 0.4 (Fig. 1). Fifty-nine patients (75%) needed spherical refraction of ±1 D and 74 patients (94%) needed ±2 D (Fig. 2).

The second group comprised 145 patients with PC IOL. Axial length ranged from 21.1 mm to 25.5 mm and corneal radius ranged from 7.17 to 8.58. The range of power PC IOLs used in the measured group were from 15.5 D to 24 D. The largest number of IOLs inserted into posterior chamber

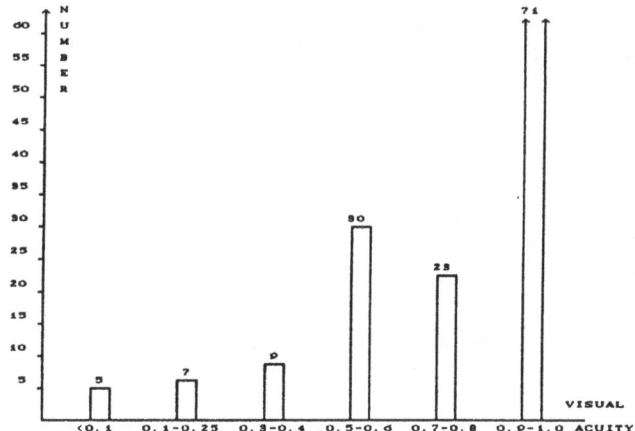

Fig. 3. Postoperative visual acuity after 6 months for PC IOL group.

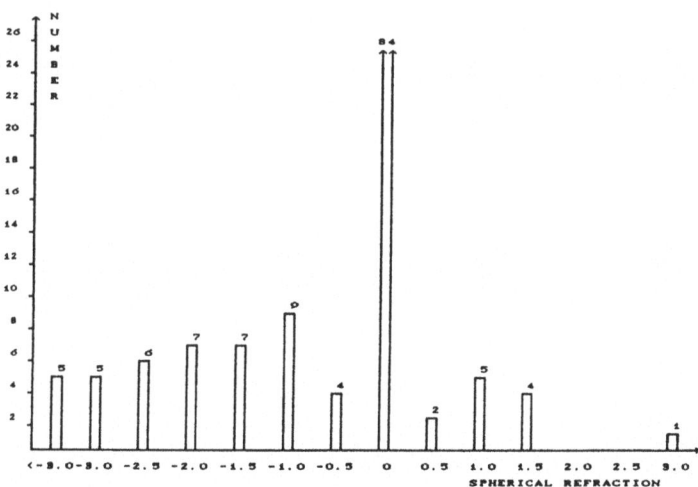

Fig. 4. Postoperative spherical refraction after 6 months for PC IOL group.

were in the group with power between 21 D and 20 D. After six months 124 patients (85.5%) had corrected or uncorrected visual acuity of more than 0.5 and 21 patients (14.5%) had corrected or uncorrected visual acuity of less than 0.4 (Fig. 3).

One hundred five patients (75%) needed spherical refraction of ±1 D and 123 patients (87.8%) needed ±2 D (Fig. 4).

The reasons for bad visual acuity for patients – 14.3% from AC IOL group: 8 eyes – macular degeneration; 3 eyes – corneal degeneration (here 1 eye had suffered after virus infection); and 1 eye – diabetic retinopathy. The reasons for poor visual acuity for 11 patients (7.6%) from PC IOL

510

group, 7 eyes – macular degenerations, 3 eyes – secondary cataracts, and 1 eye – luxation of IOL.

Conclusion

In our situation, when we implanted different models of IOL from different firms, the Binkhorst formula for IOL power calculation was good. Postoperative results of good visual acuity depend on:
1. AXL measurments and K-readings.
2. Surgical techniques and the surgeon's experience.
3. Postoperative complications.

Address for correspondence: Ophthalmic Clinic, Medical Academy, ul. Lindleya 4, 02-005 Warsaw, Poland

64. Ultrasound biometry and deprivation myopia

H.C. FLEDELIUS & E. GOLDSCHMIDT

(Hillerød, Denmark)

Abstract. Lid-suture has been demonstrated as a myopia-inducing mechanism in young experimental animals, and deprivation myopia is now considered a keyword in myopia pathogenesis. As human counterparts we might expect the development of many cases of axial myopia in patients with obstacles to clear retinal image formation in early life, although there have been few such reports in the literature. Against this background we present and discuss 11 cases observed in our own clinics. Evidently ultrasound measurements are indispensable in studies of this sort.

Introduction

A new dimension was added to the classical discipline of physiological optics when ultrasound measurement techniques became available. The presumed variation of optical components [16, 17] could be confirmed, as well as one of the main parameters, axial eye length. Ultrasonography has also become an indispensable tool in studies of refraction, such as in those pertaining to myopia pathogenesis. Ultrasound meaurements were thus performed in a series of lid-suture studies in monkeys [14, 20], which were also used as documentation for eye elongation in other experimental animals [18, 19].

The presumed trigger in experimental myopia is a blurred retinal image. A deprivation myopia theory has been advanced, and this is now the most favoured working hypothesis at myopia conferences. For obvious reasons similar experiments on human subjects cannot be conducted, other than those initiated by nature. Here we may point to clinical states which impair the clear retinal image that is regarded as essential for the correlated growth and refractive adjustment of the eye.

As a possible bridge between experimental and human myopia research we present some clinical examples documented by ultrasound biometry in our departments during the 1980s. First, there is a report of eyelid hemangiomas, previously published from the Odense University Eye Clinic [11]. Second, we describe selected cases from the Hillerød eye clinic.

Eyelid hemangiomas (*n* = 5)

Five children with periods of partial or total occlusion during infancy due to unilateral eye-lid hemangiomas were followed-up to the age of 8–15 years.

P. Till (ed.), Ophthalmic Echography 13, pp. 511–514.

Table 1. Axial eye elongation possibly related to optical imperfections in infancy or childhood, with unilateral occurrence in five of the six patients

		Axial length (mm)	
		Deprived eye	Control eye
Male 78	Lesion of right eye, probably at delivery. +L, squint	26.0	23.5
Male 67	Congenital leucoma of left eye, presumed microphthalmos. +L	29.0	22.6
Female 74	Phlyctenular keratitis of right eye, leucoma, at age 5 years	27.8	22.7
Male 51	Perforating lesion of left eye, age 9, aphakia with membrane	29.0	23.8
Male 51	Perforating lesion of left eye, age 9, aphakia.	23.9	23.1
Female 68	Bilateral keratitis, age 4–6 years (both eyes deprived)	31.0	28.0

With the fellow-eye as reference, a relative axial elongation was demonstrated in two of the five (side difference 0.8 and 3.1 mm). Further, the axis of the astigmatic cylinder depended on the initial location of the tumour, prior to its clinical cure. Refraction had thus been permanently influenced by the presence of early tumour pressure, possibly combined with obstacles to image formation. The ocular growth response, however, was not uniform; the three remaining children showed no axial elongation.

Early clouding of media (*n* = 6)

Five patients with a documented unilateral blurred image situation in early life had recent ultrasound evaluation. The underlying diseases and the axial length measurements are given in Table 1. Summing up the five selected cases, unilateral axial elongation of the eye was established with infancy or childhood obstacles to clear retinal image formation. In patient 6 both eyes had been affected in childhood; the remaining corneal opacities appeared denser in the longer (more myopic) eye.

Discussion

In 1928 our compatriot Ejler Holm [7] wrote an excellent survey about myopia and corneal opacities, apparently a frequent association in the early part of this century. In contrast, in our own series of high myopes born in 1948 [3, 5] there were no such cases. In this context we should mention the significant reduction in the prevalence of high myopia in Denmark over this century [4], possibly due to the elimination of some of the factors previously operating. One of these could be keratitis, whatever the mode of action.

As a possible parallel to experimental deprivation myopia, Raviola drew our attention to a report on Italian cases of high myopia and corneal disease [9]. Information regarding the period of eye disease indicated that it tended to occur at age 7–10 years, a stage when eye growth has not stopped yet. Obviously it is harder to imagine elongation in a fully grown eye.

Another relevant eye disease is congenital cataract. There are a few clinical studies [10, 12, 13], but in general such studies including ultrasound measurements have not gained priority. By the way, eyes with congenital or early cataract are often small eyes, but admittedly many such cases are not pure cases but part of syndromes.

Recently, a myopia-inducing role of long-standing vitreous hemorrhage during infancy was reported by Miller-Meeks et al. [8]. From Denmark we have no similar experience [1, 2], except for one or two of Brændstrup's six cases where myopia might also be ordinary juvenile or associated with prematurity. Further, in the study of Miller-Meeks and co-workers [8], axial eye elongation could not be demonstrated in cases in which ultrasound measurements had been performed.

All considered, with several years' focus on visual deprivation and image degradation in myopia research, we feel that fresh clinical reports should now have appeared in much higher numbers. They could be from established centres in the old world, or from developing countries with their high incidences of ocular problems due to infection and malnutrition.

The few series available and our own sporadic cases neither prove nor refute the myopia pathogenesis under debate. For instance, for every case reported that fits with the theory, we can find as many cases with identical disease history but without enlargement of the globe.

Let us further emphasize that in ordinary juvenile myopia, only exceptionally is there reason to suggest optical imperfection in recent or previous stages of life. Finally, one may add that low myopia appears most frequently in families living under better social and nutritional conditions than the average population, so that corneal disease is less likely to be a mechanism of general importance, nowadays at least.

Concluding remarks

From the clinical evidence available, the answer to the question regarding human counterparts to deprivation myopia seems to be negative. At present

514

at least, it is hard to suggest obstacles to image formation in the bulk of cases of myopia in Denmark. Nor is it suggested from Taiwan or other parts of Asia, where the incidence of teenage myopia is now showing an enormous increase. Finally we should stress that the above 'negative' attitude is clinically founded and that it by no means reduces the value of the important experimental myopia research going on. Thus we agree with the view of Raviola [15] that the bio- and cytochemical search for *the* myopia-generating substances can only continue using experimental animals. Following the results so far achieved, the next step will be an implication for human myopia in general.

References

1. Brændstrup, P. Vitreous hemorrhage in the newborn. Acta Ophthalmol. (Copenh) 47: 502–13 (1969).
2. Fledelius, H.C. Ocular features other than retinopathy of prematurity in the pre-term infant. Acta Ophthalmol. 68: 214–17 (1990).
3. Fledelius, H.C., Goldschmidt, E. & Stubgaard, M. Oculometric features of high myopia, around the age of 35. A 10-year follow-up. In: Thijssen, J.M. et al. (eds.), Doc. Ophthalmol. Proc. Ser. 51: 345–350 (1988).
4. Goldschmidt, E. On the etiology of myopia (thesis). Copenhagen: Munksgaard (1968).
5. Goldschmidt, E., Fledelius, H.C. & Erlin Larsen, F. Clinical features in high myopia. In: Fledelius, H.C. et al. (eds.), Doc. Ophthalmol. Proc. Ser. 28: 233–244 (1981).
6. Holden, A.L., Hodos, W., Yayes, B.P. & Fitzke, F.W. Myopia: Induced, normal and clinical. Eye 2 (Suppl.): 242–256 (1988).
7. Holm, E. Myopia and maculae corneae. Acta Ophthalmol. (Copenh) 6: 157–164 (1928).
8. Miller-Meeks, M.J., Benett, S.R., Keech, R.V. & Blodi, C.F. Myopia induced by vitreous hemorrhage. Am. J. Ophthalmol. 109: 199–203 (1990).
9. Morone, G. Macchie corneali & miopia. Boll. Soc. Med-chir. Pavia 57(3): 1–25 (1944).
10. von Noorden, G.K. & Lewis, R.A. Ocular axial length in unilateral congenital cataracts and blepharoptosis. Invest. Ophthalmol. Vis. Sci. 28: 750–752 (1987).
11. Plesner-Rasmussen, H.J., Marushak, K. & Goldschmidt, E. Capillary hemangiomas of the eye lids and orbit. Acta Ophthalmol. (Copenh) 61: 645–654 (1983).
12. Rabin, J. van Sluyters, R.C. & Malach, R. Emmetropization: A vision-dependent phenomenon. Invest. Ophthalmol. Vis. Sci. 20: 561–564 (1981).
13. Rasooly, R. & BenEzra, D. Congenital and traumatic cataract, the effect on ocular axial length. Arch. Ophthalmol. 106: 1066–1068 (1988).
14. Raviola, E. & Wiesel, T.N. An animal model of myopia. N. Engl. J. Med. 312: 1609–1616 (1985).
15. Raviola, E. & Wiesel, T.N. The mechanism of lid-suture myopia. Acta Ophthalmol. (Copenh) 66 (Suppl) 185: 91–92 (1988).
16. Sorsby, A. The nature of spherical refractive errors. Modern Ophthalmology 3: 3–20. London: Butterworths (1964).
17. Steiger, A. Die Entstehung der sphärischen Refraktionen des menschlichen Auges (1913).
18. Wallman, J., Rosenthal, D., Adams, J.I. Trachtman, J.N. & Romagnano, L. Role of accommodation and developmental aspects of experimental myopia in chicks. In: Fledelius, H.C. et al. (eds.), Doc. Ophthal. Proc. Ser. 28: 197–206 (1981).
19. Wallman, J. & Adams, J.I. Developmental aspects of experimental myopia in chicks. Vision Res. 27: 1139–1163 (1987).
20. Wiesel, T.N. & Raviola, E. Myopia and eye enlargement after neonatal lid-fusion in monkeys. Nature 226: 66 (1977).

Address for correspondence: Eye Department, Central Hospital, DK-3400 Hillerød, Denmark.

65. Postoperative disappointment in emmetropic patients

H.J. SHAMMAS
(Los Angeles, California)

Abstract. Two previously emmetropic patients experienced postoperative disappointment and induced anisometropia caused by an error in axial length measurement.

Emmetropes undergoing cataract and implant surgery usually expect good uncorrected postoperative distant vision. Disappointment occurs when these patients require postoperative myopic or hyperopic correction to restore vision. In this paper I present two such cases caused by errors in axial length measurement.

Case 1: A 64-year-old male was seen in consultation three months after his cataract surgery to the left eye, due to a disappointment in his postoperative results. The patient did not wear distance glasses prior to his surgery and had a refractive error of plano-0.50 × 82° in the right eye and plano-0.75 × 103° in the left eye.

The preoperative axial length measured in his surgeons office was 24.1 mm in the left eye and the K readings were 41.50/42.50 diopters. No measurements from the right eye were taken.

Examination at the time of the consultation revealed a refraction in the left eye of −3.00−1.25 × 121°. The axial length measured 25.4 mm in the right eye and 25.5 mm in the left eye. The K readings were 42.00/42.50 D in the right eye and 42.00/43.00 D in the left eye. The patient could not tolerate the induced anisometropia. He was referred to his surgeon for a lens exchange.

Case 2: A 62-year-old male was seen in consultation five months after his cataract surgery to the right eye due to blurring of vision in his operated dominant eye. On examination, his visual acuity in the right eye was corrected to 20/25 with +1.50 spheres and to 20/30 in the left eye with +0.25 spheres. The patient was disappointed with the postoperative result; he had always been emmetropic and could not understand why he now had to wear glasses to achieve clear distant vision.

Bilateral axial length measurements revealed a 23.4 mm in each eye while the keratometric readings were 44.75 sph in the right eye and 45.00 sph in the left eye. Information obtained from the surgeon revealed a preoperative

P. Till (ed.), Ophthalmic Echography 13, pp. 515–516.

axial length of 24.0 mm in the right eye; no measurement was taken from the left eye; the *K* readings were the same.

The methods of correction were presented to the patient with my order of preference for his case: glasses, contact lenses or lens exchange. He opted for the glasses.

Comments

Errors in axial length measurement are responsible for postoperative refractive surprises ranging from 1 to 18 D [1]. In an emmetropic eye, an error of 1 mm produces a 2.5 D change in the postoperative refraction.

The original axial length measurements were shorter by 1.4 mm in Case 1 and longer by 0.6 mm in Case 2. Shorter axial length measurements are produced by inadvertent corneal compression or by an off-axis measurement when the ultrasound beam is not properly aligned with the optical axis of the eye [2]. On the other hand, the occasional presence of an excessive tear flow will cause the transducer tip and the cornea to lose contact, giving artifactually long readings. Longer measurements can also be taken between the corneal and scleral echospikes in the presence of a poorly displayed retinal echospike. Errors in axial length measurement can be minimized by carefully evaluating the ultrasound pattern to insure the accuracy of its reading and by comparing measurements from both eyes; in both cases, measurements were only taken from the eye to be operated on. A discrepancy of over 0.3 mm between the two eyes should be suspicious enough to warrant a repeat measurement of the axial length [3].

In myopes and hyperopes who have always worn glasses for distant vision, an error in axial length measurement is covered up by a postoperative change in the lens prescription, and unless there is a large anisometropia, it rarely causes a postoperative disappointment to the patient. Our patients were both emmetropic and had expectations of postoperative emmetropia; the errors in axial length measurement resulted in a noticeable anisometropia and postoperative dissatisfaction.

References

1. Salz, J.J. & Reader, A.L. Lens implant exchanges for incorrect power: Results of an informal survey. J. Cat. Refract Surg. 14: 221–224 (1988).
2. Shammas, H.J. A comparison of immersion and contact techniques for axial length measurement. Am. Intra-Ocular Implant Soc. J. 10: 444–447 (1984).
3. Holladay, J.T., Prager, T.C. Ruiz, R.S., Lewis, J.W. & Rosenthal, H. Improving the predictability of intraocular lens power calculations. Arch. Ophthalmol. 104: 529–541 (1986).

Address for correspondence: 3510 M.L. King Jr. Blvd., Lynwood, CA 90262, Los Angeles, USA

66. Biometric measurement in the evaluation of pathological myopia

L. PIERRO, F.I. CAMESASCA, M. MISCHI & R. BRANCATO

(*Milan, Italy*)

Abstract. Pathologic myopia (greater than 6 D) is known to be associated with increased axial length and peripheral retinal changes. In order to study the frequency of peripheral retinal changes in eyes with pathological myopia and the possible influence of sex and age, we studied 513 eyes with axial length equal to or greater than 24 mm, measured with 8 MHZ T-20 standardized A-scan probe and immersion technique. Biomicroscopic examination of the periphery was performed in each eye, and the presence of the following lesions was reported: lattice degeneration, pavingstone degeneration, pigmentary degeneration, white with and without pressure, retinal holes and tears, posterior vitreous detachment, retinal detachment.

Introduction

Myopia is generally divided into two major types: simple, not progressive myopia and pathological degenerative myopia, characterized by a progressive course [1]. Chorioretinal lesions observed in degenerative myopia are commonly related to the mechanical stretching of the globe consequent to its excessive axial length increase [2, 3]. However, it is not proper to relate the severity of retinal lesions with the amount of dioptrically measured myopia. The aim of the present study was to determine the possible relationships existing between peripheral retinal degenerations and ocular axial myopia (determined with ultrasonography), as well as age and sex.

Materials and methods

We studied 513 patients with no known undergoing ocular or systemic diseases, each one having a transparent lens in both eyes allowing a proper visualization of peripheral retina. Ocular axial length was equal to or greater than 24 mm in both eyes of all patients. One eye of each patient was randomly chosen for examination, and the axial length was measured with an Ophthascan S (Biophysic Medical) ultrasonographer, standardized A-scan 8 MHz frequency probe at T-20 and immersion technique. After pharmacological dilatation of the pupil, each eye underwent 360 degrees biomicroscopic inspection of fundus periphery with Goldmann three-mirror lens and scleral indentation. We reported the presence of the following peripheral retinal lesions: lattice degeneration, pavingstone degeneration, white with and with-

P. Till (ed.), Ophthalmic Echography 13, pp. 517–521.

Table 1. Statistical comparison (student's T-test) between the average age of patients with and without certain retinal lesions in the examined eye, respectively (n.s. = not significant)

	Average age (years)		
Type of lesion	Eyes without lesions	Eyes with lesions	*p*
All retinal peripheral degenerations	49.41 ± 15.93	47.59 ± 17.01	n.s.
Lattice degeneration	48.84 ± 16.86	45.86 ± 15.69	n.s.
White with or without pressure	50.62 ± 16.74	39.89 ± 13.69	0.000
Pavingstone degeneration	46.78 ± 17.76	52.91 ± 14.63	0.000
Pigmentary degeneration	48.15 ± 16.46	49.88 ± 17.96	n.s.
Retinal holes and/or tears	49.07 ± 16.72	43.85 ± 16.16	0.021
Retinal detachment	48.21 ± 16.52	52.41 ± 19.70	n.s.
Posterior vitreous detachment	47.52 ± 16.35	49.52 ± 17.13	n.s.

out pressure, and pigmentary degeneration. Furthermore, we also reported the presence of retinal holes and/or tears, retinal detachment and posterior vitreous detachment. All data were subjected to statistical analysis to evaluate possible correlations between the above mentioned lesions and, respectively, axial length, age and sex. The significance of such correlation for each of the considered lesions was tested with the student's T-test.

Results

The age of the examined 513 patients ranged from 13 to 82 years (average age 48.44 ± 16.72), 64.7% were females (*n* = 332) and 28.3% were males (*n* = 181). The patients were divided into seven classes according to age. Axial length ranged from 24.1 mm to 36.3 mm (average 28.89 ± 2.61 mm) and the patients were divided into ten groups according to their ocular axial length. The most commonly observed lesions were pavingstone degeneration (26%) and white with or without pressure (23.2%), while retinal detachment resulted to be the less frequent change (5.6%). Posterior vitreous detachment was observed in 44% of cases. Eyes longer than 33 mm showed the highest frequency of lattice degeneration and white without pressure. In the older age classes (over 50 years) the most frequently observed changes were pavingstone degeneration (60–69 years), posterior vitreous detachment (>70 years) and pigmentary degeneration (>70 years). In the age classes below 50 years the most frequently observed changes were retinal detachment (10–19 years), retinal holes and/or tears (10–19 years), white with or without pressure (30–39 years), lattice degeneration (40–49 years).

A statistical comparison between the average age of the patients with and without the above ocular changes is presented in Table 1. We could demonstrate a significantly higher frequency in elderly patients only for pavingstone degeneration. Only white with or without pressure and retinal holes and/or tears showed a significant correlation with younger age groups.

Table 2. Statistical comparison (student's T-test) between the average axial length value of eyes with and without a certain retinal lesion (n.s. = not significant)

Type of lesion	Average axial length (mm)		
	Eyes without lesions	Eyes with lesions	*p*
All retinal peripheral degenerations	28.56 ± 2.59	29.19 ± 2.59	0.006
Lattice degeneration	28.81 ± 2.56	29.41 ± 2.78	0.0006
White with or without pressure	28.71 ± 2.55	29.63 ± 2.70	0.001
Pavingstone degeneration	28.69 ± 2.58	29.43 ± 2.61	0.004
Pigmentary degeneration	28.82 ± 2.63	29.24 ± 2.47	n.s.
Retinal holes and/or tears	28.87 ± 2.59	29.09 ± 2.71	n.s.
Retinal detachments	28.88 ± 2.61	29.12 ± 2.59	n.s.
Posterior vitreous detachment	28.60 ± 2.55	29.25 ± 2.63	0.005

A statistical comparison of the average axial length of eyes with peripheral retinal degenerations, retinal holes and/or tears, retinal detachment and posterior vitreous detachment, versus the average axial length of those eyes in which no change could be observed, is shown in Table 2. This comparison was made for all the lesions and then individually for each lesion. Affected eyes showed a statistically significant greater axial length than unaffected eyes. This was true for all the considered changes except for retinal detachment and retinal holes and/or tears. We could not demonstrate a significant relationship between sex and the presence of any lesion.

Discussion

A precise correlation between axial length and ocular refraction has been demonstrated by several authors [7, 8]. Other studies showed a correlation between the antero-posterior diameter of the eye and pathological myopia [5, 9]. A determining factor in the occurrence of peripheral retinal changes is the histological configuration of the retina-choroid complex with its possible degenerative processes. Mechanical tissue strain and vascular changes occur secondary to the antero-posterior stretching present in high myopia [10]. In very long eyes both the retina and the vitreous are responsible for the high number of posterior vitreous detachments observed in long eyes, as well as for some peripheral retinal degenerations (pigmentary, lattice, white with or without pressure and retinal tears).

The present study confirms a precise relationship between greater axial length and a higher frequency of peripheral retinal lesions. In contrast with previous studies, we performed ultrasound measurements of the ocular axial length adopting the immersion technique, which allows a more precise and reliable estimate in very long eyes [12]. Moreover, in order to permit a better statistical evaluation, we randomly chose and examined only one eye of each patient. It is well known that longer eyes are at a high risk of developing retinal lesions, thus we evaluated only the eyes with axial lengths equal to or longer than 24 mm, a value considered as the inferior axial length limit of myopic eyes [4]. All retinal lesions were more frequent in eyes with axial length equal to or greater than 27 mm. This is in line with other reports in the literature [5, 9, 13].

A significative association with a greater axial length was observed for all the considered changes, with the exception of retinal detachment and retinal holes and/or tears. In fact, retinal detachment was observed more frequently in eyes with axial length between 27 and 27.9 mm. The relationship between retinal lesions and age in our series is similar to that reported in the literature [3, 8, 9, 15]. The retinal lesions we observed more frequently in younger patients (white with or without pressure, retinal holes/tears) are almost constantly associated with the presence of vitreo-retinal traction. A healthier and not yet degenerated vitreous may exert a greater traction on the retina. Furthermore, the increased incidence of white with or without pressure in young patients can be explained considering this lesion either as an early stage or as a transient phase of another lesion [9].

Therefore, although certain lesions are more frequent in young patients and other lesions in older ones, the results of this study do not indicate a correlation between a specific lesion and a specific age group that could be constantly used in everyday practice. Certain lesions represent an evolutive stage of other ones, and their presence in the retinal periphery is therefore limited in time. Furthermore, retina-vitreous interactions may substantially alter the course of some of these lesions. Nevertheless, the present study indicates that biometric measurements may be clinically useful for the assessment of the severity of myopia. We recommend a careful biomicroscopic evaluation of the retinal periphery in eyes with increased axial length, especially if above 27 mm.

References

1. Avila, M.P., Weiter, J.J. Jalkh, A.E. et al. Natural history of choroidal neovascularization in degenerative myopia. Ophthalmol. 91: 1573–1581 (1984).
2. Bec, P., Ravault, M., Arnè, J.L. & Trepsat, L. La périphérie du fond d'oeil et myopie. La périphérie du fond d'oeil. Rapport de la Societé Française d'Ophtalmologie, pp. 425–430. Paris: Masson (1980).
3. Black, R.K., Jay, B. & MacFaul, P. The concept of degenerative myopia. Proc. Royal Soc. Med. 58: 109–112 (1965).
4. Byer, N.E. The natural history of asymptomatic retinal breaks. Ophthalmol. 89: 1033–1039 (1982).
5. Curtin, B.J. & Karlin, D.B. Axial length measurements and fundus changes of the myopic eye. Am. J. Ophthalmol. 71: 42–53 (1971).
6. Curtin, B.J. Physiologic vs pathological myopia: genetics vs environment. Ophthalmol. 86: 681–691 (1979).
7. Curtin, B.J. The myopias. Basic science and clinical management. Philadelphia: Harper & Row 13: 333–348 (1985).
8. François, S. & Goes, F. Biometrie de la myopie. Ophthalmologica 167: 49–65 (1973).

9. Grosvernor, T. High axial length/corneal radius ratio as a risk factor in the development of myopia. Am. J. Optom. Physiol. Optom. 65: 689–696 (1988).
10. Karlin, D.B. & Curtin, B.J. Peripheral chorioretinal lesions and axial length of the myopic eye. Am. J. Ophthalmol. 81: 625–635 (1976).
11. Meyer-Schwickerath, G. & Gerke, E. Biometric studies of the eyeball and retinal detachment. Br. J. Ophthalmol. 68: 29–31 (1984).
12. O'Malley, P., Allen, R. A., Straatsma, B.R. et al. Pavingstone degeneration of the retina. Arch. Ophthalmol. 73: 169–174 (1965).
13. Percival, S.P.B. Redefinition of high myopia: the relationship of axial length measurement to myopic pathology and its relevance to cataract surgery. Dev. Ophthal. 14: 42–46 (1987).
14. Shammas, H.J. A comparison of immersion and contact techniques for axial measurements. Am. Intraocul. Implant. Soc. J. 10: 444–447 (1984).
15. Sorsby, A., Benjamin, B. &d Sheridan, M. Refraction and its components during the growth of the eye from the age of three. Special report Series No 301. pp. 1–67. London: Medical Research Council. (1961).
16. Sorsby, A., Leary, G.A., Richards, M.J. & Chasten, J. Ultrasonic measurement of the components of ocular refraction during life, 2: Clinical procedures. Vision Res. 3: 499–505 (1963).
17. Tso, M.O.M. & Friedman, E. The retinal pigment epithelium, 3: Growth and development. Arch. Ophthalmol. 80: 214–220 (1968).

Address for correspondence: Department of Ophthalmology, University of Milan, H S. Raffaele, Via Olgettina 60, I-20132 Milan, Italy.

PART EIGHT

Doppler methods

67. Analysis of ocular circulatory kinetics in glaucoma using the ultrasonic Doppler method

S. TANE, M. HIRATA & M. HASHIMOTO

(*Kawasaki, Japan*)

Abstract. In order to analyze ocular circulatory kinetics related to stage progression of primary open-angle glaucoma, we studied the pulse wave of blood flow velocity in the main trunk of the central retinal artery of the fundus using the ultrasonic Doppler method. An advantage of examining the pulse wave of blood flow velocity by this method is that it enables completely harmless and exact external determination of the physiological condition of blood flow, without the exposure of any vessels.

Using the Vasoflow III-type spectrum analyser of the ultrasonic Doppler apparatus (Fig. 1), blood flow pulse waves were detected for the central retinal artery and the medial frontal artery corresponding to the periphery of the ophthalmic artery.

Fig. 2 shows our method of determining the blood flow velocity of the medial frontal artery (OA) and Fig. 3 shows how we determined the blood flow velocity of central retinal artery of the fundus (FA). We studied 100 eyes in 60 patients with open-angle glaucoma and favorably controlled intraocular pressure, whose ages ranged from 20 to 70 years. Sixty normal eyes in 30 persons, whose respective ages were the same as in the patient group, were used as controls.

The glaucoma group was called Group G and the normal group, Group N. The eyes in Group G were further classified according to Kosaki's classification of the stage of progression of the visual field, into Groups G1, G2, G3 and G4, and the same eyes were subclassified according to the C/D ratio of the optic nerve disc; eyes with values greater than or equal to 0.3 and greater than 0.6 were assigned to Group g_1 and those with values ≤ 0.6 were assigned to Group g_2.

Fig. 4 is a three-dimensional diagram of the pulse wave of blood flow velocity. The solid line indicates the simple line of maximum deviation frequency displayed in real time. The dotted line indicates the ratio of velocity components of erythrocytes flowing in the vessels, and is displayed in color in the determination.

Fig. 5 shows the mean deviation frequency of the pulse wave of blood flow velocity for two heartbeats. The solid line indicates the deviation frequency corresponding to maximum blood flow velocity in real time. The dotted line indicates the deviation frequency corresponding to mean blood flow velocity.

In Fig. 6 we see the period between the pulse wave of blood flow velocity

P. Till (ed.), Ophthalmic Echography 13, pp. 525–532.
© 1993 *Kluwer Academic Publishers*.

526

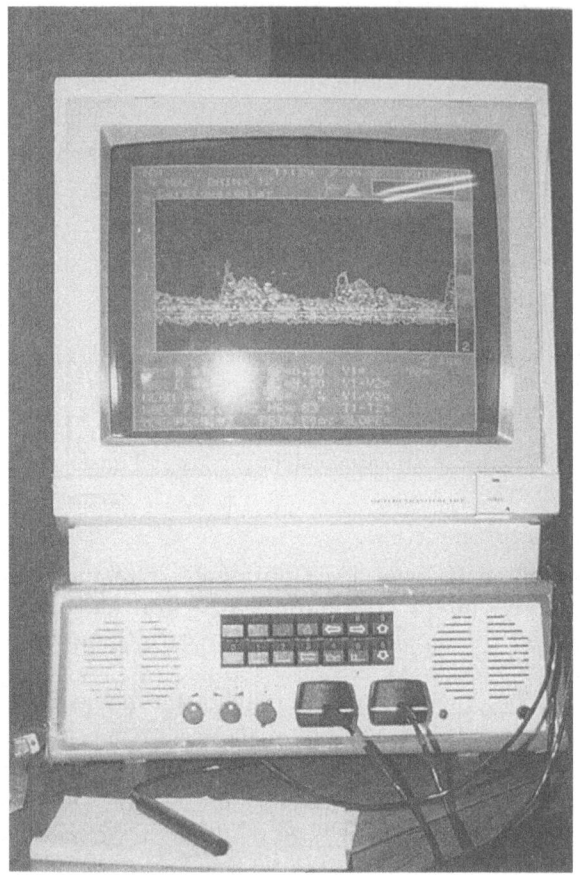

Fig. 1. The Vasoflow III-type spectrum analyser (ultrasonic Doppler apparatus).

at the terminal diastolic stage of heart dilatation (T_1) and that at maximum diastole (T_2), called the pulse rise time (PRT). In this experiment the period $T_1 - T_2$ was found to show a tendency to decrease in the presence of a constriction of the relevant vessel.

Clinical Doppler wave forms

Fig. 7 (*left*) is the fundus in a 53-year-old man with open-angle glaucoma. The C/D ratio of the optic nerve disc was 0.6, and the visual field was determined to be at stage 3 of Kosaki's progression. Fig. 7 (*right*) is the fluorescein angiogram in this case.

Fig. 8 shows the pulse waves of blood flow velocity of the FA and OA, respectively. These revealed that the blood flow velocity pulse wave of the

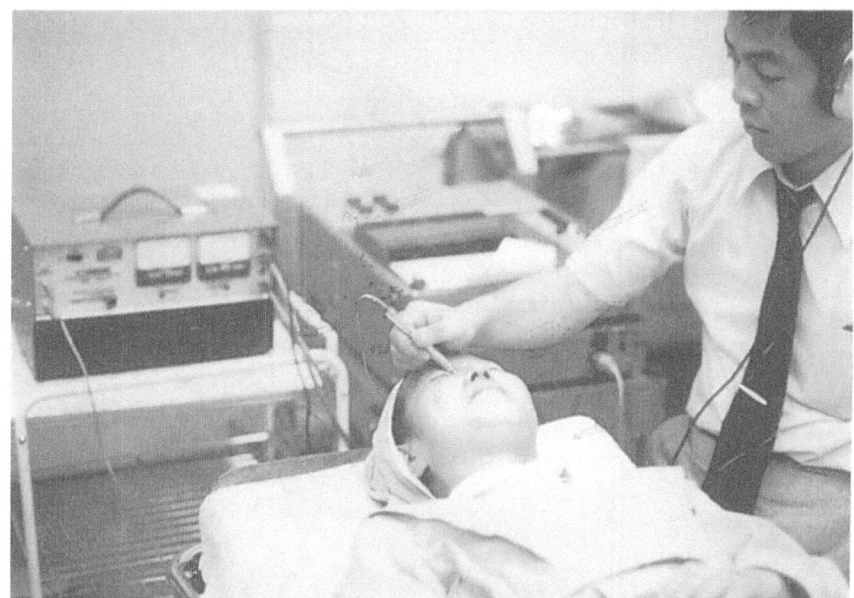

Fig. 2. The determination of the blood flow velocity of the medial frontal artery (OA).

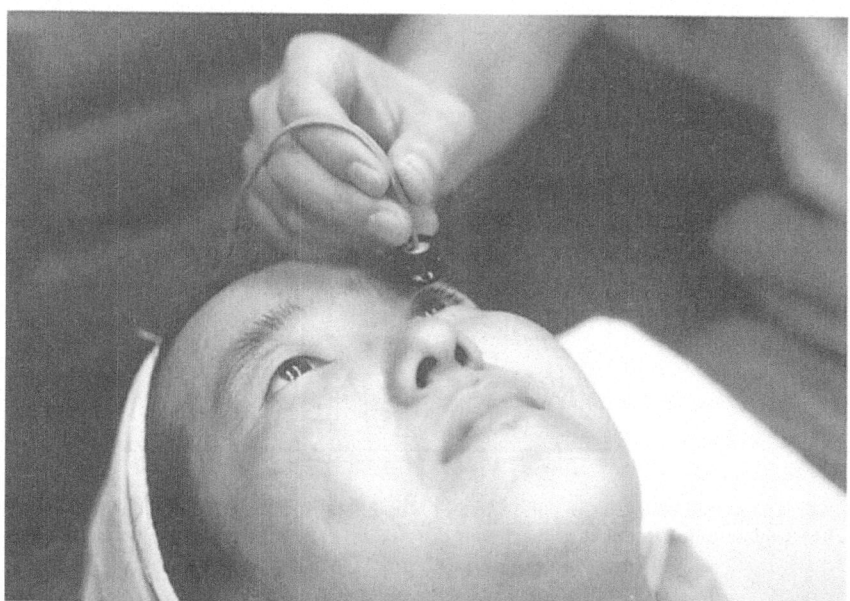

Fig. 3. The determination of the blood flow velocity of the central retinal artery (FA).

528

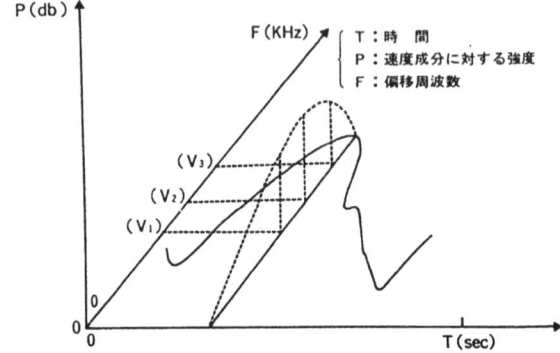

Fig. 4. A three-dimensional diagram of the pulse wave of blood flow velocity.

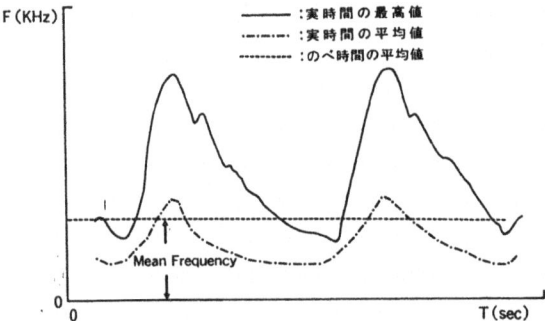

Fig. 5. The mean deviation frequency of the pulse wave of blood flow velocity for two heart beats (mean-F).

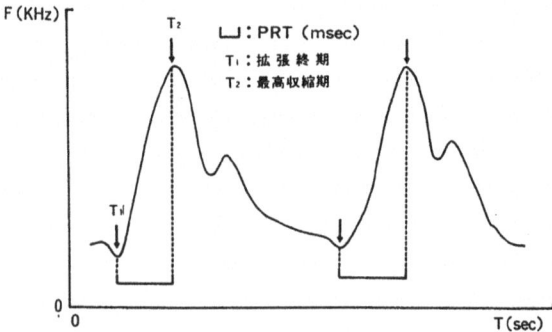

Fig. 6. The period between the pulse wave of blood flow velocity at the terminal diastolic stage of heart dilatation, T_1, and at at maximum distole, T_2, called the pulse rise time (PRT).

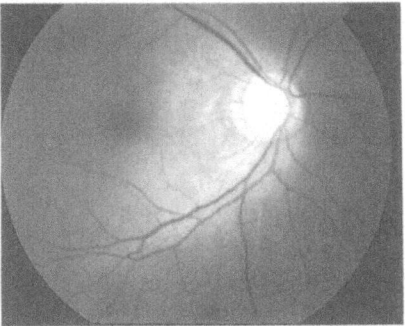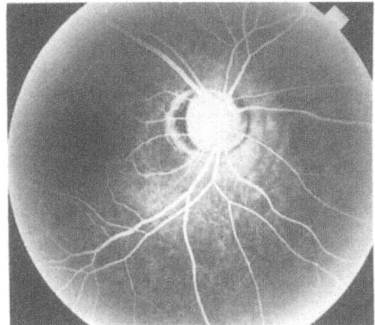

Fig. 7. *Left:* The fundus in a 53-year-old man with primary open-angle glaucoma. *Right:* The fluorescein angiogram in this case (C/D ratio = 0.6).

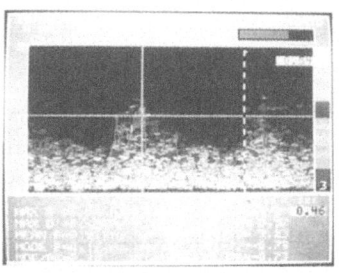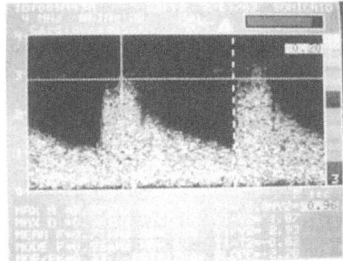

Fig. 8. The pulse waves of blood flow velocity of the FA (*left*) and OA (*right*).

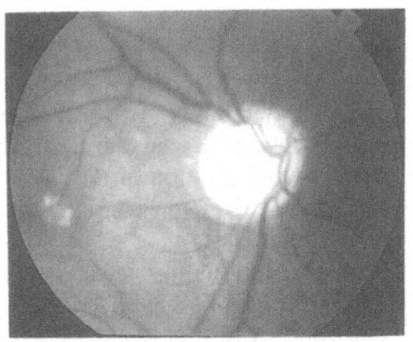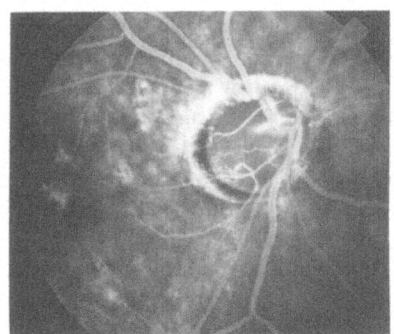

Fig. 9. The fundus (*left*) and a fluorescein angiogram (*right*) from a 61-year-old woman with primary open-angle glaucoma (C/D ratio = 0.8).

FA was decreased and the PRT of the pulse wave curve was reduced, along with progression of restriction of visual field and aggravation of C/D ratio.

Fig. 9 shows a display of the fundus and a fluorescein angiogram from a 61-year-old woman with open angle glaucoma. The C/D ratio was 0.8, and the degree of deterioration of the visual field was designated as stage 5 of

530

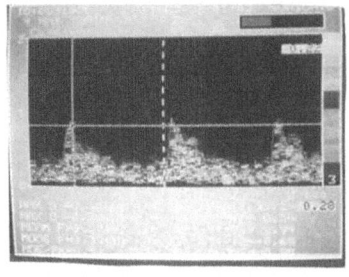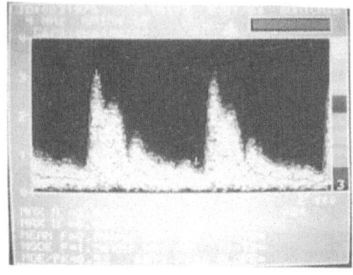

Fig. 10. The pulse waves of blood flow velocity of FA (*left*) and OA (*right*).

Table 1. The mean ratios of blood flow velocity at each stage of visual field deterioration

Case groups	Fundus blood flow ratio at each stage
	V(FA/OA) (%)
Group N	69.3 ± 11.6
Group G	54.5 ± 14.2
Group G_1	69.0 ± 15.0
Group G_2	60.8 ± 13.8
Group G_3	54.1 ± 9.2
Group G_4	47.9 ± 10.5

Mean ± SD (%).

Kosaki's progression. The fluorescein angiogram shows deficiency of the capillary vessel filling in the optic nerve disc.

Fig. 10 shows pulse waves of blood flow velocity of the FA and OA, respectively, in this patient. These revealed that decreases in the PRT and in blood flow velocity of the FA were more marked than in the OA. The blood flow velocity of the FA decreased with the progression of the disturbance of the visual field, and the PRT was reduced with the aggravation of the C/D ratio.

The mean ratios of blood flow velocity in the fundus in each group are shown according to stage of visual field deterioration in Table 1. V(FA/OA) represents the ratio of blood flow velocity of the FA to that of the OA. Fig. 11 shows the finding that V(FA/OA) decreased with the progression of glaucoma; that is, FA blood flow velocity was significantly decreased with increasing progression of stage. The relationship between the increase in the C/D ratio and the PRT of blood flow in the fundus can be seen in Table 2, and in the representative diagram in Fig. 12.

There was a statistically significant difference in PRT with a risk rate of 1% between Group N and Group G. The PRT decreased with an increase in the C/D ratio.

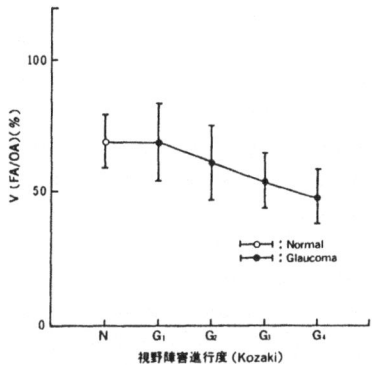

Fig. 11. V(FA/OA) decreased as the stage of glaucoma progressed.

Table 2. The relationship between increases in the C/D ratio and the PRT of blood flow in the fundus

Case groups	Pulse rise time ratio at each stage
	T(FA/OA) (%)
Group N	137.1 ± 35.2
Group G	98.1 ± 14.0
Group g_1	137.7 ± 42.0
Group g_2	76.9 ± 21.0

Mean ± SD (%).

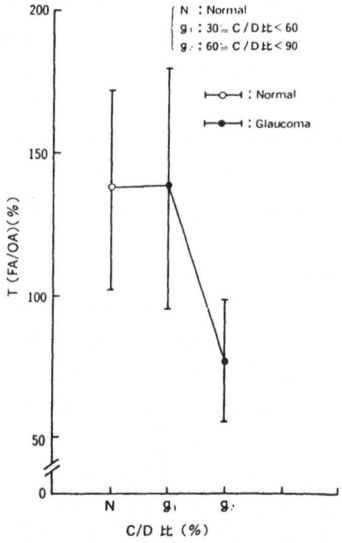

Fig. 12. The representative diagram between C/D ratio increasing and PRT of the blood flow in the fundus.

Conclusions

As a result of an investigation using the ultrasonic Doppler method, eyes with glaucoma showed a decrease in blood flow velocity of the FA with a deterioration of the visual field, and showed a tendency in PRT toward decrease. As the stages progress, this tendency becomes increasingly evident.

References

1. Hyman, B.N. Doppler sonography. A beside nonivasive method for assessment of carotid artery disease. Am. J. Ophthalmol. 77: 227–231 (1974).
2. Schwartz, B., Rieser, J.C. & Fishbein, S.L. Fluorescein angiographic defects of the optic disc in glaucoma. Arch. Ophthalmol. 95: 1961–1974 (1977).
3. Hirata, M., Hashimoto, M. & Tane, S. Analysis of ocular circulatory kinetics in glaucoma by the ultrasonic Doppler method. Acta Soc. Ophthalmol. Jpn. 93: 1054–1061 (1989).

Address for correspondence: Department of Ophthalmology, St. Marianna University, 2-16-1, Sugao, Miyamae-ku, J-213 Kawasaki-shi, Japan.

68. Angiodinography
Ultrasound technique for the study of normal and abnormal vascularization of the eye and orbit

L. FALCO, S. ESENTE, F. FANFANI & S. FANFANI
(Florence, Italy)

Abstract. Angiodinography is a new ultrasound technique. The association of B-scan images, Doppler and false color techniques adapted to both is the technique known as angiodinography. This technique is commonly used in the study of cardiovascular and vascular diseases. We have applied it to the normal and abnormal vascularization of the eye and orbit. This paper presents preliminary results and images.

Introduction

The development of echophthalmology has definitely reached a turning point. The current level of sensitivity and specificity of echographic examinations is very high. Over the years many authors have dedicated themselves to the echographic study of ocular-orbital diseases and have produced excellent results which have been and still are a fertile school for all echographists.

In this paper we report on a new and interesting potential use for this diagnostic technique in ophthalmology. In this last decade of the century, both scientific research and industry propose new and more sophisticated instruments, different image presentation systems, and new image processing systems with the aims of improving the accuracy of echophthalmologic diagnosis and increasing repeatability.

We are convinced that the 'echographic castle' built over such a long period will 'stand' for many years to come. We are also convinced, however, that the new developments in echography as applied to other disciplines will also have their impact on echophthalmology. The time in which 'special' equipment was needed for echophthalmology has perhaps passed. We do not believe that the ultrasonographs for ophthalmology will be replaced by those used for internal medicine; rather, we feel that the technology of those machines is being and will be 'transferred' to those used for ophthalmology. At the same time we also believe that some 'special' machines used in internal medicine may also be used in the diagnosis of diseases of the eye and orbit. Furthermore, we are aware that each innovation must be subjected to critical evaluation and scientifically tested in order to understand its full and real potential.

P. Till (ed.), Ophthalmic Echography 13, pp. 533–536.

Materials and methods

We used a Philips (Quantum) angiodinograph, a new, computer-based vascular imaging technology in which the signal is processed according to the phase indicating the direction of flow by colors (red or blue). The flow speed is indicated by the frequency, and the amplitude provides a digitized B-scan echographic image presented according to a grey scale.

The device is equipped with two linear probes of 5 and 7.5 MHz, respectively. The image appears on a 13-inch screen with 120 tones of grey to show over 40 dB of signals from the tissues and 64 shades of red/blue in addition to a shade of green used to process the image. At 6 dB the echographic image has at a maximum axial resolution of 0.26 mm and a lateral resolution of 0.8 mm (with the 7.5 MHz probe we used), while the volume of Doppler sampling, with the same probe, is 0.6 per 1.5 mm.

The maximum Doppler frequency that can be measured is 16 KHz and the minimum is 150 KHz. Resolution of the frequency spectrum can be selected as 126 or 256 points, with a resolution of the frequency components equal to 120 tones of grey. From the spectrum analysis menu we can gain access, in real time, to the vessel volume, maximum, minimum, mean and modal velocity and subsequently we can calculate flow, the percentage window, acceleration, pulsation, Pourcelot's index and the values of the various velocities.

There are other specifics that are of minor interest to this paper, and we skip them here. However, we wish to recall that the Philips model is an instrument for general internal medicine with great potential for vascular diseases. Therefore, although it has all the 'negative' features of an instrument that was not specifically designed for ophthalmology, it is still very effective and reliable. Our study covered the normal anatomy of the eye prior to evaluating its clinical potential with specific reference to vascular pathologies and tumors.

Discussion

The literature contains many reports of the use of color Doppler in cardiology and vascular disorder. Ophthalmologic applications are much more recent, and thus the literature is not as rich [1]. Only a few studies, carried out with various instruments have demonstrated the utility of this diagnostic technique in ophthalmology with particular reference to vascular diseases and tumors of the eye and orbit [2–6].

We have had the opportunity of beginning a study with this type of instrument to evaluate possible applications. The first 'anatomical' approach was astounding. In cardiology, the angiodinography has been compared to an 'angiocardiogram', which permits direction observation of valve stenosis, the magnitude of a reflux and the site and size of an intra- and extracardiac shunt through extraordinarily clear color images.

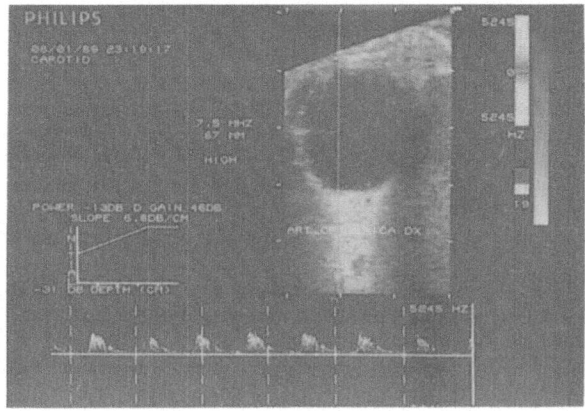

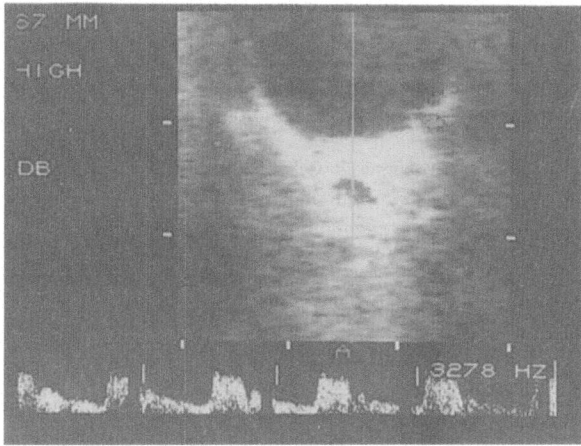

Fig. 1.

Our study of a 'normal' eye bulb surprised us by the possibility of defining all the arterial and venous branches of the eye bulb. In fact, the first pictures show that this instrument is capable of revealing even the smallest afferent branches of the eye orbit; that is, those branches which are compatible with the instrument's axial and lateral resolution (Fig. 1). The ease of visualizing both the large and small branches allows us to forecast useful applications in the field of retinal-coroidal vascular diseases. The possibility of being easily able to see the vascular component inside a neoformation, suggests a great potential in cancer diagnosis, especially in the field of differential diagnosis of vascular forms. The criteria of evaluating the vascular component and its flow permits us to forecast useful applications in the follow-up of treated and untreated tumoral lesions.

References

1. Berger, R.W., Guthoff, R., Helmke, K. & Winkle, P. Doppler ultrasonography in the follow-up of malignant melanoma of the choroid. In: Sampaolesi, R. (ed.), Ultrasonography in Ophthalmology 12. Doc. Ophthalmol. Proc. Ser. 53: 327–331. Dordrecht: Kluwer Acad. Publ. (1990).
2. Cardia, L., Reibaldi, A., Avitabile, T., Guerriero, S., Veneziani, N. & Distante, A. First results about echographical ocular tissue characterization by false color. Poster, VII Congress Eur. Soc. Ophthal., Helsinki (1984).
3. Coleman, D.J., Lizzi, F.L. & Jack, R.L. Color coding of B-Scan ultrasonograms. Arch. Ophthalmol. 91: 429–431 (1974).
4. Falco, L., Esente, S. & Passarelli, N. La nuova tecnologia degli strumenti per ecografia oftalmica: vantaggi e svantaggi. Il Sonomed B3000. Congr. SIEO 1987. Clin. Ocul. 4: 261–264 (1988).
5. Reibaldi, A., Avitabile, T., Guerriero, S. & Veneziani, N. Primi risultati sulla possbilità di differenziazione ecografica tissutale mediante falso colore. 8th Cong. SISUM 1983. Clin. Ocul. (Suppl.) 6: 9–12 (1984).
6. Reibaldi, A., Avitabile, T. & Cascone, C. Vitreous membranes up date echographical diagnosis. In: Sampaolesi, R. (ed.), Ultrasonography in Ophthalmology 12. Doc. Ophthalmol. Proc. Ser. 53: 225–231. Dordrecht: Kluwer Acad. Publ.

Address for correspondence: Ophthalmology Centre, Corso Italia 2, I-50123 Florence, Italy.

69. The effect of intracranial diseases on ophthalmic artery circulation

E. BALÁZS, L. RÓZSA & S. SZABÓ

(Debrecen, Hungary)

Introduction

Some intracranial diseases may also influence orbital blood circulation. Transcranial Doppler sonography (TDS) is a simple, noninvasive method for the follow up of these hemodynamic changes [1–3].

Materials and method

Blood flow velocity in the main basal cerebral arteries and in the ophthalmic artery, measured through the temporal and orbital window, is examined using transcranial Doppler sonography (EME TC2-64) in various intracranial diseases. These include intracranial tumours where the ophthalmic artery also contributes to the blood supply, in intracranial hypertension, in cases of vasospasm following aneurysmal subarachnoid hemorrhage, and in carotid-cavernous fistulae.

Results

1. Intracranial tumours fed partly by the ophthalmic artery. First, intracranial tumours fed partly by the ophthalmic artery were examined. It is well known that the ophthalmic artery feeds not only orbital tumours but also some intracranial tumours via some of its branches. Thus it takes part in the blood supply of subfrontal tumours by the ethmoidal arteries, of falx meningiomas by the anterior falcis artery, and of lateral sphenoid wing meningiomas by its recurrent meningial branch.

In each of our 11 cases where the branches of the ophthalmic artery contributed to the blood supply of an intracranial tumour, angiography demonstrated the dilatation of the feeding artery and TDS revealed an increase in blood flow velocity. These two sets of data were proof of an increased

P. Till (ed.), Ophthalmic Echography 13, pp. 537–542.

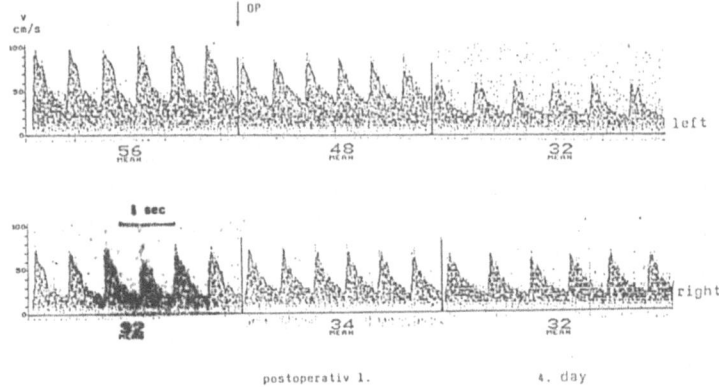

Fig. 1. Doppler recordings of a left intra- and retro-orbital meningioma.

blood supply or hyperemia which gradually decreased after tumour removal (Fig. 1).

2. Intracranial hypertension. By increasing vascular resistance, the intracranial space-occupying processes decrease cerebral perfusion pressure so that mean blood flow velocity decreases, especially in the diastolic phase,

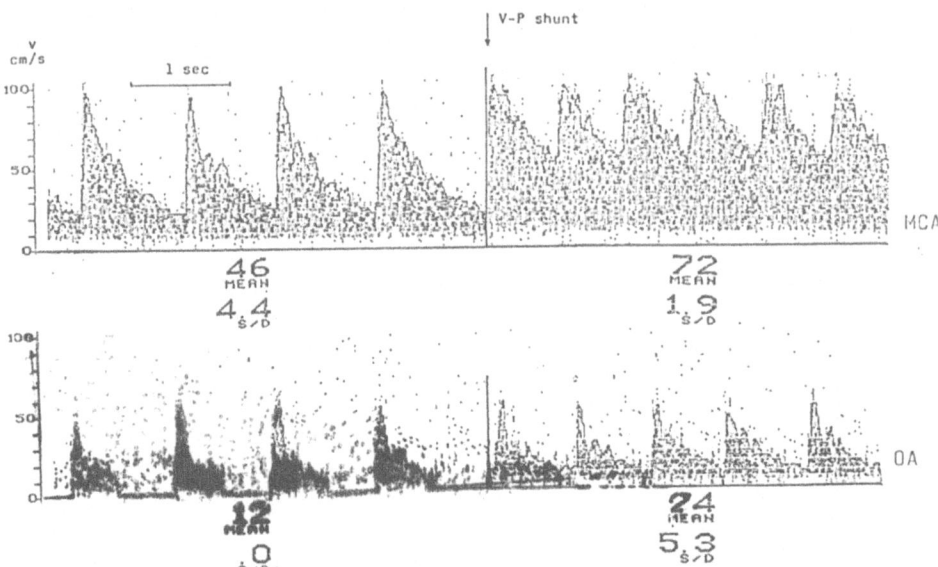

Fig. 2. Doppler recordings of middle cerebral and ophthalmic arteries in the case of intracranial hypertension caused by occlusive hydrocephalus and following ventriculo-atrial shunting. In both arteries intracranial hypertension tended to reduce flow velocity mainly during the diastolic phase. After shunting the flow velocity returned to normal.

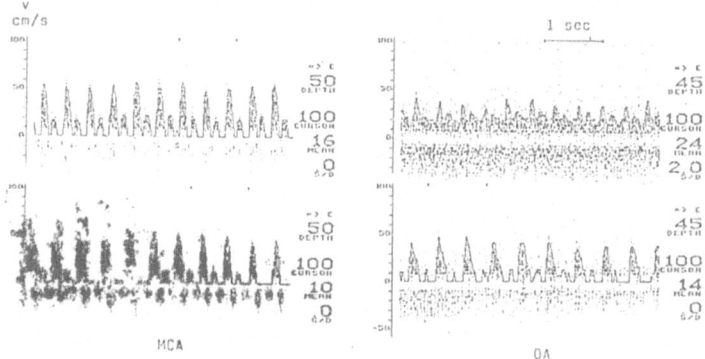

Fig. 3. Blood flow velocity in the middle cerebral (MCA) and ophthalmic artery (OA) in the case of severe diffuse brain swelling. Prior to brain death (upper curve) systolic peaks can be detected in the MCA while flow velocity in the OA remains normal. In the state of brain death (lower curve) oscillating flow in the MCA and systolic peaks in the OA can be measured.

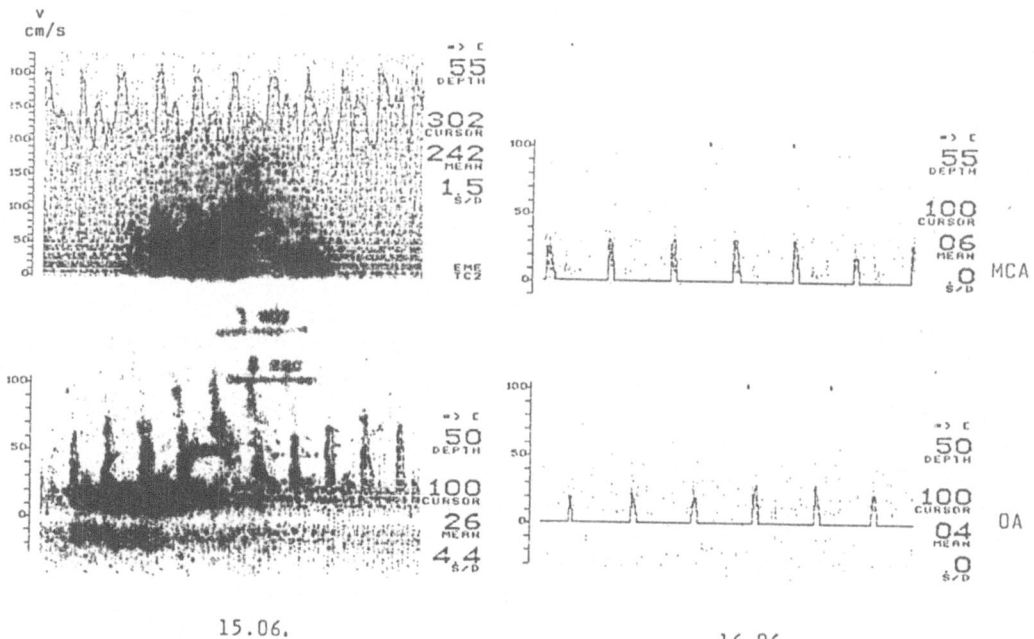

Fig. 4. Blood flow velocity in the right middle cerebral artery (MCA) and ophthalmic artery (OA) in vasospasm following subarachnoid hemorrhage and in brain death. Increased flow velocity (242 cm/s) in the MCA is characteristic of vasospasm, at the same time flow velocity in the OA is normal (*left*). The next day, in the state of brain death only systolic spikes can be detected in both arteries.

540

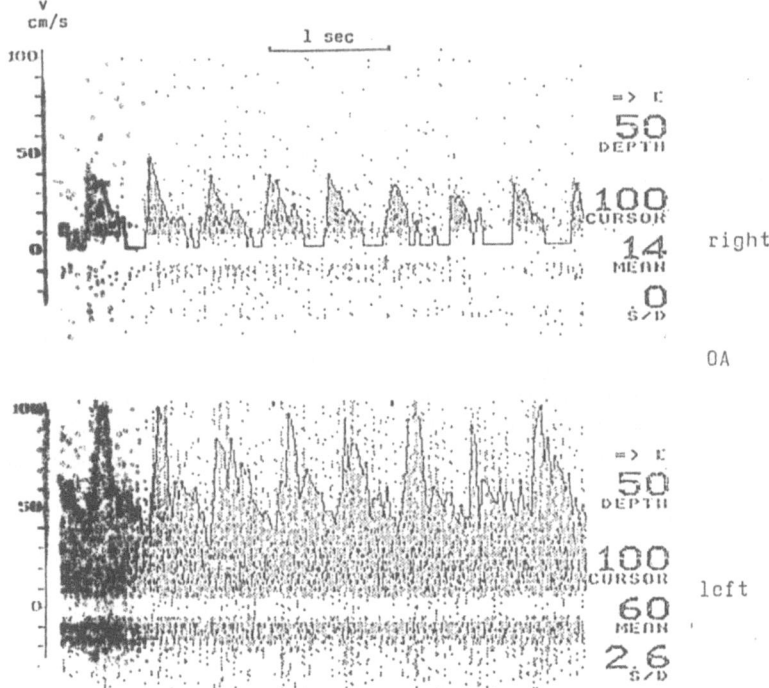

Fig. 5. Blood flow velocity in the ophthalmic arteries following left internal carotid aneurysmal subarachnoid hemorrhage. Vasospasm results in flow velocity increase in the left ophthalmic artery. Recordings of the right OA suggest increasing intracranial pressure.

the systolic/diastolic ratio (S/D) increases, and the shape of the velocity-pulse curve shows characteristic changes (Fig. 2).

In severe cases when intracranial pressure reaches the average value of the arterial blood pressure, the so-called oscillation flow or pendel flow is characteristic, the blood supply to the brain practically ceases. During the systolic phase some blood reaches the brain, but during the diastolic phase it flows back. In the case of a further increase in ICP, the cerebral perfusion pressure drops to zero, the blood flow in the brain ceases, and brain death ensues. In this case no blood flow can be detected either in the basal cerebral arteries or in the ophthalmic artery (Fig. 3). The cessation of cerebral blood flow is followed by the cessation of orbital blood flow only in a later phase.

3. Vasospasm. In the course of examinations of vasospasms following subarachnoidal hemorrhages of different origins, we wanted to determine whether the spasm of the main basal arteries spreads on to the ophthalmic artery or not. According to our examinations this is rarely the case. Out of 25 patients with vasospasms of the intracranial arteries proved by TDS, only three had increased blood flow velocities in the ophthalmic artery (Figs 4 and 5). In

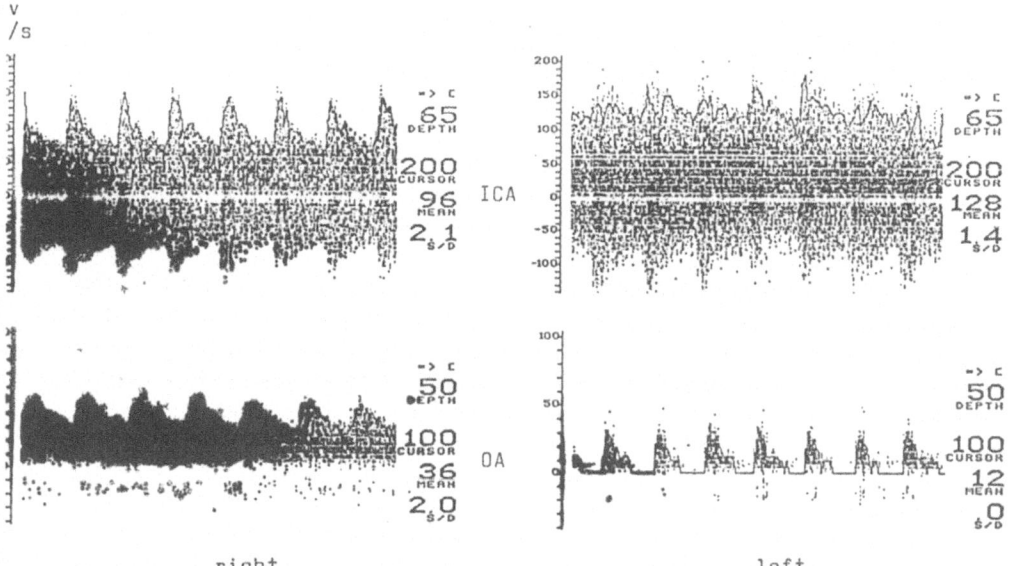

Fig. 6. Blood flow velocity in both internal carotid and ophthalmic arteries in the left carotid-cavernous fistula. In the left internal carotid artery the flow velocity increased because of reduced peripheric vascular resistance (128 cm/s). On the contrary, left OA shows decreased flow velocity caused by intraorbital hypertension (IOP: 85 mm Hg), compared to the opposite side.

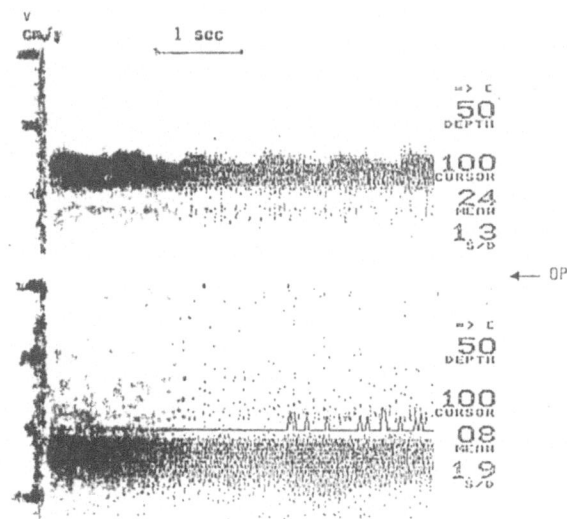

Fig. 7. Doppler recordings of the superior ophthalmic vein (SOV) before and after surgery of the carotid-cavernous fistula. Before surgery (upper curve) the flow in SOV is directed against the probe (→□), it has an arterial-pulsating character, after surgery the direction returned to normal and regained its venous feature (lower curve).

addition to high blood flow, the irregularity of the velocity-pulse curve is also characteristic of vasospasm because of turbulent flow.

4. Carotid-cavernous fistulae. Carotid-cavernous fistulae may also cause important hemodynamic changes in arterial and venous circulation of the orbit. In the ophthalmic artery the blood flow velocity may remain normal but it can also be reduced due to the steal-phenomenon of the fistula and orbital hypertension (Fig. 6).

In the case of carotid-cavernous fistulae the blood flow direction in the superior ophthalmic vein (SOV) is reversed, and the shape of the velocity–pulse curve will have an arterial character (Fig. 7, upper curve). After elimination of the fistula, SOV flow is directed again towards the cavernous sinus and regains its venous characteristics (Fig. 7, lower curve).

Conclusion

We believe that these examinations provide important information concerning the circulation in the ophthalmic artery. Its practical value is that we can draw conclusions regarding changes in intracranial blood flow on the basis of circulatory conditions in the ophthalmic artery if the temporal window cannot be used because of the thickening of the temporal bone.

References

1. Aaslid, R. Transcranial Doppler sonography. Wien: Springer (1986).
2. Harders, A. Neurosurgical applications of transcranial Doppler sonography. Wien: Springer (1986).
3. Vinken, P.J. & Bruyn, G.W. Handbook of clinical neurology: injuries of the brain and skull, Part II. pp. 399–439. Amsterdam/Oxford: North-Holland Publishing Company (1976).

Address for correspondence: Institute of Ophthalmology, University Medical School, Nagyerdei Krt. 98, H-4012 Debrecen, Hungary.

Authors Index

Addabbo G. 495
Andreuccetti F. 399
Anile, C. 101
Atta H.R. 199
Auricchio G. 405
Avitabile T. 337, 345, 483

Baba Y. 439, 489
Balázs E. 537
Bell J. A. 333
Bergamo L. 233
Bonaccorsi O. 483
Bosanquet R.C. 333
Brabant P. 257
Brancato R. 297, 517
Buccheri C. 483
Burroni M. 495
Busse H. 361

Camesasca F.I. 517
Cantalloube A. 205
Capoferri C. 297
Cardia L. 459
Cascone G. 345, 483
Casiraghi J.F. 247
Cennamo F. 405
Cennamo G. 277, 355, 405, 415
Chiarelli M. 251, 285
Clemens S. 361, 375, 393, 431

Damjanovich J. 291
D'Aniello B. 495
De Laey J.J. 257
Dell'Eva G. 495
Doro D. 233, 319

Emmerich K.-H. 431
Esente S. 399, 533

Falco L. 399, 533
Falsini, B. 101
Fanfani F. 533
Fanfani S. 533
Fledelius H.C. 307, 511
Foà T. 277
Franco L. 337, 345
Frieling E. 211
Fukiyama J. 161, 439, 489

Garcia-Reza P. 411
Gagliano C. 483
Gerding H. 375
Ghirlanda R. 337
Goes F. 257
Goldschmidt E. 511
Gosalbez R.R. 395.
Guerriero S. 459
Guida E. 415

Hasenfratz G. 135, 265
Hashimoto M. 445, 475, 525
Held K.S. 185
Henč-Petrinovic L. 179
Hidasi V. 385
Hirata M. 525
Huyghe J.P. 257

Iaccarino G. 405
Ito M. 451

Janáky M. 123
Janev K. 217
Jayyousi G. 501
Juvan V. 127

Kennerdell J.S. 209
Kimura Y. 445

Kolozsvári L. 291, 351, 381, 385

Lampé Zs. 381
Lewan U. 135
Lewandowski P. 507
Lian J. 209
Libondi T. 405
Loffredo A. 415
Lohmeyer M. 239
Longo A. 337

Magni R. 297
Mangiola, A. 101
Mantovani E. 233, 319
Marano F. 483
Marino C. 337, 483
Marchini G. 313
Marti R.B. 395
Maruiwa F. 161, 439, 489
Mazzeo V. 251, 285, 329
McAdam J. 185
Mele A. 277
Mellin K.B. 239
Midena E. 319
Minerva G. 459
Mischi M. 517
Mo Y. 209
Monari P. 251, 285
Moragrega E. 411
Moro F. 319
Motolese E. 495
Murakami K. 451

Nagy Z. 385
Nao-i N. 161
Németh J. 123, 193, 369
Nirchio F. 459

Ossoinig K.C. 3

Palma, P. 101
Pang Y. 209
Pappalardo A. 337, 345
Pasquariello G. 459
Peterra N. 495
Pelle Zs. 123
Perović-Stamenković D. 217
Perri P. 251, 285, 329
Pezone A. 415
Pierro L. 297, 517
Poujol J. 205

Prause J.U. 307

Rademacher P. 393
Radig Ch. 393
Ravalli L. 251, 285, 329
Reibaldi A. 337, 345
Riedel K.G. 265
Rodriguez F.A. 395
Rosa N. 277, 355, 405, 415
Rózsa L. 537

Sala M. 319
Salihu N. 217
Sampaolesi R. 247, 301
Sawada A. 161, 439, 489
Sayegh N. 501
Scherfig E. 307
Shaheen A. 501
Shamayleh Z. 501
Shammas H.J. 515
Shiina T. 451
Sileci S. 345
Skurczyński M. 507

Spahiu K. 217
Stanowsky A. 117, 145, 221, 273
Stefani F.H. 265
Sugata Y. 451
Szabó Á. 123
Szabó S. 537

Tamburelli C. 101, 111
Tane S. 445, 475, 525
Till P. xi, 151, 227
Tosi R. 313

Van Heuven W.A.J. 185
Végh M. 193
Velasco C. 411
Veneziani N. 459
Verbeek A.M. 421
Verbraeken H. 257

Wolff-Kormann P.G. 265
Wu Z. 209

Yamamoto Y. 451

Zarate J.O. 247, 301
Zeng Q. 209
Ziosi M. 285

Subject index

adenoid-cystic carcinomas 151
Alagille's syndrome 47
amyloidosis (lacrimal gland) 145
  bilateral
anterior eye segment 421
  immersion technique
  mode information
a.v. malformation 209

biometry 501
  extraocular muscles 111

carotid cavernous fistulas 209
  fast flow, low flow 212
  traumatic 211, 217
cataractogenesis 405
choroidal thickness 393
  in generalanesthesia
Coats' disease 291
congenital orbital cyst 239
corneal graft 415
  thickness 411
cryopexy 375
CFS 101
  dynamic parameters

Doppler methods 525
  angiodinography 533
  transcranial (TDS) 537
dysplastic retina 301
  simulating retinoblastoma

episcleral reabsorbable explants 397
epithelial tumours 151

forceps delivery (eye, orbit) 221

glomus tumour (eyelid, orbit) 233

immersion scleral shells 411, 415
immersion technique 421
instrumentation
  3 D – display (outprints) 451
  3 D – echography 495
  area and volume calculation
  false colour B-scan 483
  multielement linear curtain 459
    ultrasonic system
  simultaneous display 489
  of four B-scan images
  stored B-scan 439
    with variation of dynamic range
  telediagnosis (faxed echograms) 475

lacrimal gland 145, 161
lacrimal sac disease 193
lens capsule rupture 427
  posterior (trauma) 431
  defects 433
lymphoma (intraocular) 179, 319

melanocytosis 227
  oculodermal with orbital melanoma
melanoma (malignant) 247
  masquerading as posterior scleritis
    265
  Ruthenium-treated 257
  small sized 251
metastatic choroidal lesions 277
microphthalmus 239
  with congenital orbital cyst
minor salivary gland 151
  epiglottis, lacrimal sac, parasinuses
mucocele (unusual, orbit) 185
myositis 127
  chronic, bilateral

546

ocular wall volume 369
  intraocualar pressure
optic disk 5 ff
  coloboma 8
  drusen, pseudodrusen 9
  excavation (glaucoma) 5
  morning glory syndrome 9
  optic pit 9
  trauma 17
  tumours/pseudotumors 15
optic nerve
  AION/PION 76
  anomalies (childhood) 123
  BIH 43
  CON 61
  examination technique 17 ff
    echograms (normal)
    A-scan
  exercise 32
    30 degree test
  glioma 80
  Graves' orbitopathy 17
    muscle index
  hypoplasia 61
  leucemic cells 89
  leucemic meningeosis 117
  meningeoma (sheath) 83
  metastatic carcinoma 89
  optical atrophy 57
  optic neuritis 75
  orbital congestion 78
    hyperemia
  papilledema 50
    development
  subarachnoidal fluid (increased)
    A-scan proof (30 degree test) 47
    B-scan signs 45
    determination of amount 31
    dynamics 30
    sheath fenestration 52
  surfaces 27
    dural, arachnoidal, pial
  wet and dry 28

osteoma (bilateral) 273

pachymetry 411, 415
persistent primary vitreous 301
  simulating retinoblastoma
phlebectasy 205
phthisis bulbi 381
pigmentepithelium (retina) 361
posterior pole configuration 385
prescleral layer 355
progressive myopia 385

refraction 20
  cross section of optic nerve
  proof 20
retinoblastoma 297
retinoschisis 351
  prescleral layer 355

small choroidal solid lesions 313
spectrum analysis 445
  ultrasonic RI-signals of cataracts
Standardized Echography
  adenoid-cystic carcinomas 151
  amyloidosis (lacrimal gland) 145
  congenital orbital cyst 239
  epithelial tumours 151
  lymphoma (intraocular) 319
  metastatic lesions (choroidal) 277
  minor salivary gland 151
  optic nerve 3–99
  osteoma (choroidal, bilateral) 273
  pleomorphic adenoma 151
  prescleral layer 355
  results in orbital diseases 135
  retinoschisis 351

tamponade substances 345
  in vitreo-retinal surgery

Valsalva test 199
varix (orbit) 199
vitreal interfaces 329
  hemorrhagic, degenerative
vitreo-retinal interface 337
  pathology

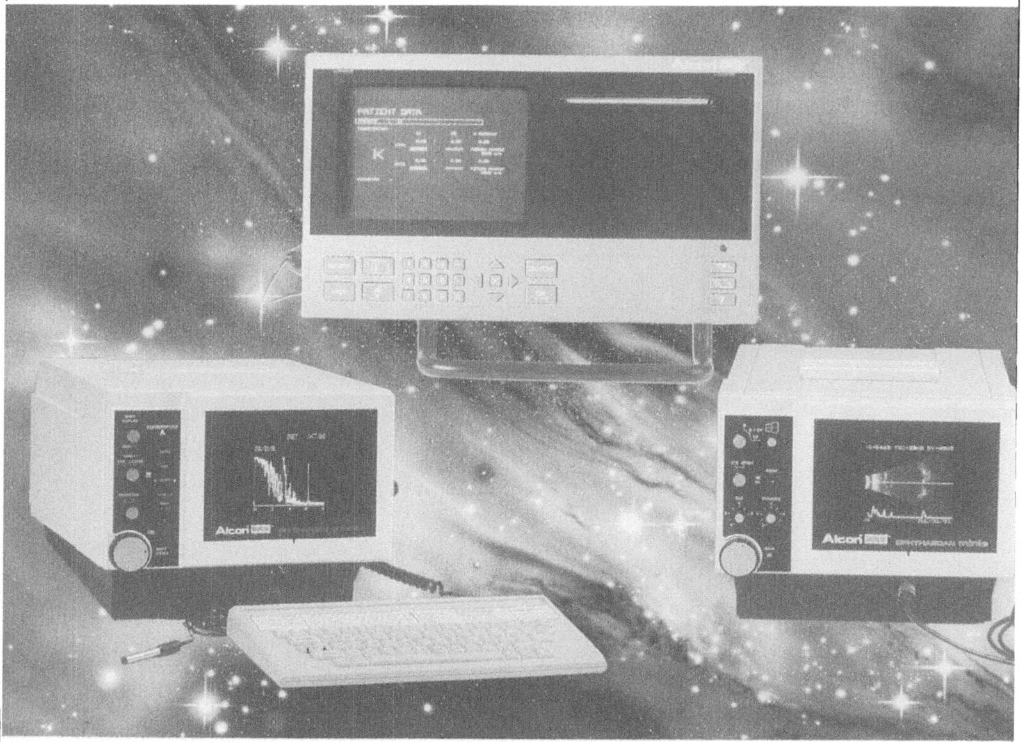

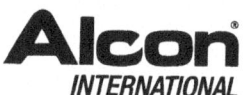

Documenta Ophthalmologica Proceedings Series

53. R. Sampaolesi (ed.): *Ultrasonography in Ophthalmology 12*. Proceedings of
     the 12th SIDUO Congress (Iguazú Falls, Argentina, 1988). 1990
     ISBN 0-7923-0765-8
54. B. Drum, J.D. Moreland & A. Serra (eds.): *Colour Vision Deficiencies X*.
     Proceedings of the 10th Symposium of the International Research Group on
     Colour Vision Deficiencies (Cagliari, Italy, 1989). 1991   ISBN 0-7923-0948-0
55. P. Till (ed.): *Ophthalmic Echography 13*. Proceedings of the 13th SIDUO
     Congress (Vienna, Austria, 1990). 1993   ISBN 0-7923-1808-0
56. B. Drum (ed.): *Colour Vision Deficiencies XI*. Proceedings of the 11th
     Symposium of the International Research Group on Colour Vision
     Deficiencies (Sydney, Australia, 1991). 1993   ISBN 0-7923-1864-1

KLUWER ACADEMIC PUBLISHERS – DORDRECHT / BOSTON / LONDON

The manufacturer's authorised representative in the EU is Springer
Nature Customer Service Centre GmbH, Europaplatz 3, 69115 Heidelberg,
Germany. If you have any concerns regarding our products, please
contact ProductSafety@springernature.com

Printed and bound by CPI Group (UK) Ltd, Croydon, CR0 4YY
29/04/2026
02099527-0003